Nutrigenetics: Advanced Principles

Nutrigenetics: Advanced Principles

Edited by Arthur Willis

hayle medical

New York

Hayle Medical,
750 Third Avenue, 9th Floor,
New York, NY 10017, USA

Visit us on the World Wide Web at:
www.haylemedical.com

ISBN: 978-1-63241-891-3

Cataloging-in-Publication Data

Nutrigenetics : advanced principles / edited by Arthur Willis.
p. cm.
Includes bibliographical references and index.
ISBN 978-1-63241-891-3
1. Nutrition--Genetic aspects. 2. Nutritionally induced diseases--Genetic aspects. 3. Dietetics.
4. Diet in disease. I. Willis Arthur.
QP144.G45 N88 2020
612.3--dc23

Table of Contents

Preface

There exists a strong correlation between human nutrition and health, and the human genome. Each individual responds differently to diet. This is due to genetic variations in each individual. Nutritional imbalances during lactation and gestation can contribute to cardiovascular disease, obesity, diabetes, cancer and hypertension. Certain diseases that have genomic anomalies can have consequences on appetite, such as the Prader-Willi syndrome which is characterized by insatiable appetite. Such studies are explored in the domain of nutritional genomics and nutriepigenomics. A crucial area in the study of these fields is obesity. By understanding the interaction between genetic factors and dietary patterns, management of obesity can be possible with targeted dietary changes. This book brings forth some of the most innovative concepts and elucidates the unexplored aspects of genes and their effect on human nutrition. It presents researches and studies performed by experts across the globe on nutritional genomics and nutriepigenomics. With state-of-the-art inputs by acclaimed experts of this field, this book targets students and professionals.

This book is the end result of constructive efforts and intensive research done by experts in this field. The aim of this book is to enlighten the readers with recent information in this area of research. The information provided in this profound book would serve as a valuable reference to students and researchers in this field.

At the end, I would like to thank all the authors for devoting their precious time and providing their valuable contribution to this book. I would also like to express my gratitude to my fellow colleagues who encouraged me throughout the process.

Editor

1

Expression of cardiac insulin signalling genes and proteins in rats fed a high-sucrose diet: effect of bilberry anthocyanin extract

Shamjeet Singh[1], Thomas Netticadan[2] and D. Dan Ramdath[1,3*]

Abstract

Scope: Insulin resistance is associated with impaired cardiac function, but the underlying molecular abnormalities are largely unexplained. Bilberry anthocyanin (BAcn) may be protective, as it appears to potentiate insulin action.

Methods: Rats were randomly allocated to control, sucrose-fed (SF) or sucrose-fed + BAcn diets (SF-A) for 15 weeks. Cardiac insulin signalling genes and proteins were quantified using reverse transcription quantitative real-time polymerase chain reaction and western blots.

Results: Glucose tolerance was not different with treatment. SF showed lower ($p < 0.05$) ferric reducing antioxidant power, which increased with BAcn. SF resulted in significantly decreased ($p < 0.05$) expression of 10 genes: acetyl-coenzyme A carboxylase alpha; V-Akt murine thymoma viral oncogene homolog 1; Bcl2-like 1; cytosine-cytosine-adenosine-adenosine-thymidine/enhancer binding protein; FK506 binding protein 12-rapamycin associated; glycerol-3-phosphate dehydrogenase 1 (soluble); solute carrier family 2 (facilitated glucose transporter), member 1, 4; hexokinase 2; and thyroglobulin. SF-A prevented these changes. Compared to SF-A, SF up-regulated ($p < 0.05$) complement factor D and phosphoinositide-3-kinase, regulatory subunit1 (α); sterol regulatory element binding transcription factor 1 was down-regulated ($p < 0.05$). SF increased ($p < 0.05$) cardiac phospholamban and decreased phosphorylated troponin I, which were not attenuated by BAcn. Compared to control or SF, SF-A resulted in significantly lower ($p < 0.05$) 5′-AMP-activated protein kinase.

Conclusions: SF lowered antioxidant capacity and changed the expression of insulin signalling genes, which were modulated by BAcn.

Keywords: Anthocyanins, Heart, Insulin resistance, PCR array, Type 2 diabetes mellitus

Introduction

Increased consumption of diets high in refined carbohydrates has been linked to the growing prevalence of type 2 diabetes mellitus (T2DM) (Eckel 2005; Mellor et al. 2010). Current estimates suggest that approximately 6.6 % of the world's adult population is diabetic with the majority having T2DM (IDF 2009). Of greater concern is that about 7.9 % show impaired glucose tolerance (IGT) or prediabetes (IDF 2009). One of the main underlying cellular defects associated with the diabetic and prediabetic state is insulin resistance (IR) (Abdul-Ghani and DeFronzo 2009; Reaven 1988), which is the inability of cells to respond to the action of insulin and can exist several years prior to the onset of T2DM (Lebovitz 1999).

IR can induce debilitating effects on various organs such as the kidneys, brain, liver and especially the heart (Sharma and McNeill 2006). In fact, epidemiological and clinical studies suggest that a large percentage of diabetics succumb to cardiac complications (Asghar

* Correspondence: dan.ramdath@agr.gc.ca
[1]Department of Pre-Clinical Sciences, Faculty of Medical Sciences, The University of the West Indies, St. Augustine Campus, St. Augustine, Trinidad and Tobago, West Indies
[3]Guelph Food Research Centre, Agriculture and Agri-Food Canada, 93 Stone Road West, Guelph, ON N1G 5C9, Canada
Full list of author information is available at the end of the article

et al. 2009), and this is largely attributed to myocardial infarction resulting from atherosclerotic build-up (DeFronzo 2010). However, the existence of a distinct disease of the heart muscle known as diabetic cardiomyopathy (DCM) has also been demonstrated (Galderisi et al. 1991). Although much is unknown about the aetiology of DCM, it can play a significant role in heart failure and in the recovery of cardiac tissue after an ischemic insult (Boudina and Abel 2007; Maisch et al. 2011). It is therefore crucial to examine the underlying cellular defects that accompany the very early stages of the development of IR and its contribution to the aetiology of DCM.

In the normal heart, binding of insulin to its receptors on cardiac cells elicits a series of downstream signal transduction pathways, which results in tight regulation of glucose and fatty acid uptake and utilization, glycogen and protein production, and vascular function (Muniyappa et al. 2007). However, when cells become resistant to the actions of insulin, lipotoxicity (An and Rodrigues 2006) and systemic hyperglycemia ensue; this results in a compensatory increase in insulin secretion (Chavez 2006). As such, persistent hyperinsulinemia resulting from IR can promote dyslipidemia and the proliferation of inflammatory factors (Kasuga 2006), which probably contribute to the onset of overt T2DM and DCM. However, the underlying molecular mechanisms and metabolic changes associated with these abnormalities are largely unknown, but could involve modulation of gene and protein expression.

In diabetic rodent models, DCM is associated with reduced glucose uptake and lipotoxicity, and adverse changes in calcium handling and contractile variables (Belke et al. 2000; Vasanji et al. 2006). In particular, the calcium handling protein sarco(endo)plasmic reticulum Ca^{2+}ATPase (SERCA), its regulator phospholamban (PLN), and the contractile protein cardiac Troponin I (cTnI), which have pivotal roles in the control of cardiac contraction and relaxation (Bers 2002), are significantly affected in DCM. Many of these studies have found that DCM-like cardiac complications are accompanied by significant changes in the expression and function of these proteins (Frank et al. 2002; Kranias and Bers 2007; Li et al. 2000; Ramirez-Correa and Murphy 2007).

Given the magnitude of the burden of T2DM and DCM, numerous approaches are being explored to prevent and/or reverse the associated metabolic effects. One such approach is in the use of plant-based products, such as anthocyanins, to influence cell signalling mechanisms. Anthocyanins are naturally occurring, pigmented compounds from fruits and vegetables, regularly consumed in fruits and vegetables and represent a major subclass of flavonoids (Mazza and Miniati 1993). Estimates on human intakes vary widely from 3 to 215 mg/day (de Pascual-Teresa et al. 2010). Purple corn anthocyanin has been shown to be protective towards IR, weight gain, elevated serum lipids and the production of tumour necrosis factor-α (TNF-α) in C57BL/6J rats fed a high-fat diet (Tsuda et al. 2003). Anthocyanins extracted from bilberry effectively improved hyperglycemia and insulin sensitivity in a genetic rodent model of T2DM (KK-A^y mice). This was associated with higher levels of AMP-activated protein kinase (AMPK) activity (Takikawa et al. 2010), which is also the target of metformin, a pharmacological agent routinely used in the management of T2DM (Hawley et al. 2002). Given these findings, it appears that anthocyanins can modulate intermediary metabolic pathways and perhaps influence the outcomes of risk factors for T2DM. However, the extent to which anthocyanins are able to reverse or modulate the molecular mechanisms of cardiac IR is unknown, although it is reasonable to assume that changes in the insulin signalling pathway are likely to occur.

We hypothesized that a high-sucrose diet leads to changes in the expression of insulin signalling genes and proteins as well as cardiac contractile proteins, and that these changes can be modulated by treatment with an anthocyanin extract. Our objectives were to reproduce the sucrose-fed insulin-resistant animal model, ascertain changes in gene and protein expression in the insulin signalling pathway in rat hearts and attempt to modulate these changes with an anthocyanin treatment.

Materials and methods

Bilberry anthocyanin

Commercially available dried bilberry powder, prepared using a low-temperature technique (Natural Newfoundland Nutraceuticals, Newfoundland, Canada) and containing 29.60 mg GAE/g total phenolics and 24.05 mg C3GE/g anthocyanins was double-extracted with acidified methanol (85 % MeOH: 14 % H_2O: 1 % HOAc) and partially purified using flash chromatography (Isolera One, Biotage, Sweden, AB). The latter treatment also resulted in the removal of free sugars. Methanol was removed by rotary evaporation, and the resulting extracts were freeze-dried and stored at −20 °C until use. Total anthocyanin concentration (TAC) was determined in triplicate using a modified pH differential method using a cyanidin-3-glucoside standard (Li et al. 2012).

Bilberry extract was solubilized in 2 N HCl solution at 1 mg/mL and hydrolyzed by incubation in a boiling water bath for 2 h and further characterized using an UHPLC system (Accela-Thermal Technologies Co., Ltd., USA) equipped with a diode array detector. Separation was achieved with a Phenomenex® Kinetex PFP, 4.6 × 150 mm, a 2.6-μm column (100 × 2.1 mm, Phenomenex, Torrance, CA, USA) attached to a Phenomenex® PFP guard column (4 × 3 mm). The column was thermostatically controlled at 30 °C and the flow rate was set to 1 mL/min. The mobile phase consisted of water-formic acid (A, 95:5, *v*/*v*) and methanol-formic acid (B, 95:5, *v*/*v*) with the following solvent gradient: 0–25 min, 0–50 % B; 25–27.5 min, 50–100 % B, and held at 100 % B for additional 2.5 min. The column was then re-equilibrated at 100 % A for 5 min. Peak absorbance was collected between 200 and 620 nm using DAD, and the chromatogram output was set at 520 nm. Stock solutions of the standards were prepared by dissolving 10 mg of each compound in 5 mL DMSO and then topped up to 100 mL in a volumetric flask with 50 % methanol (final concentration 100 μg/mL).

Petunidin was confirmed using a Finnigan LCQ DECA ion trap mass spectrometer (ThermoFnnigan, San Jose, CA, USA) equipped with electrospray ionization (ESI) source. Separation was performed with the same binary solvent system as in the HPLC method, but a different column (Luna 3-μm PFP (2) (4.6 mm × 100 mm; Phenomenex, Torrance, CA, USA)) and gradient programme: 0–26 min, 10–100 % B; 26–28.5 min, 100–10 % B, then the gradient was held at 10 % A for an additional 5 min. The flow rate was set at 1.0 mL/min. Positive mode was selected for data collection. The instrument was tuned by using cyanidin standard to reach its optimum performance. Other analytical conditions have been previously described by (Li et al. 2012).

Experimental design

Male Sprague Dawley rats, approximately 200 g and 6 weeks of age, were randomly divided into three experimental groups (four rats/cage): control (C), sucrose-fed (SF) and sucrose-fed anthocyanin treated (SF-A) as shown in Table 1. Control animals were fed a basal AIN-93 diet while the SF and SF-A animals were fed a high-sucrose diet. The diets were isocaloric; however, the high-sucrose diet contained 55 % of energy as sucrose, whereas in the basal diet, energy was mainly from cornstarch. All diets were formulated by Dyets Incorporated (PA, USA), and the compositions are shown in Table 1.

The animals were all fed the control diet for 3 days, after which a tail vein blood sample was taken for baseline measurements. All the groups were fed and watered ad libitum. Anthocyanin was supplemented (SF-A) by addition to drinking water (0.2 mg/mL anthocyanin) which was stored in dark bottles and replaced every 2 days. Chow intake and body weight were measured weekly and fluid intake every 2 days. Based on the weekly chow intake and the energy content of the diet (Table 1), the average energy intake per rat for each week was calculated and standardized according to body weights. At 3-week intervals, the animals were fasted overnight and ~1.0 mL blood was drawn into freshly prepared heparinized tubes (3 units/0.5 mL blood) using the tail clip method. Plasma was separated and stored at −70 °C pending batch analyses for glucose, insulin and triglycerides. After 14 weeks, an intraperitoneal glucose tolerance test (IPGTT) was performed on the fasted animals by intraperitoneal injection of a glucose solution (2 g/kg body weight). Blood was then drawn and analysed for glucose using a Hemocue 201 Analyzer (Hemocue AB, Ängelholm, Sweden) at baseline and at 30, 60 and 120 min following glucose administration. One week after the IPGTT, the animals were terminally anaesthetized; the heart was harvested, flash-frozen in liquid nitrogen and stored at −80 °C pending biochemical analyses.

Biochemical analyses

Commercially available analytical kits were used to measure plasma levels of triglycerides (Human Diagnostics, Wiesbaden, Germany) and insulin (Linco Research, MO, USA). The oxygen radical absorbance capacity (ORAC) (Prior et al. 2003) and ferric reducing antioxidant power (FRAP) (Benzie and Strain 1996) assays were used to determine total antioxidant capacity of serum. The homeostasis assessment model (HOMA) was used to

Table 1 Experimental treatments and diet composition

Experimental group	Water	Diet[a]	Diet composition[b] (g/kg)	
Control (C); $n = 8$	No treatment	Control	Sucrose	100
			Cornstarch	466
			Dyetrose	155
			Protein	140
			Fat	40
			Energy 3602 kcal/kg	
Sucrose-fed (SF); $n = 12$	No treatment	High sucrose	Sucrose	550
Sucrose-fed/anthocyanin supplemented (SF-A); $n = 12$	0.2 mg/mL anthocyanin	High sucrose	Cornstarch	130
			Protein	140
			Fat	40
			Energy 3604 kcal/kg	

[a]Diets were formulated by Dyets Incorporated, PA, USA
[b]Both diets contained the recommended concentrations of vitamins, minerals and fibre

calculate HOMA-IR. This was calculated by multiplying fasting plasma insulin (FPI) by fasting plasma glucose (FPG), then dividing by 22.5 (Diabetes Trials Unit, University of Oxford, UK).

For gene expression studies, RNA was isolated from heart tissue using TRI Reagent (Sigma-Aldrich, CA, USA). Impurities were removed using RNeasy Mini Kit (Qiagen, Valencia, CA), and RNA quality was assessed using the absorbance ratios at 260 nm/230 nm and 260 nm/280 nm. Purified RNA was then used to quantify gene expression for 84 genes along the insulin signalling pathway utilizing the 7500 ABI Fast Real Time PCR System (Applied Biosystems, CA, USA) with the RT^2 Profiler PCR Array System (SABiosciences, Frederick, MD, USA). C_t (cycle threshold) values were generated by the 7500 ABI Fast Real Time PCR System and used to calculate fold changes in gene expression. Fold change differences between experimental groups were calculated for each gene as follows: Fold Δ (GOI) = Ave [C_t (TEST) – C_t (HKG)]/Ave [C_t (CONTROL) – C_t (HKG)], where GOI is gene of interest and HKG is housekeeping gene.

Proteins were prepared by dicing and homogenizing left ventricular tissue with a hand-held homogenizer in cold lysis buffer: 50 mM Tris-HCl pH 7.5, 150 mM NaCl, 0.1 % SDS, 1 mM EGTA, containing protease inhibitors (1:250) (Roche Diagnostics Corporation, IN, USA), phosphatase inhibitor cocktails I and II (1 mL/100 mL buffer, Sigma-Aldrich, CA, USA) and protein kinase inhibitor H-7 (1 mL/100 mL buffer, Sigma-Aldrich, CA, USA). This homogenate was then centrifuged at 10,000×*g* for 10 min at 4 °C. The supernatant was removed, aliquoted and stored at –70 °C pending sodium dodecyl sulphate polyacrylamide gel electrophoresis (SDS-PAGE). Proteins were electrophoresed on 12 % polyacrylamide gels at 150 V for 1.5 hr under denaturing conditions (Laemmli 1970) and subsequently transblotted onto polyvinyl difluoride membrane (Towbin et al. 1979) and probed with antibodies for PLN, SERCA, cTnI, the insulin receptor, Akt, AMPK and the phosphorylated forms of these proteins (Badrilla, Leeds, UK; Affinity Bioreagents, CO, USA; Cell Signalling Technology MA, USA; Abcam, MA, USA). Primary antibodies were diluted at a ratio of 1:1000, and secondary antibodies were diluted at a ratio of 1:2000. Blots were then quantified using Image J (NIH, MD, USA) and normalized using the protein glyceraldehyde-3-phosphate dehydrogenase (GAPDH) (Cell Signalling Technology MA, USA). The protein expression ratios of PLN/SERCA and phosphorylated to unphosphorylated protein for cTnI, the insulin receptor, Akt and AMPK were calculated and compared between experimental groups to gauge the functionality of these proteins.

Statistical analyses

The study was designed using a power analysis based on an expected difference of 50 % in the area under the glucose response curve following an IPGTT, a type I error of 0.05 and a power of 90 %. The required sample size was calculated to be at least eight. Statistical analyses were performed using the SPSS 12 software for Windows (SPSS Inc., Chicago, IL, USA). Differences in insulin, glucose and triglyceride levels and blood glucose during the IPGTT, between control and SF animals, were evaluated using repeated measures ANOVA. The differences in ORAC, FRAP, C_t values, AUC from the IPGTT and western blotting results were compared using one way ANOVA. A p value of less than 0.05 was regarded as being significant.

Results

The bilberry extract had a total anthocyanin content of 204.24 ± 2.17 mg CyGE/100 g DW and was consistent with other studies (Bakowska-Barczak et al. 2007; Zhang et al. 2004), the major anthocyanidin aglycones being delphinidin, cyanidin, petunidin, peonidin and malvidin (Fig. 1). Among the study groups, there were no significant differences in body weight (Fig. 2) or energy consumption (Fig. 3). After 15 weeks on the experimental diet, neither HOMA-IR (Fig. 4) nor plasma triglyceride concentration (Fig. 5) was significantly different among the study groups at any time point. The IPGTT also showed no significant differences among the groups for blood glucose levels at any time point or in the incremental area under the blood glucose response curve (Fig. 6). The FRAP assay showed significantly lower values for SF when compared to control, and significantly higher values for SF-A when compared to SF animals (Fig. 7a). However, ORAC values were not significantly different among the experimental groups (Fig. 7b).

When SF treatment was compared to control, PCR array gene analyses of left ventricular tissues showed that the expression of several genes were significantly down-regulated ($p < 0.05$; Table 2) and included acetyl-coenzyme A carboxylase alpha (ACC1), V-Akt murine thymoma viral oncogene homolog 1 (Akt), Bcl2-like 1 (Bcl2), CCAAT/enhancer binding protein (C/EBP), beta (C/EBPβ), FK506 binding protein 12-rapamycin associated (mTOR), glycerol-3-phosphate dehydrogenase 1 (soluble) (GPDH1), hexokinase 2 (HK2), solute carrier family 2 (facilitated glucose transporter), member 1 (GLUT1), solute carrier family 2 (facilitated glucose transporter), member 4 (GLUT4) and Thyroglobulin (Tg). These changes were not observed when SF-A animals were compared with control, indicating that anthocyanin supplementation prevented these changed in gene expression. Further, when SF was compared with SF-A treatment, complement factor D (adipsin) and phosphoinositide-3-kinase, regulatory subunit 1 (α) (PI3Kα) were significantly up-regulated ($p < 0.05$), while sterol regulatory element binding transcription factor 1

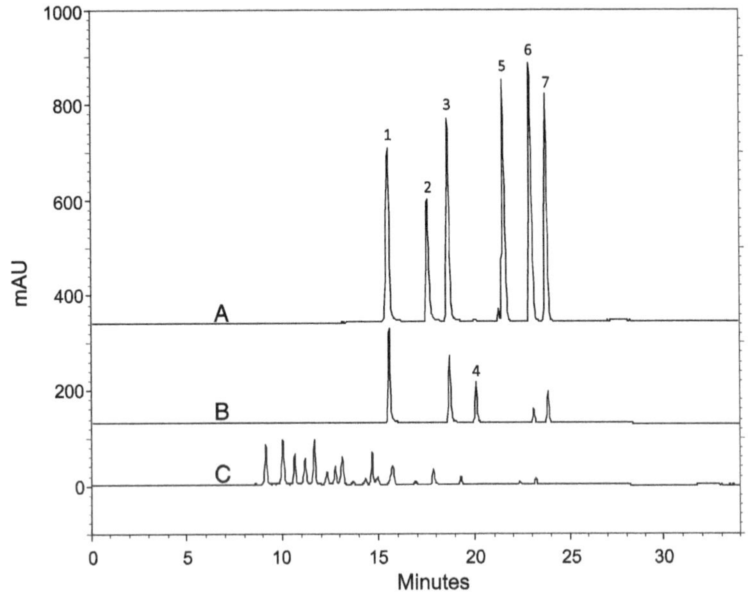

Fig. 1 UHPLC-DAD chromatograms of mixed standards (*A*) and bilberry extract before (*C*) and after acid hydrolysis (*B*). Mobile phase A—95 %:5 % water-formic acid; mobile phase B—95 % methanol:5 % formic acid (*v/v*); flow rate 1.0 mL/min; column: Phenomenex Kinetex PFP, 4.6 × 150 mm, 2.6 μm; detection at 520 nm; injection: 10 μL. *A* = standards: *1* delphinidin, *2* luteolinidin, *3* cyanidin, *4* petunidin, *5* pelargonidin, *6* peonidin, *7* malvidin; *B* = hydrolyzed bilberry extract; *C* = bilberry extract

(SREBF1) was significantly down-regulated ($p < 0.05$) (Table 3).

Compared to control, PLN levels were significantly increased ($p < 0.05$) and p*-cTnI levels were significantly decreased ($p < 0.05$) in the heart of SF-treated rats (Fig. 8a, d, respectively); these changes were not attenuated by anthocyanin supplementation. However, total AMPK expression was significantly lower ($p < 0.05$) in SF-A when compared to both control and SF hearts (Fig. 8i), while protein expression for SERCA, cTnI, IRec, p*-IRec, Akt, p*-Akt and p*-AMPK were not different (Fig. 8b, c, e–h, j, respectively). The ratio of SERCA/PLN was significantly higher ($p < 0.05$) in SF-A rats when compared to that in SF (Fig. 9a), whereas the ratio of p*-cTnI/cTnI was significantly decreased in both SF and SF-A animals (Fig. 9b).

Discussion

We found that feeding male Sprague Dawley rats a solid high-sucrose diet for 15 weeks did not result in the animals becoming insulin resistant, hypertriglyceridemic or obese, although others have been able to achieve these metabolic abnormities using sucrose diets (Davidoff et al. 2004; Vasanji et al. 2006). In our laboratory, when these animals are fed sucrose (32 %, *w/v*) in drinking

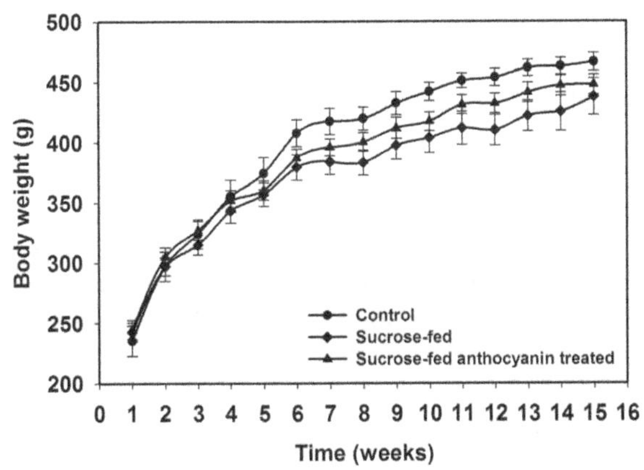

Fig. 2 Body weights (mean ± SE) for control (*n* = 8), sucrose-fed (*n* = 12) and sucrose-fed anthocyanin treated (*n* = 12) rats over 15 weeks

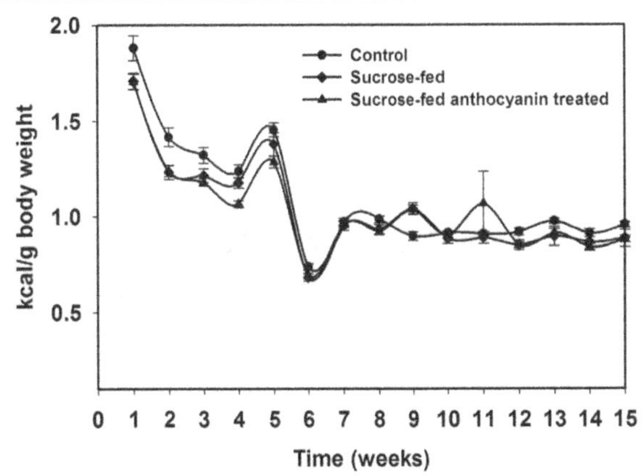

Fig. 3 Energy consumption in kcal/g body weight (mean ± SE) for control (*n* = 8), sucrose-fed (*n* = 12) and sucrose-fed anthocyanin treated (*n* = 12) rats over 15 weeks

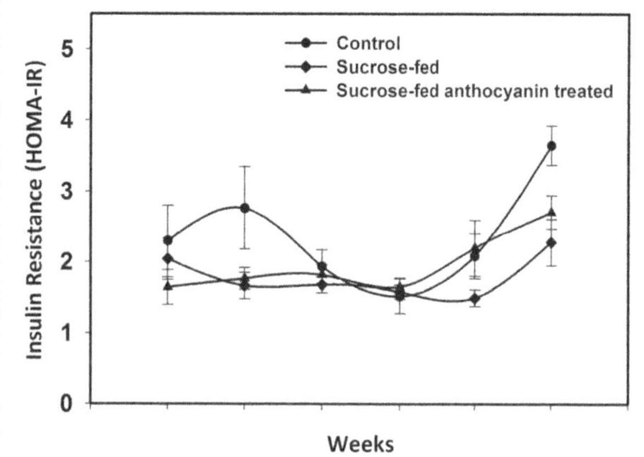

Fig. 4 HOMA-IR (mean ± SE) for control ($n = 8$), sucrose-fed ($n = 12$) and sucrose-fed anthocyanin treated ($n = 12$) rats over 15 weeks

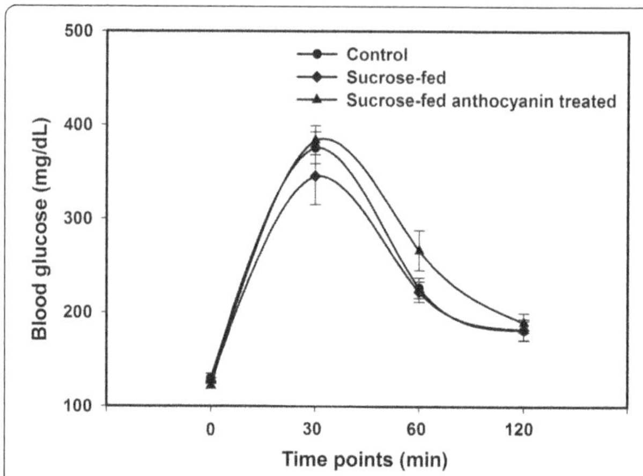

Fig. 6 IPGTT test (mean ± SE) for control ($n = 8$), sucrose-fed ($n = 12$) and sucrose-fed anthocyanin treated ($n = 12$) rats after 15 weeks

water (presumably absorbed primarily in the small intestine), they become obese and insulin resistant after 8–10 weeks of feeding. However, they consume less solid food and increase water consumption, so that their nutrient intake profile becomes altered (Singh and Ramdath unpublished); this would be a concern in efforts to establish a diet-induced rodent model of T2DM. Recent studies have suggested that the gut microbiota might play a crucial role in the onset of diabetes (Everard and Cani 2013; Turnbaugh et al. 2008). As such, it is possible that our animals, obtained from the local animal house, might have acquired a microbiota that is different from animals obtained from a central breeding source, and this could account for their resistance to developing a diabetic/prediabetic condition when fed orally with a solid high-sucrose diet. Others have shown that both Sprague Dawley and Wistar rats failed to become obese on a high-fat diet (Perez de Heredia et al. 2006) and may have different rates of weight gain which is associated with hyperglycaemia (Lauterio et al. 1994). It seems reasonable to expect that

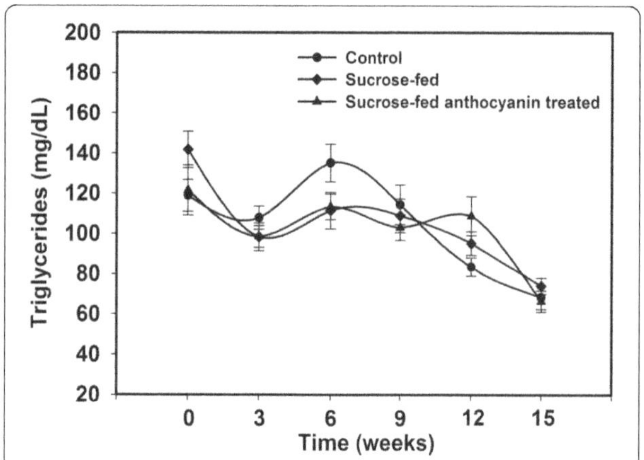

Fig. 5 Plasma triglycerides (mean ± SE) for control ($n = 8$), sucrose-fed ($n = 12$) and sucrose-fed anthocyanin treated ($n = 12$) rats over 15 weeks

there is inherent metabolic variation (metabolic plasticity) among rodents that allows them to resist changes in glucose and lipid metabolism (Chang et al. 1990).

Clearly, the fact that our animals showed no abnormal metabolic changes or signs of DCM on a high-sucrose diet is not unique. We contend that our results from gene and protein expression assays are indicative of very early cellular changes in insulin signalling and cardiac function resulting from a high-sucrose diet. It is likely that these will eventually lead to phenotypic changes and result in overt metabolic changes. However, the length of time between these events is likely to be influenced by cellular adaptation and metabolic plasticity, as mentioned above. Moreover, identification of very early changes in the expression of genes and proteins associated with insulin signalling and cardiac function could allow for a better understanding of DCM aetiology and facilitate early intervention.

Using the multiple gene profiling feature of microarray analysis with real-time PCR quantitation techniques, we showed that expression of GLUT1, GLUT4, HK2, GLUT4 and Akt were down-regulated. Decreased expression of GLUT1 and GLUT4 may be indicative of reduced glucose transport into cardiomyocytes, which could impair cardiac muscle contractility (Abel 2004). However, in mice with cardiac-specific inactivation of the GLUT4 gene, there is modest ventricular hypertrophy with no contractile changes (Abel et al. 1999). In contrast, decreased expression of HK2 in sucrose-fed rats, as found on our study, has been linked to a reduction glucose phosphorylation and possibly a reduction in ATP production and contractility (Ye et al. 2005). Further, cardiac contractility might have been slightly impaired in our SF animals, given the small but significant decrease in Akt gene expression observed. In a similar study, Roberts et al. 2005 showed that a high-fat, high-sugar diet resulted in decreased Akt protein expression

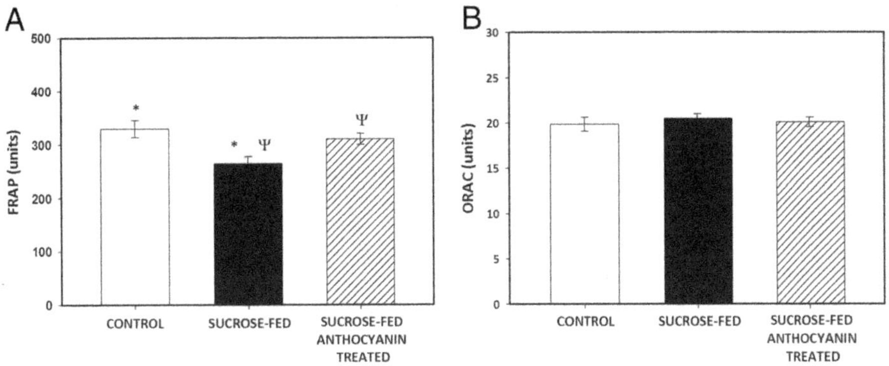

Fig. 7 a Ferric reducing antioxidant power (FRAP) values (mean ± SE) for control ($n = 8$), sucrose-fed ($n = 12$) and sucrose-fed anthocyanin treated ($n = 12$) rats after 15 weeks. (*, Ψ significantly different at $p < 0.05$). **b** Oxygen radical absorbance capacity (ORAC) values (mean ± SE) for control ($n = 8$), sucrose-fed ($n = 12$) and sucrose-fed anthocyanin treated ($n = 12$) rats after 15 weeks (1 ORAC unit equals to the net antioxidant protection produced by 1 μM Trolox (the water-soluble vitamin E analogue used as a positive control))

in aorta and heart tissue; they suggested that eNOS activation by Akt and therefore endothelial function may be impaired by HFS. Akt phosphorylates a wide range of substrates in the proximal part of the insulin signalling pathway, and impairment of this function has been shown to result in downstream contractile abnormalities, similar to those associated with IR and DCM. However, the ratio of p-Akt/Akt, which is the activation status of Akt, was unaltered, suggesting that sucrose feeding did not affect Akt activation. As such, the metabolic effects of decreased Akt protein expression require further investigation (Roberts et al. 2005).

Taken together, changes in the expression of genes along the insulin signalling pathway as well as those involved in cellular energy utilization (ACC1, mTOR and GPDH1) suggest that glucose transport and usage is decreased in the heart of SF-fed rats, and this may result in impaired cardiac contractility. This is consistent with observations in diabetic rats: they exhibit cardiac dysfunction and IR associated with decreased glucose and increased fatty acid utilization, decreased mRNA and protein levels of GLUT4 (van den Brom et al. 2009). Furthermore, defects in GLUT4 translocation has been demonstrated in the skeletal muscle of Goto-Kakizaki rats and in type 2 diabetic patients (Zdychova and Komers 2005). Collectively, reductions in the expression of C/EBPβ and Bcl2 and genes that play a critical role in cellular energy homeostasis may provide an aetiological mechanism for the onset of DCM following high-sucrose feeding (Bosch et al. 1995; Cory and Adams 2002; Hage et al. 2011).

Our protein expression data further suggests that high-sucrose feeding might have resulted in impaired cardiac contractility. We found that SF led to increase levels of PLN, while SERCA/PLN ratio, p*-cTnI and p*cTnI/cTnI ratio were decreased. An increase in PLN is likely to increase inhibition of SERCA and prolong

Table 2 Mean (±SE) C_t values for cardiac genes that showed different expression levels when SF samples were compared to control samples

Description	Control ($n = 5$)	Sucrose-fed ($n = 5$)	p value	[a]Fold Δ
Acetyl-coenzyme A carboxylase alpha	26.71 ± 0.13	27.21 ± 0.16	0.038	−1.12
V-Akt murine thymoma viral oncogene homolog 1	25.65 ± 0.10	26.03 ± 0.11	0.027	−1.04
Bcl2-like 1	23.61 ± 0.12	24.20 ± 0.22	0.047	−1.19
CCAAT/enhancer binding protein (C/EBP), beta	23.45 ± 0.16	24.14 ± 0.23	0.037	−1.28
MTOR- FK506 binding protein 12-rapamycin associated	25.08 ± 0.09	25.60 ± 0.17	0.026	−1.13
Glycerol-3-phosphate dehydrogenase 1 (soluble)	24.61 ± 0.24	25.42 ± 0.14	0.019	−1.38
Hexokinase 2	26.37 ± 0.13	27.25 ± 0.29	0.022	−1.46
Solute carrier family 2 (facilitated glucose transporter), member 1	29.45 ± 0.19	30.49 ± 0.36	0.034	−1.64
Solute carrier family 2 (facilitated glucose transporter), member 4	23.21 ± 0.09	24.07 ± 0.20	0.005	−1.44
Thyroglobulin	29.88 ± 0.18	30.40 ± 0.09	0.037	−1.12

All were significant at $p < 0.05$
– represent downregulation
[a]Fold changes; calculated after C_t values were normalized using housekeeping genes

Table 3 Mean (±SE) C_t values for cardiac genes that showed different expression levels when SF-A samples were compared to SF samples

Description	Sucrose-fed ($n = 5$)	Sucrose-fed anthocyanin treated ($n = 5$)	p value	[a]Fold Δ
Complement factor D (adipsin)	26.05 ± 0.29	25.31 ± 0.13	0.045	+1.48
Phosphoinositide-3-kinase, regulatory subunit 1 (alpha)	24.23 ± 0.19	23.62 ± 0.14	0.030	+1.35
Sterol regulatory element binding transcription factor 1	34.25 ± 0.21	34.82 ± 0.15	0.056	−1.66

All were significant at $p < 0.05$
− represents downregulation, + represent upregulation
[a]Fold changes; calculated after C_t values were normalized using housekeeping genes

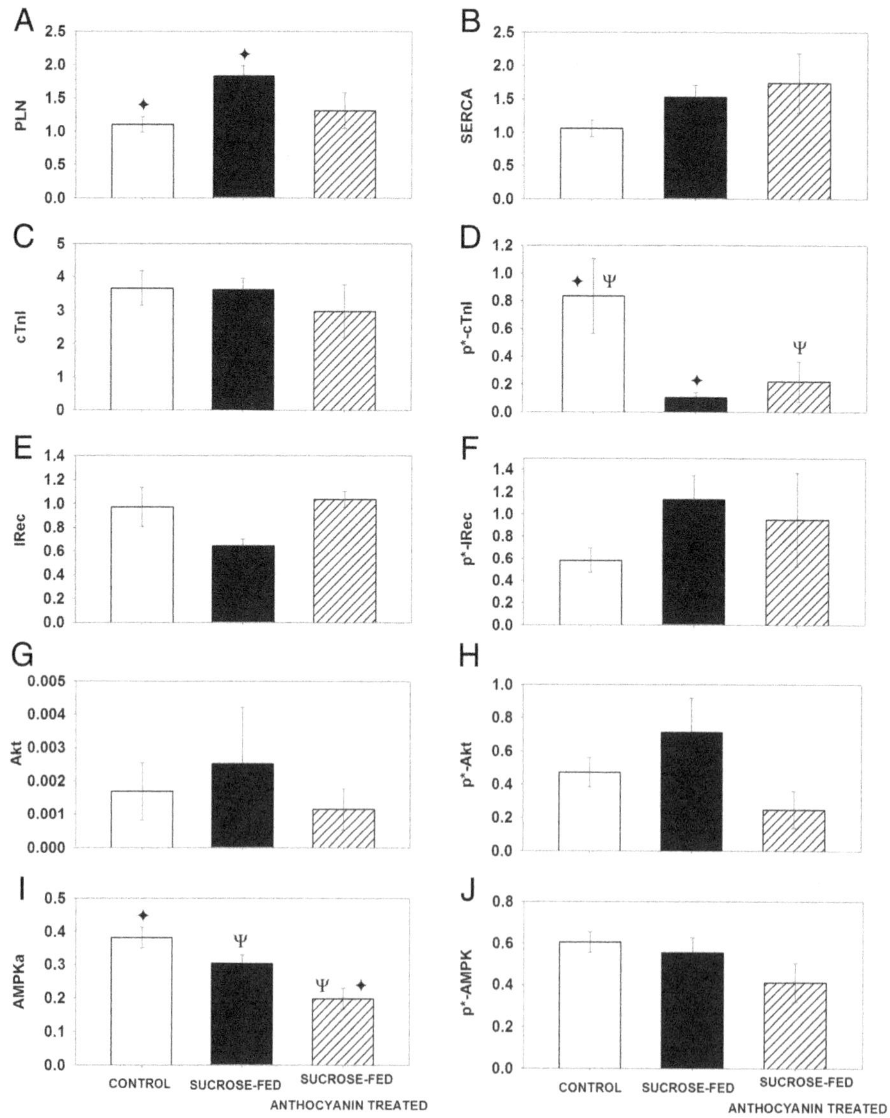

Fig. 8 Protein expression for PLN (**a**), SERCA (**b**), cTnI (**c**), p*-CTnI (**d**), IRec (**e**), p*-IRec (**f**), Akt (**g**), p*-Akt (**h**), AMPK (**i**) and p*-AMPK (**j**) in control, sucrose-fed and sucrose-fed anthocyanin treated rat heart homogenates. All densitometric measurements were normalized using GAPDH before comparisons were made (p* phosphorylated; ♦, Ψ significantly different at $p < 0.05$; $n = 5$)

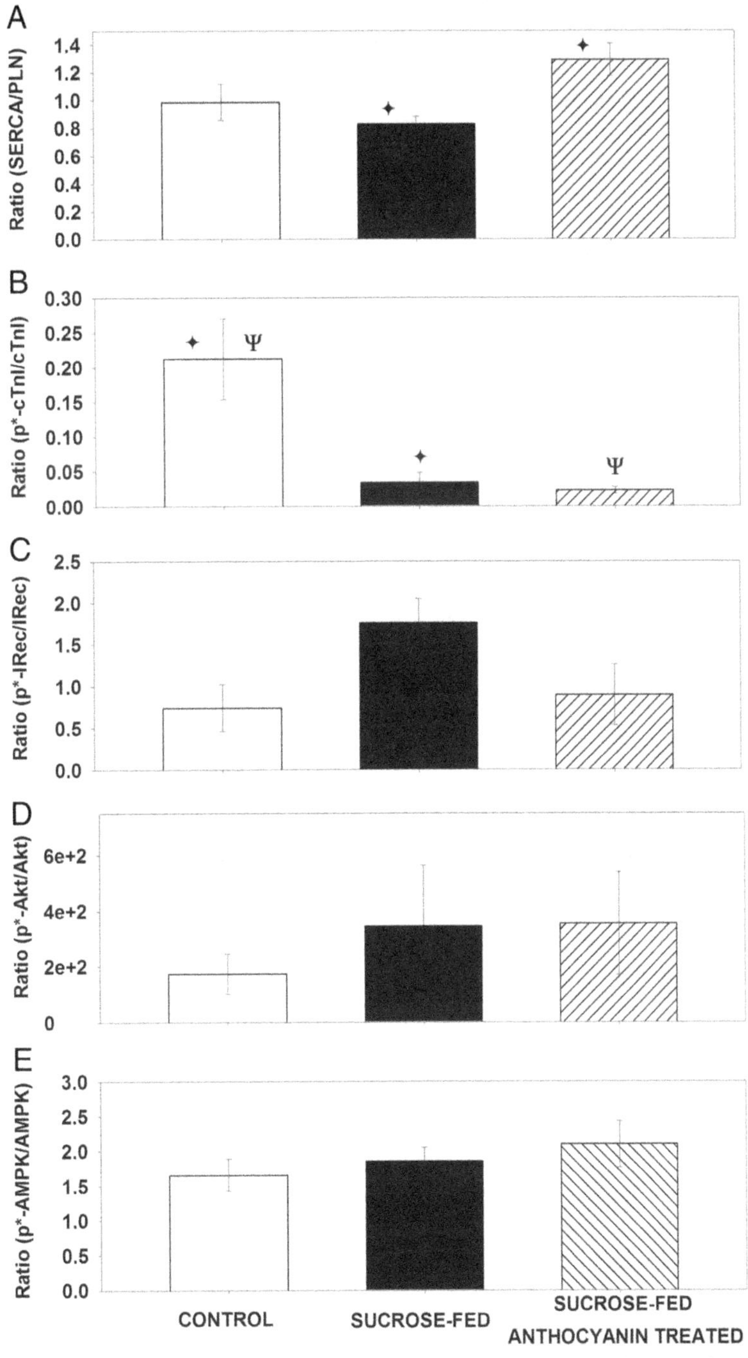

Fig. 9 Ratios of SERCA/PLN (**a**), p*-cTnI/cTnI (**b**), p*-IRec/IRec (**c**), p*-Akt/Akt (**d**) and p*-AMPK/AMPK (**e**) in control, sucrose-fed and sucrose-fed anthocyanin treated rat heart homogenates (p* phosphorylated; ♦, ψ significantly different at $p < 0.05$; $n = 5$)

relaxation rates of cardiac muscles (Koss et al. 1997); decreased p*-cTnI and p*cTnI/cTnI ratio could also contribute to lengthen rates of relaxation via a depression of cross-bridge cycling (Zhang et al. 1995). An analysis of the expression and activity of PKA, CaMKII and the other Tn subunits may be required in order to fully interpret these results. AMPK is regarded as a metabolic sensor since it upregulates catabolic pathways that generate ATP and down-regulates anabolic pathways that consume ATP (Hardie 2008). In the present study, expression of AMPK protein was decreased with sucrose feeding. However, the ratio of p-AMPK/AMPK, which is the activation status of AMPK was unaltered, suggesting that sucrose feeding did not affect AMPK activation.

Anthocyanin supplementation of the high-sucrose diet augmented the changes in gene expression induced by the SF diet. SF-A further led to an increased expression of adipsin and PI3Kα and decreased the expression of SREBF1. PI3Kα has a central role in the proximal part of the insulin signalling pathway and increased expression may represent a compensatory mechanism to decreased expression of GLUT1, GLUT2 and HK2. SREBF1 expression, shown to be reduced in T2DM (Sewter et al. 2002), represents a series of transcription factors that responds to both Akt and MAPK pathways and influences lipogenesis and TAG deposition in skeletal muscle (Lecomte et al. 2010). As such, downregulation of SREBF1 by anthocyanin supplementation could result in the prevention of lipid accumulation in the heart. Indeed, anthocyanins have been shown to prevent the onset of obesity in animal models (Lee et al. 2014; Wu et al. 2013). An increase in ratio of SERCA/PLN, as seen in SF-A rats, has been shown to promote contractile efficiency (Currie and Smith 1999), and therefore supplementation with anthocyanins may improve heart function.

In our study, we used both ORAC and FRAP assays to estimate the antioxidant potential of serum and found that ORAC was not different among treatment groups, but FRAP was decreased with SF, and SF-A prevented this decrease. These findings are likely due to the fact that FRAP and ORAC assess different antioxidant potentials. ORAC measures the ability of antioxidants in a sample to quench one type of free radical (probably peroxyl) and is influenced by material with and without lag phases of their antioxidants (Cao and Prior 1998). On the other hand, FRAP measures the reducing power of plasma and has been shown to increase with polyphenol supplementation (Benzie et al. 1999). Others have found that sucrose feeding results in depressed level of antioxidants (Diniz et al. 2008; Fang et al. 2005), possibly resulting from oxidative stress which is associated with disrupted insulin signalling and obesity (Styskal et al. 2012). The bilberry anthocyanin supplement used in our study provided a rich source of polyphenols which would likely account for the increase in FRAP, but not ORAC.

In the present study, feeding Sprague Dawley rats a high-sucrose diet did not result in IR. However, the collective evidence from gene expression and protein quantitation studies suggest that the animals experience very early cellular changes in insulin signalling and cardiac function, which may be some of the earliest cellular adaptations to a high-sucrose diet. Importantly, anthocyanins appear capable of modulating some of these changes and may represent a possible therapeutic adjunct in the management of T2DM.

Abbreviations

ACC1: acetyl-coenzyme A carboxylase alpha; Akt: V-Akt murine thymoma viral oncogene homolog 1; AMPK: 5'-AMP-activated protein kinase; BAcn: bilberry anthocyanin; Bcl2: Bcl2-like 1; CCAAT/EBP: cytosine-cytosine-adenosine-adenosine-thymidine/enhancer binding protein; cTnI: cardiac troponin I; FRAP: ferric reducing antioxidant power; GLUT1: solute carrier family 2 (facilitated glucose transporter), member 1; GLUT4: solute carrier family 2 (facilitated glucose transporter), member 4; GPDH1: glycerol-3-phosphate dehydrogenase 1 (soluble); HK2: hexokinase 2; HOMA-IR: homeostasis model assessment-estimated insulin resistance; IPGTT: intraperitoneal glucose tolerance test; IR: insulin resistance; mTOR: FK506 binding protein 12-rapamycin associated; ORAC: oxygen radical absorbance capacity; p*: phosphorylated; PI3Kα: phosphoinositide-3-kinase, regulatory subunit 1 (α); PLN: phospholamban, SREBF1, sterol regulatory element binding transcription factor 1; RT-qPCR: reverse transcription quantitative real-time polymerase chain reaction; SERCA: sarco(endo)plasmic reticulum Ca^{2+}ATPase; SF: sucrose-fed; SF-A: sucrose-fed + BAcn; Tg: thyroglobulin; T2DM: type 2 diabetes mellitus.

Competing interests

The authors declare that they have no competing interests.

Author's contributions

DDR and SS conceptualized the study and obtained funding. SS conducted the experiments, cleaned the data and performed initial statistical analysis and reporting. TN supervised the identification of cardiac contractile proteins. All authors interpreted the data and contributed to the final manuscript.

Acknowledgements

This work was supported in part by the A-base research programme of Agriculture & Agri-Food Canada (RBPI #1343) and The University of the West Indies, St. Augustine, Trinidad and Tobago (CRP.5.NOV08.5). We thank Aileen Hawke and Dr. Rong Tsao for the assistance in preparing the anthocyanin extract from bilberry and Dr. Ronghua Liu for the assistance with the polyphenol, anthocyanin and antioxidant analyses.

Author details

[1]Department of Pre-Clinical Sciences, Faculty of Medical Sciences, The University of the West Indies, St. Augustine Campus, St. Augustine, Trinidad and Tobago, West Indies. [2]Canadian Centre for Agri-Food Research in Health and Medicine, 351 Taché Avenue, Winnipeg, Manitoba, Canada. [3]Guelph Food Research Centre, Agriculture and Agri-Food Canada, 93 Stone Road West, Guelph, ON N1G 5C9, Canada.

References

Abdul-Ghani MA, DeFronzo RA (2009) Plasma glucose concentration and prediction of future risk of type 2 diabetes. Diabetes Care 32 Supple 2:S194–S198. doi:10.2337/dc09-S309

Abel ED (2004) Glucose transport in the heart. Front Basic 9:201–215

Abel ED et al (1999) Cardiac hypertrophy with preserved contractile function after selective deletion of GLUT4 from the heart. J Clin Invest 104:1703–1714. doi:10.1172/JCI7605

An D, Rodrigues B (2006) Role of changes in cardiac metabolism in development of diabetic cardiomyopathy. Am J Physiol Heart Circ Physiol 291:H1489–H1506. doi:10.1152/ajpheart.00278.2006

Asghar O et al (2009) Diabetic cardiomyopathy. Clin Sci (Lond) 116:741–760. doi:10.1042/CS20080500

Bakowska-Barczak AM, Marianchuk M, Kolodziejczyk P (2007) Survey of bioactive components in Western Canadian berries. Can J Physiol Pharmacol 85:1139–1152. doi:10.1139/Y07-102

Belke DD, Larsen TS, Gibbs EM, Severson DL (2000) Altered metabolism causes cardiac dysfunction in perfused hearts from diabetic (db/db) mice. Am J Physiol Endocrinol Metab 279:E1104–E1113

Benzie IF, Strain JJ (1996) The ferric reducing ability of plasma (FRAP) as a measure of "antioxidant power": the FRAP assay. Anal Biochem 239:70–76. doi:10.1006/abio.1996.0292

Benzie IF, Szeto YT, Strain JJ, Tomlinson B (1999) Consumption of green tea causes rapid increase in plasma antioxidant power in humans. Nutr Cancer 34:83–87. doi:10.1207/S15327914NC340112

Bers DM (2002) Cardiac excitation-contraction coupling. Nature 415:198–205. doi:10.1038/415198a

Bosch F, Sabater J, Valera A (1995) Insulin inhibits liver expression of the CCAAT/enhancer-binding protein beta. Diabetes 44:267–271

Boudina S, Abel ED (2007) Diabetic cardiomyopathy revisited. Circulation 115: 3213–3223. doi:10.1161/CIRCULATIONAHA.106.679597

Cao G, Prior RL (1998) Comparison of different analytical methods for assessing total antioxidant capacity of human serum. Clin Chem 44:1309–1315

Chang S, Graham B, Yakubu F, Lin D, Peters JC, Hill JO (1990) Metabolic differences between obesity-prone and obesity-resistant rats. Am J Physiol 259:R1103–R1110

Chavez BEHRR (2006) Type 2 diabetes: insulin resistance, beta cell dysfunction, and other metabolic and hormonal abnormalities. In: Clinical Diabetes. Saunders Elsevier, PA, USA, pp 21–34

Cory S, Adams JM (2002) The Bcl2 family: regulators of the cellular life-or-death switch. Nat Rev Cancer 2:647–656. doi:10.1038/nrc883

Currie S, Smith GL (1999) Enhanced phosphorylation of phospholamban and downregulation of sarco/endoplasmic reticulum Ca2+ ATPase type 2 (SERCA 2) in cardiac sarcoplasmic reticulum from rabbits with heart failure. Cardiovasc Res 41:135–146

Davidoff AJ et al (2004) Sucrose-induced cardiomyocyte dysfunction is both preventable and reversible with clinically relevant treatments. Am J Physiol Endocrinol Metab 286:E718–E724. doi:10.1152/ajpendo.00358.2003

de Pascual-Teresa S, Moreno DA, Garcia-Viguera C (2010) Flavanols and anthocyanins in cardiovascular health: a review of current evidence. Int J Mol Sci 11:1679–1703. doi:10.3390/ijms11041679

DeFronzo RA (2010) Insulin resistance, lipotoxicity, type 2 diabetes and atherosclerosis: the missing links. The Claude Bernard Lecture 2009. Diabetologia 53:1270–1287. doi:10.1007/s00125-010-1684-1

Diniz YS et al (2008) Conjugated linoleic acid and cardiac health: oxidative stress and energetic metabolism in standard and sucrose-rich diets. Eur J Pharmacol 579:318–325. doi:10.1016/j.ejphar.2007.11.008

Eckel RH (2005) Obesity. Circulation 111:e257–e259. doi:10.1161/01.CIR.0000163653.38992.E5

Everard A, Cani PD (2013) Diabetes, obesity and gut microbiota best practice & research. Clin Gastroenterol 27:73–83. doi:10.1016/j.bpg.2013.03.007

Fang CX, Dong F, Ren BH, Epstein PN, Ren J (2005) Metallothionein alleviates cardiac contractile dysfunction induced by insulin resistance: role of Akt phosphorylation, PTB1B, PPARgamma and c-Jun. Diabetologia 48:2412–2421. doi:10.1007/s00125-005-1940-y

Frank KF, Bolck B, Brixius K, Kranias EG, Schwinger RH (2002) Modulation of SERCA: implications for the failing human heart. Basic Res Cardiol 97 Suppl 1:I72–I78

Galderisi M, Anderson KM, Wilson PW, Levy D (1991) Echocardiographic evidence for the existence of a distinct diabetic cardiomyopathy (the Framingham Heart study). Am J Cardiol 68:85–89

Hage M, Zantout MS, Azar ST (2011) Thyroid disorders and diabetes mellitus. J Thyroid Res 2011:439463. doi:10.4061/2011/439463

Hardie DG (2008) AMPK: a key regulator of energy balance in the single cell and the whole organism. Int J Obes 32 Suppl 4:S7–S12. doi:10.1038/ijo.2008.116

Hawley SA, Gadalla AE, Olsen GS, Hardie DG (2002) The antidiabetic drug metformin activates the AMP-activated protein kinase cascade via an adenine nucleotide-independent mechanism. Diabetes 51:2420–2425

International Diabetes Federation (2015) IDF Diabetes, 7 ed. International Diabetes Federation, Brussels, Belgium. http://www.diabetesatlas.org. Assessed 5 Oct 2015.

Kasuga M (2006) Insulin resistance and pancreatic beta cell failure. J Clin Invest 116:1756–1760. doi:10.1172/JCI29189

Koss KL, Grupp IL, Kranias EG (1997) The relative phospholamban and SERCA2 ratio: a critical determinant of myocardial contractility. Basic Res Cardiol 92 Suppl 1:17–24

Kranias EG, Bers DM (2007) Calcium and cardiomyopathies. Subcell Biochem 45:523–537

Laemmli UK (1970) Cleavage of structural proteins during the assembly of the head of bacteriophage T4. Nature 227:680–685

Lauterio TJ, Bond JP, Ulman EA (1994) Development and characterization of a purified diet to identify obesity-susceptible and resistant rat populations. J Nutr 124:2172–2178

Lebovitz HE (1999) Type 2 diabetes: an overview. Clin Chem 45:1339–1345

Lecomte V et al (2010) A new role for sterol regulatory element binding protein 1 transcription factors in the regulation of muscle mass and muscle cell differentiation. Mol Cell Biol 30:1182–1198. doi:10.1128/MCB.00690-09

Lee IC, Kim DY, Choi BY (2014) Antioxidative activity of blueberry leaf extract prevents high-fat diet-induced obesity in C57BL/6 mice. J Cancer Prev 19: 209–215. doi:10.15430/JCP.2014.19.3.209

Li L, Desantiago J, Chu G, Kranias EG, Bers DM (2000) Phosphorylation of phospholamban and troponin I in beta-adrenergic-induced acceleration of cardiac relaxation. Am J Physiol Heart Circ Physiol 278:H769–H779

Li H, Deng Z, Zhu H, Hu C, Liu R, Young JC, Tsao R (2012) Highly pigmented vegetables: anthocyanin compositions and their role in antioxidant activities. Food Res Int 46:250–259

Maisch B, Alter P, Pankuweit S (2011) Diabetic cardiomyopathy—fact or fiction? Herz 36:102–115. doi:10.1007/s00059-011-3429-4

Mazza G and Miniati E (1993) Anthocyanins in fruits, vegetables and grains. CRC Press Inc., Boca Raton

Mellor KM, Ritchie RH, Davidoff AJ, Delbridge LM (2010) Elevated dietary sugar and the heart: experimental models and myocardial remodeling. Can J Physiol Pharmacol 88:525–540. doi:10.1139/y10-005

Muniyappa R, Montagnani M, Koh KK, Quon MJ (2007) Cardiovascular actions of insulin. Endocr Rev 28:463–491. doi:10.1210/er.2007-0006

Perez de Heredia F, Garaulet M, Portillo MP, Zamora S (2006) Resistance to dietary obesity in rats given different high-energy diets. International journal for vitamin and nutrition research Internationale Zeitschrift fur Vitamin- und Ernahrungsforschung Journal international de vitaminologie et de nutrition 76:271–279. doi:10.1024/0300-9831.76.5.271

Prior RL et al (2003) Assays for hydrophilic and lipophilic antioxidant capacity (oxygen radical absorbance capacity (ORAC(FL))) of plasma and other biological and food samples. J Agric Food Chem 51:3273–3279. doi:10.1021/jf0262256

Ramirez-Correa GA, Murphy AM (2007) Is phospholamban or troponin I the "prima donna" in beta-adrenergic induced lusitropy? Circ Res 101:326–327. doi:10.1161/CIRCRESAHA.107.158873

Reaven GM (1988) Banting lecture 1988. Role of insulin resistance in human disease. Diabetes 37:1595–1607

Roberts CK, Barnard RJ, Sindhu RK, Jurczak M, Ehdaie A, Vaziri ND (2005) A high-fat, refined-carbohydrate diet induces endothelial dysfunction and oxidant/antioxidant imbalance and depresses NOS protein expression. J Appl Physiol 98:203–210. doi:10.1152/japplphysiol.00463.2004

Sewter C et al (2002) Human obesity and type 2 diabetes are associated with alterations in SREBP1 isoform expression that are reproduced ex vivo by tumor necrosis factor-alpha. Diabetes 51:1035–1041

Sharma V, McNeill JH (2006) Diabetic cardiomyopathy: where are we 40 years later? Can J Cardiol 22:305–308

Styskal J, Van Remmen H, Richardson A, Salmon AB (2012) Oxidative stress and diabetes: what can we learn about insulin resistance from antioxidant mutant mouse models? Free Radic Biol Med 52:46–58. doi:10.1016/j.freeradbiomed.2011.10.441

Takikawa M, Inoue S, Horio F, Tsuda T (2010) Dietary anthocyanin-rich bilberry extract ameliorates hyperglycemia and insulin sensitivity via activation of AMP-activated protein kinase in diabetic mice. J Nutr 140: 527–533. doi:10.3945/jn.109.118216

Towbin H, Staehelin T, Gordon J (1979) Electrophoretic transfer of proteins from polyacrylamide gels to nitrocellulose sheets: procedure and some applications. Proc Natl Acad Sci U S A 76:4350–4354

Tsuda T, Horio F, Uchida K, Aoki H, Osawa T (2003) Dietary cyanidin 3-O-beta-D-glucoside-rich purple corn color prevents obesity and ameliorates hyperglycemia in mice. J Nutr 133:2125–2130

Turnbaugh PJ, Backhed F, Fulton L, Gordon JI (2008) Diet-induced obesity is linked to marked but reversible alterations in the mouse distal gut microbiome. Cell Host Microbe 3:213–223. doi:10.1016/j.chom.2008.02.015

van den Brom CE et al (2009) Altered myocardial substrate metabolism is associated with myocardial dysfunction in early diabetic cardiomyopathy in rats: studies using positron emission tomography. Cardiovasc Diabetol 8:39. doi:10.1186/1475-2840-8-39

Vasanji Z, Cantor EJ, Juric D, Moyen M, Netticadan T (2006) Alterations in cardiac contractile performance and sarcoplasmic reticulum function in sucrose-fed rats is associated with insulin resistance. Am J Physiol Cell Physiol 291:C772–C780. doi:10.1152/ajpcell.00086.2005

Wu T, Tang Q, Gao Z, Yu Z, Song H, Zheng X, Chen W (2013) Blueberry and mulberry juice prevent obesity development in C57BL/6 mice. PLoS One 8, e77585. doi:10.1371/journal.pone.0077585

Ye G, Donthi RV, Metreveli NS, Epstein PN (2005) Overexpression of hexokinase protects hypoxic and diabetic cardiomyocytes by increasing ATP generation. Cardiovasc Toxicol 5:293–300

Zdychova J, Komers R (2005) Emerging role of Akt kinase/protein kinase B signaling in pathophysiology of diabetes and its complications. Physiol Res 54:1–16

Zhang R, Zhao J, Mandveno A, Potter JD (1995) Cardiac troponin I phosphorylation increases the rate of cardiac muscle relaxation. Circ Res 76:1028–1035

Zhang Z, Kou X, Fugal K, McLaughlin J (2004) Comparison of HPLC methods for determination of anthocyanins and anthocyanidins in bilberry extracts. J Agric Food Chem 52:688–691. doi:10.1021/jf034596w

2

Effect of high carbohydrate diet on elongase and desaturase activity and accompanying gene expression in rat's liver

Jagoda Drąg[1,4*], Anna Goździalska[2], Małgorzata Knapik-Czajka[1], Anna Gawędzka[1], Katarzyna Gawlik[3] and Jerzy Jaśkiewicz[2]

Abstract

Background: Hepatic fatty acids (FAs) are modified through different metabolic pathways including elongation and desaturation. These processes are catalyzed by elongases and desaturases, respectively. Glucose, by transcription factors, regulates these processes. The aim of the study was to evaluate the influence of high carbohydrate diet (68%) on the expression of elongase (Elovl-2, Elovl-5, and Elovl-6) and desaturase (Δ5D, Δ6D, Scd 1, Scd 2) genes and the activity of the enzymes. The changes in serum lipid profile (triglycerides (TG), total cholesterol (TC), HDL cholesterol) and glucose concentration were measured. Male Wistar rats were randomized into two study groups: animals fed with high carbohydrate diet ($n = 6$; HiCHO) and a control group fed with a standard diet ($n = 6$; ST). The expression of mRNA was determinate using reverse transcription PCR (RT-PCR). Hepatic FA composition was determined by gas chromatography, and FA ratios were used to estimate the activity of enzymes. Serum lipid profile and glucose concentration were measured using spectrophotometric methods.

Results: The mean values of transcript expression of all examined elongases and desaturases in liver HiCHO rats were higher as compared to ST. Higher expression did not always correspond to higher activity (as index). More monounsaturated FAs (MUFAs) were detected in the liver of HiCHO rats as compared to ST. Serum TG level was higher in the HiCHO than in ST.

Conclusions: These studies support the notion that the regulation of both Elovl and desaturase expression may play an important role in managing hepatic lipid composition in response to changes in dietary status.

Keywords: Elongases, Desaturases, Fatty acids, High carbohydrate diet

Background

In mammals, the liver is responsible for the conversion of excess dietary carbohydrates into triglycerides (TG), through de novo lipogenesis (DNL). Fatty acids (FAs) derived from a diet as well as synthesized from carbohydrates are modified through different metabolic pathways including elongation and desaturation [1]. FAs are then used mainly for TG synthesis, then incorporated into lipoproteins (mainly VLDL), and released to plasma [2–4]. Parts of FAs are the components of phospholipids (PL) and neutral lipids [5].

FA elongation is performed in four steps, catalyzed by the following enzymes: ketoacyl-CoA synthase (elongase, EC 2.3.1.), 3-ketoacyl-CoA reductase (KAR; EC 1.1.1.-), 3-hydroxyacyl-CoA dehydratase (EC 4.2.1.134), and 2,3-transenoyl-CoA reductase (TER; EC 1.3.1.38). Elongation occurs in the membrane of the endoplasmic reticulum (ER) with malonyl-CoA as two-carbon donor, mitochondria with acetyl-CoA as two-carbon donor and peroxisomes [2, 6–8]. Based on different substrate specificity, elongases (Elovl) can be divided into four groups. The first group are isoforms that elongates saturated (SFA) and monounsaturated fatty acids (MUFA) (Elovl-1, Elovl-3, Elovl-6, and Elovl-7); the second group includes

* Correspondence: jagoda.drag@gmail.com
[1]Department of Analytical Biochemistry, Faculty of Pharmacy, Jagiellonian University Medical College, Krakow, Poland
[4]Andrzej Frycz Modrzewski Krakow University, 1 G. Herlinga-Grudzińskiego St., 30-705 Krakow, Poland
Full list of author information is available at the end of the article

elongase 2 (Elovl-2) that is involved in polyunsaturated fatty acid (PUFA) synthesis; the third group is elongase 5 (Elovl-5) catalyzing elongation of 18–22 carbons of PUFA as well as 16:1 n-7, and the last one is elongase 4 (Elovl-4) that elongates saturated as well as unsaturated very long chain FAs [4, 7–10].

FAs are also products in the oxidative desaturation process. The introduction of a double bond into a carbon chain occurs in the endoplasmic reticulum and requires molecular oxygen, NAD(P)H, flavoprotein cytochrome b5 reductase, and the electron acceptor cytochrome b5 and is catalyzed by a specific desaturase. In mammals, FA desaturases (EC 1.14.19) are acyl-CoA desaturases, which include mainly Δ5 desaturase (Δ5D), Δ6 desaturase (Δ6D), and Δ9 desaturase (Δ9D) (also known as stearoyl-CoA-desaturase or SCD). Δ5D and Δ6D catalyze the biosynthesis of PUFA. Their most common substrates are C16–C24, mainly exogenous nutrients as α-linoleic acid and linolenic acid. Δ9D catalyzes introduction of a double bond into SFA with the preferred substrates as C16:0-CoA and 18-CoA. Two isoforms of Δ9D called Scd1 and Scd2 exist in rats [2, 5, 11, 12].

Physiological control of FA elongation and desaturation remains poorly defined. It is known that the elongases and desaturases appear to be mainly regulated on the transcriptional level. It was proposed that transcriptional factors such as carbohydrate-responsive element-binding protein (ChREBP) [3, 13–17], liver X receptor α (LXRα) [2, 18, 19], and sterol regulatory element-binding proteins 1c (SREBP-1c) [3, 8, 20–23] are key mediators in elongases and desaturases messenger RNA (mRNA) levels regulation. These transcription factors are modified by different nutritional factors and metabolic states. It has been shown that glucose as a substrate for FA synthesis induces lipogenesis and expressions of lipogenic genes [24]. In primary hepatocytes, Elovl-6 and SCD mRNAs were induced by glucose [3]. Expression of the murine liver stearoyl-CoA desaturase gene (SCD1) is induced upon feeding fasted mice a fat-free, high carbohydrate diet [25]. Expression and activity of elongases and desaturases was changed in adult male rats by HiCHO diet supplemented with olive oil (10%, *w/w*), fish oil (10%, *w/w*), or the PPAR-agonist WY14, 643 (0.1%, *w/w*) [1]. In the liver of diabetic rats (diabetes induced with streptozotocin), declined Elovl-6 and SCD mRNA abundance were shown [1]. Treatment of rat insulinoma (INS)-1 cells with elevated glucose increased de novo FA synthesis by modification of elongases and desaturases expression and enhanced production of monounsaturated fatty acids [4].There are no studies showing the changes of mRNA levels for many elongases and desaturases together with their activities (expressed as indexes) in Wistar's rat livers after the carbohydrate diet (68% sucrose).

The aim of the present study was to evaluate the influence of high carbohydrate diet (68%) on the expression of elongase (Elovl-2, Elovl-5, and Elovl-6) and desaturases' (Δ5D, Δ6D, Scd 1, and Scd 2) genes. The activities of the Δ5D (20:4n-6/20:3n-6), Δ6D (18:3n-6/18:2n-6), stearoyl-CoA desaturase 1 (SCD-1; 16:1n-7/16:0, SCD-16 and 18:1n-9/18:0, SCD-18), DNL (16:0/18:2n-6), Elovl-6 (18:0/16:0) and FA elongation (18:0 + 18:1 n-9/16:0) was expressed as FA ratios. For the first time, the ratio 20:3 n-6/18:3 n-6 was used as the activity of Elovl-5 (Elovl-5 index). FA composition in rat livers was determined. We have also measured the changes in serum lipid profile (TG, total cholesterol (TC), HDL cholesterol) and glucose concentration.

Methods

Animals

Animal experiments were conducted in accordance with the guidelines for animal experiments of Animal Research Committee and were approved by the Jagiellonian University Ethic Committee.

Male Wistar rats weighing 151 ± 3 g were purchased from the breeding facility of the Jagiellonian University Faculty of Pharmacy. Animals were multi-caged and maintained under standardized conditions of artificial 12-h light/dark cycle and constant room temperature (21–23 °C). Animals were given ad libitum access to food and water. Animals were randomized into two study groups: (1) standard diet-fed controls (ST) ($n = 6$, control) (Murigran, Concentrate and Mix Feed Factory AGROPOL, Motycz) and (2) high-carbohydrate diet-fed study group (HiCHO) ($n = 6$) (containing 68% carbohydrates, MP Biomedicals, 960236), until rats achieved 250 g (25 days ST vs. 21 days HiCHO). Then rats were sacrificed, and liver tissues were excised and freeze-clamped with aluminum tongs precooled in liquid nitrogen. From each rat, the blood was collected to obtain serum, which was stored at −80 °C until analysis. All samples were stored immediately at −80 °C and kept frozen until further analysis.

Determination of elongases and desaturases mRNA expression

Relative levels of specific mRNA for Elovl-2, Elovl-5, and Elovl-6 and Δ5D, Δ6D, Scd 1, and Scd 2 in rat's liver were assessed by semi-quantitative reverse transcription polymerase chain reaction (RT-PCR). Each gene was amplified together with a housekeeping gene β-actin (Actb; internal control). Total RNA was isolated from the liver using TRI reagent (Sigma-Aldrich, Germany), and complementary DNA (cDNA) was subsequently synthesized using 1 μg total RNA, reverse-transcriptase, and oligo dT primers (RevertAid™ H Minus First Strand cDNA Synthesis Kit, Fermentas, Lithuania). cDNA was amplified with OptiTaq DNA polymerase (Eurx, Poland) following manufacturer's instructions. Each PCR reaction was performed with 1.2 μl cDNA and 1.6 μl of specific primers for each gene (Table 1) that were designed using Primer3 v.0.4.0 (Table 1). Mastercycler gradient EP 5331 (Eppendorf, Germany) was used. The PCR products were then subjected to agarose gel electrophoresis (1.5% agarose gel), stained with ethidium bromide and analyzed by densitometry using the Quantity One 4.2.1. software (Bio Rad). Obtained data were calculated to the mean value of the 200-bp band marker first (GeneRuler™ 1 kb Plus DNA, Fermentas, Lithuania) and then normalized to β-actin (in the same sample).

Lipid extraction and quantitation of hepatic FA composition

Total lipid extraction from the liver was carried out using a solution of chloroform/methanol (2:1) [26]. The synthesis of FA methyl esters (FAME) was carried out with 14% BF3 in methanol [27]. FAME were analyzed using gas chromatography (Agilent 6890 N) with FID and a DB-23 (60 m, 0.25 mm) column as described earlier [28, 29]. Fatty acid methyl esters were identified according to standards Supelco® 37 Component FAME Mix (Sigma, Supelco). The data were analyzed using ChemStation. Results were expressed in relative percentage of the sum of saturated (SAT), unsaturated (UNSAT), monounsaturated (MUFA), and polyunsaturated fatty acids (PUFA). The group of SAT includes 12:0, 14:0, 16:0, 17:0, 18:0, 21:0, and 22:0. The group of UNSAT includes 16:1 n-7, 18:1 n-9, 18:2 n-6, 18:3 n-6, 20:3 n-6, 20:4 n-6, 20:5 n-3, and 22:6 n-3. The group of MUFA includes 16:1 n-7 and 18:1 n-9. The group of PUFA includes 18:2 n-6, 18:3 n-6, 20:3 n-6, 20:4 n-6, 20:5 n-3, and 22:6 n-3.

Desaturation, elongation, and de novo lipogenesis indexes

Particular FA ratios were used to estimate relative activities of the Δ5D (20:4n-6/20:3n-6), Δ6D (18:3n-6/18:2n-6), stearoyl-CoA desaturase 1 (SCD-1; 16:1n-7/16:0, SCD-16 and 18:1n-9/18:0, SCD-18), DNL (16:0/18:2n-6), Elovl-6 (18:0/16:0), and FA elongation (18:0 + 18:1 n-9/16:0) as described earlier [4, 30–32]. For the first time, the ratio 20:3 n-6/18:3 n-6 was used as activity of Elovl-5 (Elovl-5 index).

Determination of rat's serum lipid profile and glucose concentration

Serum lipid parameters including total cholesterol, HDL cholesterol, triglycerides, and glucose concentration were measured spectrophotometrically using standard kits (AQUA-MED, Poland and BioMaxima, Poland). Tests were performed according to manufacturer's instructions. Results were presented as mmol/L.

Statistics

Statistical calculations were performed using STATISTICA 12.0 and GraphPad Prism v. 5.02. Shapiro-Wilk test was used for normality assessing. Student's t test for unpaired samples (data are presented as mean ± SD) was used to analyze mRNA expression for all elongases and desaturases, with indicators such as PUFA and MUFA, composed of 14:0, 16:0, 16:1 n-7, 17:0, 18:0, 18:1 n-9, 18:2 n-6, 18:3 n-6, 21:0, 22:0, 20:3 n-6, and 20:5 n-3, and indexes for Δ5D, Scd 1 (C16), DNL, Elovl-5, Elovl-6, elongation FAs, and glucose concentration and serum lipid profile. Mann-Whitney U test (data are presented as median and range) was used to analyze the indicators SAT and UNSAT, composed of 12:0, 20:4 n-6, 22:6 n-3, and indexes for Δ6D and Scd 1 (C18). Acceptable significance level was set at $p < 0.05$.

Results

mRNA expression of elongases and desaturases

In the liver of HiCHO and ST rats, mRNA expression of Elovl-2, Elovl-5, and Elovl-6 was obtained (Fig. 1). The mean values of transcript expression of all examined elongases in liver HiCHO rats were higher than in ST. In HiCHO group, mRNA levels were increased for Elovl-2, Elovl-5, and Elovl-6 by 1, 25, and 15% as compared to ST, respectively. The difference in expression for Elovl-5 and Elovl-6 were statistically significant ($p < 0.05$).

Table 1 The primers sequences used for PCR

Gene name (symbol)	Left primer sequence	Right primer sequence	Concentration; left/right primer	Length of product
Elovl-2	TCAACAATGGCAGCTCAAAG	GGGGGATTTACTTGGGAAAA	4 μm/4 μm	249
Elovl-5	GAGGCATCCTGGTGGTGTAT	ACGTGCAGGACTGTGATCTG	4 μm/4 μm	247
Elovl-6	GCTACAACGGAGCAGAGGAC	CCATTTTCAAGCCAACCAGT	4 μm/4 μm	247
Δ5D	GAAGGAACAGCAGTCCAAGC	GTCTGGACTCGTGGAAGAGC	4 μm/4 μm	185
Δ6D	ATCTGCCCTACAACCACCAG	TGTGACCCACACAAACCAGT	4 μm/4 μm	248
Scd 1	CTGTTAGCCCAGCCTCACTC	GTCTGCAGGAAAACCTCTGC	2 μm/2 μm	668
Scd 2	CCAGAGCGTACCAGCTTTTC	GGCTGTCACCCAATCAGAAT	4 μm/4 μm	342
β-actin (Actb)	AGCCATGTACGTAGCCATCC	CTCTCAGCTGTGGTGGTGAA	4 μm/4 μm	228

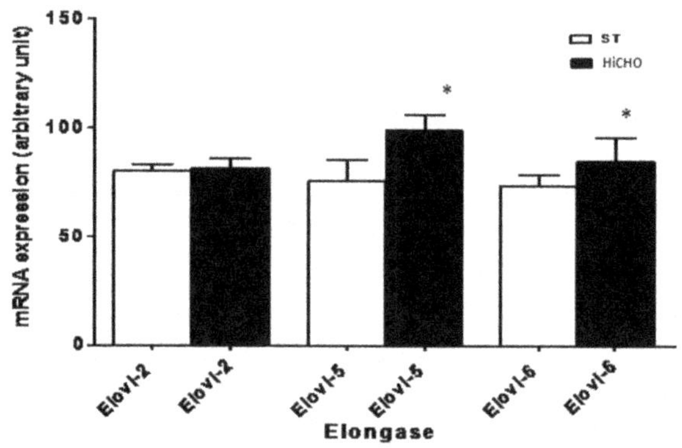

Fig. 1 Relative levels of specific mRNA for Elovl-2, Elovl-5, and Elovl-6 in the liver of HiCHO and control groups. *HiCHO* high-carbohydrate (68%) diet-fed study group ($n = 6$), *ST rats* standard diet-fed controls ($n = 6$). Male Wistar rats weighing 151 ± 3 g were fed until achieved 250 g (21 days HiCHO vs. 25 days ST). The expression was determined by RT-PCR. Each gene was amplified together with a housekeeping gene β-actin (Actb; internal control). PCR products were separated on 1.5% agarose gel, stained with ethidium bromide, and analyzed by densitometry using the Quantity One 4.2.1. software. Obtained data were calculated to the mean value of the 200-bp band marker first and then normalized to β-actin (in the same sample). Shapiro-Wilk test was used for normality assessing. Student's *t* test for unpaired samples; $*p < 0.05$

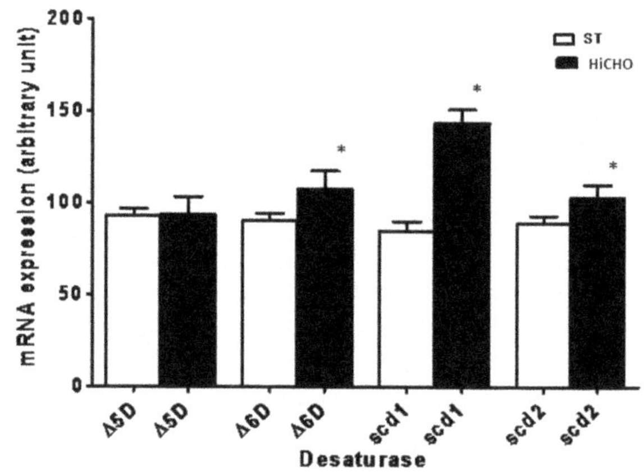

Fig. 2 Relative levels of specific mRNA for Δ5D, Δ6D, Scd 1, and Scd 2 in the liver of the HiCHO and control groups. *HiCHO* high-carbohydrate (68%) diet-fed study group ($n = 6$); *ST rats* standard diet-fed controls ($n = 6$). Male Wistar rats weighing 151 ± 3 g were fed until achieved 250 g (21 days HiCHO vs. 25 days ST). Each gene was amplified together with a housekeeping gene β-actin (Actb; internal control). The expression was determined by RT-PCR. $*p < 0.05$. PCR products were separated on 1.5% agarose gel, stained with ethidium bromide, and analyzed by densitometry using the Quantity One 4.2.1. software. Obtained data were calculated to the mean value of the 200-bp band marker first and then normalized to β-actin (in the same sample). Shapiro-Wilk test was used for normality assessing. Student's *t* test for unpaired samples; $*p < 0.05$

In the liver of HiCHO and ST rats, mRNA expression of Δ5D, Δ6D, Scd 1, and Scd 2 desaturases was obtained (Fig. 2). The mean values of transcript expression of all examined desaturases in liver HiCHO rats were higher than in ST. In HiCHO group, mRNA expression levels increased by 5, 19, 69, and 16% as compared to ST for desaturases Δ5D, Δ6D, Scd 1, and Scd 2, respectively. The difference in expression for Δ6D, Scdl, and Scd2 desaturases was statistically significant ($p < 0.05$).

Hepatic fatty acid composition

The mean values of SAT, UNSAT, PUFA, and MUFA in the liver of HiCHO and ST rats were calculated (Fig. 3). In the liver of HiCHO rats, the value of SAT increased by 4% and UNSAT decreased by 2.5% as compared to ST group. In liver of HiCHO group, the mean value of MUFA increased by 83% while the mean value of PUFA decreased by 26% as compared to ST. The difference in hepatic fatty acid composition for MUFA and PUFA indicators were statistically significant ($p < 0.05$).

Fifteen fatty acids were determined using gas chromatography. In the liver of HiCHO and ST rats, groupwise, the relative percentage of individual fatty acids differed (Fig. 4). The relative percentage of 12:0, 14:0, 16:0, 16:1 n-7, 18:1 n-9, and 18:3 n-6 in rat liver of HiCHO group increased by 4.5, 99, 32, 207, 71, and 203%, respectively, as compared to ST. The relative percentage of 17:0, 18:0, 18:2 n-6, 22:0, 20:3 n-6, 20:4 n-6, 20:5 n-3, and 22:6 n-3 decreased by 51, 50, 3.8, 75, 50, 81%, 85.5, and 71%,

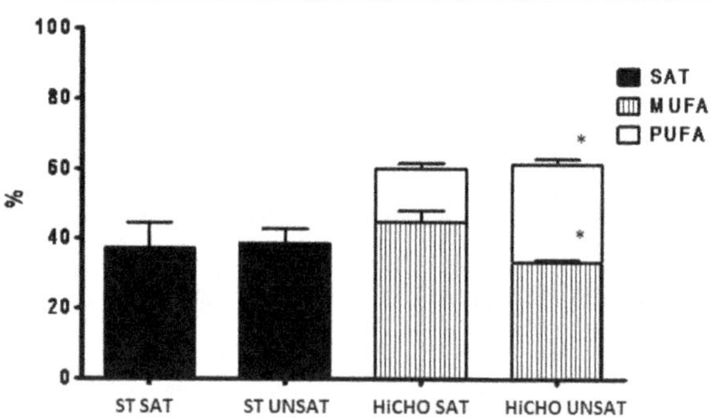

Fig. 3 The mean values of indicators *SAT*, *UNSAT*, *PUFA*, and MUFA in the liver of the HiCHO and control groups. *HiCHO* high-carbohydrate (68%) diet-fed study group ($n = 6$); *ST rats* standard diet-fed controls ($n = 6$). Male Wistar rats weighing 151 ± 3 g were fed until achieved 250 g (21 days HiCHO vs. 25 days ST). Fatty acid composition was determined using gas chromatography. Results were expressed in relative percentage of the sum of saturated (SAT), unsaturated (UNSAT), monounsaturated (MUFA), and polyunsaturated fatty acids (PUFA). The group of SAT includes 12:0, 14:0, 16:0, 17:0, 18:0, 21:0, and 22:0. The group of UNSAT includes 16:1 n-7, 18:1 n-9, 18:2 n-6, 18:3 n-6, 20:3 n-6, 20:4 n-6, 20:5 n-3, and 22:6 n-3. The group of MUFA includes 16:1 n-7 and 18:1 n-9. The group of PUFA includes 18:2 n-6, 18:3 n-6, 20:3 n-6, 20:4 n-6, 20:5 n-3, and 22:6 n-3. Shapiro-Wilk test was used for normality assessing. Student's *t* test for unpaired samples (data are presented as mean ± SD) was used to analyze indicators such as PUFA and MUFA; Mann-Whitney *U* test (data are presented as median and range) was used to analyze the indicators SAT and UNSAT. $*p < 0.05$

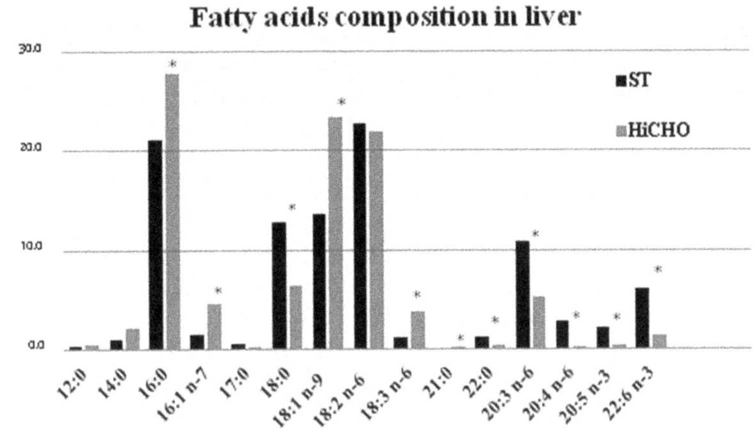

Fig. 4 The relative percentage of individual fatty acids in the liver of the HiCHO and control groups. *HiCHO* high-carbohydrate (68%) diet-fed study group ($n = 6$); *ST rats* standard diet-fed controls ($n = 6$). Male Wistar rats weighing 151 ± 3 g were fed until achieved 250 g (21 days HiCHO vs. 25 days ST). Fatty acid composition was determined using gas chromatography. Shapiro-Wilk test was used for normality assessing. Student's *t* test for unpaired samples (data are presented as mean ± SD) was used to analyze the composition of 14:0, 16:0, 16:1 n-7, 17:0, 18:0, 18:1 n-9, 18:2 n-6, 18:3 n-6, 21:0, 22:0, 20:3 n-6, and 20:5 n-3, and Mann-Whitney *U* test (data are presented as median and range) was used to analyze the composition of 12:0, 20:4 n-6, and 22:6 n-3; $^*p < 0.05$

respectively, as compared to ST group. Heneicosanoic acid (21:0) was detected only in the liver of HiCHO group not in ST group. The difference in the relative percentage of individual fatty acids for 16:0, 16:1 n-7, 18:0, 18:1 n-9, 18:3 n-6, 21:0, 22:0, 20:3 n-6, 20:4 n-6, 20:5 n-3, and 22:6 n-3 was statistically significant ($p < 0.05$).

Desaturation, elongation, and DNL indexes

In the rat's liver, the differences in the value of indexes for desaturation, elongation, and DNL were observed (Table 2). In HiCHO group, indexes for Δ5D, Elovl-5, Elovl-6, and FA elongation decreased by 80, 84, 62, and 17%, respectively, as compared to ST group. In HiCHO group, indexes for Δ6D, SCD1(16), SCD1(18), and DNL increased by 153, 137, 311, and 27% as compared to ST group. The differences in the indexes for Δ5D, Δ6D, SCD1 (16), SCD1 (18), Elovl-5, and Elovl-6 were statistically significant ($p < 0.05$).

Table 2 The mean values of indexes for desaturation, elongation, and DNL. Data are presented as mean ± SD or median (range)

Name	Index	ST	HiCHO
Δ5D	20:4 n-6/20:3 n-6	0.25 ± 0.11	0.05 ± 0.06*
Δ6D	18:3 n-6/18:2 n-6	0.07 (0.02–0.07)	0.17 (0.14–0.19)*
Scd 1 (C16)	16:1 n-7/ 16:0	0.07 ± 0.02	0.17 ± 0.02*
Scd 1 (C18)	18:1 n-9/18:0	0.92 (0.71–2.56)	3.79 (3.13–4.34)*
DNL	16:0/18:2 n-6	1.02 ± 0.36	1.29 ± 0.22
Elovl-5	20:3 n-6/18:3 n-6	9.27 ± 1.98	1.49 ± 0.43*
Elovl-6	18:0/16:0	0.60 ± 0.16	0.23 ± 0.02*
Elongation FA	18:0 + 18:1 n-9/16:0	1.3 ± 0.1	1.07 ± 0.06*

$^*p < 0.05$

Analysis of serum lipid profile and glucose concentration

Parameters of serum lipid profile and glucose concentration differed in two study groups (Fig. 5). In HiCHO group, glucose, TG, TC, and HDL cholesterol increased by 11, 241, 23, and 7.4%, respectively, as compared to ST. Significantly higher concentration was only for TG ($p < 0.05$).

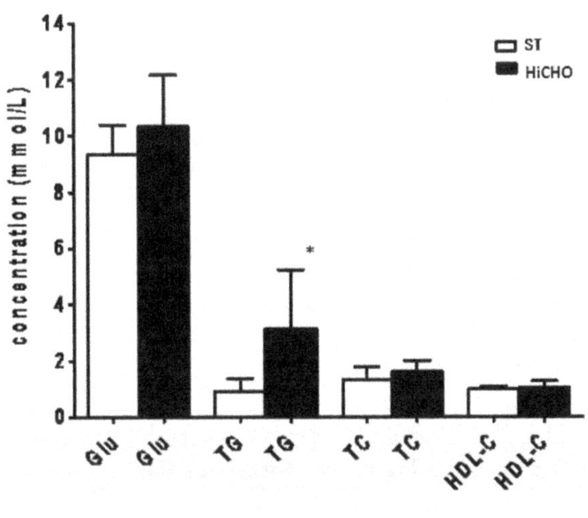

Fig. 5 The mean concentrations of glucose, TG, TC, and HDL cholesterol in the serum of the HiCHO and control groups. *HiCHO* high-carbohydrate (68%) diet-fed study group ($n = 6$); *ST rats* standard diet-fed controls ($n = 6$). Male Wistar rats weighing 151 ± 3 g were fed until achieved 250 g (21 days HiCHO vs. 25 days ST). Shapiro-Wilk test was used for normality assessing. Student's *t* test for unpaired samples (data are presented as mean ± SD) was used to analyze glucose concentration and serum lipid profile. $^*p < 0.05$. Results are expressed as millimolar per liter

Discussion

De novo FA synthesis and MUFA

Diets enriched in carbohydrates are well established to alter FA metabolism and increase TG accumulation [4]. In our study, we observed the active DNL and the influence of the HiCHO diet on increased expression of all studied enzymes resulting in increased production of MUFAs. The most important changes concern metabolism of 16:0 and 18:0 as a dominant products of DNL [30]. Both FAs are subjects to elongation or desaturation processes [33]. On the basis of our observation, the desaturation is a main process of 16:0 and 18:0 metabolism in liver of rat fed HiCHO diet because of a higher expression of mRNA for Scd1 (Fig. 2), a higher content of 16:1 n-7 and 18:1 n −9 (Fig. 4), and a higher activity of desaturases as indexes for Scd1 (C16) and Scd1 (C18) (Tab. 2) as compared to control group. The index for Scd1 (C16) is proposed as an indirect biomarker of DNL [30]. Scd 1 is the main isoform in MUFAs synthesis with 16:0 and 18:0 as main substrates [34]. As Scd1 plays a crucial role in this synthesis, the role of Scd2 remains unclear. Our findings indicate that 16:0 and 18:0 metabolism is directed to MUFAs synthesis as 16:1 n-7 and 18:1 n-9, respectively, that are main components of TG and PL. Especially, 18:1 n-9 is the preferred substrate for TG storage of excess FAs [4]. In our study, it was observed that in HiCHO group, liver tissues contain statistically more MUFAs (with prevalence 16:1 n-7 and 18:1 n-9 fatty acids; Figs. 3 and 4) and less PUFAs than control. The study by Wang et al. [1] indicates that 16:0, 18:0, 18:1 n-9, and 18:2 n-6 acids represent the major fatty acids and 16:1 n-7 is an end product of DNL and Scd. The results from our study (Fig. 4) are consistent with the results obtained by Wang et al. [1]. The last but not the least, in our study, serum level of TG was higher in HiCHO than in control (Fig. 5) that may indicate that newly synthesized FAs as TG incorporated into lipoproteins were released to plasma.

The glucose is converted into FAs in DNL process by the induction of genes transcription that increase glucose metabolism and lipogenesis in the liver [4]. According to substrate specific, Elovl-6, Scd1, and Scd2 desaturases might be responsible for these changes [2, 8]. Genes of Elovl-6, Scd1, and Scd2 desaturases contain the response element for transcriptional factors such as SREBP, LXR, and ChREBP, in their promoter [1]. Wang et al. [1] indicate that in primary hepatocytes glucose regulates both Elovl-6 and Scd expression by mechanisms that control the nuclear abundance of ChREBP and MLX. It is known that during carbohydrates excess, glucose/insulin stimulates hepatic lipogenesis via LXR and SREBP-1 [18, 35, 36]. Glucose as natural ligand for LXR may induce FA and TG synthesis as it was seen in our study, where rat fed with HiCHO diet had higher serum TG level than control group. ChREBP, a central transcriptional regulator of hepatic DNL, is also regulated by glucose itself, increasing expression of mRNA for elongase 6 and Scd desaturases [1, 2].

PUFA synthesis

Metabolism of PUFAs depends on the content of 18:2 n-6 and 18:3 n-3 as essential FAs derived from a diet. These FAs are substrates for elongases and desaturases. In our study, we observed that liver tissues of HiCHO group contain statistically less PUFAs than control group (Fig. 3). In the current study, it was observed that the diet enriched in glucose increased expression of Elovl-5, Δ5D, and Δ6D mRNA (Figs. 1 and 2) but relative activities of these enzymes were different (Tab. 2). The result of these processes is reduction of PUFA synthesis. Because of the low activity of Elovl-5 and Δ5D, we observed the lower content of 20:3 n-6, 20:4 n-6, and 22:6 n-3 PUFAs in HiCHO group than in control group. The control mechanism of decreasing activity of these two enzymes remains unresolved. Moon et al. [10] reported that ablation of Elovl5 increases hepatic lipid content, at least in part by inducing SREBP-1, a key transcription factor controlling de novo lipogenesis. Tissues of Elovl5(−/−) mice accumulated the C18 substrates of ELOVL5 and the levels of C20:4 n-6 and C22:6 n-3 were decreased [10]. The same changes in the content of FAs were observed in our study but mainly as a result of lower relative activity of Elovl-5 than the lower level of expression. It cannot be excluded that high expression of SREBP-1c decrease activity of Elovl-5. It may explain the results achieved in the current study because of glucose as a strong inducer of SREBP-1. Recently, Wang et al. [37] reported the metabolic effects of adenoviral-mediated overexpression of Elovl-5. The relative levels of 20:4 n-6 and 22:6 n-3 in mouse livers that overexpressed Elovl-5 were decreased despite an increase in 20:3 n-6. Thus, it is possible that the Δ5 desaturase becomes rate-limiting in case of Elovl-5 overexpression [37]. Δ5D a rate-limiting enzyme, as it was suggested by Wang, can explain only low levels for 20:4 n-6 and 22:6 n-3. More research is needed to clarify the cause of Elovl-5 and Δ5D low activity.

In the current study, only two members of n-3 PUFA family were determined (20:5 n-3 and 22:6 n-3; Fig. 4). It is difficult to explain changes in content of these FAs in the liver because of the lack of 18:3 n-3 precursor. We may conclude that the hypothesis stated by Wang [37] (Δ5 desaturase is a rate-limiting enzyme) may explain lower hepatic levels of 20:5 n-3 and 22:6 n-3 in HiCHO group compares to ST.

The expressions of Elovl-5, Δ5D, and Δ6D involved in PUFA metabolism are under control of transcription factors such as PPAR, LXR, and SREBP-1c [1, 19, 35, 38]. Genes of Elovl-5, Δ5D, and Δ6D contain the response element for these transcriptional factors in their promoter. Only elongase 2 is not regulated in this way. In our study, expression of elongase 2 did not change in liver of rats fed high carbohydrate diet in comparison to control group. Our results complements data obtained by Wang et al. [3], who investigated the influence of different diets (high carbohydrate diet supplemented with olive oil, fish oil, or olive oil plus WY14,643) on mRNA expression for elongase 2. None of them changed the mRNA expression of elongase 2 [3]. Hepatic Elovl-5 is regulated by LXRα-SREBP-1c [19]. Mitro et al. [18] showed that glucose binds and stimulates the transcriptional activity of LXR. These findings may suggest the regulation of Elovl-5 expression by these factors in liver of rats fed high carbohydrate diet. The problem of low activity of Elovl-5 remains unresolved. Wang et al. [1] suggest that the induction of Δ5D and Δ6D by insulin and T1317 (the LXR agonist) is attributable to increased SREBP-1 nuclear abundance. These findings, altogether, may explain higher expression of Δ5D and Δ6D in livers of rats of HiCHO group as compared to control group. PPAR-α expressed primarily in the liver is essential for metabolic adaptation to starvation by inducing genes for β-oxidation and ketogenesis and by downregulating energy expenditure [39]. It can confirm that this transcriptional factor through a high carbohydrate diet given ad libitum plays a minor role in regulation of lipogenic gene transcription. To sum up, increased hepatic glucose flux activates SREBP and LXR, which act to couple increased carbohydrate intake with induction of lipogenic genes as Δ5D and Δ6D.

Conclusions

In this study, we have established that hepatic fatty acid elongases (Elovl-5 and Elovl-6) and desaturases (Δ5D, Δ6D, Scd-1, and Scd-2) are regulated by high carbohydrate diet. Additionally, we have indicated that changes in activity do not always correspond to changes of Elovl and desaturases mRNA levels. We have demonstrated that elevated intake of glucose modified FAs composition in liver with prevalence of MUFA as well as increased serum level of TG, of which MUFA are main components. The changes might be connected with unfavorable lipogenesis in liver. These studies support the notion that the regulation of both Elovl and desaturase expression may play an important role in managing hepatic lipid composition in response to changes in dietary status.

Abbreviations

Δ5D: Δ5 desaturase; Δ6D: Δ6 desaturase; Δ9D or SCD: Δ9 desaturase; ChREBP: Carbohydrate-responsive element-binding protein; DNL: De novo lipogenesis; Elovl: Elongases; ER: Endoplasmic reticulum; FAME: Fatty acid methyl esters; FAs: Fatty acids; KAR: 3-ketoacyl-CoA reductase; LXRα: Liver X receptor α; MUFA: Monounsaturated fatty acids; PL: Phospholipids; PUFA: Polyunsaturated fatty acids; RT-PCR: Reverse transcription polymerase chain reaction; SAT or SFA: Saturated fatty acids; SCD1: Stearoyl-CoA desaturase isoform 1; SREBP-1c: Sterol regulatory element-binding proteins 1c; TC: Total cholesterol; TER: 2,3-transenoyl-CoA reductase; TG: Triglycerides; UNSAT: Unsaturated fatty acids

Acknowledgements

Authors would like to thank Katarzyna Wadowska for her excellent technical support.

Authors' contributions

JD and JJ conceived and designed the experiment. AG, AG, and MKC provided the technique. JD performed the animal experiment. JD, AG, MKC, AG, and JJ analyzed the data. JD, MKC, and KG wrote the paper. All authors read and approved the final manuscript.

Competing interests

The authors declare that they have no competing interests.

Author details

[1]Department of Analytical Biochemistry, Faculty of Pharmacy, Jagiellonian University Medical College, Krakow, Poland. [2]Faculty of Health and Medical Sciences, Andrzej Frycz Modrzewski Krakow University, Krakow, Poland. [3]Department of Diagnostics, Chair of Clinical Biochemistry, Jagiellonian University Medical College, Krakow, Poland. [4]Andrzej Frycz Modrzewski Krakow University, 1 G. Herlinga-Grudzińskiego St., 30-705 Krakow, Poland.

References

1. Wang Y, Botolin D, Xu J, Christian B, Mitchell E, Jayaprakasam B, Nair MG, Peters JM, Busik JV, Olson LK, Jump DB. Regulation of hepatic fatty acid elongase and desaturase expression in diabetes and obesity. J Lipid Res. 2006;47(9):2028–41.
2. Miyazaki M, Ntambi JM. Fatty acid desaturation and chain elongation in mammals. In: Vance JE, Vance DE, editors. Biochemistry of lipids lipoproteins and membranes. 5th ed. Amsterdam: Elsevier; 2008. p. 191–211.
3. Wang Y, Botolin D, Christian B, Busik J, Xu J, Jump DB. Tissue-specific nutritional and developmental regulation of rat fatty acid elongases. J Lipid Res. 2005;46:706–15.
4. Green CD, Ozguden-Akkoc CG, Wang Y, Jump DB, Olson LK. Role of fatty acid elongases in determination of de novo synthesized monounsaturated fatty acid species. J Lipid Res. 2010;7(51):1871–7.
5. Paton CM, Ntambi JM. Biochemical and physiological function of stearoyl-CoA desaturase. Am J Physiol Endocrinol Metab. 2009;297(1):E28–37.
6. Leonard AE, Pereira SL, Sprecher H, Yung-Sheng H. Elongation of long-chain fatty acids. Prog Lipid Res. 2004;43:36–54.
7. Kihara A. Very long-chain fatty acids: elongation, physiology and related disorders. J Biochem. 2012;152(5):387–95.
8. Jakobsson A, Westerberg R, Jacobsson A. Fatty acid elongases in mammals: their regulation and roles in metabolism. Prog Lipid Res. 2006;45:237–49.
9. Matsuzaka T, Shimano H, Yahagi N, Yoshikawa T, Amemiya-Kudo M, Hasty AH, Okazaki H, Tamura Y, Iizuka Y, Ohashi K, Osuga J, Takahashi A, Yato S, Sone H, Ishibashi S, Yamada N. Cloning and characterization of a mammalian fatty acyl-CoA elongase as a lipogenic enzyme regulated by SREBPs. J Lipid Res. 2002;43(6):911–20.
10. Moon YA, Hammer RE, Horton JD. Deletion of ELOVL5 leads to fatty liver through activation of SREBP-1c in mice. J Lipid Res. 2009;50(3):412–23.
11. Cho HP, Nakamura MT, Clarke SD. Cloning, expression, and nutritional regulation of the mammalian delta-6 desaturase. J Biol Chem. 1999;274(1):471–7.
12. Mihara K. Structure and regulation of rat liver microsomal stearoyl-CoA desaturase gene. J Biochem. 1990;108(6):1022–9.
13. Ma L, Robinson LN, Towle HC. ChREBP*Mlx is the principal mediator of glucose-induced gene expression in the liver. J Biol Chem. 2006;281(39):28721–30.
14. Ma L, Tsatsos NG, Towle HC. Direct role of ChREBP.Mlx in regulating hepatic glucose-responsive genes. J Biol Chem. 2005;280(12):12019–27.
15. Uyeda K, Yamashita H, Kawaguchi T. Carbohydrate responsive element-binding protein (ChREBP): a key regulator of glucose metabolism and fat storage. Biochem Pharmacol. 2002;63(12):2075–80.

16. Dentin R, Denechaud PD, Benhamed F, Girard J, Postic C. Hepatic gene regulation by glucose and polyunsaturated fatty acids: a role for ChREBP. J Nutr. 2006;136:1145–9.
17. Yamashita H, Takenoshita M, Sakurai M, Bruick RK, Henzel WJ, Shillinglaw W, Arnot D, Uyeda K. A glucose-responsive transcription factor that regulates carbohydrate metabolism in the liver. Proc Natl Acad Sci U S A. 2001;98(16): 9116–21.
18. Mitro N, Mak PA, Vargas L, Godio C, Hampton E, Molteni V, Kreusch A, Saez E. The nuclear receptor LXR is a glucose sensor. Nature. 2007;445:219–23.
19. Qin Y, Dalen KT, Gustafsson JA, Nebb HI. Regulation of hepatic fatty acid elongase 5 by LXR alpha-SREBP-1c. Biochim Biophys Acta. 2009;1791:40–7.
20. Jazurek M, Dobrzyń P, Dobrzyń A. Regulation of gene expression by long-chain fatty acids. Postepy Biochem. 2008;54(3):242–50.
21. Jump DB. Fatty acid regulation of gene transcription. Crit Rev Clin Lab Sci. 2004;41(1):41–78.
22. Moon YA, Shah NA, Mohapatra S, Warrington JA, Horton JD. Identification of a mammalian long chain fatty acyl elongase regulated by sterol regulatory element-binding proteins. J Biol Chem. 2001;276:45358–66.
23. Kumadaki S, Matsuzaka T, Kato T, Yahagi N, Yamamoto T, Okada S, Kobayashi K, Takahashi A, Yatoh S, Suzuki H, Yamada N, Shimano H. Mouse Elovl-6 promoter is an SREBP target. Biochem Biophys Res Commun. 2008; 368(2):261–6.
24. Zhang GH, Lu JX, Chen Y, Guo PH, Qiao ZL, Feng RF, Chen SE, Bai JL, Huo SD, Ma ZR. ChREBP and LXRα mediate synergistically lipogenesis induced by glucose in porcine adipocytes. Gene. 2015;565(1):30–8.
25. Ntambi JM. Dietary regulation of stearoyl-CoA desaturase 1 gene expression in mouse liver. J Biol Chem. 1992;267(15):10925–30.
26. Folch J, Lees M, Stanley GHS. A simple method for the isolation and purification of total lipids from animal tissues. J Biol Chem. 1957;226:497–509.
27. Metcalfe LD, Schmitz AA. The rapid preparation of fatty acid esters for gas chromatographic analysis. Anal Chem. 1961;33:363–4.
28. Li Y, Watkins BA. Conjugated linoleic acids alter bone fatty acid composition and reduce ex vivo prostaglandin E2 biosynthesis in rats fed n-6 or n-3 fatty acids. Lipids. 1998;33:417–25.
29. Chaves Das Neves HJ, Vasconcelos AMP. Capillary gas chromatography of amino acids, including asparagine and glutamine: sensitive gas chromatographic-weight spectrometric and selected ion monitoring gas chromatographic-weight spectrometric detection of the N,O (S)-test-butyldimethylsilyl deri. J Chromatogr. 1987;392:249–58.
30. Lee JJ, Lambert JE, Hovhannisyan Y, Ramos-Roman MA, Trombold JR, Wagner DA, Parks EJ. Palmitoleic acid is elevated in fatty liver disease and reflects hepatic lipogenesis. Am J Clin Nutr. 2015;101(1):34–43.
31. Cedernaes J, Alsiö J, Västermark A, Risérus U, Schiöth HB. Adipose tissue stearoyl-CoA desaturase 1 index is increased and linoleic acid is decreased in obesity-prone rats fed a high-fat die. Lipids Health Dis. 2013;12:2.
32. Harding SV, Bateman KP, Kennedy BP, Rideout TC, Jones PJ. Desaturation index versus isotopically measured de novo lipogenesis as an indicator of acute systemic lipogenesis. BMC Res Notes. 2015;8:49.
33. Moon YA, Ochoa CR, Mitsche MA, Hammer RE, Horton JD. Deletion of ELOVL6 blocks the synthesis of oleic acid but does not prevent the development of fatty liver or insulin resistance. J Lipid Res. 2014;55: 2597–605.
34. Marks KA, Kitson AP, Stark KD. Hepatic and plasma sex differences in saturated and monounsaturated fatty acids are associated with differences in expression of elongase 6, but not stearoyl-CoA desaturase in Sprague-Dawley rats. Genes Nutr. 2013;8(3):317–27.
35. Chen G, Liang G, Ou J, Goldstein JL, Brown MS. Central role for liver X receptor in insulin-mediated activation of Srebp-1c transcription and stimulation of fatty acid synthesis in liver. Proc Natl Acad Sci U S A. 2004; 101(31):11245–50.
36. Shimano H. Sterol regulatory element-binding proteins (SREBPs): transcriptional regulators of lipid synthetic genes. Prog Lipid Res. 2001;40:439–52.
37. Wang Y, Torres-Gonzalez M, Tripathy S, Botolin D, Christian B, Jump DB. Elevated hepatic fatty acid elongase-5 activity affects multiple pathways controlling hepatic lipid and carbohydrate composition. J Lipid Res. 2008;49: 1538–52.
38. Guillou H, Zadravec D, Martin PG, Jacobsson A. The key roles of elongases and desaturases in mammalian fatty acid metabolism: Insights from transgenic mice. Prog Lipid Res. 2010;49(2):186–99.
39. Nakamura MT, Yudell BE, Loor JJ. Regulation of energy metabolism by long-chain fatty acids. Prog Lipid Res. 2014;53:124–44.

3

Transcriptomic profile adaptations following exposure of equine satellite cells to nutriactive phytochemical gamma-oryzanol

K. A. Szcześniak, A. Ciecierska, P. Ostaszewski and T. Sadkowski*

Abstract

Background: Adult skeletal muscle myogenesis depends on the activation of satellite cells that have the potential to differentiate into new fibers. Gamma-oryzanol (GO), a commercially available nutriactive phytochemical, has gained global interest on account of its muscle-building and regenerating effects. Here, we investigated GO for its potential influence on myogenesis, using equine satellite cell culture model, since the horse is a unique animal, bred and exercised for competitive sport. To our knowledge, this is the first report where the global gene expression in cultured equine satellite cells has been described.

Methods: Equine satellite cells were isolated from *semitendinosus* muscle and cultured until the second day of differentiation. Differentiating cells were incubated with GO for the next 24 h. Subsequently, total RNA from GO-treated and control cells was isolated, amplified, labeled, and hybridized to two-color *Horse Gene Expression Microarray* slides. Quantitative PCR was used for the validation of microarray data.

Results: Our results revealed 58 genes with changed expression in GO-treated vs. control cells. Analysis of expression changes suggests that various processes are reinforced by GO in differentiating equine satellite cells, including inhibition of myoblast differentiation, increased proliferation and differentiation, stress response, and increased myogenic lineage commitment.

Conclusions: The present study may confirm putative muscle-enhancing abilities of GO; however, the collective role of GO in skeletal myogenesis remains equivocal. The diversity of these changes is likely due to heterogenous growth rate of cells in primary culture. Genes identified in our study, modulated by the presence of GO, may become potential targets of future research investigating impact of this supplement in skeletal muscle on proteomic and biochemical level.

Keywords: Gamma-oryzanol, Equine satellite cells, Differentiation, Muscle, Gene expression

Background

Since horses were domesticated on the Eurasian Steppe over 6000 years ago, they had been selected for strength, speed, and endurance exercise [23]. Nowadays in Europe, working horses are very seldom used for farming purposes; they became exclusively domestic animals exercised for competitive sport. In both equine and human athletes, nutritional ergogenic aids have been used to improve physical ability with an appropriate training regimen. Although training increases physical condition, the ease of taking a nutritional additive to improve training results explains the demand for supplementation, which may increase mechanical energy of work, delay onset of fatigue, and improve neuromuscular coordination [26].

Gamma-oryzanol (GO) is a unique mixture of triterpene alcohol and sterol ferulates present in rice bran oil, a by-product of rice processing. GO has a wide range of

* Correspondence: tomasz_sadkowski@sggw.pl
Department of Physiological Sciences, Faculty of Veterinary Medicine, Warsaw University of Life Sciences - SGGW, Nowoursynowska 159, 02-776 Warsaw, Poland

potential therapeutically useful activities including prevention of coronary atherosclerosis and anticancerogenic and antidiabetic action [28]; however, in our study, we focused on the anabolic properties of GO.

GO has been shown to be very safe with no major side effects being reported in either animal or human studies and is a popular ergogenic aid approved for commercial use in the USA [17]. Moreover, GO is often used by veterinary practitioners in order to improve muscle mass gain and recovery in horses. It was temporarily accounted as a prohibited substance by the Federation Equestre Internationale (FEI) unit governing rules of fair play in equestrian competition (FEI Veterinary Regulations 11th edition, 1st January 2009) [44].

Despite this, only a few studies of ergogenic use of GO were described in the peer-reviewed literature. In one study, authors looked on the resistance-weight-trained male athletes supplemented with 500 mg of GO daily [19]. However, this study failed to demonstrate any effect of GO on training performance. In a recent study, Eslami et al. [17] revealed that 600 mg/day of GO supplementation changed muscular strength in young healthy males in the 9-week resistance training without any significant alteration in anthropometric measurements. Ostaszewski et al. [49] showed that GO supplementation prevented exercise-induced muscle damage in thoroughbred race horses during 16 weeks of training. Animals received 3 g of GO a day. However, no paper describing GO's influence on equine satellite cells was published.

Skeletal muscle satellite cells (SC) are mononucleated cells located under the basal lamina of myofiber. They play an indispensable role during adult skeletal muscle regeneration and hypertrophy. SC are quiescent during most of their normal adult life. Upon activation, they proliferate, differentiate, and finally fuse with adjacent muscle fiber or with other satellite cells to form new multinucleated fibers [40]. The procedure of harvesting satellite cells from equine muscles was first described in 1992 [22], but until now, except for that single report, studies concerning equine satellite cells in vitro are scarce. Previous transcriptomic analyses in horses were conducted on peripheral blood cells and muscle samples obtained by muscular biopsy; thus, our report is the first trial where the global gene expression in cultured equine satellite cells has been described [51]. Satellite cells require an activation signal to proliferate and differentiate and can be controlled by a variety of hormones, growth factors, and metabolites. In vitro reports suggest that satellite cells may also be regulated directly by specific dietary components including ergogenic aids [18, 50, 62]. Determining the factors that independently regulate satellite cells is important to understand overall mechanisms involved in muscle growth and regeneration.

This study focused on revealing possible molecular mechanism underlying GO's influence on skeletal myoblasts. For this purpose, transcriptomic profile analysis of primary culture of equine satellite cells incubated with GO was performed. This in vitro model can help to identify and better understand potential therapeutic to promote muscle regeneration in mammals, among them also in sport horses.

Methods

Cell culture media and reagents

The following reagents/materials were used during cell culture: GO powder was purchased from TCI Chemicals, USA; *Penicillinum crystalicum* was purchased from Polfa Tarchomin, Poland; and Dulbecco's Modified Eagle's medium (DMEM) (1×) with Glutamax, fetal bovine serum (FBS), horse serum (HS), and antibiotics (AB), penicillin-streptomycin and amphotericin B, were purchased from Gibco, Life Technologies, USA. Phosphate-buffered saline (PBS), protease from *Streptomyces griseus*, and DMSO were purchased from Sigma-Aldrich, USA. Primaria tissue culture flasks (25 and 75 cm^2) and Collagen I Cellware six-well plates were purchased from Becton Dickinson, USA.

Animals and muscle samples

Samples of *semitendinosus* muscle were collected from six horses (6-month-old, healthy colts), aseptically in a commercial abattoir during routine slaughter. Next, they were dissected free of connective and adipose tissues to minimize contamination with adipocytes and fibroblasts. The tissue was sliced to pieces, washed four times in PBS with gradually decreasing antibiotic concentration (40,000 units (U) *Penicillinum crystalicum*/100 ml PBS, 20,000 U *Penicillinum crystalicum*/100 ml PBS), suspended in sterile FBS with addition of 10 % DMSO, gradually cooled down to −80 °C, and then stored in liquid nitrogen until isolation.

Satellite cell isolation, cell culture, and experimental design

Since the purpose of the study was to evaluate the impact of GO on in vitro differentiation, primary satellite cell cultures from *semitendinosus* muscle of all horses were isolated and assessed for cell viability (MTT assay) and fusion index (data not shown). For further analysis, the cell line with the best scores was chosen.

To isolate equine satellite cells, six samples of *semitendinosus* muscle were thawed in water bath in 37 °C, centrifuged, and washed three times with PBS with *Penicillinum crystalicum*. Then, each sample was incubated (1.5 h) with DMEM/AB/protease from *S. griseus* (pH 7.3) and sieved in order to separate tissue debris. The filtrates were centrifuged three times, resuspended in proliferation medium (10 % FBS/10 % HS/DMEM/AB), and transferred to polypropylene Petri culture disks. To minimize possible fibroblast contamination, 1.5-h pre-plating was used. Subsequently, supernatant containing myoblasts was transferred to Primaria culture flasks. The growth medium was changed every 2 days. On the 10th day of proliferation, cells were trypsinized and counted by Scepter Cell Counter (Merck Millipore, Germany). Equal number of cells (30,000) from each isolation was transferred to separate the well of Collagen I Cellware six-well plates. After obtaining 80 % of confluence, proliferation medium was replaced by differentiation medium (2 % HS/DMEM/AB). Figure 1 presents equine SC at various stages of growth. At the 48th hour of differentiation, 0.125 μM GO was added and cells were incubated for 24 h. Because GO is insoluble in water, DMSO (0.04 μl/ml) was used as a vehicle. The concentration of GO has been chosen on the basis of assessing cell viability with 3-(4,5-dimethylthiazol-yl)-2-5-diphenyltetrazolium bromide (MTT) colorimetric assay (data not shown). Control medium contained DMSO in the same dose as in GO-treated cells. Following the GO treatment, medium from each plate was discarded and plates were stored at −80 °C until further analysis. Cell culture's schema is illustrated in Fig. 2.

RNA isolation, validation, labeling, and hybridization

Total RNA (from GO-treated and control groups, $n = 6$) was isolated according to the protocol supplied with the miRNeasy Mini Kit (Qiagen, USA). RNA quantity was measured spectrophotometrically using NanoDrop (NanoDrop Technologies, USA). The analysis of the final RNA quality and integrity was performed with BioAnalyzer 2100 (Agilent Technologies, USA). To ensure optimal microarray data quality, four RNA samples with the highest RIN ≥ 9.2 were included into the analysis.

Analysis of gene expression profile was performed using *Horse Gene Expression Microarray*, 4 × 44 K ($n = 4$) (Agilent Technologies, USA). Low Input Quick Amp Labeling Kit (Agilent Technologies, USA) was used to amplify and label total RNA (100 ng) to generate complementary RNA (cRNA). On each two-color microarray, 825 ng of cRNA from GO-exposed cells (labeled by Cy5, $n = 4$) and 825 ng of cRNA from control cells (labeled by Cy3, $n = 4$) were hybridized to the arrays (Gene Expression Hybridization Kit, Agilent Technologies, USA) according to the manufacturer's protocol.

RNA Spike-In Kit (Agilent Technologies, USA) was used as an internal control to efficiently monitor microarray workflow for linearity, sensitivity, and accuracy. Acquisition and analysis of hybridization intensities were performed using the Agilent DNA microarray scanner and Agilent Feature Extraction software 10.7.3.1 according to the standard manufacturer's procedures and Linear Lowess normalization (Cy5/Cy3 dye bias compensation).

The statistical analysis was performed using Gene Spring 13 software (Agilent Technologies, USA) with default setting for two-color microarrays. The estimated significance level (p value) was corrected for multiple hypotheses testing using Benjamini and Hochberg false discovery rate (FDR) adjustment. Messenger RNAs (mRNAs) with FDR ≤ 0.05 and fold change (FC) ≥1.3 were selected as significantly differentially expressed.

The microarray experiment was performed according to MIAME guidelines [6]. The data discussed in this publication have been deposited in NCBI's Gene Expression Omnibus [16] and are accessible through GEO Series accession number GSE73730 (http://www.ncbi.nlm.nih.gov/geo/query/acc.cgi?acc=GSE73730).

cDNA synthesis and quantitative real-time PCR

To verify microarray results, the quantitative real-time polymerase chain reaction (qPCR) method was applied. The sequences of verified genes, complementary to those on microarrays, were obtained from Ensembl database. Primers were designed using Primer-Blast software (NCBI database) and then checked for secondary structures using Oligo Calculator (http://www.basic.northwestern.edu/biotools/oligocalc.html). The secondary structures of the amplicon were examined using m-fold Web Server (http://mfold.rna.albany.edu/?q=mfold). The sequences of the primers are listed in Table 1. The primers were purchased from Oligo IBB (Polish Academy of Science, Warsaw, Poland). Each primer pair was quality tested to ensure that a single product was amplified (dissociation curve analysis) and that there was no primer-dimer coupling.

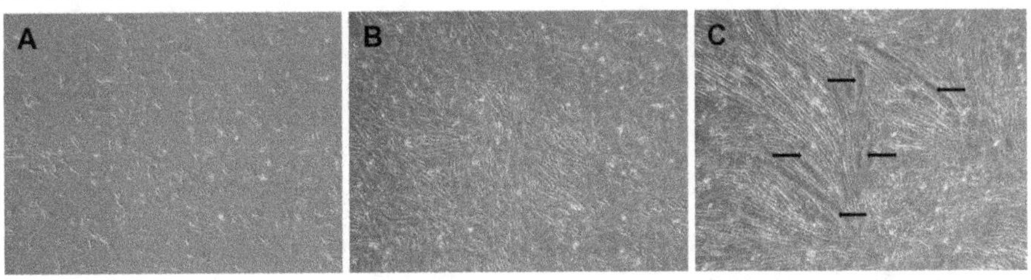

Fig. 1 Cultured equine satellite cells: sixth day of proliferation, 30 % confluence (**a**); 10th day of proliferation, 80 % confluence (**b**); and 48 h of differentiation (**c**). Myotubes are marked with *arrows*

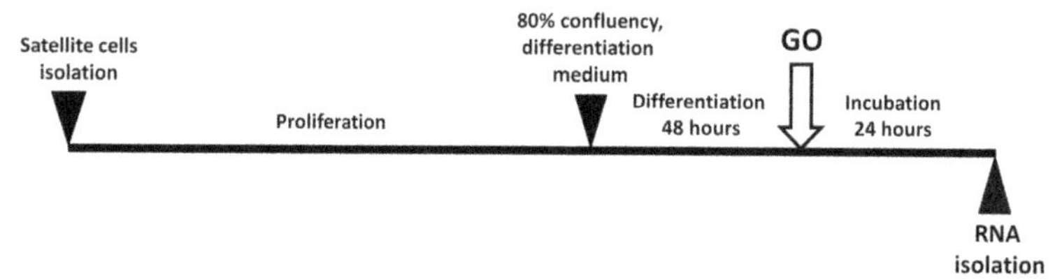

Fig. 2 Experiment design. Equine SC were cultured until reaching 80 % of confluence, and then proliferation medium was replaced by differentiation medium. After the second day of differentiation, cells were incubated for 24 h with GO. Following the GO treatment, differentiating cells were scraped and stored at −80 °C until further analysis

One microgram of total RNA from GO-treated and control samples ($n = 6$) was reverse transcribed using Trancription First-Strand cDNA Synthesis Kit (Roche, USA). All analyses were performed on individual samples of total RNA using a SensiFAST SYBR lo-ROX Kit (Blirt, Bioline, Poland) following the manufacturer's protocol. Assays for each gene were conducted in duplicate in a Stratagene Mx3005p thermal cycler according to the following protocol: pre-incubation for 2 min at 95 °C and amplification (40 cycles) containing denaturation at 95 °C for 5 s and annealing at a temperature specified in Table 1 for 15 s. Dissociation curve setting was as follows: denaturation at 95 °C for 0 s, annealing at a temperature specified in Table 1, continuous melting up to 95 °C for 0 s (slope = 0.1 °C/s), and cooling at 40 °C for 30 s. *Gapdh* was used as a reference gene. The relative expression of the target gene was calculated according to the following formula:

$$\Delta\Delta CT = \Delta CT(\text{sample}) - \Delta CT(\text{control})$$

where ΔCT is the difference in CT between the targeted gene and reference control. Results were calculated as $2^{-\Delta\Delta CT}$ [38] using GenEx 6.0 (MultiD Analyses, Sweden). The amplification efficiency ($E = 10^{(-1/\text{slope})} - 1$) was determined by performing a comparative quantitation standard curve and was >0.9 for each target gene and the reference gene. Standard curves were generated using a four-point 1:10 dilution series starting with cDNA representing 10 ng of input total RNA. qPCR analysis has been conducted according to a standardized approach [10].

Functional analysis

The list of significantly modulated by GO genes was analyzed by Functional Analysis tool in the Database for Annotation, Visualization and Integrated Discovery (DAVID version 6.7) (da Huang et al. 2009) in order to identify their annotations in gene ontology divided into three functional classes: biological processes, cellular components, and molecular functions. Gene ontology enrichment was calculated by EASE score corrected for multiple hypotheses testing using Benjamini and Hochberg FDR.

Relationships between all differentially expressed genes (microarray and RT-PCR) were visualized with Pathway Studio's Build Pathway functionality (Elsevier, USA) which is based on the wave-propagation algorithm developed for the navigation through complex networks.

Table 1 Primers used for real-time qPCR; full names of genes are available in Table 2

No.	Gene symbol	Forward primer	Reverse primer	Annealing temperature (°C)	Product length (bp)
1.	*bdnf*	CCCCATGAAAGAAGCAAACG	TACAAGTCCGCGTCCTTACT	60	213
2.	*btg1*	GGCTCCATCTGTGTGCTGTA	GCCCACCCAAAGCAAAACTC	60	227
3.	*gja1*	TGCTGCGAACCTACATCATC	CGATGACGTTCAAGGCAAGA	60	255
4.	*igf1*	CAGAAGCAATGGGAAAAATCA	CGTGGGCTTGTTGAAATAAAA	62	242
5.	*itpr2*	CTGTGGGTATTCGGCCATTT	GCCACGATTTCCGACAAAAC	60	143
6.	*mllt3*	GGAACCGAAACCCATGTCAA	GGGCTTTTTGTCAGCAGAAC	60	220
7.	*mstn*	GCCTGGAAACAGCTCCTAAC	GTCGTCGCGTGGTAATCATC	60	151
8.	*myf5*	GGAGACGCCTGAAGAAAGTC	CCGGCAGGCTGTAGTAATTC	60	171
9.	*myog*	CTCGCTCACCTCCATTGTG	CAGTTGGGCATGGTTTCATC	60	78
10.	*tgfb2*	AGTACTACGCCAAGGAGGTT	TAGGCGGGATGGCATTTTCC	60	72
11.	*gapdh*	GTTTGTGATGGGCGTGAACC	GTCTTCTGGGTGGCAGTGAT	60	198

In this analysis, Find Direct Links/All Objects Directions Algorithm was used. Protein entity type and direct regulation, regulation, expression, and promoter-binding relationships were selected in the analysis. Such created graph was expanded with five muscle-related biological processes.

Results

The number of differentially expressed genes

Comparison of gene expression between GO-treated and control cells revealed statistically significant (FDR ≤ 0.05, FC ≥ 1.3) differences in the expression of 97 transcripts. Sequences of differentially expressed probes not annotated by microarray manufacturer were compared with the NCBI nucleotide databases (using blastn) to assign a gene name. Probes not matching in 100 % with any eukaryotic mRNA/gene were excluded from gene lists used for functional analysis. That resulted in 58 identified, unduplicated, transcript IDs including 17 up- and 41 down-regulated genes in GO vs. control group. The list of identified transcripts can be found in Table 2. All array data are plotted and shown in Additional file 1.

In this paper, symbols of genes and their protein products have been presented in their original form referring to specificity of the cited paper, as lowercase italic or uppercase letters, when they refer to transcriptomic or proteomic research, respectively. In the following discussion, arrows indicate up- (↑) or down-regulation (↓) of gene expression. Validated (from microarray) or tested (*mstn, myog, igf1*) by qPCR genes are marked with hash (#).

Real-time qPCR

According to the ontological classification and available literature, seven genes involved in the skeletal muscle development, sarcomere development, actin binding, and regulation of cell proliferation and differentiation were selected for qPCR validation. Except for gap junction protein alpha 1 (*gja1*), all expression changes from qPCR overlapped microarray results (Table 3, Fig. 3). In our study, we focused on the impact of GO on muscle development; thus, we also measured mRNA levels of three genes from muscle development profile *myog*, *igf1*, and *mstn*, which did not reach the FC ≥ 1.3 threshold (Fig. 4).

Functional analysis

Significantly enriched gene ontologies retrieved from DAVID output files are presented in Additional file 2. In Table 4, selection of most significant biological processes is shown (EASE score <0.001), providing a comprehensive overview of important processes possibly induced by GO in differentiating ESC.

Using Pathway Studio's Build Pathway algorithm, we identified 116 relationships within selected entities, which are displayed in a graph view on Fig. 4. Seventy of identified relationships had the highest (third) confidence level which means that the number of references confirming this relationship was ≥3. Detected types of regulation were regulation (86), expression (28), direct regulation (1), and promoter binding (1). Fifty-five relations were positive, 22 negative, and 39 not defined. Chosen relationships are further discussed in the following chapter.

Discussion

According to Fernyhough et al. [18], oral supplements may affect myofibers in five potential ways: (1) by direct interaction, (2) by direct influence and producing paracrine agents that affect SC, (3) by affecting SC, (4) by producing hormones that exert indirect effects in muscle cells, and (5) by protecting all cell types against oxidative damage. Although, the exact mode of GO action on muscles was not revealed, GO has been previously postulated to act through mechanisms 4 [12, 44] and 5 [17, 49]. In further discussion, we suggest that the direct interaction of GO with SC (3) may be a part of its skeletal muscle-enhancing mechanism [63]. For this purpose, genes important for myogenesis have been selected and are discussed in four functional groups.

Ontology of differentially expressed genes

According to functional analysis, the five most significant biological processes induced by 24-h incubation of differentiating equine SC with 0.125 μmol GO are related to skeletal muscles; however, muscle organ development is the only record showing significance after FDR correction (Table 4). Moreover, GO influenced genes associated with contractile apparatus development (Additional file 2; CC and MF sheet). All this together indicates that GO, indeed, may directly influence SC activity and in vitro differentiation. Other significantly enriched processes referred to macromolecule metabolism and positive regulation of transcription (Table 4). The last has also a confirmation in enriched molecular functions: transcription regulator activity and transcription cofactor activity (Additional file 2; MF sheet). Functional analysis revealed also that GO influenced growth factor activity (Additional file 2; MF sheet). Axon and neuron projection-related genes (Additional file 2; CC sheet) could be connected with recent in vivo findings by Eslami et al. [17] who suggested that GO-induced increase in muscle strength may arise from neural adaptations without altering muscle mass.

Table 2 List of differentially expressed genes in GO-treated vs. CTRL equine satellite cells—microarray analysis (FDR ≤ 0.05, fold change ≥1.3, $n = 4$)

No.	Gene symbol	Regulation	FC	Corr. *p* value	Description	Accession number
1.	*il-1r2*	Up	3.1	0.040	Interleukin-1 receptor type II	[NM_001081816]
2.	*efhc2*	Up	3.0	0.049	EF-hand domain (C-terminal) containing 2	[ENSECAT00000017638]
3.	*tcrd*	Up	2.2	0.050	T cell receptor delta	[L38389]
4.	*tfap2e*	Up	1.8	0.039	Transcription factor AP-2 epsilon (activating enhancer-binding protein 2 epsilon)	[ENSECAT00000003183]
5.	*cdca7*	Up	1.7	0.027	Cell division cycle associated 7	[ENSECAT00000012017]
6.	*f2rl2*	Up	1.6	0.048	Coagulation factor II (thrombin) receptor-like 2	[ENSECAT00000010830]
7.	*rcor2*	Up	1.5	0.026	REST corepressor 2	[ENSECAT00000024786]
8.	*lrrc16a*	Up	1.5	0.049	Leucine-rich repeat containing 16A	[ENSECAT00000026357]
9.	*mapk14*	Up	1.5	0.037	Mitogen-activated protein kinase 14	[XM_005604060]
10.	*fezf2*	Up	1.4	0.029	FEZ family zinc finger 2	[ENSECAT00000022391]
11.	*colec12*	Up	1.4	0.026	Collectin subfamily member 12	[XM_005604060]
12.	*pir*	Up	1.4	0.038	Pirin (iron-binding nuclear protein)	[ENSECAT00000014292]
13.	*gja1*	Up	1.4	0.048	Gap junction protein 1	[ENSECAT00000005498]
14.	*itpr2*	Up	1.4	0.05	Inositol 1,4,5-trisphosphate receptor, type 2	[ENSECAT00000009891]
15.	*tmem107*	Up	1.3	0.045	Transmembrane protein 107	[ENSECAT00000014966]
16.	*steap1*	Up	1.3	0.045	6 transmembrane epithelial antigen of the prostate (metalloreductase)	[ENSECAT00000024982]
17.	*alcam*	Up	1.4	0.045	Activated leukocyte cell adhesion molecule	[XM_005602026]
18.	*musk*	Down	−1.3	0.042	Muscle, skeletal, receptor tyrosine kinase	[ENSECAT00000010687]
19.	*exoc6*	Down	−1.3	0.044	Exocyst complex component 6	[ENSECAT00000025821]
20.	*sept6*	Down	−1.3	0.036	Septin 6	[XM_005614469]
21.	*mdh2*	Down	−1.3	0.039	Malate dehydrogenase 2, NAD (mitochondrial)	[NM_001195526]
22.	*nexn*	Down	−1.3	0.039	Nexilin (F-actin-binding protein)	[ENSECAT00000016039]
23.	*setd7*	Down	−1.3	0.026	SET domain containing lysine methyltransferase 7	[ENSECAT00000020466]
24.	*tmem47*	Down	−1.3	0.045	Transmembrane protein 47	[XM_008544808]
25.	*bdnf*	Down	−1.3	0.027	Brain-derived neurotrophic factor	[NM_001081787]
26.	*snca*	Down	−1.3	0.038	Synuclein, alpha (non A4 component of amyloid precursor)	[ENSECAT00000016509]
27.	*actg2*	Down	−1.4	0.045	Actin, gamma 2, smooth muscle, enteric	[ENSECAT00000020181]
28.	*btg1*	Down	−1.4	0.039	B cell translocation gene 1, antiproliferative	[ENSECAT00000022009]
29.	*znf423*	Down	−1.5	0.045	Zinc finger protein 423	[ENSECAT00000000207]
30.	*aqp1*	Down	−1.5	0.027	Aquaporin 1	[XM_003364834]
31.	*bcl2l11*	Down	−1.5	0.035	BCL2-like 11 (apoptosis facilitator)	[ENSECAT00000023850]
32.	*nr2f2*	Down	−1.5	0.040	Nuclear receptor subfamily 2, group F, member 2	[ENSECAT00000008488]
33.	*pak1*	Down	−1.5	0.050	CDC42 effector protein (Rho GTPase binding) 3	[ENSECAT00000019645]
34.	*cryab*	Down	−1.5	0.035	Crystallin, alpha B	[ENSECAT00000012936]
35.	*abra*	Down	−1.5	0.045	Actin-binding Rho-activating protein	[ENSECAT00000016765]
36.	*capn6*	Down	−1.5	0.038	Calpain 6	[ENSECAT00000011583]
37.	*herpud1*	Down	−1.5	0.045	Homocysteine-inducible, endoplasmic reticulum stress-inducible (ubiquitin-like domain member 1)	[JL623642]
38.	*tmcc3*	Down	−1.6	0.033	Transmembrane and coiled-coil domain family 3	[ENSECAT00000012141]
39.	*tbc1d8*	Down	−1.6	0.027	TBC1 domain family, member 8 (with GRAM domain)	[ENSECAT00000013116]
40.	*kiaa1958*	Down	−1.6	0.045	Protein-coding gene	[ENSECAT00000008002]
41.	*neo1*	Down	−1.6	0.038	Neogenin 1	[ENSECAT00000026822]

Table 2 List of differentially expressed genes in GO-treated vs. CTRL equine satellite cells—microarray analysis (FDR ≤ 0.05, fold change ≥1.3, *n* = 4) *(Continued)*

42.	*lrrn1*	Down	−1.6	0.045	Leucine-rich repeat neuronal 1	[ENSECAT00000002791]
43.	*ctrc*	Down	−1.6	0.044	Chymotrypsin C (caldecrin)	[XM_008540961]
44.	*itgb1bp2*	Down	−1.6	0.048	Integrin beta 1-binding protein (melusin) 2	[ENSECAT00000016364]
45.	*stk17b*	Down	−1.6	0.039	Serine/threonine kinase 17b (apoptosis-inducing)	[JL616416]
46.	*hist1h4a*	Down	−1.6	0.045	Chromosome 4 open reading frame 21	[ENSECAT00000006145]
47.	*camta1*	Down	−1.6	0.039	Calmodulin binding transcription activator 1	[ENSECAT00000022451]
48.	*kcnk12*	Down	−1.7	0.033	Potassium channel, subfamily K, member 12	[XM_008530912]
49.	*phactr3*	Down	−1.7	0.035	Phosphatase and actin regulator 3	[ENSECAT00000008448]
50.	*mllt3*	Down	−1.7	0.044	Myeloid/lymphoid or mixed-lineage leukemia (trithorax homolog, *Drosophila*)	[ENSECAT00000025395]
51.	*tgfb2*	Down	−1.8	0.038	Transforming growth factor, beta 2	[ENSECAT00000017826]
52.	*scd5*	Down	−2.0	0.038	Stearoyl-CoA desaturase 5	[ENSECAT00000015537]
53.	*myf5*	Down	−2.0	0.039	Myogenic factor 5	[ENSECAT00000021416]
54.	*garem*	Down	−2.0	0.039	GRB2 associated, regulator of MAPK1	[ENSECAT00000012124]
55.	*duoxa2*	Down	−2.2	0.026	Dual oxidase maturation factor 2	[ENSECAT00000015499]
56.	*ncald*	Down	−2.2	0.044	Neurocalcin delta	[XM_005613237]
57.	*kcnmb2*	Down	−2.5	0.036	Potassium large conductance calcium-activated channel, subfamily M, beta member 2	[ENSECAT00000009305]
58.	*hla-dqb1*	Down	−5.0	0.028	Major histocompatibility complex, class II, DQ beta I	[XM_008506652]

Interaction of GO with myogenic regulatory factors

Pre- and postnatal skeletal muscle development depends on the expression of four basic helix-loop-helix transcription factors called myogenic regulatory factors (MRFs). This group shares the ability to induce myogenic differentiation when expressed in non-muscle cells [43]. Three MRFs, *myf5*, myogenin (*myog*), and *myod*, were investigated in our study, but only two of them possessed significant changes in expression.

In adult skeletal muscle, the highest expression of *myf5* is present in committed satellite cells and decreases when progression to myocytes and myotubes occurs [4]. Likewise, in cultured equine SC, qPCR showed that *myf5* mRNA levels were highest during intensive proliferation and decreased dramatically at the onset of differentiation [25]. Compared to control cells, 24-h incubation of equine SC with GO induced down-regulation of *myf5* (↓#). According to this observation, we suggest that GO could potentially advance equine SC differentiation.

Table 3 Results of real-time qPCR analysis (*n* = 6)

GO vs. CTRL	Fold change	*p* value
myf5	−2.6	3.9E-07
mllt3	−2.3	1.3E-07
tgfb2	−1.6	3.7E-07
gja1	−1.3	6.8E-04
bdnf	−1.3	7.3E-03
itpr2	1.5	9.8E-03
bdnf	−1.3	7.3E-03
btg1	−1.3	2.4E-02
myog	−1.5	3.3E-04
mstn	−2.6	5.4E-04
igf1	−1.8	3.4E-03
myod	−1.1	1.6E-01

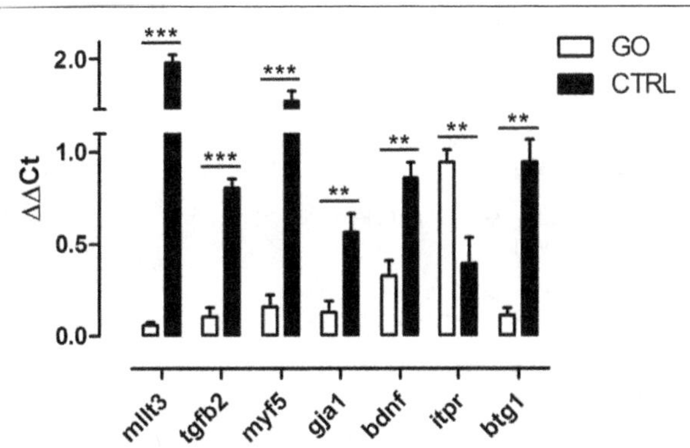

Fig. 3 Results of qPCR validation of selected genes revealed in microarray experiment (FDR ≤ 0.05). *Asterisks* indicate the following criteria of significance: **p* ≤ 0.05; ***p* ≤ 0.01; and ****p* ≤ 0.001; (*n* = 6)

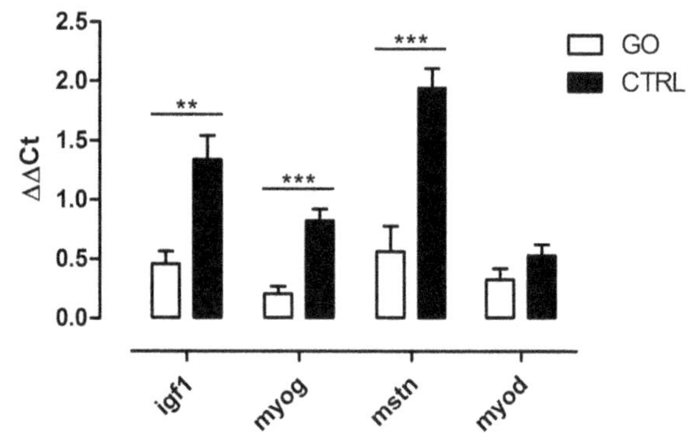

Fig. 4 Results of qPCR analysis of additional genes important for myogenic differentiation of equine SC (FDR > 0.05). *Asterisks* indicate the following criteria of significance: $^{*}p \leq 0.05$; $^{**}p \leq 0.01$; and $^{***}p \leq 0.001$; ($n = 6$)

It was shown that up-regulation of MYF5 triggers the expression of myogenin (*myog*). That contributes to the withdrawal of myoblasts from the cell cycle [55]. Undetectable during proliferation, *Myog* expression level is highest when myocytes differentiate and fuse into myotubes [25] and remains at a slightly lower level in adult skeletal muscle cells [4]. Disregarded of this, additional qPCR showed down-regulation of *myog* (↓#) mRNA in experimental cells. Down-regulation of both MRFs may indicate that GO actually inhibits myogenic differentiation. Our experiment was performed, 48 h after changing proliferation medium to differentiation medium. At this stage, proliferating myocytes begin to differentiate and fuse. However, the exact cell cycle of experimental cells remains unequal and undefined. Thus, it is possible that GO has multiple ways of action and by down-regulation of *myog*, it delays terminal differentiation and simulates proliferation of equine SC. Moreover, transcription factors involved in myogenic lineage progression are not strictly acting in a linear manner but are organized in complex feedback and feed-forward networks with other muscle development genes [4]. These relationships will be discussed further in this paper.

Genes belonging to the transforming growth factor β superfamily

Transforming growth factor β2 (*tgf-β2*) (↓#) belongs to a subset of transforming growth factor β superfamily members, which exert strong control over proliferation, migration, and adhesion of satellite cells [35]. TGF-β2 delays myoblast differentiation while increasing cellular proliferation. Molecular mechanism of TGF-β2 includes an increased rate of degradation of *myod* (Schabort et al. 2009). However, it has not been examined whether a similar relationship exists in equine skeletal muscle. In a recent study, de Mello et al. [41] showed *tgf-β2* mRNA levels were high only in proliferative C_2C_{12} cells and began to decrease after differentiation induction. *Tgf-β2* mRNA levels were 10-fold lower after 3 days of differentiation that strongly agrees with our observations, which indicate that GO down-regulated *tgf-β2* (↓#) in equine myoblast during the third day of differentiation, when compared to control cells.

This result encouraged us to investigate another member of transforming growth factor superfamily, playing a key role in the negative regulation of muscle growth in mammals: myostatin (*mstn*). Although microarray analysis did not passed FDR correction test, additional

Table 4 Selected significantly enriched (EASE score *p* value <0.001) gene ontologies, DAVID

No.	Name	# of genes	p value	Genes	Bonferroni	Benjamini	FDR
1.	GO:0007517—muscle organ development	10	6.6E-8	*musk, cryab, mapk14, itgb1bp2, myf5, mstn, igf1, myog, nr2f2, tgfb2*	5.92E-5	5.92E-5	1.03E-4
2.	GO:0014706~striated muscle tissue development	6	7.5E-5	*musk, mapk14, myf5, myog, nr2f2, tgfb2*	0.06	0.03	0.12
3.	GO:0060537—muscle tissue development	6	9.4E-5	*musk, mapk14, myf5, myog, nr2f2, tgfb2*	0.08	0.03	0.15
4.	GO:0007519—skeletal muscle tissue development	5	1.0E-4	*musk, mapk14, myf5, myog, nr2f2*	0.08	0.02	0.16
5.	GO:0060538—skeletal muscle organ development	5	1.0E-4	*musk, mapk14, myf5, myog, nr2f2*	0.09	0.02	0.16
6.	GO:0010604—positive regulation of macromolecule metabolic process	12	2.4E-4	*mapk14, snca, myf5, gja1, mstn, igf1, abra, myog, nr2f2, tfap2e, znf423, tgfb2*	0.19	0.047	0.37
7.	GO:0010557—positive regulation of macromolecule biosynthetic process	10	5.8E-4	*mapk14, myf5, mstn, igf1, abra, myog, nr2f2, tfap2e, znf423, tgfb2*	0.40	0.08	0.89
8.	GO:0009891—positive regulation of biosynthetic process	10	8.9E-4	*mapk14, myf5, mstn, igf1, abra, myog, nr2f2, tfap2e, znf423, tgfb2*	0.55	0.11	1.38
9.	GO:0045941—positive regulation of transcription	9	9.9E-4	*mapk14, myf5, mstn, igf1, abra, myog, nr2f2, tfap2e, znf423*	0.59	0.10	1.5

qPCR demonstrated decreased *mstn* (↓#) mRNA level in GO vs. control cells. The deletion of myostatin in mice induces dramatic and widespread increase in skeletal muscle mass due to both muscle hypertrophy and hyperplasia [32], and it also cause double-muscling phenotype of some cattle and sheep breeds [57]. Wicik et al. [67] showed inhibitory effect of exogenous MSTN on differentiating C_2C_{12} myoblasts.

We suggest that decreased expression of these two genes could contribute to the putative GO-mediated muscle growth enhancement, by increasing differentiation process. However, this needs to be reconciled with decreased expression of differentiation marker *myog*.

Other genes involved in cell proliferation and differentiation processes

Our interest was also focused on genes involved in cell proliferation and differentiation, described in the literature as important for myogenesis.

Mitogen-activated protein 14 (*mapk*14) (↑) also called p-38α belongs to one of the major regulators of gene transcription and metabolism in response to oxidative, energetic, and mechanical stress in skeletal muscle. Chronic activation of MAPK14 signaling pathway has been implicated in the development of adaptive and maladaptive response in skeletal muscle pathologies, such as diabetes [7] and protein catabolism [53], and physiological states, such as growth and differentiation [34]. Mapk14 expression coincides with *myog* expression during differentiation [8], which could potentially indicate the role of GO in muscle differentiation; however, in our study, expression of this genes was opposite.

According to the qPCR analysis, exposition of SC to GO induced significant down-regulation of insulin-like growth factor 1 (*igf-1*) (↓#). *Igf-1* is, up to date, the only known growth factor positively regulating proliferation and differentiation of these cells [60]. IGF-1 can indirectly affect satellite cells, by increasing the expression of *myf5*, *myog*, and *myod*, and embryonic myosin heavy chain [70] and decreasing expression of *mstn* [56]. Analysis of the relationships between the abovementioned genes places *igf-1* on the top of the signaling cascade hypothetically induced by GO (Fig. 5). Thus, it may be suggested that GO decreases expression of MRF through the inhibition of *igf-1* signaling. These findings are in contrast with presumed abilities of GO.

Haddad and Adams [24] indicated that intact signaling through MAPK is necessary for the development of IGF-I-induced skeletal muscle hypertrophy in vivo. However, in our study, this relationship was not observed, as indicated by different changes in the expression of these two molecules. In contrast, Trendelenburg et al. [66] showed that pro-inflammatory cytokines may inhibit myoblast growth via p38 signaling activity. This observation corresponds with up-regulation of interleukin 1 receptor type II (*il1r2*) (↑) expression and MRF's down-regulation in our culture cells, suggesting that GO can activate stress-related signaling in cultured cells.

Another gene deserving attention is *gja1* (↓#) gene encoding gap junction protein alpha 1—component of intercellular channels that provides a route for the diffusion of low molecular weight particles from cell to cell. Except for that, GJA1 affects cell proliferation and differentiation in various tissues. Although not present in normal adult skeletal muscle, GJA1 is necessary during regenerative myogenesis in rodents [1, 21]. The relationship between *gja1* and MRF expression was observed in the L6 myogenic cell line; pharmacological gap junction blockers were found to inhibit myogenin expression and myotube formation, reversibly [3]. Likewise, delayed expression of *myog* was found in myoblast cultures prepared from mice with an inducible deletion of *gja1* [1]. Similar function in differentiating myoblasts was reported for B cell translocation gene 1 (*btg1*) (↓#). The *btg1* overexpression inhibited proliferation of several cell lines including NIH3T3, PC12, and QM7 quail myoblast lines [52]. Therefore, it was initially believed that these proteins possess antiproliferative properties. However, other studies demonstrated that *btg1* up-regulation is crucial at the onset of myoblast differentiation [54]. More recently, Busson et al. [9] described the molecular basis of *btg1* action and proved that it stimulates the activity of not only MRFs but also nuclear receptors already known as positive myogenic regulators (T3 and all-*trans* retinoic acid receptors).

From all these studies, it becomes evident that the outcome of *gja1* and *btg1* expression in muscle cells is associated with the onset of differentiation while irreversible withdrawal from the cell cycle occurs. Thus, the context of the signal is essential for understanding their role in GO signaling. Taking into account that GO was added to differentiating myoblasts, *gja1* and *btg1* down-regulation indicate that GO may decrease equine myoblast fusion and could suggest pro-proliferative action of *btg1* and *gja1* in equine SC exposed to GO, which agrees with the reduced levels of MRF's expression.

Herein, we demonstrate down-regulation of brain-derived neurotrophic factor (*bdnf*) (↓#). *Bdnf* is a member of the mammalian family of neurotrophins, studied for their roles in the nervous system function [13]. Further expression-profiling studies have shown that *bdnf* is differentially expressed in skeletal muscle under various physiological and pathological conditions [11] but *bdnf* expression pattern in certain physiological states remained elusive. Mousavi and Jasmin [45] showed that *bdnf* expression during myogenic differentiation has been significantly reduced. Moreover, siRNA knockdown of *bdnf* expression evoked precocious differentiation of

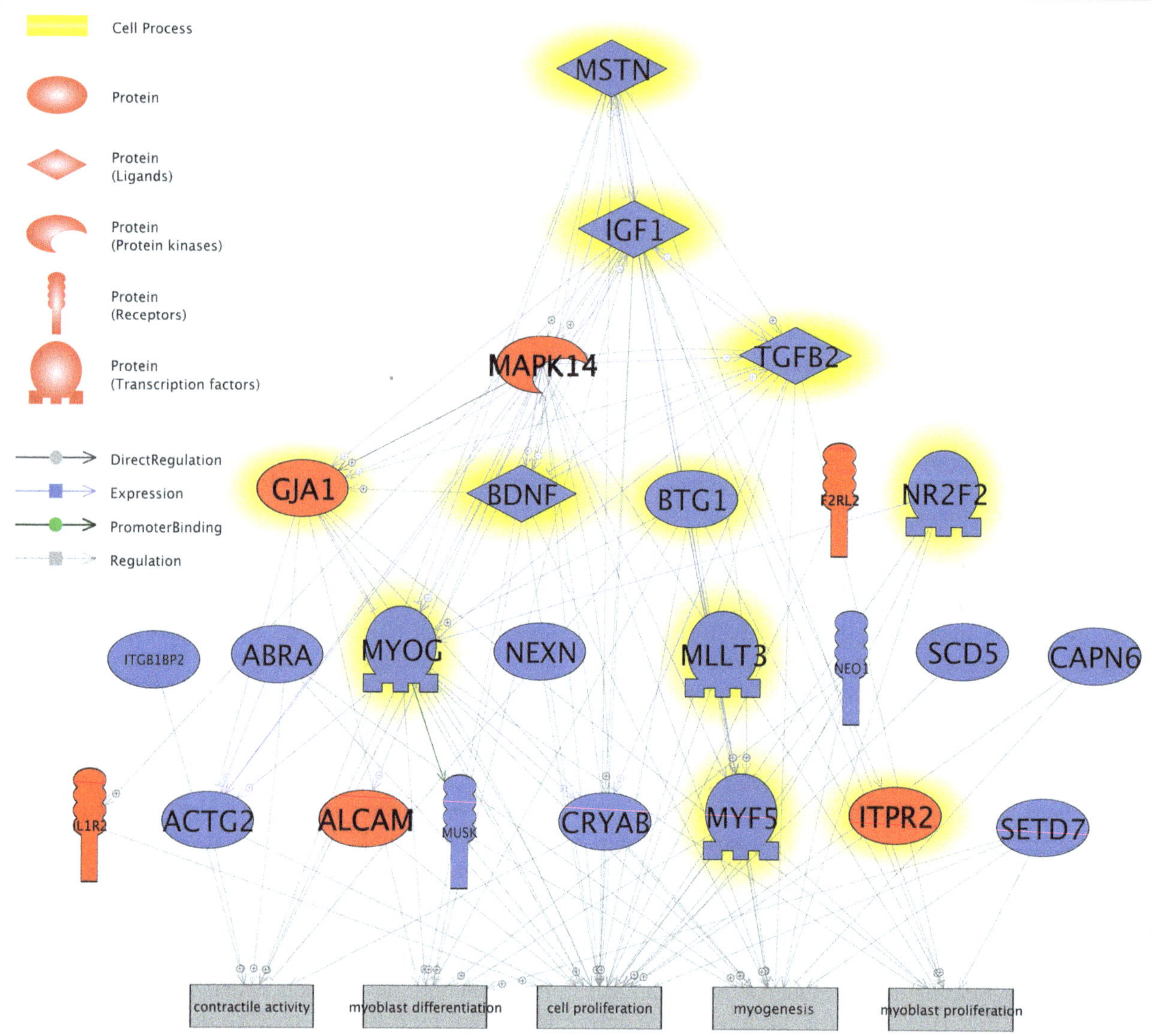

Fig. 5 Relationships between differentially expressed genes, based on Pathway Studio. Genes are marked with *red* and *blue colors* for up- and down-regulation, respectively. The pathway was enriched with myogenesis-related biological processes and additional qPCR-tested genes of muscle development profile (*mstn, igf1, myog*). Genes validated or tested by qPCR are *highlighted*

myoblasts. This effect was inhibited by the administration of recombinant *bdnf.* However, more recently, Clow and Jasmin [13] indicated that instead of its inhibitory role, bdnf$^{-/-}$ mice demonstrated impaired induction of several molecular markers of regeneration, including *pax7, myod,* and *myog* when proliferating myoblasts began to differentiate and fuse to repair damaged myofibers. The role of *bdnf* remains questionable; however, attenuated MRF's expression in our culture may confirm that expression of this gene is required for normal myogenic differentiation. This finding can also be applied to the next specified molecule down-regulated by GO: αβ-crystallin (*cryab*), (↓) a small heat shock protein involved in preventing protein aggregation. Expression of *cryab* was induced selectively in myoblasts during an early stage of their differentiation in vitro [33]. Moreover, mice lacking αβ-crystallin died prematurely with extensive muscle wastage [59] which indicates its essential role during myogenesis. Indeed, the αβ-crystallin promoter contains canonical skeletal muscle-specific E-box element that binds MRFs [20]. On the other hand, overexpression of *cryab* inhibits myogenic differentiation by negatively regulating differentiation-related apoptosis, inhibiting caspase-3 activation and altering *myod* levels [33, 59].

Next, gene affected by the presence of GO which deserves attention is nuclear receptor 2F2 (*nr2f2*) (↓#) alias chicken ovalbumin upstream promoter transcription factor II (*coup-tfII*). It encodes nuclear orphan receptor of the steroid-thyroid hormone receptor superfamily. Recently, growing evidence suggests the pivotal role of COUP-TFs in mesenchymal stem cell (MSC) regulation and development [69]. As illustrated both in vitro and in vivo, loss of COUP-TFII reprograms the precursors by shifting the cell identity to osteogenic and myogenic lineages at the expense of adipogenic and chondrogenic programs, supporting the notion that COUP-TFII is essential for fate choice and commitment [68]. The molecular mechanism by which COUP-TFII affects MSC development is, at least partially, through the down-regulation of Wnt cascade substrate: Wnt10b. This phenomenon resulted in reduced fat tissue and enhanced glucose tolerance and insulin sensitivity, as well as increased bone mineralization and muscle mass in COUP-TFII-deficient mice [68]. Moreover, previous reports indicated that COUP-TFII inhibits myogenesis by the transcriptional and posttranscriptional regulation of *myod* [2, 46]. In conclusion, down-regulation of this gene may indicate that GO stimulates in vitro myogenesis.

Finally, in our study, increased expression (↑) of activated leukocyte cell adhesion molecule (*alcam*), also known as cluster of differentiation 166 (CD166), has been detected. *Alcam* plays an important role in cell proliferation and the differentiation of mesenchymal tissues in multiple species [61]. Moreover, *alcam* may increase cell survival in several tumor types as well as monocytes [61]. These abilities may result from the anti-apoptotic capacity of this protein [39]. Other authors speculate that ALCAM-ALCAM interactions, in cooperation with other adhesion molecules, facilitate stroma progenitor cell contact, resulting in proliferation of progenitor cell subsets [47]. It may be presumed that expression of *alcam* could mediate GO action on SC, but the functional roles in muscle physiology of this marker remains unknown and needs further investigation.

Other genes positively regulating muscle differentiation, whose expression was changed by GO, include neogenin (*Neo1*) (↓), actin-binding Rho-activating protein (*Abra*) (↓), actin γ-2 (*actg2*) (↓), integrin beta-1-binding protein 2 (melusin 2, *Itgb1bp2*) (↓), muscle-specific tyrosine kinase receptor (*Musk*) (↓), nexilin (*nexn*) (↓), histone H3-K4 methyltransferase (*setd7*) (↓), and calpain 6 (*capn6*) (↓)-myogenesis-suppressing gene [5, 14, 27, 36, 37, 42, 64, 65]. Down-regulation of these genes may suggest that 24-h incubation with 0.125 μM of GO decreased differentiation of equine satellite cells.

Other gamma-oryzanol treatment-related genes

GO has been reported to possess strong antioxidant activity; thus, it is postulated that GO might enhance endurance and muscle-building capacity by hindering the production of free radicals, which in theory could lessen muscle exhaustion and fatigue in reaction to anaerobic exercise [17]. Consistent with this, significantly lower post-exercise total antioxidant status and thiobarbituric acid-reactive substance level were observed in racing horses receiving GO compared to horses from other groups [49]. GO's influence on oxidative stress-related genes has been shown in other tissues [30, 31]. However, in our study, gene ontology analysis did not show any significant involvement of differentially expressed genes in antioxidative processes. It will be important in future studies to determine if antioxidant activity is involved in the protective effects of GO under oxidative stress conditions.

Lowered expression of stearoyl-CoA desaturase and isoform 5 gene (*scd5*) (↓) as well as of *coup-tfII* (↓) may reflect positive influence of GO on energy homeostasis in skeletal muscle. As mentioned before, *Coup-tfII*-deficient mice demonstrated reduced fat tissue and enhanced glucose tolerance and insulin sensitivity [68]. Likewise, SCD deficiency is evidenced to activate metabolic pathways which promote β-oxidation and decrease lipogenesis both in the liver and skeletal muscles. SCD mutation results also in general changes in the expression of genes involved in lipid metabolism. SCD1-deficient mice have increased energy expenditure and reduced body adiposity and are resistant to diet-induced obesity (Dobrzyn and Ntambi 2005). These results may confirm GO utility in the treatment of diabetes (Ohara et al. 2009) as well as positive effect on lean body mass gain.

Conclusions

In conclusion, we demonstrated for the first time that GO can affect the transcriptomic profile of equine satellite cells in vitro. Many of differentially expressed genes are reported to be crucial for skeletal muscle development. Analysis of expression changes proves that various processes are reinforced by GO in equine SC (Fig. 6); however, inhibition of myoblast differentiation is prevailing observation. Incubation with GO was performed at the onset of differentiation; thus, decreased expression of differentiation markers may indicate that GO delays this process in cultured equine SC that may contribute to increased field of cells that will later differentiate into myotubes. This could be explained in further investigation of GO's influence on satellite cells in proliferation stage. Beyond this, 24-h incubation with GO induced different expression of genes responsible for stress response, increased myogenic lineage commitment, cell proliferation and differentiation, and finally positive influence on energy homeostasis. Our study may confirm putative muscle-enhancing abilities of GO; however,

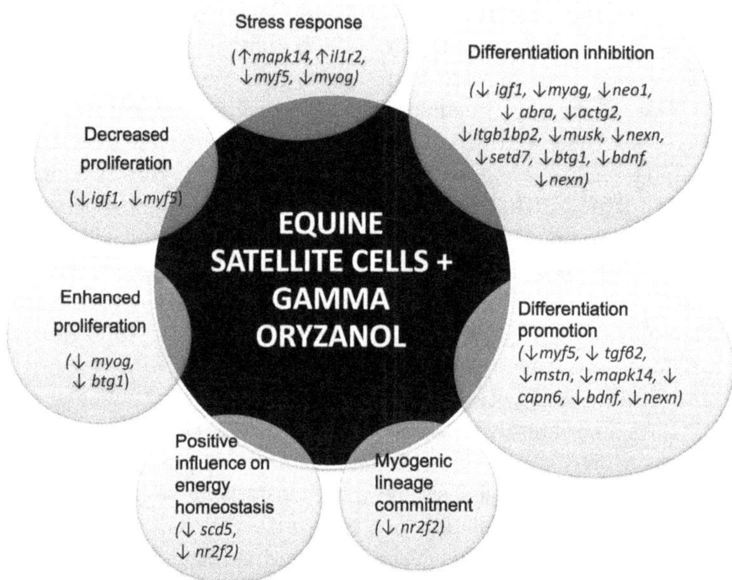

Fig. 6 Processes reinforced in equine satellite cells incubated with 0.125 μM of GO for 24 h

analysis of changes in gene expression did not give equivocal results. Gene transcription is only one step in the regulatory pathway that leads to the functional protein synthesis. Our results encourage for investigation of GO-skeletal muscle relation in proteomic and biochemical level in the future. The collective role of GO in skeletal myogenesis remains unclear and needs further investigation.

Compliance with ethics guidelines

This article does not contain any studies with human or animal subjects performed by the any of the authors.

Competing interests

The authors declare that they have no competing interests.

Authors' contributions

KS carried out the muscle sampling, QPCR validation of microarray results, ontological analysis, and interpretation of the obtained data and drafted the manuscript. AC carried out the equine satellite cell isolation and culture, RNA isolation, and microarray analysis. PO participated in the study design and helped in the manuscript preparation. TS designed the study, supervised the project, performed the muscle sampling and statistical analysis of the microarray and QPCR data, and assisted in the manuscript preparation and revision. All authors read and approved the final manuscript.

Funding

This research was funded by National Science Centre (Poland), Grant No. 2011/03/B/NZ5/05697. Publication of this manuscript was supported by KNOW (Leading National Research Centre) Scientific Consortium "Healthy Animal - Safe Food," decision of the Ministry of Science and Higher Education No. 05-1/KNOW2/2015.

References

1. Araya R, Eckardt D, Maxeiner S, Krüger O, Theis M, Willecke K, et al. Expression of connexins during differentiation and regeneration of skeletal muscle: functional relevance of connexin43. J Cell Sci. 2005;118(1):27–37.
2. Bailey P, Muscat GE, Sartorelli V, Hamamori Y. The orphan nuclear receptor, COUP-TF II, inhibits myogenesis by post-transcriptional regulation of MyoD function: COUP-TF II directly interacts with p300 and myoD. Nucleic Acids Res. 1998;26(23):5501–10.
3. Balogh S, Naus CC, Merrifield PA. Expression of gap junctions in cultured rat L6 cells during myogenesis. Dev Biol. 1993;155(2):351–60.
4. Bentzinger CF, Wang YX, Rudnicki MA. Building muscle: molecular regulation of myogenesis. Cold Spring Harbor Perspect Biol. 2012;4(2):a008342.
5. Brancaccio M, Guazzone S, Menini N, Sibona E, Hirsch E, De Andrea M, et al. Melusin is a new muscle-specific interactor for β1 integrin cytoplasmic domain. J Biol Chem. 1999;274(41):29282–8.
6. Brazma A, Hingamp P, Quackenbush J, Sherlock G, Spellman P, Stoeckert C, et al. Minimum information about a microarray experiment (MIAME)—toward standards for microarray data. Nat Genet. 2001;29(4):365–71.
7. Brown AE, Palsgaard J, Borup R, Avery P, Gunn DA, De Meyts P, et al. p38 MAPK activation upregulates proinflammatory pathways in skeletal muscle cells from insulin-resistant type 2 diabetic patients. Am J Physiol Endocrinol Metab. 2015;308(1):E63–70.
8. Brown D, Hikim APS, Kovacheva EL, Sinha-Hikim I. Mouse model of testosterone-induced muscle fiber hypertrophy: involvement of p38 mitogen-activated protein kinase-mediated Notch signaling. J Endocrinol. 2009;201(1):129–39.
9. Busson M, Carazo A, Seyer P, Grandemange S, Casas F, Pessemesse L, et al. Coactivation of nuclear receptors and myogenic factors induces the major

BTG1 influence on muscle differentiation. Oncogene. 2005;24(10):1698–710.

10. Bustin SA, Benes V, Garson JA, Hellemans J, Huggett J, Kubista M, et al. The MIQE guidelines: minimum information for publication of quantitative real-time PCR experiments. Clin Chem. 2009;55(4):611–22.
11. Chevrel G, Hohlfeld R, Sendtner M. The role of neurotrophins in muscle under physiological and pathological conditions. Muscle Nerve. 2006;33(4): 462–76.
12. Cicero AFG, Gaddi A. Rice bran oil and γ-oryzanol in the treatment of hyperlipoproteinaemias and other conditions. Phytother Res. 2001;15(4): 277–89.
13. Clow C, Jasmin BJ. Brain-derived neurotrophic factor regulates satellite cell differentiation and skeletal muscle regeneration. Mol Biol Cell. 2010;21(13): 2182–90.
14. DeChiara TM, Bowen DC, Valenzuela DM, Simmons MV, Poueymirou WT, Thomas S, et al. The receptor tyrosine kinase MuSK is required for neuromuscular junction formation in vivo. Cell. 1996;85(4):501–12.
15. Dobrzyn A, & Ntambi JM. (2005). The role of stearoyl-CoA desaturase in the control of metabolism. Prostaglandins, leukotrienes and essential fatty acids, 73(1), 35-41.
16. Edgar R, Domrachev M, Lash AE. Gene Expression Omnibus: NCBI gene expression and hybridization array data repository. Nucleic Acids Res. 2002; 30(1):207–10.
17. Eslami S, Esa NM, Marandi SM, Ghasemi G, Eslami S. Effects of gamma oryzanol supplementation on anthropometric measurements & muscular strength in healthy males following chronic resistance training. Indian J Med Res. 2014;139(6):857.
18. Fernyhough ME, Helterline DL, Vierck JL, Dodson MV, Bucci LR, Feliciano JEFF. Myogenic satellite cell proliferative and differentiative responses to components of common oral ergogenic supplements. Res Sports Med. 2004;12(3):161–90.
19. Fry AC, Bonner E, Lewis DL, Johnson RL, Stone MH, Kraemer WJ. The effects of gamma-oryzanol supplementation during resistance exercise training. Int J Sport Nutr. 1997;7(4):318–29.
20. Gopal-Srivastava R, Haynes J, Piatigorsky J. Regulation of the murine alpha B-crystallin/small heat shock protein gene in cardiac muscle. Mol Cell Biol. 1995;15(12):7081–90.
21. Gorbe A, Krenacs T, Cook JE, Becker DL. Myoblast proliferation and syncytial fusion both depend on connexin43 function in transfected skeletal muscle primary cultures. Exp Cell Res. 2007;313(6):1135–48.
22. Greene EA, Raub RH. Procedures for harvesting satellite cells from equine skeletal muscle. J Equine Vet Sci. 1992;12(1):33–5.
23. Gu J, Orr N, Park SD, Katz LM, Sulimova G, MacHugh DE, et al. A genome scan for positive selection in thoroughbred horses. PLoS One. 2009;4(6):e5767.
24. Haddad F, Adams GR. Inhibition of MAP/ERK kinase prevents IGF-I-induced hypertrophy in rat muscles. J Appl Physiol. 2004;96(1):203–10.
25. Hansen, Abigail. (2014). Myostatin mRNA expression in cultured equine satellite cells. Retrieved from the University of Minnesota Digital Conservancy, http://hdl.handle.net/11299/163114
26. Harris PA, Harris RC. Ergogenic potential of nutritional strategies and substances in the horse. Livest Prod Sci. 2005;92(2):147–65.
27. Hong M, Schachter K, Jiang G, Krauss R. Neogenin regulates Shh pathway activity during digit patterning. Dev Biol. 2011;356(1):147.
28. Huang CCJ. Potential functionality and digestibility of oryzanol as determined using in vitro cell culture models. Doctoral dissertation, Louisiana State University. 2003: http://etd.lsu.edu/docs/available/etd-0609103-135757/.
29. da Huang DW, Sherman BT, Lempicki RA. Systematic and integrative analysis of large gene lists using DAVID Bioinformatics Resources. Nat Protoc. 2011;4(1):44–57.
30. Ismail M, Al-Naqeeb G, Mamat WA, Ahmad Z. Gamma-oryzanol rich fraction regulates the expression of antioxidant and oxidative stress related genes in stressed rat's liver. Nutr Metab. 2010;7(23):1–13.
31. Ismail N, Ismail M, Imam MU, Azmi NH, Fathy SF, Foo JB. Mechanistic basis for protection of differentiated SH-SY5Y cells by oryzanol-rich fraction against hydrogen peroxide-induced neurotoxicity. BMC Complement Altern Med. 2014;14(1):467.
32. Jank M, Zwierzchowski L, Siadkowska E, Budasz-Świderska M, Sadkowski T, Oprządek J, et al. Polymorphism in the 5'flanking region of the myostatin gene affects myostatin and TGF-β. J Anim Feed Sci. 2006;15:381–91.
33. Kamradt MC, Chen F, Sam S, Cryns VL. The small heat shock protein αB-crystallin negatively regulates apoptosis during myogenic differentiation by inhibiting caspase-3 activation. J Biol Chem. 2002;277(41):38731–6.
34. Keren A, Tamir Y, Bengal E. The p38 MAPK signaling pathway: a major regulator of skeletal muscle development. Mol Cell Endocrinol. 2006;252(1): 224–30.
35. Kollias HD, McDermott JC. Transforming growth factor-β and myostatin signaling in skeletal muscle. J Appl Physiol. 2008;104(3):579–87.
36. Lamon S, Wallace MA, Léger B, Russell AP. Regulation of STARS and its downstream targets suggest a novel pathway involved in human skeletal muscle hypertrophy and atrophy. J Physiol. 2009;587(8):1795–803.
37. Lee A, Hakuno F, Northcott P, Pessin JE, Adcock MR. Nexilin, a cardiomyopathy-associated F-actin binding protein, binds and regulates IRS1 signaling in skeletal muscle cells. PLoS One. 2013;8(1):e55634.
38. Livak KJ, Schmittgen TD. Analysis of relative gene expression data using real-time quantitative PCR and the 2− ΔΔCT method. Methods. 2001;25(4): 402–8.
39. Ma L, Lin J, Qiao Y, Weng W, Liu W, Wang J, et al. Serum CD166: a novel hepatocellular carcinoma tumor marker. Clin Chim Acta. 2015;441:156–62.
40. Mauro A. Satellite cell of skeletal muscle fibers. J Biophys Biochem Cytol. 1961;9(2):493–5.
41. de Mello F, Streit DP, Sabin N, Gabillard JC. Dynamic expression of tgf-β2, tgf-β3 and inhibin βA during muscle growth resumption and satellite cell differentiation in rainbow trout (Oncorhynchus mykiss). Gen Comp Endocrinol. 2015;210:23–9.
42. Miwa T, Manabe Y, Kurokawa K, Kamada S, Kanda N, Bruns G, et al. Structure, chromosome location, and expression of the human smooth muscle (enteric type) gamma-actin gene: evolution of six human actin genes. Mol Cell Biol. 1991;11(6):3296–306.
43. Mok GF, Sweetman D. Many routes to the same destination: lessons from skeletal muscle development. Reproduction. 2011;141(3):301–12.
44. Mösseler A, Licht S, Wilhelm L, Kamphues J, Ellis AD et al. Can oral intake of gamma-oryzanol (experimentally given orally as pure substance) result in doping relevant testosterone levels in the urine of mares and geldings?. The Impact of Nutrition on the Health and Welfare of Horses, Wageningen Academic Publishers. 2010; 128;293-296.
45. Mousavi K, Jasmin BJ. BDNF is expressed in skeletal muscle satellite cells and inhibits myogenic differentiation. J Neurosci. 2006;26(21):5739–49.
46. Muscat GE, Rea S, Downes M. Identification of a regulatory function for an orphan receptor in muscle: COUP-TF II affects the expression of the myoD gene family during myogenesis. Nucleic Acids Res. 1995;23(8): 1311–8.
47. Nelissen JM, Torensma R, Pluyter M, Adema GJ, Raymakers RA, van Kooyk Y, et al. Molecular analysis of the hematopoiesis supporting osteoblastic cell line U2-OS. Exp Hematol. 2000;28(4):422–32.
48. Ohara K, Uchida A, Nagasaka R, Ushio H, Ohshima T. The effects of hydroxycinnamic acid derivatives on adiponectin secretion. Phytomedicine. 2009;16(2):130–7.
49. Ostaszewski P, Kowalska A, Szarska E, Szpotański P, Cywinska A, Bałasińska B, et al. Effects of β-hydroxy-β-methylbutyrate and γ-oryzanol on blood biochemical markers in exercising thoroughbred race horses. J Equine Vet Sci. 2012;32(9):542–51.
50. Powell DJ, McFarland DC, Cowieson AJ, Muir WI, Velleman SG. The effect of nutritional status and muscle fiber type on myogenic satellite cell fate and apoptosis. Poult Sci. 2014;93(1):163–73.
51. Ramery E, Closset R, Art T, Bureau F, Lekeux P. Expression microarrays in equine sciences. Vet Immunol Immunopathol. 2009;127(3):197–202.
52. Rodier A, Marchal-Victorion S, Rochard P, Casas F, Cassar-Malek I, Rouault MJP, et al. BTG1: a triiodothyronine target involved in the myogenic influence of the hormone. Exp Cell Res. 1999;249(2):337–48.
53. Rom O, Kaisari S, Reznick AZ, & Aizenbud D. Peroxynitrite induces degradation of myosin heavy chain via p38 MAPK and muscle-specific E3 ubiquitin ligases in C2 skeletal myotubes. Advs. Exp. Medicine, Biology. 2014;832:1-8.
54. Rouault JP, Rimokh R, Tessa C, Paranhos G, Ffrench M, Duret L, et al. BTG1, a member of a new family of antiproliferative genes. EMBO J. 1992;11(4):1663.
55. Rudnicki MA, Schnegelsberg PN, Stead RH, Braun T, Arnold HH, Jaenisch R. MyoD or Myf-5 is required for the formation of skeletal muscle. Cell. 1993; 75(7):1351–9.

56. Sadkowski T, Jank M, Zwierzchowski L, Oprzadek J, Motyl T. Comparison of skeletal muscle transcriptional profiles in dairy and beef breeds bulls. J Appl Genet. 2009;50(2):109–23.
57. Sadkowski T, Jank M, Zwierzchowski L, Siadkowska E, Oprządek J, Motyl T. Gene expression profiling in skeletal muscle of Holstein-Friesian bulls with single-nucleotide polymorphism in the myostatin gene 5′-flanking region. J Appl Genet. 2008;49(3):237–50.
58. Schabort EJ, van der Merwe M, Loos B, Moore FP, Niesler CU. TGF-β's delay skeletal muscle progenitor cell differentiation in an isoform-independent manner. Exp Cell Res. 2009;315(3):373–84.
59. Singh BN, Rao KS, Rao CM. Ubiquitin–proteasome-mediated degradation and synthesis of MyoD is modulated by αB-crystallin, a small heat shock protein, during muscle differentiation. Biochim Biophys Acta. 2010;1803(2): 288–99.
60. Suleiman MS, Singh RJR, Stewart CEH. Apoptosis and the cardiac action of insulin-like growth factor I. Pharmacol Ther. 2007;114(3):278–94.
61. Swart GW. Activated leukocyte cell adhesion molecule (CD166/ALCAM): developmental and mechanistic aspects of cell clustering and cell migration. Eur J Cell Biol. 2002;81(6):313–21.
62. Szcześniak KA, Ostaszewski P, Fuller JC, Ciecierska A, Sadkowski T. Dietary supplementation of β-hydroxy-β-methylbutyrate in animals—a review. J Anim Physiol Anim Nutr. 2015;99(3):405–17.
63. Szcześniak KA, Ostaszewski P, Ciecierska A, & Sadkowski T. Investigation of nutriactive phytochemical–gamma-oryzanol in experimental animal models. J Anim Physiol Animal Nutr. 2015: doi:10.1111/jpn.12428.
64. Tao Y, Neppl RL, Huang ZP, Chen J, Tang RH, Cao R, et al. The histone methyltransferase Set7/9 promotes myoblast differentiation and myofibril assembly. J Cell Biol. 2011;194(4):551–65.
65. Tonami K, Hata S, Ojima K, Ono Y, Kurihara Y, Amano T, et al. Calpain-6 deficiency promotes skeletal muscle development and regeneration. PLoS Genet. 2013;9:e1003668. doi:10.1371/journal.pgen.1003668.
66. Trendelenburg AU, Meyer A, Jacobi C, Feige JN, Glass DJ. TAK-1/p38/nNF B signaling inhibits myoblast differentiation by increasing levels of Activin A. Skelet Muscle. 2012;2(1):3.
67. Wicik Z, Sadkowski T, Jank M, Motyl T. The transcriptomic signature of myostatin inhibitory influence on the differentiation of mouse C_2C_{12} myoblasts. Pol J Vet Sci. 2011;14(4):643–52.
68. Xie X, Qin J, Lin SH, Tsai SY, Tsai MJ. Nuclear receptor chicken ovalbumin upstream promoter-transcription factor II (COUP-TFII) modulates mesenchymal cell commitment and differentiation. Proc Natl Acad Sci. 2011;108(36):14843–8.
69. Xie X, Tang K, Yu CT, Tsai SY, Tsai MJ. Regulatory potential of COUP-TFs in development: stem/progenitor cells. Semin Cell Dev Biol. 2013;24(10):687–93. Academic Press.
70. Zhang L, Wang XH, Wang H, Du J, Mitch WE. Satellite cell dysfunction and impaired IGF-1 signaling cause CKD-induced muscle atrophy. J Am Soc Nephrol. 2010;21(3):419–27.

4

Moderately decreased maternal dietary energy intake during pregnancy reduces fetal skeletal muscle mitochondrial biogenesis in the pigs

Tiande Zou, Bing Yu, Jie Yu, Xiangbing Mao, Ping Zheng, Jun He, Zhiqing Huang, Yue Liu and Daiwen Chen*

Abstract

Background: Mitochondria are of major importance in oocyte and early embryo, playing a key role in maintaining energy homeostasis. Epidemiological findings indicate that maternal undernutrition-induced mitochondrial dysfunction during pregnancy is associated with the development of metabolic disorders in offspring. Here, we investigated the effects of moderately decreased maternal energy intake during pregnancy on skeletal muscle mitochondrial biogenesis in fetal offspring with pig as a model.

Methods: Pregnant Meishan sows were allocated to a standard-energy (SE) intake group as recommended by the National Research Council (NRC; 2012) and a low-energy (LE) intake group. Fetal umbilical vein serum and longissimus muscle samples were collected for further analysis on day 90 of pregnancy.

Results: Sow and fetal weights and the concentrations of serum growth hormone (GH) and glucose were reduced in LE group. Maternal LE diet decreased the messenger RNA (mRNA) expression of genes involved in mitochondrial biogenesis and function such as peroxisome proliferator-activated receptor gamma coactivator 1α (PPARGC1A), nuclear respiratory factor 1 (NRF1), mitochondrial transcription factor A (TFAM), β subunit of mitochondrial H^+-ATP synthase (ATB5B), sirtuin 1 (Sirt1), and citrate synthase (CS). The protein expression of PPARGC1A and Sirt1, intracellular NAD^+-to-NADH ratio, and CS activity was reduced in LE group, and accordingly, mitochondrial DNA (mtDNA) content was decreased. Moreover, copper/zinc superoxide dismutase (CuZn-SOD) expression at both mRNA and protein levels and SOD and catalase (CAT) activities were reduced in LE group as well.

Conclusions: The observed decrease in muscle mitochondrial biogenesis and antioxidant defense capacity suggests that moderately decreased maternal energy intake during pregnancy impairs mitochondrial function in fetal pigs.

Keywords: Maternal energy intake, Skeletal muscle, Mitochondrial biogenesis, Oxidative stress, Fetal pig

Background

Obesity, characterized by an imbalance between energy intake and expenditure, is increasing at an alarming rate in most parts of the world. In particular, human epidemiological and animal experimental studies have demonstrated that hormonal, metabolic, and nutritional disturbances at crucial prenatal time periods may also determine the predisposition to deleterious health outcomes in adult life, including obesity and associated metabolic disorders [3, 12, 20]. Thus, maternal undernutrition during pregnancy has been reported to have persistent effects on offspring metabolic energy regulatory systems [42, 45], although the underlying mechanisms of this process are still unclear.

Mitochondria are of major importance in oocyte and early embryo, playing a key role in maintaining energy homeostasis [26, 40]. Deregulation of energy homeostasis is a common underlying characteristic of metabolic

* Correspondence: dwchen@sicau.edu.cn
Key Laboratory for Animal Disease-Resistant Nutrition of the Ministry of Education of China, Animal Nutrition Institute, Sichuan Agricultural University, Cheng du, China

syndrome, and many studies have demonstrated that prenatal maternal undernutrition programs offspring mitochondrial function in various tissues of different animal models, such as the pancreatic islet [41] and kidney [9] of rat and the skeletal muscle of sheep [17]. The skeletal muscle composes about 40–50 % of body mass and is the major site of glucose and fatty acid utilization, playing an important role in preventing obesity and type 2 diabetes (T2D) [36, 47]. There is growing evidence that increased mitochondrial function may be essential for skeletal myogenesis [33]. Moreover, mitochondrial dysfunction in the skeletal muscle is been implicated in the development of T2D [2, 19]. Studies in mice have shown that maternal exposure to a low-protein diet during pregnancy and lactation decreases mitochondrial DNA content and citrate synthase activity and leads to mitochondrial gene expression changes in the offspring liver and skeletal muscle [18, 27]. However, currently, to our knowledge, no studies have addressed the effects of maternal low-energy (LE) diets on fetal offspring skeletal muscle mitochondrial biogenesis and function.

Compared with sheep and rodents, pigs share a number of anatomical and physiological similarities with humans making them an excellent experimental model for metabolic studies [31, 39]. However, there is no data in the pig skeletal muscle on how maternal LE intake during pregnancy may affect mitochondrial number and function. In addition, prenatal skeletal muscle development is particularly susceptible to environmental factors in mammalians [8]. Thus, understanding the effect of maternal LE diet on mitochondrial biogenesis and function in the skeletal muscle of the pig fetuses may provide important insights into the fetal origins of the metabolic syndrome. In the present study, our objective was to investigate the effects of moderately decreased maternal dietary energy intake during pregnancy on skeletal muscle mitochondrial biogenesis in pig fetuses on day 90 of pregnancy.

Methods

Animals and diets

The experimental procedures were approved by the Animal Care and Use Committee of Sichuan Agricultural University. Eight primiparous, purebred Meishan sows (initial body weight 72.8 ± 4.0 kg) were artificially inseminated three times, at the third observation of estrus, with the semen of purebred Meishan boars. The day of the last insemination constituted the first day of pregnancy. The pregnant sows were randomly assigned to one of the two experimental groups differing in daily digestible energy (DE) intake: standard-energy (SE) and low-energy (LE) groups. Based on the consideration that Meishan pigs, being raised with modern commercial diets composed following NRC standards, were traditionally raised on LE diets, we fed the sows in SE group with diets containing 12.90 MJ of DE/kg, while those in LE group were fed diets containing 11.24 MJ of DE/kg to mimic the energy levels in traditional diets during pregnancy. During early pregnancy (days 1 to 35 of pregnancy), sows were fed with rations of 2.0 kg/day because lower feed intake level is beneficial to embryo survival during early pregnancy [16], supplying 25.80 and 22.48 MJ DE per day for SE and LE sows, respectively. Additionally, considering the rapid increasing demand of maternal weight gain and fetal growth during mid-late pregnancy (days 36 to 90 of pregnancy) [25], sows were fed on diets with the rations of 2.4 kg/day, supplying 30.96 and 26.98 MJ DE per day for SE and LE sows, respectively (Fig. 1). The isoprotein corn-wheat bran-soybean meal-based diets were used, and the LE diet was formulated to allow the sow to ingest approximately 13 % less DE than the SE group (Table 1). Although the additional dietary fiber was added to the LE diet to decrease energy concentration, crude fiber (CF) intake was only 1.52 % higher in LE sows than in SE sows. Danielsen and Vestergaard [6] reported that even excess dietary fiber intake (CF, 4.6 vs 12.7 %) of pregnant sows influenced neither fetal survival nor litter size at birth. Consequently, it is quite unlikely in this experiment that the dietary fiber supplementation affected the fetal survival rate directly. The dietary treatments were introduced from mating to day 90 of pregnancy. During pregnancy, sows were housed in individual feed stalls in a breeding facility. Sows were fed discretely twice daily (08:00 and 14:00 h) with 50 % of the daily ration each time and had free access to drinking water.

Sample collection

After a 12-h overnight fast, pregnant sows of both groups (SE/LE) were weighed and anesthetized with an intramuscular injection of Zoletil (Zoletil 50, Virbac; 4 mg/kg body weight) on day 90 of pregnancy ($n = 4/4$). The maternal abdomen was opened, and the reproductive tracts were removed immediately. Blood from the umbilical vein of each fetus was collected and coagulated for 30 min and then centrifuged at 3500×g for 10 min to separate serum which was stored at −20 °C until analysis. The body weight of each fetus was recorded. Two female fetuses and two male fetuses, with weight close to the average level, were selected from each sow for muscle sample collection. The longissimus muscles (LMs) were collected from the fetuses, snap-frozen in liquid nitrogen, and stored at −80 °C until subsequent analysis.

Measurement of metabolites and hormone

The malondialdehyde (MDA) concentration in the skeletal muscle was measured using an assay kit (Jiancheng Institute of Bioengineering, Nanjing, Jiangsu, China). The concentrations of triglyceride and glucose in umbilical vein serum were determined using commercial kits

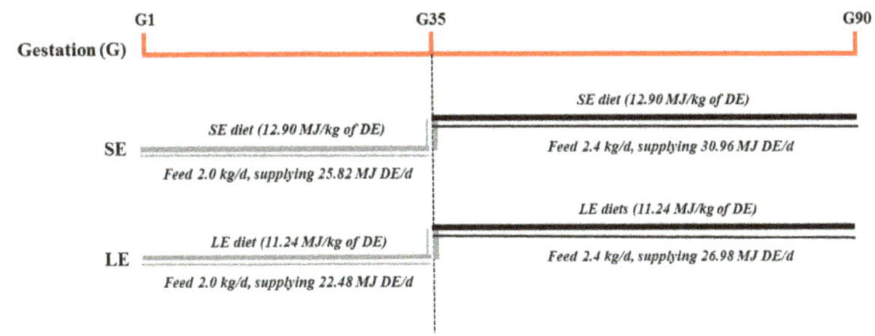

Fig. 1 The experimental design and the timing of the different treatments and procedures. *SE* maternal standard-energy diet, *LE* maternal low-energy diet, *DE* digestible energy

Table 1 Ingredients and composition of the experimental diets (as-fed basis)

Items	SE	LE
Ingredient (%)		
Maize	45.00	45.00
Soybean meal	13.60	13.60
Wheat bran	27.80	27.80
Soybean oil	4.50	–
Wheat bran fiber	2.54	5.02
Soyabean fiber	1.10	2.17
Corn fiber	0.96	1.91
Salt	0.40	0.40
L-Lys·HCl, 75 %	0.10	0.10
L-Thr	0.10	0.10
Limestone	1.23	1.23
Monocalcium phosphate	1.99	1.99
Choline chloride, 50 %	0.14	0.14
Vitamin premix[a]	0.04	0.04
Mineral premix[b]	0.50	0.50
Total	100.00	100.00
Nutritional composition		
Digestible energy, MJ/kg	12.90	11.24
Crude protein (%)	13.92	14.35
Crude fiber (%)	4.97	6.49
Lys (%)	0.69	0.69
Met + Cys (%)	0.35	0.35
Thr (%)	0.46	0.46
Ca (%)	0.96	0.96
Available P (%)	0.48	0.48
Total P (%)	0.79	0.79

[a]Provided the following per kilogram of diet: 1.2 mg retinol, 0.02 mg cholecalciferol, 44 mg α-tocopherol, 0.5 mg phylloquinone, 1 mg thiamin, 3.75 mg riboflavin, 1 mg pyridoxine, 0.015 mg cyanocobalamin, 10 mg niacin, 12 mg pantothenic acid, 1.3 mg folic acid, and 0.2 mg biotin

[b]Provided the following per kilogram of diet: 80 mg Fe (as $FeSO_4.7H_2O$), 10 mg Cu (as $CuSO_4.5H_2O$), 100 mg Zn (as $ZnSO_4.7H_2O$), 25 mg Mn (as $MnSO_4.H_2O$), 0.15 mg Se (as Na_2SeO_3), and 0.14 mg I (as KI)

(Jiancheng Institute of Bioengineering, Nanjing, Jiangsu, China) according to the provided instructions. Growth hormone (GH) concentration in umbilical vein serum was measured using a commercially available radioimmunoassay kits purchased from Beijing North Institute of Biotechnology (Beijing, China). Insulin was determined with porcine ELISA kit (R&D Systems, Minneapolis, MN, USA). Sensitivities of the assays were 0.02 ng/ml and 2.15 pmol/l for GH and insulin, respectively. Intra- and inter-assay coefficients of variation were 4.3 and 6.6 % for GH and 3.9 and 7.4 % for insulin, respectively.

Measurement of enzyme activities

The activities of superoxide dismutase (SOD), glutathione peroxidase (GPx), and catalase (CAT) in the skeletal muscle were measured using assay kits (Jiancheng Institute of Bioengineering, Nanjing, Jiangsu, China). Citrate synthase (CS) activity in the skeletal muscle was measured spectrophotometrically using a commercial kit (GenMed Scientifics Inc, USA).

NAD^+-to-NADH ratio measurement

The NAD^+-to-NADH ratio in the skeletal muscle was measured using a colorimetric assay kit (BioVision, Milpitas, CA, USA) according to the manufacturer's instructions. Briefly, muscle samples were washed with cold PBS followed homogenization using NAD^+/NADH extraction buffer. To decompose NAD^+, 200 μl of extract was heated to 60 °C for 30 min. Under this condition, all NAD^+ were decomposed but keeping NADH intact. Both heated and unheated extract from each sample, together with the NADH standard solutions, were transferred into 96-well plates, added with 100 μl of NAD cycling mix into each well, mixed, and incubated at room temperature for 5 min to convert NAD^+ to NADH. Then, 10 μl of NADH developer was added into each well and incubated at room temperature for 2 h. Read the plate at OD 450 nm. The amount of NAD^+ from each sample was calculated as total NAD (values from the unheated extracts) minus NADH (values from the heated extracts) and then divided by the protein concentration.

Mitochondrial DNA copy number

Total DNA was extracted from LM muscle using QIAamp DNA extraction kit (QIAGEN, Valencia, CA, USA). The mitochondrial DNA (mtDNA) copy number was determined using quantitative real-time PCR as previously described with some modifications [5]. mtDNA was amplified using primers specific for the mitochondrial cytochrome b (*MT-CYB*) and normalized to genomic DNA by amplification of the *18S rRNA*. The sequence of primers was presented in Table 2.

Quantitative real-time PCR

Total RNA was extracted from frozen muscle tissues using RNAiso Plus reagent (Takara, Dalian, China), and complementary DNA (cDNA) was synthesized from 0.5 μg of the total RNA using the PrimeScript™ RT reagent kit (Takara). Real-time quantitative PCR was carried out in the final volume of 10 ul containing 5 ul of SYBR® Premix Ex TaqTM II, 0.8 ul of the primer pair, 0.2 ul of ROX Reference Dye, 1 ul of cDNA template, and 3 ul of dH_2O using the ABI Prism® 7900HT Sequence Detection System (Applied Biosystems, Foster city, CA, USA). The thermal cycling parameters comprised an initial denaturation step at 95 °C for 30 s, 40 cycles of PCR reaction at 95 °C for 5 s, and 60 °C for 34 s, followed by a dissociation step at 95 °C for 15 s, 60 °C for 1 min, and 95 °C for 15 s. To confirm specific product amplification, melt curve analysis was conducted. Primers for individual genes were designed using Primer Express 3.0 (Applied Biosystems) and are shown in Table 2. For normalization, *ACTB* was chosen as the reference gene since no variation in its expression was observed between treatments. The messenger RNA (mRNA) level of each target gene for SE group was set to 1.0.

Table 2 Primer sequences of the target and reference genes

Gene	Primer sequence (5′–3′)	Product size (bp)	GeneBank no.
PPARGC1A	F: CCCGAAACAGTAGCAGAGACAAG R: CTGGGGTCAGAGGAAGAGATAAAG	111	NM_213963
SIRT1	F: TGACTGTGAAGCTGTACGAGGAG R: TGGCTCTATGAAACTGCTCTGG	143	EU030283.2
NRF1	F: GCCAGTGAGATGAAGAGAAACG R: CTACAGCAGGGACCAAAGTTCAC	166	AK237171.1
TFAM	F: GGTCCATCACAGGTAAAGCTGAA R: ATAAGATCGTTTCGCCCAACTTC	167	NM_001130211
ATP5B	F: CATGAAGCAGGTGGCAGGTA R: CAGACGAACACCACGACTCA	127	NM_001185142
POLG	F: CTTTGAGGTTTTCCAGCAGCAG R: GCTCCCAGTTTTGGTTGACAG	119	XM_005653521.1
SSBP1	F: CTTTGAGGTAGTGCTGTGTCG R: CTCACCCCTGACGATGAAGAC	142	XM_005673118.1
COX4	F: CCAAGTGGGACTACGACAAGAAC R: CCTGCTCGTTTATTAGCACTGG	131	Liu et al. [22]
CYCS	F: TAGAAAAGGGAGGCAAACACAAG R: GGATTCTCCAGGTACTCCATCAG	154	Liu et al. [22]
CS	F: CCTTTCAGACCCCTACTTGTCCT R: CACATCTTTGCCGACTTCCTTC	127	Liu et al. [22]
CuZn-SOD	F: AACATGGTGGGCCAAAGGAT R: CGGCCAATGATGGAATGGTC	136	NM_001190422.1
ACTB	F: TCTGGCACCACACCTTCT R: TGATCTGGGTCATCTTCTCAC	114	DQ178122
MT-CYB	F: ATGAAACATTGGAGTAGTCCTACTATTTACC R: CTACGAGGTCTGTTCCGATATAAGG	149	NC_000845.1
18S rRNA	F: GGTAGTGACGAAAAATAACAATACAGGAC R: ATACGCTATTGGAGCTGGAATTACC	141	NC_010448.3

ACTB β-actin, *COX* cytochrome c oxidase, *CS* citrate synthase, *CuZn-SOD* copper/zinc superoxide peroxidase, *MT-CYB* mitochondrially encoded cytochrome b, *CYCS* cytochrome c, somatic, *ATP5B* β subunit of mitochondrial H^+-ATP synthase, *NRF1* nuclear respiratory factor 1, *PPARGC1A* peroxisome proliferator-activated receptor gamma coactivator 1α, *POLG* gamma DNA polymerase, *SIRT1* sirtuin 1, *SSBP1* mitochondrial single-strand DNA-binding protein, *TFAM* mitochondrial transcription factor A

Immunoblotting analysis

Total protein was extracted from frozen muscle tissue using the protein extraction kit (Beyotime Biotechnology, Jiangsu, China) according to the manufacturer's guide. The protein content of lysates was measured with the Pierce BCA protein Assay kit (Thermo, Waltham, MA, USA). Immunoblotting analysis was performed as previously described [29]. The primary antibodies included PPARGC1A (ab54481, Abcam, Cambridge, MA, USA), Sirt1 (sc-19857, Santa Cruz Biotechnology, CA, USA), CuZn-SOD (sc-271014, Santa Cruz Biotechnology), and β-tubulin (sc-9104, Santa Cruz Biotechnology). The density of bands was quantified using the Gel Doc XR System (Bio-Rad, Hercules, CA, USA) and then normalized to β-tubulin content. The normalized values were used for comparison of the expression of target protein between SE and LE groups.

Statistical analysis

Results were presented as least square means with their standard errors. Data were analyzed using the MIXED procedures of Statistical Analysis System (version 8.1, SAS Institute, Inc.) with treatment, gender, and the two-way interactions as the fixed effect and with sow as the random effect. However, none of the gender and interactions were statistically significant. Therefore, they were removed from the model, and data from female and male fetuses were pooled together for analysis. The least square means were separated using the PDIFF option with the Turkey adjustment. The $2^{-\Delta\Delta Ct}$ method was used to analyze the relative changes in each gene expression [23]. Statistical significance was considered as $P < 0.05$, and a tendency towards difference was considered as $P < 0.10$.

Results

Pregnancy performance

On day 90 of pregnancy, the maternal body weight and fetal weight were reduced in LE group ($P < 0.05$; Table 3). However, no significant differences were observed for litter size and variation in fetal weight within a litter (as indicated by the coefficient of variation) between SE and LE groups ($P > 0.05$).

Table 3 Sow body weight, litter size, fetal weight, and variation in fetal weight within a litter on day 90 of pregnancy

Item	SE	LE	SEM	*P* value
Sow BW (kg)				
At insemination	72.7	72.9	0.9	0.840
At day 90 of pregnancy	127.9	117.0	1.9	0.002
Litter size	12.0	11.8	0.9	0.856
Fetal weight (g)	574.4	507.7	17.9	0.039
CV, %	14.86	12.72	1.48	0.345

$n = 4$ for each group

SE maternal standard-energy diet, *LE* maternal low-energy diet, *BW* body weight, *CV* coefficient of variation, values determined from fetal weights within each litter

Serum concentrations of metabolites and hormone

As shown in Table 4, the glucose concentration tended to be reduced ($P = 0.091$) in umbilical vein serum of LE fetuses. Serum GH concentration was significantly decreased ($P < 0.05$) in LE fetuses compared with SE group, whereas maternal diet had no effect on the concentrations of triglyceride and insulin ($P > 0.05$).

Mitochondrial DNA contents, CS activity, and the NAD^+-to-NADH ratio

As shown in Fig. 2a, the mtDNA copy number in the skeletal muscle was significantly lower ($P < 0.05$) in LE fetuses than in SE fetuses. Furthermore, CS activity was also reduced ($P < 0.05$) in LE fetuses (Fig. 2b). Though NADH level was not changed ($P > 0.05$), the NAD^+ level and NAD^+-to-NADH ratio were significantly decreased ($P < 0.05$) in the skeletal muscle of LE fetuses compared with SE fetuses (Fig. 2c).

Expression of genes implicated in mitochondrial biogenesis and function

To clarify the mechanisms involved in the reduction of mitochondrial density in the muscle of LE fetuses, we measured the expression of genes implicated in mitochondrial biogenesis and function. As shown in Fig. 3a, b, the mRNA and protein levels of PPARGC1A and Sirt1 in LE fetuses were decreased ($P < 0.05$) when compared with SE group. In addition, the mRNA abundance of nuclear respiratory factor 1 (NRF1), mitochondrial transcription factor A (TFAM), β subunit of mitochondrial H^+-ATP synthase (ATP5B), and CS were significantly decreased in the skeletal muscle of LE fetuses as well ($P < 0.05$, Fig. 3c). Meanwhile, the mRNA abundance of gamma DNA polymerase (POLG) and single-stranded DNA-binding protein 1 (SSBP1) responsible for mtDNA replication were lower ($P < 0.05$, Fig. 3d) in LE fetuses.

Table 4 Concentrations of metabolites and hormones in fetal umbilical vein serum on day 90 of pregnancy

Item	SE	LE	SEM	*P* value
Glucose (mmol/l)	4.07	3.55	0.19	0.091
Triglyceride (mmol/l)	0.30	0.26	0.02	0.275
GH (ng/ml)	20.06	17.57	0.72	0.021
Insulin (pmol/ml)	134.98	130.16	2.80	0.227

$n = 16$ for each group

SE maternal standard-energy diet, *LE* maternal low-energy diet, *GH* growth hormone

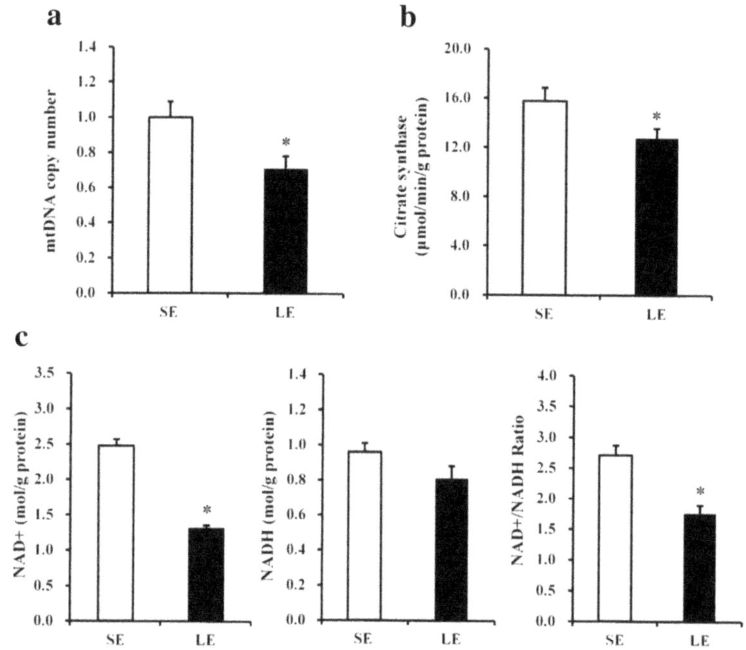

Fig. 2 mtDNA copy number (**a**), citrate synthase activity (**b**), and the NAD^+-to-NADH ratio (**c**) in the fetal longissimus muscles of SE and LE sows. Values are least squares means ± SEMs, $n = 16$. *SE* maternal standard-energy diet, *LE* maternal low-energy diet, *mtDNA* mitochondrial DNA. *$P < 0.05$ compared with SE group

MDA level, CuZn-SOD gene expression, and antioxidant enzyme activities in the skeletal muscle

We further measured the MDA level, CuZn-SOD expression, and the activities of three major antioxidative enzymes in the skeletal muscle to determine the effects of maternal energy restriction on reactive oxygen species (ROS) defense system. As shown in Table 5 and Fig. 4, the LE fetuses had markedly lower activities of SOD and CAT ($P < 0.05$) and mRNA and protein expression of CuZn-SOD ($P < 0.05$) in the skeletal muscle compared to the SE fetuses. No significant changes in MDA level and GPx activity were found between treatments ($P > 0.05$).

Discussion

Epidemiological data demonstrate that low birth weight due to maternal malnutrition is associated with increased rates of metabolic diseases in adulthood [1, 11]. This study used the domestic pig as an animal model for the study of maternal nutrition and is of interest for human health and livestock science. Consistent with previous reports [15, 32], the maternal LE diets decreased fetal weight, which was linked to significantly lower serum GH concentration. Cumulative evidence have shown that mitochondrial dysfunction in the skeletal muscle is implicated in the developmental origins of metabolic syndrome [3, 43]. Mitochondria are inherited through the maternal lineage and easily affected by the environment because of its position outside the nucleus [37]. It was reported that maternal low-protein diets during gestation affect mtDNA transcription regulation through changing the DNA methylation and hydroxymethylation on the promoter of mtDNA in the liver of newborn piglets [15]. Previous studies in rodents also suggest that maternal nutritional stress causes changes to skeletal muscle mitochondrial function and oxidative metabolism that persist into adult offspring, increasing the risk of T2D [4, 21]. Moreover, because mitochondrial biogenesis accompanies skeletal myogenesis [34], and we previously reported that maternal LE diets attenuate fetal skeletal muscle development [48], thus, we hypothesized that the impairment of mitochondrial biogenesis may contribute to maternal LE diet-induced delayed skeletal myogenesis in pig fetuses. In the present study, we found that maternal LE diets during pregnancy decreased the mtDNA copy number in the skeletal muscle of LE fetuses, indicating a decrease in mitochondrial density. Similar results have been reported previously in rats' offspring of dams fed with a low-protein diet [30, 41]. However, some studies have shown no consistent effects, and even advantageous effects, on mtDNA copy number when prenatal exposure to maternal low-protein diets in various tissues of different animal models, including the muscle in sheep [17] and muscle [4] and kidney [9] in rats, as well as fat in mice [18]. Thus, there are contradictory results on how maternal nutritional limitation during pregnancy affects mitochondrial biogenesis in the offspring. These findings imply that the time period and duration of treatment during pregnancy, the type and amount of nutrient changes, and the different

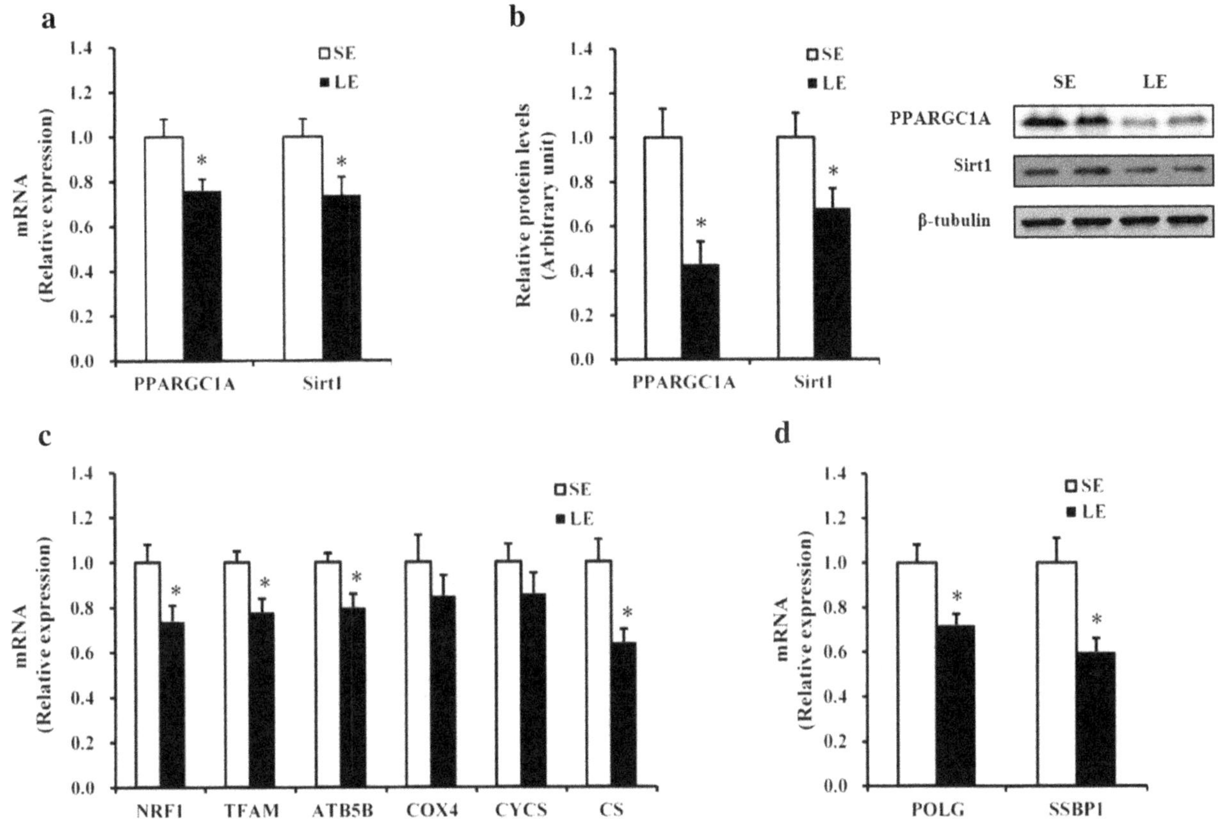

Fig. 3 PPARGC1A and Sirt1 mRNA (**a**) and protein (**b**) levels and relative mRNA expression of the selected genes responsible for mitochondrial biogenesis and function (**c**) and mtDNA replication (**d**) in the fetal longissimus muscles of SE and LE sows. Values are least squares means ± SEMs, *n* = 16. *SE* maternal-standard energy diet, *LE* maternal low-energy diet. **P* < 0.05 compared with SE group

animal models and tissues tested seem to be important factors resulting in variation between studies. To our knowledge, this is the first report regarding the effect of maternal LE diets on mtDNA content in the skeletal muscle of pig fetuses.

The decrease in muscle mtDNA content indicates disrupted mitochondrial biogenesis. The control of mitochondrial biogenesis is a complex biological process that needs the coordinated regulation of multiple transcriptional factors, including nuclear and mitochondrial-encoded genes [10]. It is well established that the NAD^+-dependent deacetylase Sirt1 plays an important role in numerous fundamental cellular processes including gene silencing, DNA repair, and metabolic regulation [14]. In our study, the expression of Sirt1 at both the mRNA and protein levels was reduced in the skeletal muscle of LE fetuses. Because Sirt1 deacetylase activity is driven by NAD^+ levels, we examined whether maternal LE diets suppress Sirt1 by altering the intracellular NAD^+/NADH ratio. Supporting this hypothesis, the NAD^+/NADH ratio was decreased in LE fetuses. However, NADH content was not changed by maternal LE diets, implying that, apart from the interconversion of NAD^+ and NADH during redox reactions, the concentration of both partners of this redox pair may be controlled by other mechanisms as well. Previous study in astrocytes has shown that both NAD^+ and NADH contents are controlled independently from each other [44]. Sirt1 deacetylates and activates PPARGC1A [10, 13], the master regulator of mitochondrial biogenesis that coactivates the NRF-1, which induce the expression of genes involved in mitochondrial biogenesis [46]. In the present study, we found that the mRNA and protein expression of PPARGC1A were reduced in the skeletal muscle of LE fetuses. Consistently, the mRNA

Table 5 Malondialdehyde content and antioxidant enzyme activities in the fetal longissimus muscle of SE and LE sows

Item	SE	LE	SEM	*P* value
MDA (nmol/mg protein)	2.18	2.05	0.13	0.468
SOD (U/mg protein)	32.39	28.59	0.51	0.008
GPx (U/mg protein)	40.32	36.17	2.05	0.169
CAT (U/mg protein)	8.35	6.41	0.45	0.006

n = 16 for each group
SE maternal standard energy diet, *LE* maternal low energy diet, *MDA* malondialdehyde, *SOD* superoxide dismutase, *GPx* glutathione peroxidase, *CAT* catalase

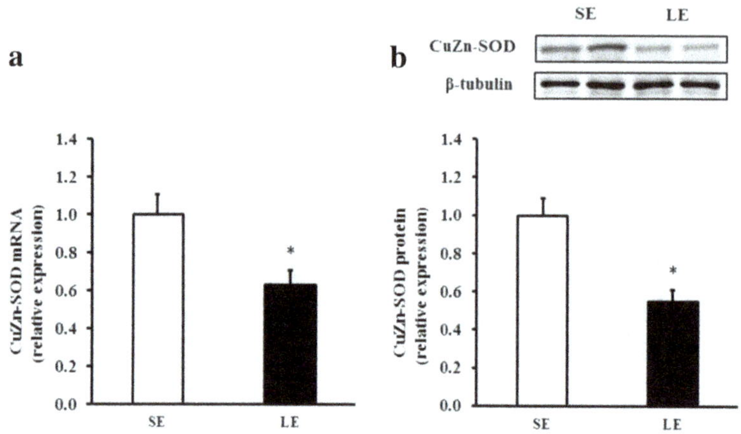

Fig. 4 CuZn-SOD mRNA (**a**) and protein (**b**) expression in the fetal longissimus muscles of SE and LE sows. Values are least squares means ± SEMs, $n = 16$. *SE* maternal standard-energy diet, *LE* maternal low-energy diet. $^{*}P < 0.05$ compared with SE group

expression of NRF1 were decreased in LE fetuses. With further investigation, the mRNA expression of TFAM, a direct regulator of mtDNA replication and transcription that could be regulated by PPARGC1A and NRF1 [46], was reduced in LE fetuses as well. Similar with previous reports in rats [30, 41], abnormal expression patterns of genes implicated in mtDNA biogenesis in the offspring liver or pancreatic islets of malnourished dams were observed. Additionally, because ATP5B is a critical molecule required for mitochondrial ATP synthesis [7], the decrease of mitochondrial biogenesis in LE fetuses was also reflected by down-regulated expression of ATP5B. Gamma DNA polymerase (POLG) and SSBP1 play a key role in mtDNA replication and repair [35]. As expected, we observed a decrease in POLG and SSBP1 in the skeletal muscle of LE fetuses. Together, these data show that maternal LE diets significantly reduced intracellular NAD^{+} levels and as a result decreased Sirt1 expression that subsequently decreased mtDNA replication and mitochondrial biogenesis in the skeletal muscle of LE fetuses.

Maternal malnutrition is associated with a depressed mitochondrial function and respiration in offspring [4, 9, 17]. In this study, although the mRNA expression levels of genes, such as COX4 and CYCS, responsible for mitochondrial function were not changed in LE fetuses, CS mRNA expression and activity were markedly decreased. Because it has been suggested a role for oxidative stress in skeletal muscle mitochondrial dysfunction [2], we speculate that oxidative stress may be implicated in undernutrition-associated mitochondrial alterations. ROS removal is regulated by many antioxidant enzymes, including SOD, GPx, and CAT [24]. In the present study, the mRNA and protein expression of CuZn-SOD and activities of SOD and CAT were reduced in the skeletal muscle of LE fetuses, suggesting the failure of ROS defense system, which is also an evidence of mitochondrial function changes [28]. However, muscle GPx activity was not changed by maternal LE diets. Thus, changes in the antioxidant system seem to occur in an enzyme-specific manner in prenatal energy-restricted fetal pigs. Similarly, previous study showed that maternal protein malnutrition significantly reduced SOD activity while GPx activity was not significantly affected in the liver of rat offspring [30]. Therefore, the enhanced oxidative stress may not explain completely the mitochondrial changes in the fetal muscle as a whole. Previous studies have shown that acute GH action promotes muscle mitochondrial function by stimulating mitochondrial oxidative capacity and transcript abundance of mitochondrial genes [38]. It is here shown

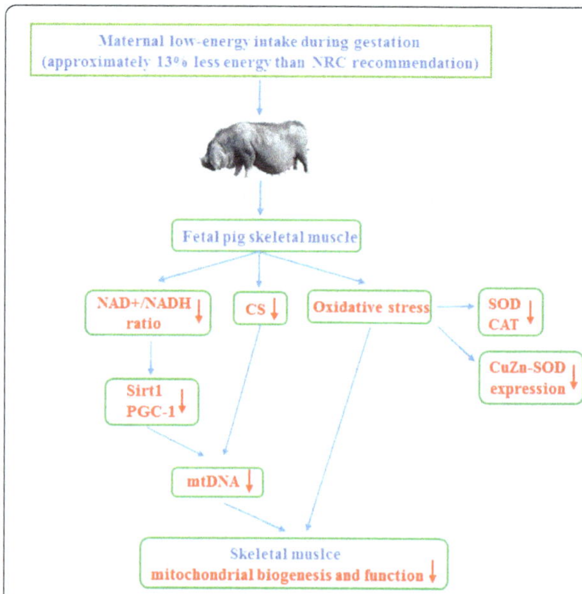

Fig. 5 Diagram explains the effect of moderately decreased maternal energy intake during gestation on skeletal muscle mitochondrial biogenesis and function in fetal pigs

that GH concentrations in umbilical vein serum of LE fetuses were reduced, which could, at least partly, explain the decreases in skeletal muscle mitochondrial biogenesis and function.

Conclusions

This study provides evidence that moderately decreased maternal dietary energy intake in pregnant sows during pregnancy impairs fetal development on day 90 of pregnancy, through decreased mitochondrial biogenesis and function in the skeletal muscle (Fig. 5). The mitochondrial changes during fetal life may further contribute to the disorder of energy homeostasis in adulthood. Consequently, understanding the molecular mechanisms underlying the effect of maternal undernutrition on fetal development may give access to useful knowledge regarding the onset of metabolic diseases.

Acknowledgements

This study was supported by the National Basic Research Program of China (2012CB124701) and the National Natural Science Foundation of China (31372323).

Authors' contributions

TZ, BY, JY, XM, PZ, JH, and ZH participated in the design of the study and performed the statistical analysis. DC conceived and designed the study and helped in drafting the manuscript. TZ and YL carried out the animal experiments and performed the laboratory work. TZ wrote the manuscript. All authors read and approved the final manuscript.

Competing interests

The authors declare that they have no competing interests.

References

1. Barker D. The developmental origins of adult disease. J Am Coll Nutr. 2004;23:588S–95.
2. Bonnard C, Durand A, Peyrol S, Chanseaume E, Chauvin M-A, Morio B, et al. Mitochondrial dysfunction results from oxidative stress in the skeletal muscle of diet-induced insulin-resistant mice. J Clin Invest. 2008;118:789–800.
3. Bruce KD, Hanson MA. The developmental origins, mechanisms, and implications of metabolic syndrome. J Nutr. 2010;140:648–52.
4. Claycombe KJ, Roemmich JN, Johnson L, Vomhof-DeKrey EE, Johnson WT. Skeletal muscle Sirt3 expression and mitochondrial respiration are regulated by a prenatal low-protein diet. J Nutr Biochem. 2015;26:184–9.
5. D'Antona G, Ragni M, Cardile A, Tedesco L, Dossena M, Bruttini F, et al. Branched-chain amino acid supplementation promotes survival and supports cardiac and skeletal muscle mitochondrial biogenesis in middle-aged mice. Cell Metab. 2010;12:362–72.
6. Danielsen V, Vestergaard E-M. Dietary fibre for pregnant sows: effect on performance and behaviour. Anim Feed Sci Tech. 2001;90:71–80.
7. de Heredia ML, Izquierdo JM, Cuezva JM. A conserved mechanism for controlling the translation of β-F1-ATPase mRNA between the fetal liver and cancer cells. J Biol Chem. 2000;275:7430–7.
8. Du M, Yan X, Tong JF, Zhao J, Zhu MJ. Maternal obesity, inflammation, and fetal skeletal muscle development. Biol Reprod. 2010;82:4–12.
9. Engeham S, Mdaki K, Jewell K, Austin R, Lehner AN, Langley-Evans SC. Mitochondrial respiration is decreased in rat kidney following fetal exposure to a maternal low-protein diet. J Nutr Metab. 2012;2012:989037.
10. Fernandez-Marcos PJ, Auwerx J. Regulation of PGC-1α, a nodal regulator of mitochondrial biogenesis. Am J Clin Nutr. 2011;93:884S–90.
11. Fernandez-Twinn D, Ozanne S. Mechanisms by which poor early growth programs type-2 diabetes, obesity and the metabolic syndrome. Physiol Behav. 2006;88:234–43.
12. Garcia A, Palou M, Priego T, Sanchez J, Palou A, Pico C. Moderate caloric restriction during gestation results in lower arcuate nucleus NPY-and αMSH-neurons and impairs hypothalamic response to fed/fasting conditions in weaned rats. Diabetes Obes Metab. 2010;12:403–13.
13. Gerhart-Hines Z, Rodgers JT, Bare O, Lerin C, Kim SH, Mostoslavsky R, et al. Metabolic control of muscle mitochondrial function and fatty acid oxidation through SIRT1/PGC-1α. EMBO J. 2007;26:1913–23.
14. Haigis MC, Guarente LP. Mammalian sirtuins—emerging roles in physiology, aging, and calorie restriction. Genes Dev. 2006;20:2913–21.
15. Jia Y, Li R, Cong R, Yang X, Sun Q, Parvizi N, et al. Maternal low-protein diet affects epigenetic regulation of hepatic mitochondrial DNA transcription in a sex-specific manner in newborn piglets associated with GR binding to its promoter. PloS one. 2013;8:e63855.
16. Jindal R, Cosgrove J, Aherne F, Foxcroft G. Effect of nutrition on embryonal mortality in gilts: association with progesterone. J Anim Sci. 1996;74:620–4.
17. Jørgensen W, Gam C, Andersen JL, Schjerling P, Scheibye-Knudsen M, Mortensen OH, et al. Changed mitochondrial function by pre-and/or postpartum diet alterations in sheep. Am J Physio-Endoc Metab. 2009;297:E1349–57.
18. Jousse C, Muranishi Y, Parry L, Montaurier C, Even P, Launay J-M, et al. Perinatal protein malnutrition affects mitochondrial function in adult and results in a resistance to high fat diet-induced obesity. Plos one. 2014;9:e104896.
19. Kelley DE, He J, Menshikova EV, Ritov VB. Dysfunction of mitochondria in human skeletal muscle in type 2 diabetes. Diabetes. 2002;51:2944–50.
20. King JC. Maternal obesity, metabolism, and pregnancy outcomes. Annu Rev Nutr. 2006;26:271–91.
21. Latouche C, Heywood SE, Henry SL, Ziemann M, Lazarus R, El-Osta A, et al. Maternal overnutrition programs changes in the expression of skeletal muscle genes that are associated with insulin resistance and defects of oxidative phosphorylation in adult male rat offspring. J Nutr. 2014;144:237–44.
22. Liu J, Chen D, Yao Y, Yu B, Mao X, He J, et al. Intrauterine growth retardation increases the susceptibility of pigs to high-fat diet-induced mitochondrial dysfunction in skeletal muscle. PloS one. 2012;7:e34835.
23. Livak KJ, Schmittgen TD. Analysis of relative gene expression data using real-time quantitative PCR and the $2^{-\Delta\Delta CT}$ method. Methods. 2001;25:402–8.
24. Mates J. Effects of antioxidant enzymes in the molecular control of reactive oxygen species toxicology. Toxicology. 2000;153:83–104.
25. McPherson R, Ji F, Wu G, Blanton J, Kim S. Growth and compositional changes of fetal tissues in pigs. J Anim Sci. 2004;82:2534–40.
26. Mitchell M, Schulz SL, Armstrong DT, Lane M. Metabolic and mitochondrial dysfunction in early mouse embryos following maternal dietary protein intervention. Biol Reprod. 2009;80:622–30.
27. Mortensen OH, Olsen HL, Frandsen L, Nielsen PE, Nielsen FC, Grunnet N, et al. A maternal low protein diet has pronounced effects on mitochondrial gene expression in offspring liver and skeletal muscle; protective effect of taurine. J Biomed Sci. 2010;17:S38.
28. Murphy MP. Mitochondrial dysfunction indirectly elevates ROS production by the endoplasmic reticulum. Cell Metab. 2013;18:145–6.
29. Pang W, Wang Y, Wei N, Xu R, Xiong Y, Wang P, et al. Sirt1 inhibits akt2-mediated porcine adipogenesis potentially by direct protein-protein interaction. PloS one. 2013;8:e71576.
30. Park KS, Kim SK, Kim MS, Cho EY, Lee JH, Lee K-U, et al. Fetal and early postnatal protein malnutrition cause long-term changes in rat liver and muscle mitochondria. J Nutr. 2003;133:3085–90.
31. Patterson JK, Lei XG, Miller DD. The pig as an experimental model for elucidating the mechanisms governing dietary influence on mineral absorption. Exp Biol Med. 2008;233:651–64.
32. Pond WG, Maurer RR, Klindt J. Fetal organ response to maternal protein deprivation during pregnancy in swine. J Nutr. 1991;121:504–9.
33. Remels A, Langen R, Schrauwen P, Schaart G, Schols A, Gosker H. Regulation of mitochondrial biogenesis during myogenesis. Mol Cell Endocrinol. 2010;315:113–20.
34. Rochard P, Rodier A, Casas F, Cassar-Malek I, Marchal-Victorion S, Daury L, et al. Mitochondrial activity is involved in the regulation of myoblast differentiation through myogenin expression and activity of myogenic factors. J Biol Chem. 2000;275:2733–44.

35. Scarpulla RC. Nuclear control of respiratory gene expression in mammalian cells. J Cell Biochem. 2006;97:673–83.
36. Schenk S, Horowitz JF. Acute exercise increases triglyceride synthesis in skeletal muscle and prevents fatty acid-induced insulin resistance. J Clin Invest. 2007;117:1690–8.
37. Schwartz M, Vissing J. New patterns of inheritance in mitochondrial disease. Biochem Bioph Res Co. 2003;310:247–51.
38. Short KR, Moller N, Bigelow ML, Coenen-Schimke J, Nair KS. Enhancement of muscle mitochondrial function by growth hormone. J Clin Endocr Metab. 2008;93:597–604.
39. Spurlock ME, Gabler NK. The development of porcine models of obesity and the metabolic syndrome. J Nutr. 2008;138:397–402.
40. Starkov AA. The role of mitochondria in reactive oxygen species metabolism and signaling. Ann NY Acad Sci. 2008;1147:37–52.
41. Theys N, Bouckenooghe T, Ahn M-T, Remacle C, Reusens B. Maternal low-protein diet alters pancreatic islet mitochondrial function in a sex-specific manner in the adult rat. Am J Physiol Regul Integr Comp Physiol. 2009;297:R1516–25.
42. Thompson NM, Norman AM, Donkin SS, Shankar RR, Vickers MH, Miles JL, et al. Prenatal and postnatal pathways to obesity: different underlying mechanisms, different metabolic outcomes. Endocrinology. 2007;148:2345–54.
43. Wells GD, Noseworthy MD, Hamilton J, Tarnopolski M, Tein I. Skeletal muscle metabolic dysfunction in obesity and metabolic syndrome. Can J Neurol Sci. 2008;35:31–40.
44. Wilhelm F, Hirrlinger J. The NAD+/NADH redox state in astrocytes: independent control of the NAD+ and NADH content. J Neurosci Res. 2011;89:1956–64.
45. Wu G, Bazer FW, Cudd TA, Meininger CJ, Spencer TE. Maternal nutrition and fetal development. J Nutr. 2004;134:2169–72.
46. Wu Z, Puigserver P, Andersson U, Zhang C, Adelmant G, Mootha V, et al. Mechanisms controlling mitochondrial biogenesis and respiration through the thermogenic coactivator PGC-1. Cell. 1999;98:115–24.
47. Youn JY, Cai H. Fueling up skeletal muscle to reduce obesity: a TrkB story. Chem Biol. 2015;22:311–2.
48. Zou T, He D, Yu B, Yu J, Mao X, Zheng P, et al. Moderate maternal energy restriction during gestation in pigs attenuates fetal skeletal muscle development through changing myogenic gene expression and myofiber characteristics. Reprod Sci. 2016. doi:10.1177/1933719116651151.

5

Tocotrienols induce endoplasmic reticulum stress and apoptosis in cervical cancer cells

Raffaella Comitato[1*], Barbara Guantario[1], Guido Leoni[2], Kalanithi Nesaretnam[3], Maria Beatrice Ronci[1], Raffaella Canali[1] and Fabio Virgili[1]

Abstract

Background: We have previously reported that γ- and δ-tocotrienols (γ- and δ-T3) induce gene expression and apoptosis in human breast cancer cells (MDA-MB-231 and MCF-7). This effect is mediated, at least in part, by a specific binding and activation of the estrogen receptor-β (ERβ). Transcriptomic data obtained within our previous studies, interrogated by different bioinformatic tools, suggested the existence of an alternative pathway, activated by specific T3 forms and leading to apoptosis, also in tumor cells not expressing ER. In order to confirm this hypothesis, we conducted a study in HeLa cells, a line of human cervical cancer cells void of any canonical ER form.

Results: Cells were synchronized by starvation and treated either with a T3-rich fraction from palm oil (10–20 μg/ml) or with purified α-, γ-, and δ-T3 (5–20 μg/ml). α-tocopherol (TOC) was utilized as a negative control. Apoptosis, accompanied by a significant expression of caspase 8, caspase 10, and caspase 12 was observed at 12 h from treatments. The interrogation of data obtained from transcriptomic platforms (NuGO Affymetrix Human Genechip NuGO_Hs1a520180), further confirmed by RT-PCR, suggested that the administration of γ- and δ-T3 associates with Ca^{2+} release. Data interrogation were confirmed in living cells; in fact, Ca-dependent signals were observed followed by the expression and activation of IRE-1α and of other molecules involved in the unfolded protein response, the core pathway coping with endoplasmic reticulum stress in eukaryotic cells, finally leading to apoptosis.

Conclusions: Our study demonstrates that γ- and δ-T3 induce apoptosis also in tumor cells lacking of ERβ by triggering signals originating from endoplasmic reticulum stress. Our observations suggest that tocotrienols could have a significant role in tumor cell physiology and a possible therapeutic potential.

Keywords: Tocotrienol, Endoplasmic reticulum stress, XBP-1, Apoptosis, IRE-1α

Background

The chemical structure of tocotrienols (T3) is very similar to that of tocopherols (TOC), only differing in the unsaturation of the phytyl chain. On the basis of a modest inhibitory effect in a fetal resorption test in rats, T3 are frequently pooled together with TOC within the family of "vitamin E," but a wide spectrum of specific biological activities has also been reported that is not exhibited by TOC [27]. For instance, several studies have demonstrated that T3, especially the γ- and δ-T3 isoforms, have inflammatory and antioxidant activities not shared with TOC and in particular with α-TOC [26, 54, 57]. Moreover, evidences exist indicating that each vitamin E isomer has a specific pharmaco-dynamic profile [3, 6].

In a study based on a transcriptomic (complementary DNA (cDNA) array) approach, we have previously reported that a T3-rich fraction (TRF) extracted from palm oil induces a significant inhibition of cell proliferation both in vitro in cultured breast cancer cells [40, 41] and in vivo in tumors caused by the inoculation of human breast cancer cells in athymic mice [40]. More recently, on the basis of a subsequent set of studies in silico, followed by in vitro binding experiments coupled with cell culture studies, we have demonstrated that the effects of specific T3 (γ- and δ-T3 forms) on gene expression are, at least in part, mediated by the binding to estrogen receptor-β (ERβ) in cultured MDA-MB-231 [16] and MCF-7 cells [15]. The transcriptomic data set

* Correspondence: raffaella.comitato@crea.gov.it
[1]Council for Agricultural Research and Economics - Food and Nutrition Research Centre (C.R.E.A.-AN), via Ardeatina 546, 00178 Rome, Italy
Full list of author information is available at the end of the article

obtained within these studies, further interrogated by means of bioinformatic tools, suggested the existence of an alternative pathway, activated by specific T3 forms, leading to apoptosis also in tumor cells not expressing any of the two canonical forms of ER (ERα and ERβ). Data interrogation suggested the hypothesis that this alternative pathway could be mainly ascribable to the induction of a cellular stress, at the level of the endoplasmic reticulum (EndoR).

We have therefore extended our previous investigation exploring a putative pathway activated at the level of EndoR by specific T3 forms. To this aim, HeLa cells, a cell line not expressing any of the canonical forms of ER, were selected as the experimental model. This paper reports the activation of EndoR stress and Ca-dependent gene expression following the administration of T3, leading to apoptosis, independently of the presence of estrogen receptors.

Results

TRF and T3 induce apoptosis in HeLa cells

As mentioned in the "Background" section, the interrogation of transcriptomic data collected in our previous investigations [15, 16], further corroborated by recent indication that appeared in the literature [61], suggested the presence of a pro-apoptotic effect of T3, independent on ERβ signaling. Therefore, HeLa cells, void of these receptors, were utilized to verify the hypothesis of a pro-apoptotic effect of T3 in the absence of ER.

First of all, we assessed if T3 and TRF could induce cell death also in tumor cells not expressing ERs. Figure 1 shows that at 48 h from TRF and γ- and δ-T3 administration, cells display DNA laddering followed by cellular death by apoptosis (morphology not shown) in HeLa cells. Noteworthy, the apoptotic effect of T3 in HeLa cells was detectable 24 h later with respect to what we observed in our previous experiments in MCF-7 cells [15], this time shift suggesting the presence of a distinct pathway modulated by T3. The presence of α-TOC and α-T3 were not associated with any detectable DNA laddering.

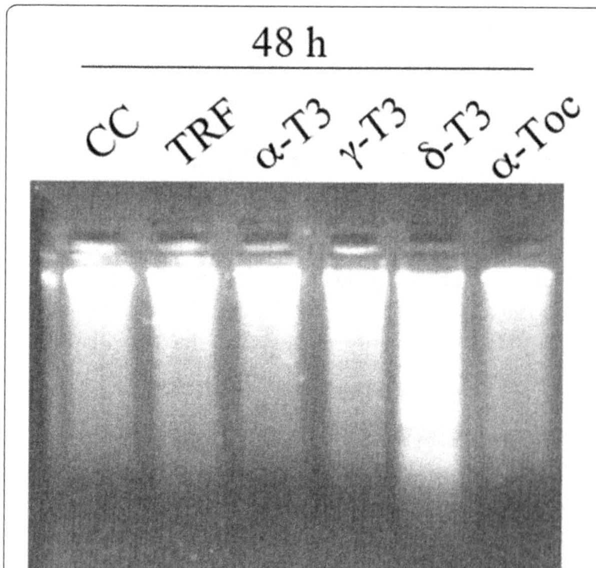

Fig. 1 T3-induced apoptosis in HeLa cells. TRF, γ-, and δ-T3 (10 μg/ml) induce apoptosis in HeLa cells as indicated by an evident DNA laddering at 48 h from treatment

Identification and characterization of alternative pathways affected by T3 in HeLa cells

On the basis of this initial observation, we characterized the changes of transcriptome expression of HeLa cells associated with 24 h of T3 treatment by a microarray approach.

The profiles of differentially expressed genes obtained by microarrays were further subjected to functional analysis with the aim of characterizing biological processes and cellular components annotated in GO and modulated by T3.

Finally, by clustering "semantic" similarities [4, 30] between enriched GO terms, we compared the transcriptomic phenotype observed in HeLa with that previously observed in our laboratories on MCF-7 cells treated with T3 [15].

Microarray analysis indicated that the treatment with 10 μg/ml γ-T3 and δ-T3 is associated with a higher number of modulated genes (177 genes and 147 genes, respectively) than that observed following α-T3 treatment (21 genes) (see Fig. 2 and Additional file 1: Table S1).

Out of 13 genes significantly modulated by all T3, 8 genes have been described to be specifically involved in sterol and steroid metabolism (DHCR24, FADS2, FDFT1, IDI1, INSIG1, LDLR, SCD, SREBF1) and 5 genes (KLF7, LPIN1, FADS2, MMAB and MYO6) have been reported to play a role in different aspects of cellular

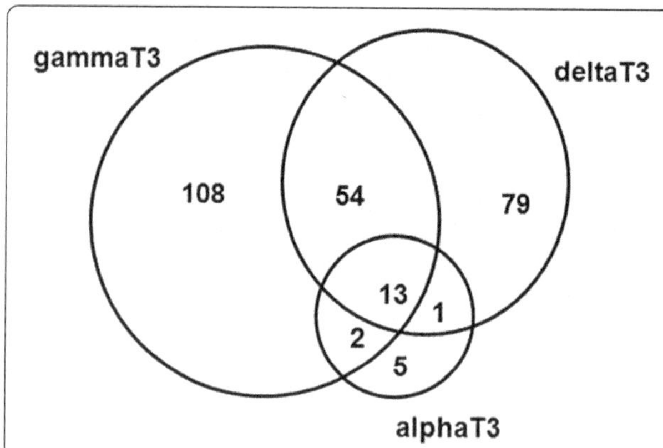

Fig. 2 Venn diagram reporting the number of differentially expressed genes observed after treatment of HeLa cells with T3. Differentially expressed genes were identified by LIMMA analysis according to a fold-change threshold (treatment vs control) of at least ±0.5 and a p value threshold above 0.05

metabolism. More specifically, KLF7 is involved into regulation of adiponectin expression in mouse embryonic fibroblast [12], LPIN1 and FADS2 are involved in the control of fatty acid metabolism at different levels [28, 58], and MYO6 mediates endocytosis within intracellular organelles [23].

In order to identify ERβ-independent pathways of apoptosis activation, we compared γ-T3-related changes in gene expression profiles, previously observed in MCF-7 with those obtained in HeLa. Figure 3 shows that the effect of T3 treatment only partially overlaps in the two cell lines. In fact, in both cell lines, we observed a significant modulation of isoprenoid metabolism and sterol and steroid biosynthetic processes. In HeLa cells, we also observed an enrichment of biological processes related to the regulation of the cell cycle, hexose, and carboxylic acid metabolism. Similarly, we observed an enrichment of the biological processes related to the regulation of apoptosis, cytokines biosynthesis, and glutathione metabolism associated with the profiles of genes differentially expressed in MCF-7. Several evidences indicated that these processes have a role in regulating a common phenotype related to cellular death [7, 13].

Conversely, the profile of differentially expressed genes in HeLa cells specifically involved processes related to tissue development and regulation of transcription, suggesting the activation of specific molecular mechanisms distinct from those activated in MCF-7.

A similar functional analysis was performed to identify cellular compartments annotated in GO and mainly enriched by the profiles resulting from gene modulation affected by T3 treatment.

In HeLa, the treatment with γ-T3 was mainly associated with the modulation of gene products located within intracellular organelles and in particular at the level of the EndoR. The same cellular compartment was identified as a target also in our previous experiments only focusing on MCF-7 cells (Additional file 2: Figure S1). However, in MCF-7, γ-T3 treatment mainly resulted in the modulation of profiles related to mitochondria and Golgi apparatus.

In both MCF-7 and HeLa cells, γ-T3 treatment induced a significant modulation of sterol and steroid biosynthetic processes and of processes related to isoprenoid metabolism.

In order to investigate the relationship between "death-committed" phenotype and the involvement of EndoR identified by the analysis of GO cellular compartment

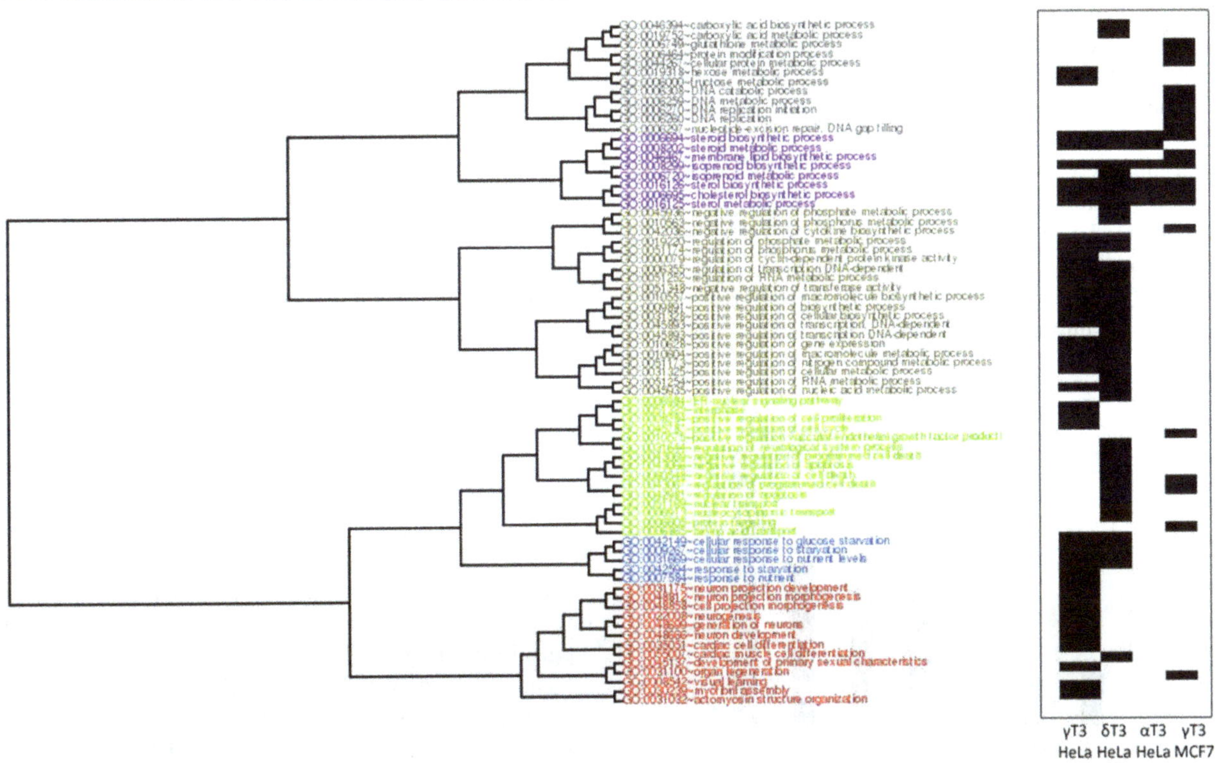

Fig. 3 Clustering analysis of biological processes modulated by T3 treatment. Biological processes enriched by differentially expressed genes in HeLa (24 h) and MCF-7 (24 h) cells treated with T3 are represented in the *plot with black blocks*. The matrix of semantic similarities between each pair of significantly enriched biological processes was estimated by Resnik measure. Hierarchical cluster analysis was performed on the obtained matrix. The optimal cluster division was estimated by the analysis of silhouette scores. Each cluster is represented by *different colors* in the dendrogram

enrichment, we performed a more specific analysis, to further characterize the gene expression profile induced by T3 treatments and specifically related to EndoR stress.

Utilizing a data-mining approach, we built a list of 568 genes, for which evidences exist in the literature that indicate an involvement in EndoR stress. This list was utilized to map the profiles of differentially expressed genes observed in HeLa experiments. This approach suggests that γ-T3 and δ-T3 have a stronger ability to modulate the expression of genes related to EndoR stress with respect to α-T3. Only three genes related to EndoR stress were downregulated by all T3 (SREBF1, SCD, LPIN1). Both γ-T3 and δ-T3 downregulated three genes (SREBF2, CDKN1A, ID2) and upregulated four genes (HSPA5, ASNS, PHLDA1, GDF15). γ-T3 specifically upregulated seven genes (CCND1, CHAC1, DNAJB9, FAS, GEM, GFPT1, XBP-1), whereas δ-T3 downregulated three genes (GSK3B, DNAJC10, JUN) and upregulated four genes (SDF2L1, BCR, TRIB3, FAM129A). Noteworthy, several genes belonging to this group are established markers of EndoR stress (ASNS, CDKN1A, FAS, XBP-1, SDF2L1, TRIB3, HSPA5) [2, 19, 24, 29, 36, 63].

T3-induced Ca^{2+} release in EndoR

T3-induced changes in gene expression profile that were obtained by microarray experiments, eventually confirmed by RT-PCR (data not shown), suggested the presence of EndoR stress upstream to the apoptosis induced by T3. We therefore tested the occurrence of one of the first, more evident signals associated with EndoR stress: the intracellular Ca^{2+} release from the endoplasmic reticulum.

Figure 4 shows that α-T3, γ-T3, and δ-T3, but not TRF, induced a marked and significant Ca^{2+} release from the endoplasmic reticulum to the cytoplasm, confirming the involvement of EndoR stress in T3-induced apoptosis. It is interesting to note that α-TOC had no significant effect on Ca^{2+} release, further indicating that the observed effects are definitively structure-specific.

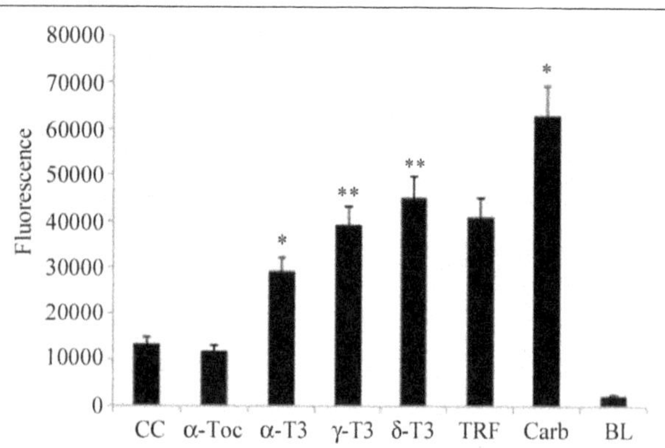

Fig. 4 T3-induced Ca^{2+} release in the cytosol. Quantitation of Ca^{2+} release by Fluo-4 NW Calcium Assay. HeLa cells were incubated in the presence of α-TOC, α-T3, γ-T3 or δ-T3, and TRF (10 μg/ml) for 15 min. As the positive control, cells were treated with 50 μM carbachol. *CC* indicates treatment with the vehicle only (DMSO)

Characterization of T3-induced EndoR stress

X-box binding protein-1 (XBP-1) and C/EBP homology protein (CHOP) are two of the major players involved in EndoR stress response. At 24 h from the administration of γ-T3 (20 μg/ml) and δ-T3 (10 μg/ml), we observed an increased expression of total XBP-1. Conversely, CHOP messenger RNA (mRNA) expression only increased in association with the treatment with the highest (20 μg/ml) concentration of γ-T3 (Fig. 5a, b). In agreement with the absence of effect on Ca^{2+} release, the treatment with α-TOC and TRF did not induce any significant changes of XBP-1 and CHOP expression (data not shown).

The proteolitic digestion with Pst1 restriction enzyme allows to discriminate between the unspliced and spliced forms of XBP-1. In fact, the splicing of this mRNA is associated with the loss of Pst1 "cutting" site within XBP-1-mRNA. Therefore, after Pst1 digestion, the unspliced form is visualized as two separate bands (at 291 and 307 kD), while the spliced form is visualized as one band only (at 572 kD), typical of EndoR stress. Figure 5c shows that TRF (10 and 20 μg/ml), γ-T3 (5, 10, and 20 μg/ml), and δ-T3 (5 μg/ml) induced the alternative splicing of XBP-1 (sXBP-1).

Also in this case, α-TOC had a different effect, only inducing the expression of the unspliced form, uXBP-1. Therefore, according to the notion that XBP-1 alternative splicing is mediated by inositol requiring enzyme-1α (IRE-1α), we hypothesized that γ- and δ-T3 treatment indirectly modulates IRE-1α activity.

The treatment with tocotrienols did not induce PERK phosphorylation and ATF-6 cleavage but only activate the IRE-1α pathway

At least three different molecular pathways have been reported to be affected by EndoR stress [5]. Therefore, together with the expression of IRE-1α, we investigated the expression of protein kinase RNA (PKR)-like ER kinase (PERK) and of the activating transcription factor-6 (ATF-6). To this aim, we selected the concentrations of α-, γ-, and δ-T3 that were associated with a more evident effect on gene expression. As positive control for EndoR stress induction, HeLa cells were treated with 5 μg/ml tunicamycin (TM).

Figure 6a (and Additional file 3: Figure S2) shows that any of T3 (10 μg/ml) induced either ATF-6 proteolytic cleavage or PERK phosphorylation at 24 h and at longer incubation times (not shown). To better characterize the effect of T3 on the IRE-1α phosphorylation, we performed a time-course observation in HeLa cells incubated with 10 μg/ml of α-, δ-, and γ-T3 and TRF at different time points (24, 26, 28, and 30 h). At 26 h incubation, only δ-T3

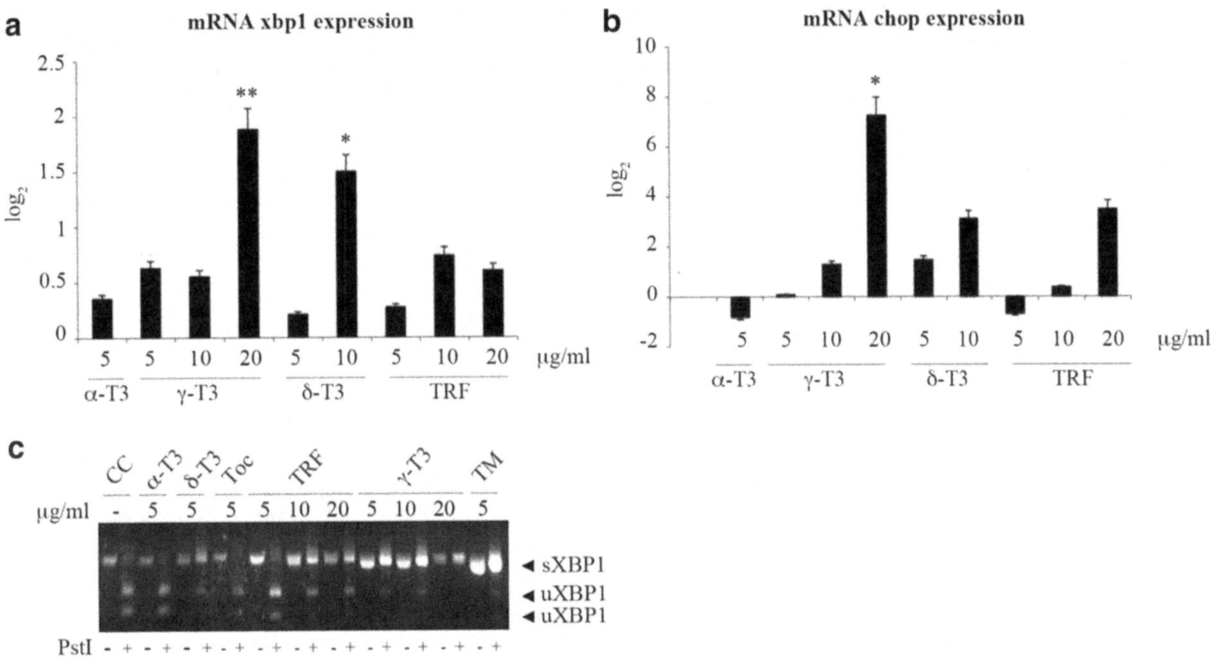

Fig. 5 γ-T3- and δ-T3-induced expression of EndoR stress genes after 24 h of treatment. **a** Effect of γ- and δ-T3 and α-T3 on XBP-1-mRNA expression. γ-T3 (20 µg/ml) and δ-T3 (10 µg/ml) induce significant mRNA expression of XBP-1. **b** Effect of γ- and δ-T3 and α-T3 on chop-mRNA expression. Only γ-T3 (20 µg/ml) induces significant mRNA expression of chop. **c** α-T3 (5 µg/ml), δ-T3 (5 µg/ml), TRF (5–20 µg/ml), and γ-T3 (5–20 µg/ml), but not α-TOC (5 µg/ml), induce the alternative splicing of XBP-1. Details about the Pst1 digestion are provided in the "Methods" section. Tunicamycin (TM) was used as a positive control of EndoR stress induction. *Asterisks* indicate significant differences (p value ≤0.05) between treated cells vs control (*CC*)

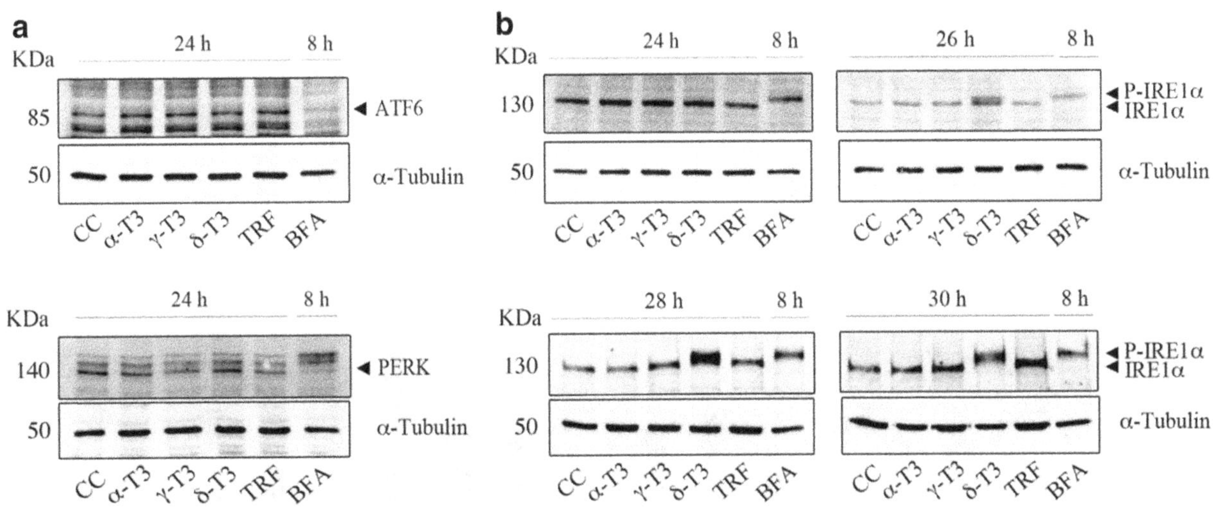

Fig. 6 Effects of TRF and purified T3 on PERK, ATF-6, and IRE-1α activity. T3 (10 µg/ml) affect the UPR intracellular pathway in HeLa cells. *CC* indicates the treatment with the vehicle only (DMSO). Brefeldin (*BFA*) (2.5 µg/ml) was used as a positive control of EndoR stress. α-Tubulin was used as the loading control. **a** T3 treatment has no effect on the expression of ATF-6 and PERK proteins at 24 h from the treatment. **b** IRE-1 protein expression and phosphorylation are significantly affected by T3 treatment. The figure shows one representative experiment out of at least three separate experiments. Densitometry and statistical analysis is showed as Additional file 3: Figure S2

treatment was associated with a shift of the electrophoretic mobility of IRE-1α (Fig. 6b and Additional file 3: Figure S2) in comparison to control (lane cc), indicating the occurrence of protein phosphorylation and, therefore, the activation of this pathway. In addition, longer exposures to δ-T3 (28 and 30 h) were associated with IRE-1α phosphorylation, indicating the presence of a long-term maintenance of protein activation only upon the treatment with δ-T3.

Effects of TRF and purified T3 on caspase activity

It is known that one of the outcomes of EndoR stress is the activation of apoptosis [11]. Twelve hours after the administration of γ-T3 or TRF (10 μg/ml), we detected a significant increase of caspase-12 and caspase-8 activity (Fig. 7b, d). Moreover, δ-T3 treatment (10 μg/ml) induced a modest but significant increase of caspase-12 activity. On the contrary, caspase-10 activity was insensitive to all the different treatments (Fig. 7c). Finally, we observed caspase-9 cleavage only in association with δ-T3 administration (Fig. 7a).

Effects of PBA on GRP78 protein expression and caspase-12 activity

Glucose-regulated protein 78 (GRP78) is a natural molecular chaperone. It is expressed as a response to EndoR stress, and it is involved in protein folding, proteasome degradation, EndoR Ca^{2+} binding, and also in the control and activation of transmembrane EndoR stress sensors. GRP78 is therefore one of the major upstream regulators of ER protein folding, directly involved in the activation of ATF-6, IRE-1, and PERK.

In order to assess the real involvement of EndoR stress in the apoptosis induced by T3, we measured the GRP78 protein level in the presence of a chemical chaperone, sodium 4-phenylbutyrate (4-PBA), that stabilizes protein structure improving cellular folding capacity, therefore reducing EndoR stress.

Firstly, we performed a dose-response curve to evaluate the appropriate 4-PBA concentration. HeLa cells were incubated with different concentrations of 4-PBA (5, 8, 10 mM) with or without TM for 4 h. Then, we utilized the lowest 4-PBA concentration (5 mM) not associated with toxic effect on HeLa proliferation (data not shown).

HeLa cells were treated with T3 and TRF (10 μg/ml) and co-incubated with or without 4-PBA (5 mM) for 24 h. Figure 8a shows that the treatment with δ- and γ-T3, and TRF is associated with an increase of GRP78 protein level. δ-T3 had a more remarkable effect in comparison with other T3 forms and TRF. 4-PBA significantly reduced GRP78 increase induced by δ-T3 and TRF treatment.

Finally, we assessed the effect of T3 on caspase-12 activity, which is the final effector of EndoR stress-induced apoptosis. Figure 8b shows that, after 24 h, co-incubation with 4-PBA significantly reduced the activity of caspase-12 with respect to γ- and δ-T3 treatment.

XBP-1 activation in MCF-7 breast cancer cells not expressing ERβ

To further confirm that T3-induced XBP-1 alternative splicing was independent of the presence of ERβ, we

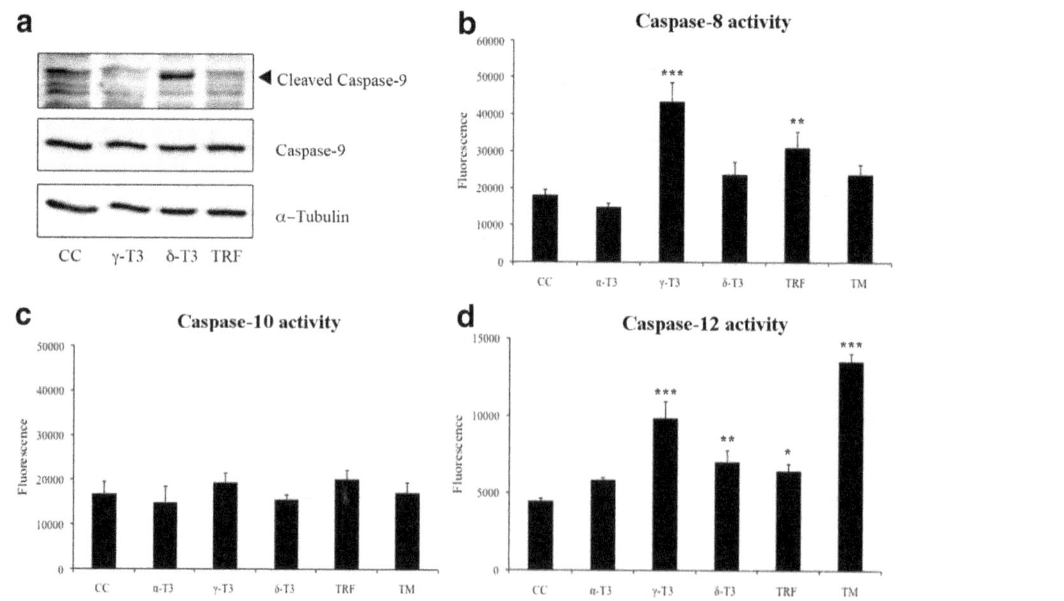

Fig. 7 Effect of T3 on caspase activity. T3 modulate caspase-9 protein levels (**a**) and caspase-8, caspase-10, and caspase-12 activity (**b**, **c**, and **d**, respectively) in HeLa cells. Cells were treated with α-T3, γ-T3, δ-T3, or TRF (10 μg/ml) for 12 h or TM (5 μg/ml) for 4 h; *CC* indicates treatment with the vehicle only (DMSO). The *panels* show one representative experiment out of at least three separate experiments. The *asterisks* indicate significant differences (p value ≤0.05) between treated cells vs control (*CC*)

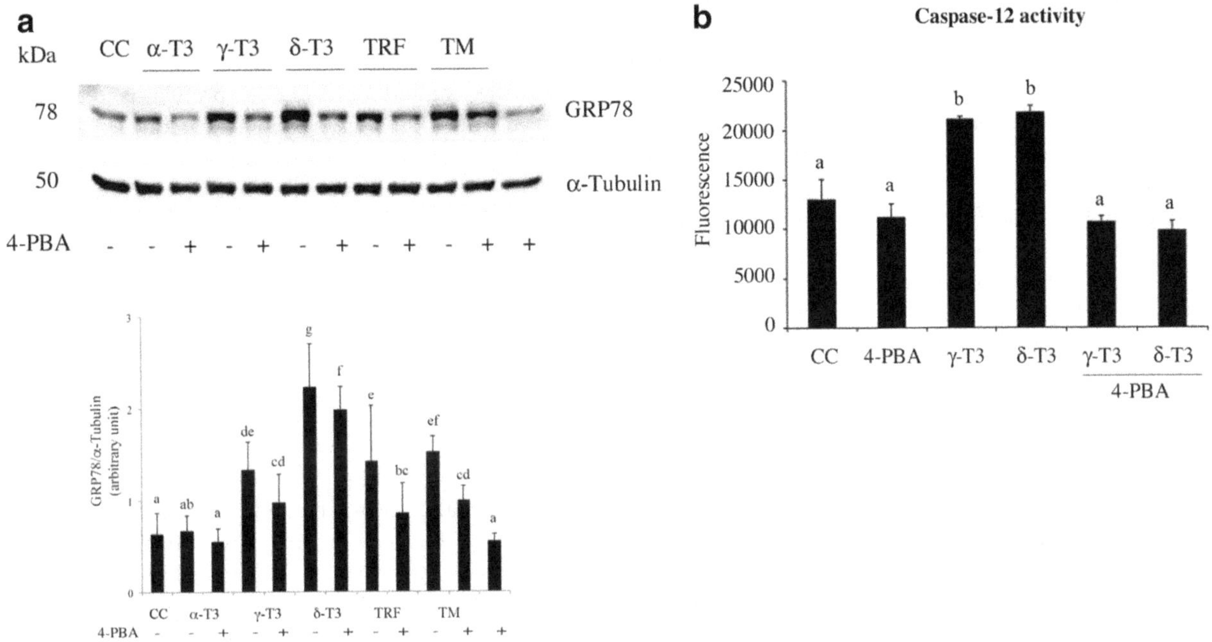

Fig. 8 Effects of PBA ER stress inhibitor on GRP78 protein levels and caspase-12 activity. T3 modulates the expression level of EndoR molecular chaperone GRP78. HeLa cells were treated with α-T3, γ-T3, δ-T3, or TRF (10 μg/ml) for 24 h. *CC* indicates the treatment with the vehicle only (DMSO). Tunicamycin (*TM*) (5 μg/ml, for 4 h) was used as a positive control of EndoR stress induction. 4-PBA was used as the specific inhibitor of EndoR stress. α-Tubulin was utilized as a loading control. **a** GRP78 protein levels are affected by T3 treatment, and the co-treatment with 4-PBA (5 mM) prevents the changes induced by T3. The figures show one representative experiment out of at least three separate experiments. Data obtained by densitometry were log_2 transformed in order to obtain data symmetrically distributed and were analyzed by one-way ANOVA with repeated measures followed by Fisher's test. *p* values ≤0.05 were considered to be statistically significant. *Different letters* indicate significant differences between groups ($p < 0.05$). **b** co-treatment with 4-PBA after 24 h significantly inhibits γ-T3- and δ-T3-induced increase of caspase-12 activity. Data were analyzed by one-way ANOVA with repeated measures followed by Fisher's test. *p* values ≤0.05 were considered to be statistically significant. *Different letters* indicate significant differences between groups ($p < 0.05$)

repeated the experiment on a specific clone of MCF-7 breast cancer cells not expressing ERβ [8].

Similar to HeLa, the administration of γ-T3 (20 μg/ml) and δ-T3 (10 μg/ml) to a clone of MCF-7 cells not expressing ERβ induced the alternative splicing of XBP-1 (sXBP-1). Also in this case, α-T3 induced only the expression of the unspliced form, uXBP-1.

Discussion

Several studies have shown that T3 inhibit cell proliferation and induce apoptosis in human and murine breast cancer cells [22, 34, 43, 55] and in many other types of tumor cells [17, 52, 59]. More recently, the beneficial effects of T3 on different human disorders have been evaluated in clinical trials [1, 33, 42, 45]. Within this context, few studies have definitively addressed the molecular mechanisms underlying T3 activity. We have previously demonstrated a novel molecular mechanism involving the interaction of γ- and δ-T3 with estrogen receptor-β [15, 16]. In these studies, we reported that the activated complex ERβ/T3 translocates into the nucleus to modulate the expression of specific genes related to the apoptotic response and containing ERE in their promoters. However, as mentioned above, the antiproliferative activity of T3 has also been observed in several other cell types, including melanoma, prostate cancer and lung and liver carcinoma, and in particular in HeLa [61], a cell type known to be void of any form of canonical ERs. Therefore, we considered the possibility of an alternative pathway for the modulation of apoptotic response, independent of ER activity.

We conducted a set of preliminary experiments, showing that T3 modulate the expression of a pro-apoptotic gene, containing ERE sequences, also in HeLa cells, where this expression is obviously not driven by the activation of ERs. In particular, we observed a significant increase of MIC-1 and cathepsin D expression in response to the administration of γ- and δ-T3 (data not shown). Starting from this background, we planned and carried out a first "problem-driven" protocol, utilizing a transcriptomic approach to identify the profile of differential gene expression associated with T3 treatment in HeLa cells. A "data-mining process" identified a significant modulation of several genes involved in EndoR stress following the treatment with γ- and δ-T3. According to the similarity between the biological processes enriched in HeLa and MCF-7 following the administration of T3, we focused our attention on their role in activating EndoR stress, a pathway identified in both MCF-7 and HeLa (see Fig. 3).

A wide spectrum of genes related to EndoR was significantly affected by T3. Among them, we observed a downregulation of SCD expression that has been reported to be associated with an increase of EndoR stress in response to palmitate and to apoptosis in pancreatic β-cells [21]. Similarly, we observed a downregulation of the LPIN gene, already reported to be induced by EndoR stress ([37]) and a downregulation of SREBF1 and SREBF2 by γ-T3 and δ-T3. The expression of these genes, in particular SREBF2, is activated within the unfolded protein response (UPR) pathway to cope with EndoR stress [14]. We could therefore conclude that both γ-T3 and δ-T3 affect the ability of UPR to react to stress stimuli. The molecular specificity of this effect is quite high, as several transcription factors related to EndoR stress are modulated by γ- and δ-T3, but not by α-T3. Interestingly, after δ-T3 and γ-T3 treatment, we also observed the upregulation of HSPA5 (or GRP78), a molecular chaperone that promotes protein folding and inhibits protein aggregation in the EndoR [35].

On the basis of the results obtained by microarray, we concluded that specific T3 forms induce apoptosis in HeLa cells via EndoR stress. The precise reason why specific isomers are more effective than others and the molecular mechanisms underlying these distinct effects are still scarcely understood.

EndoR stress has already been identified as one of the major pathways involved in the initiation of apoptosis, and it is known that EndoR stress-induced apoptosis is strictly associated with Ca^{2+} release in cytoplasm [50]. In fact, EndoR acts as an intracellular store and retains Ca^{2+} at a concentration thousands of times higher than those present in the cytosol. Ca^{2+} disposal is modulated by EndoR-located Ca^{2+} channels that, in the presence of EndoR stress, release Ca^{2+} from the lumen to activate specific Ca^{2+}-depending signals and, eventually, apoptosis [49]. In the present study, we observed Ca^{2+} release to the cytoplasm of HeLa cells immediately (15 min) after T3 treatment (Fig. 4). This observation led our focus on the three major molecular pathways that characterize EndoR stress.

As mentioned, at least three different transmembrane proteins are involved in EndoR stress, namely the following: PERK, ATF-6, and IRE-1 [49]. These proteins remain inactive and bound to glucose-regulated proteins (GRPs) and, in particular, to GRP78 also known as "immunoglobulin heavy chain-binding protein" (BiP) or HSPA5, a chaperone member of the heat-shock protein-70 (HSP70) family that plays an important role in regulating the UPR pathway. Under condition of EndoR homeostasis, GRP78 remains in its inactive form and constitutively binds to three UPR transmembrane sensors, ATF-6, PERK, and IRE-1 [51]. Following EndoR stress, the complex BiP/EndoR protein is dissociated, released from UPR sensors and activated [11].

As shown in Fig. 6, treatment with T3 (γ-T3, δ-T3, and TRF) did not induce a differential expression of proteins PERK and ATF-6, while the expression of IRE-1α phosphorylation was significantly modulated. In fact, at 24 h from T3 treatment, IRE-1α phosphorylation was faintly detectable, while the splicing of XBP-1 pre-mRNA, a downstream step to IRE-1 activity, was evident and detectable (Fig. 5c) both at shorter and longer exposure times (12 and 48 h, data not shown). We confirmed that the pathway leading to the expression of a spliced form of XBP-1, induced by γ- and δ-T3, is not cell-specific and ERβ-dependent by utilizing a specific clone of MCF-7 that has been reported to be void of ERβ [8]. Similarly, to HeLa cells, the administration of γ- and δ-T3, but not α-T3, to this cell line was associated with the expression of a truncated form of XBP-1 (see Fig. 9). The apparent discrepancy between IRE-1α phosphorylation and XBP-1 splicing at 24 h from T3 treatment could be explained by the lesser sensitivity of western blot methodology in comparison with PCR assay.

We observed an evident variability of IRE-1 phosphorylation suggesting that, in our experimental conditions, this protein is likely to oscillate between two different states, either "active" or "refractive" while maintaining its endoribonuclease activity. This interpretation is supported by a study published by Li and coworkers [31]

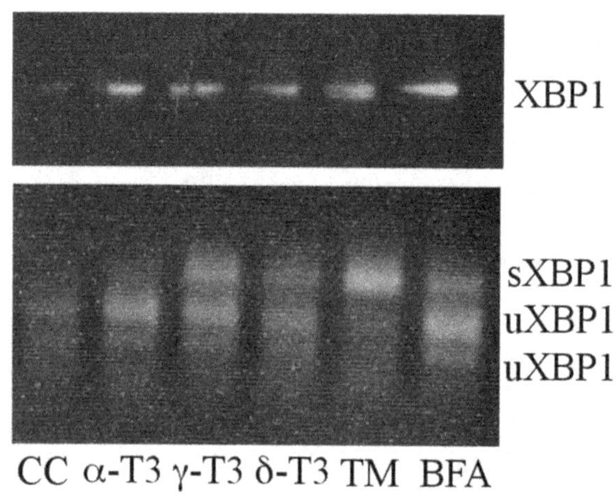

Fig. 9 XBP-1 activation in a ERβ silenced clone of breast cancer cells (MCF-7). A specific clone of MCF-7 cells, not expressing ERβ, was incubated with δ-T3 (20 μg/ml), γ-T3 (10 μg/ml), α-TOC, and α-T3 (20 μg/ml). Details about Pst1 digestion are provided in the "Methods" section. *CC* indicates treatment with the vehicle only (DMSO). Brefeldin (*BFA*) was used as a positive control of EndoR stress induction. The figure shows one representative experiment out of at least three separate experiments

that described a *three-state* model for the activation of mammalian IRE-1α: (i) an inactive state that can be "switched on" by EndoR stress; (ii) an active state characterized by IRE-1α oligomerization and XBP-1 splicing; and (iii) a refractive state in which IRE-1α enters after a prolonged activation, no longer responding to an "unresolved" EndoR stress. The same authors reported that different IRE-1α forms are not necessarily recognized by the anti-p-IRE-α antibody and suggested that de-phosphorylation has an important role for the entering into the refractive state. Other authors [25] demonstrated that, upon persistent EndoR stress (e.g., inositol depletion), IRE-1 is weakly but continuously activated in a non-clustered form through its association with BiP. The same study reports that the weak activity of IRE-1α might act as an indispensable "fine tuning" for cell adaption to chronic EndoR stress conditions. When homeostasis is not recovered, UPR signaling induces cell death by apoptosis.

Besides affecting IRE-1, we observed that treatment with T3 is associated with a significant modulation of XBP-1 and CHOP mRNA expression, starting at 24 h from administration (Fig. 5a, b).

Overall, our data indicate that specific forms of T3 are able to induce EndoR stress in HeLa cells through the activation of IRE-1α (fluctuating between active/refractive forms), which in turn mediates the alternative splicing of XBP-1 mRNA, and modulates CHOP transcription. A prolonged EndoR stress leads to an increase of CHOP expression that switches EndoR stress signaling from "pro-survival" to "pro-apoptosis" [56, 62]. We confirmed our hypothesis utilizing the EndoR stress inhibitor, 4-PBA. In fact, co-treatment with 4-PBA significantly reduced both GRP78 protein levels and caspase activity induced by γ- and δ-T3.

Finally, if cells undergoing EndoR stress do not succeed in restoring cellular homeostasis and degrade protein aggregates, UPR leads to cell cycle arrest and, subsequently, to apoptosis [48]. In other words, in our experimental conditions, T3 treatment "forced" HeLa cells toward apoptosis.

Accordingly, we have shown that specific forms of T3 activate caspase-12 and caspase-8 expression (see Fig. 7). Although T3 treatment has already been reported to activate EndoR stress [44, 60], no studies had previously addressed the role of these molecules in inducing EndoR-mediated apoptosis in a model different from breast cancer. It is interesting to note that caspase-12, an EndoR resident caspase, is specifically cleaved and activated during EndoR stress, but not following the activation of death receptors and other mitochondria-related apoptotic signals. Ca^{2+} efflux from EndoR during stress activates calpain that, in turn, activates EndoR-caspase-12 [39]. Once activated, caspase-12 can trigger the maturation cascade finally leading to the activation of caspase-3 to complete the apoptotic program [38]. In HeLa cells, we observed the activation of caspase-12 both following γ- and δ-T3 treatment, but only the latter was associated with caspase-9 cleavage (Fig. 7). Even though we could not observe any direct evidence of IRE-1α phosphorylation associated with γ-T3 treatment, the presence of evident downstream consequences to its activation lets us hypothesize that, at least in HeLa cells, also γ-T3 is involved in the UPR pathway.

In our study, we also observed a significant activation of caspase-8, even though this protease is known to play a role in death receptor-mediated apoptosis [47]. Therefore, we cannot exclude a possible involvement of a death receptor-related pathway within the spectrum of T3 activities.

Our data provide ground to speculate about the presence of a putative (orphan) receptor, possibly located at the level of the cellular membrane able to bind T3 and other estrogen mimetics such as ICI-182,730. This mechanism could be active in several cell types, independently of the presence of functional ERs. In fact, previous (unpublished) observations from our group have unexpectedly indicated that, also in HeLa, the treatment with the specific ER inhibitor ICI-182,780 weakens the effects of T3 on MIC-1 gene expression (Additional file 4: Figure S3). This evidence allows us to speculate that a hypothetical "specific" (orphan) receptor characterized by a pocket able to also bind ICI-182,780 (see Fig. 10) exists, also able to bind γ- and δ-T3. According to the chemo-physical characteristics of T3, the candidate downstream target(s) of the activity of this receptor could reasonably be located at the level of EndoR. The activation of this hypothetical (orphan) receptor would sequentially trigger EndoR stress, IRE-1 activation, and XBP-1 splicing. Once synthesized, sXBP-1 would modulate the expression of a specific set of genes, inducing apoptosis.

Conclusions

Our study demonstrates that γ- and δ-T3 activate a series of specific cellular responses leading to apoptosis also in cells lacking of ERβ. We have identified and characterized an EndoR stress-dependent pathway activated by γ- and δ-T3 that is likely to cooperate with ERβ (when present)-dependent signaling in triggering apoptosis in several tumor cell types. Further future studies must address the molecular mechanism by which γ- and δ-T3 induce EndoR stress.

Methods

Chemicals

TRF was obtained from Golden Hope Plantation (Malaysia) and purified as previously described [53]. T3 and α-TOC constituted more than 95% of the final TRF

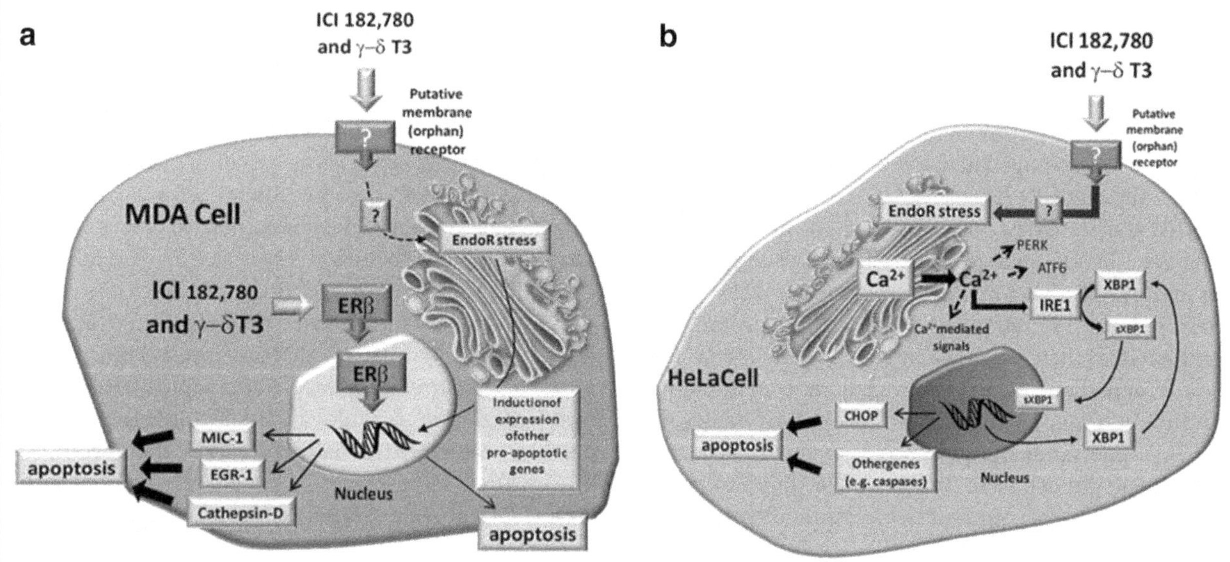

Fig. 10 **a** In tumor cells expressing ERβ (MDA-MB-231, MCF-7), γ- and δ-T3 bind to and activate the ERβ receptor, inducing the expression of pro-apoptotic genes such as MIC-1, EGR-1, and cathepsin-D, finally triggering apoptosis. More details about this mechanism are described in (6). Also in these cell types, a contribution by pro-apoptotic signals originating from EndoR is not to be excluded. **b** In tumor cells not expressing any of the canonical forms of ERs (ERα and ERβ), γ- and δ-T3 induce EndoR stress activating Ca^{2+} release in the cytoplasm. Overall, the treatment with specific forms of T3, but not α-TOC, is associated with specific Ca-dependent signals involved in the unfolded protein response (UPR), the core pathway to cope with EndoR stress in eukaryotic cells. In particular, Ca^{2+} release is followed by the activation of IRE-1, which in turn activates XBP-1 splicing, the binding of this latter to DNA, and the subsequent induction of the expression of pro-apoptotic genes. The expression of other genes associated with EndoR stress (PERK and ATF-6) is not significantly affected by T3. Our data also provide ground to speculate about the presence of a putative (orphan) receptor, possibly located at the level of the cellular membrane able to bind T3 and other estrogen mimetics such as ICI-182,730. This mechanism could be active in several cell types, independently of the presence of functional ERs

composition, the remaining being minor components (carotenoids, flavonoids). TRF typically contained 32% α-TOC, 25% α-T3, 29% γ-T3, and 14% δ-T3.

Purified T3 were provided by Dr. Hiroyuki Yoshimura at Eisai Food and Chemical Co., Ltd (Tokyo, Japan). Purity was ~99% for all T3. Pure α-TOC (≥95.5%) was purchased by Sigma-Aldrich (St. Louis, MO, USA). The real concentration of T3 and α-TOC solutions was determined spectrophotometrically from the specific extinction coefficients (ε_{292} α-TOC = 75.8; $\varepsilon_{292.5}$ α-T3 = 91; ε_{296} γ-T3 = 90.5; ε_{297} δ-T3 = 89.1) before each experiment. Stock solutions of TRF and T3 were stored at–20 °C in aliquots and diluted to the desired concentration in dimethyl sulfoxide (DMSO).

Cells lines and treatments

HeLa cells were obtained from the American Tissue Culture Collection (Manassas, VA, USA). A clone of MCF-7 breast cancer cells, not expressing ER-β [8], was a gift of Prof M. Marino.

Cells were grown in DMEM medium (Euroclone, Pero, Milan, Italy) supplemented with 10% fetal bovine serum (FBS, Sigma-Aldrich), 100 U/ml penicillin and 100 μg/ml streptomycin (Pen/Strep, Euroclone), 2 mM glutamine (Euroclone), and 1% non-essential amino acid (Sigma Aldrich). Cells were maintained at 37 °C in a humidified atmosphere of 5% CO_2/95% air.

Before any experimental session, cells were synchronized in G_1/G_0 by starvation in serum-free medium for 2 days. Once synchronized, 300.000 cells were seeded onto multi-well plates. TRF, purified T3, or α-TOC were dissolved in DMSO and individually added to the culture medium. When not differently indicated in the text, incubation time was 24 or 48 h. The final TRF concentration in culture media was 10 μg/ml. Purified α-TOC and T3 were added to the medium at the following concentrations: α-TOC was 5 μg/ml; α-T3 was 5 μg/ml; γ-T3 was 5, 10, and 20 μg/ml; and δ-T3 was 5 and 10 μg/ml. These concentrations have been selected in order to facilitate the comparison with previous published studies by our group or by others. Control cells were treated with an equal volume of DMSO alone.

Tunicamycin (TM) and brefeldin A (BFA) were utilized as inducers of EndoR stress response. Preliminary investigations indicated that they have identical effects on our cellular model. Treatments with 2.5 μg/ml BFA for 8 h or 5 μg/ml TM for 4 h were therefore utilized as a positive control for EndoR stress. Different concentrations (5, 8, and 10 mM) of sodium 4-phenylbutyrate (4-PBA, Calbiochem, USA), a specific inhibitor of EndoR stress, were administered to HeLa along with T3 or TRF.

DNA laddering

DNA extraction was performed according to Gooch and Yee [20], and with minor modifications previously described [15], extracted DNA was electrophoresed in 1.5% agarose gels containing ethidium bromide (EtBr) and visualized by UVIpro Bronze acquisition system (UVITEC, Cambridge, UK).

Calcium release assessment and free calcium assay

Free Ca^{2+} concentration was determined by the Fluo-4 NW Calcium Assay Kit (Invitrogen) according to the manufacturer's instructions. HeLa cells were incubated in the presence of TRF, α-TOC, α-T3, γ-T3, or δ-T3 (10 μg/ml), and at the end of the incubation time, fluorescence was measured (494-nm excitation/516-nm emission) by a Tecan fluorometer (TECAN Infinite® 200 PRO).

cDNA hybridization and microarray data analysis

Two micrograms of high-quality total RNA were sent to ServiceXS BV (Leiden, The Netherlands) and processed according to the Affymetrix protocol (Affymetrix Eukaryotic One-Cycle Target Labeling and Control reagents) to generate biotin-labeled antisense cRNA (Complementary RNA). Labeled cRNA was hybridized to the NuGO Affymetrix Human Genechip NuGO_Hs1a520180 (custom designed by the European Nutrigenomics Organization NuGO, consisting of 23,941 probe sets including 71 control probe sets).

Cell intensity files (*.cel) for each GeneChip processed were generated using Command Console Software.

Three biological replicates were generated for each experimental condition. Microarray statistical analysis was performed using oneChannelGUI R package.

Raw signal intensities were normalized using GCRMA method as background correction, and differentially expressed genes were identified with LIMMA analysis selecting only the genes with a fold change (T3 treatment vs control) of at least 0.5 and a p value threshold above 0.05. The analysis of differential expression by the LIMMA method is based on an empirical Bayesian approach and has been reported to be reliable also in the case of small and unequal sample sizes (ref: PMID:16646809).

Specific up- and downregulated genes from microarray analysis were selected for a technical validation by RT-qPCR technique.

Pathway and network analysis

The set of modulated genes identified by microarrays was submitted for the analysis of enrichment of gene ontology (GO) biological processes and cellular components (level 5) utilizing the DAVID web server [18]. Significant enriched GO biological processes were identified according to a p value <0.05.

Overrepresented biological processes and cellular components modulated by γ-T3 in HeLa and MCF-7 were compared utilizing the GOSim package on the basis of the Resnik method to assess their semantic similarities. The obtained matrix of similarity distances was clustered by the Ward method, and the optimal number of clusters used to identify the groups of similar GO terms was assessed choosing the number of clusters that produces the best silhouette score. Similar analysis was performed to compare overrepresented terms according to the treatment with different T3 in HeLa cells.

A specific list of genes related to EndoR stress was built by merging the annotation obtained from the UniProt database and PubMed. The search on PubMed was performed by the Agilent literature search of Cytoscape software [32], searching about 1000 papers having "endoplasmic reticulum stress" and "Homo sapiens" within the keywords.

RNA isolation and real-time PCR measurements

Total RNA and real-time PCR analysis have been performed as previously described in the detail [15]. Primers used in real-time PCR measurements (see Table 1) have been designed according to the available literature of by a specific software (Primer Express™). Quantitative differences in cDNA target among samples were measured according to the mathematical model of Pfaffl [46]. The expression ratio was determined for each sample by calculating $(E_{sample})^{\Delta Ct(sample)}/(E_{control})^{\Delta Ct(control)}$, where E is the efficiency of the primer set and $\Delta Ct = Ct_{(control)} - Ct_{(sample)}$. Different normalization options, based on a set of different "housekeeping" genes, have been tested (data not shown) and provided no significant differences at the level of differential gene expression detection. β-actin was therefore selected to normalize expression data. Finally, results have been $\log_2$ transformed in order to obtain symmetrically distributed data. The amplification efficiency of each primer set was calculated from the slope of a standard amplification curve of log μl cDNA/reaction vs Ct value over at least 4 orders of magnitude ($E = 10^{-(1/slope)}$); β-actin primers, $E = 2.15$; MIC primers, $E = 2.03$; cathepsin D primers, $E = 2.55$; CHOP primers, $E = 1.94$; XBP-1 primers, $E = 2.19$.

RT-PCR analysis of XBP-1 splicing

cDNA was synthesized from total RNA using One-Step RT-PCR SuperScript III reverse transcriptase (Invitrogen) according to manufacturer's protocol. The primers used for PCR (see Table 1) were specific for human sXBP-1 (hsXBP-1). The PCR conditions were as follows: 95 °C for 5 min, 95 °C for 1 min, 58 °C for 30 s, 72 °C for 30 s, and 72 °C for 5 min, with 35 cycles of amplification. A 289-bp

Table 1 List of genes considered on the basis of data interrogation and primers utilized in RT-PCR and PCR assay

Gene	GenBank	Primers 5′→3′	Size template
β-actin (RT-PCR)	NM_001101.3	F: AGAAGGATTCCTATGTGGGGG	101 bp
		R: CATGTCGTCCCAGTTGGTGAC	
MIC-1 (RT-PCR)	NM_004864	F: TGGTGCTCATTCAAAAGACCG	123 bp
		R: GTGGAAGGACCAGGACTGCTC	
Cathepsin D (RT-PCR)	NM_001909	F: CTGTGAGGCCATTGTGGACAC	140 bp
		R: CAGCTTGTAGCCTTTGCCTCC	
XBP-1 (RT-PCR)	NM_005080.3	F: GGAGTTAAGACAGCGCTTGGGGA	118 bp
		R: TGTTCTGGAGGGGTGACAACTGGG	
CHOP (RT-PCR)	NM_001195057.1	F: CCACACCTGAAAGCAGACTGATCCA	102 bp
		R: TCATACCAGGCTTCCAGCTCCCA	
hXBP-1 (PCR)	NM_001079539.1	F: AAACAGAGCAGCAGTCCAGACTGC	472(u)bp 448(s)bp
		R: TCCTTCTGGGTAGACCTCTGGGAG	

amplicon was generated from unspliced XBP-1 (uXBP-1) and a 263-bp amplicon from spliced XBP-1 (sXBP-1). PCR amplicons were digested by Pstl. The Pstl cleavage site is located in the 26-nt intron of uXBP-1, which allows differentiation between the uXBP-1 amplicon (cut PCR product) and sXBP-1. Digested and not-digested PCR products were resolved on 2% agarose gels, stained with EtBr. The PCR fragments were visualized with UVIpro Bronze Imaging System (UVitec, Cambridge, UK).

Protein extraction and western blot

Total protein were extracted as described according to standardized protocols. The antibody considered were the following: XBP-1 (1:5000, anti-mouse, Santa Cruz Biotechnology), PERK (1:1000, anti-rabbit, Cell Signaling Technology), IRE-1α and phospho-IRE-1α (1:1000, anti-rabbit, Cell Signaling Technology), ATF-6 (1:1000, anti-rabbit, Abcam), caspase-9 and cleaved caspase-9 (1:1000, anti-rabbit, Cell Signaling Technology), α-tubulin (1:10,000, anti-mouse, MP Biomedicals), and GRP78 (1:1000, anti-rabbit, Cell Signaling Technology).

In order to detect IRE-1α and phospho-IRE-1α (p-IRE-1α) protein levels, we carried out a cytosolic and nuclear protein extraction as described by Canali et al. [10]. Protein concentration was determined using a commercial assay kit (Bio-Rad Laboratories, Hercules, CA, USA). Protein samples (30 μg per lane) were loaded onto a SDS polyacrylamide gel, and then, proteins were transferred to a polyvinylidene difluoride (PVDF) membrane (Millipore Corp., Bedford, MA, USA). The PVDF membrane was incubated overnight at 4 °C with an appropriate concentration of specific primary antibody. After washing and incubation with 1:2000 goat anti-mouse or goat anti-rabbit peroxidase-conjugated secondary antibodies (Santa Cruz Biotechnology), specific bands were detected by chemiluminescence reagent ECL Plus (Amersham Pharmacia Biotech, Piscataway, NJ) and visualized by Image Quant LAS 4000 (GE Healthcare Life Sciences).

The band analysis tools of ImageQuant TL software (GE Healthcare Life Sciences) were used to select and determine the background-subtracted density of the bands in all the western blot gels.

Caspase assay

The activity of caspase-8, caspase-10, and caspase-12 was assessed by means of a Biovision kit (Biovision, Lyon, France) according to the manufacturer's instructions. The assay is based on the detection of cleavage of substrate IETD-AFC (AFC: 7-amino-4-trifluoromethyl coumarin) that emits blue light (λmax = 400 nm), upon cleavage of the substrate by FLICE or related caspases, which can be quantified using a fluorometer or a fluorecence microtiter plate reader. Samples were transferred into a 96-well plate, and the fluorescence assessed using a Tecan fluorometer (TECAN Infinite® 200 PRO).

Statistical analysis and data presentation

Statistical analysis was performed with R software from the R Foundation for Statistical Computing (Vienna, Austria). Data were analyzed by one-way ANOVA with repeated measures followed by Tukey's test or Fisher's test. p values ≤0.05 were considered to be statistically significant.

Data obtained by transcriptomic platform have been handled according to the MIAME guidelines (see http://www.ncbi.nlm.nih.gov/geo/info/MIAME.html). Raw data have been deposited into the Gene Expression Omnibus (GEO: http://www.ncbi.nlm.nih.gov/geo/query/acc.cgi?acc=GSE48668) publicly accessible database.

Data obtained by real-time PCR have been handled according to the MIQE guidelines [9].

Figures show one out of at least three independent experiments providing similar results. Histograms present the mean (±S.E.) of at least three experiments.

Additional files

Additional file 1: Table S1. List of genes modulated by T3 according to microarray analysis. Expression levels are represented as log_2 fold changes. The last column on the right indicates if the gene has been reported to be involved in EndoR stress.

Additional file 2: Figure S1. Clusterization of CC enriched after T3 treatment in HeLa and MCF-7 cells. The distances between enriched CC were estimated according to the *Resnik measure*. The optimal number of clusters was estimated by silhouette scores and represented with different colors within the dendrogram. The box on the right side of the figure shows CCs enriched by a specific treatment.

Additional file 3: Figure S2. Densitometric analysis of ATF-6, PERK, and IRE-1α activity. Treatments with T3 have no significant effect on the protein expression of ATF-6 and PERK at 24 h from the treatment. Conversely, IRE-1 phosphorylation is significantly affected by T3 treatment. Data were analyzed by one-way ANOVA with repeated measures followed by Fisher's test. Asterisks indicate significant differences (p value ≤0.05) between treated cells vs control (CC).

Additional file 4: Figure S3. Modulation of MIC-1 mRNA expression. MIC-1 mRNA upregulation induced by T3 was partially prevented by pre-treatment with ICI-182,780. Once synchronized, 300.000 cells were seeded onto multi-well plates and pre-incubated with ICI-182.780 (10^{-5} M) for 30 min. TRF, purified T3 or α-TOC were added to the culture medium for 24 h. Gene expression was analyzed by real-time quantitative PCR, and results were log transformed (logarithm 2) in order to obtain data symmetrically distributed [46]. Statistical significance was calculated by one-way ANOVA with repeated measures followed by Tukey's test using ΔCt value. Asterisks (*) indicate significant differences (p value ≤0.05) with respect to control. Data represent the pooled values of at least three independent experiments.

Abbreviations

ASNS: Asparagine synthetase (glutamine-hydrolyzing); BCR: Breakpoint cluster region; CCND1: Cyclin D1; CDKN1A: Cyclin-dependent kinase inhibitor 1A; CHAC1: ChaC, cation transport regulator homolog 1; DHCR24: 24-dehydrocholesterol reductase; DNAJB9: DnaJ (Hsp40) homolog, subfamily B, member 9; DNAJC10: DnaJ (Hsp40) homolog, subfamily C, member 10; FADS2: Fatty acid desaturase 2; FAM129A: Family with sequence similarity 129, member A; FAS: Fas (TNF receptor superfamily member 6); FDFT1: Farnesyl-diphosphate farnesyltransferase 1; GDF15: Growth differentiation factor 15; GEM: GTP binding protein overexpressed in skeletal muscle; GFPT1: Glutamine-fructose-6-phosphate transaminase 1; GSK3B: Glycogen synthase kinase 3 beta; HSPA5: Heat-shock 70 kDa protein 5; ID2: Inhibitor of DNA binding 2; IDI1: Isopentenyl-diphosphate delta isomerase 1; INSIG1: Insulin-induced gene 1; JUN: Jun proto-oncogene; KLF7: Kruppel-like factor 7; LDLR: Low-density lipoprotein receptor; MIC-1: Macrophage inhibitory cytokine; MMAB: Methylmalonic aciduria (cobalamin deficiency) cblB type; MYO6: Myosin VI; PHLDA1: Pleckstrin homology-like domain, family A, member 1; SCD: Stearoyl-CoA desaturase (delta-9-desaturase); SDF2L1: Stromal cell-derived factor 2-like 1; SREBF1: Sterol regulatory element binding transcription factor 1; SREBF2: Sterol regulatory element binding transcription factor 2; TRIB3: Tribbles pseudokinase 3

Acknowledgements

We wish to thank Dr. Hiroyuki Yoshimura of the Eisai Food and Chemical Co. for the generous gifts of purified T3. Moreover, we wish to thank professor Maria Marino of the University Roma Tre for the generous gift of a clone of MCF-7 breast cancer cells not expressing ERβ.

Funding

This work was supported by the Malaysian Palm Oil Board (MPOB) and by the Italian Ministry of Agricultural and Nutritional Policies and Forestry (Special Research Projects MiPAAF—NUME and MiPAAF—MEDITO). MPOB and MiPAAF did not meddle in the design or interpretation of the data.

Authors' contributions

All authors provided critical review of all drafts of the manuscript, had full editorial control of the manuscript, and provided their final approval of all content. CoR conceived of the study, carried out the molecular studies, and wrote the paper. GB carried out the western blot experiments. LG carried out the bioinformatic analysis. NK participated in the writing of the paper. RMB carried out the HeLa cell maintenance and participated in the molecular studies. CaR participated in the study design and performed the statistical analysis. VF participated in the study design and coordination and helped to draft the manuscript.

Competing interests

KN is an employee of MPOB. The other authors did not have other relationships or activities that could appear to have influenced the submitted work. The views expressed in this paper are those of the authors and do not represent the views or opinions of their affiliate bodies.

Author details

[1]Council for Agricultural Research and Economics - Food and Nutrition Research Centre (C.R.E.A.-AN), via Ardeatina 546, 00178 Rome, Italy. [2]Department of Physics, Sapienza University of Rome, Piazzale Aldo Moro 5, 00185 Rome, Italy. [3]Malaysian Palm Oil Board, 6 Persiaran Institusi, Bandar Baru Bangi, 4300 Selangor, Malaysia.

References

1. Abruzzo PM, Marini M, Bolotta A, Malisardi G, Manfredini S, Ghezzo A, Pini A, Tasco G, Casadio R. Frataxin mRNA isoforms in FRDA patients and normal subjects: effect of tocotrienol supplementation. Biomed Res Int. 2013;2013: 276808.
2. Baruch M, Hertzog BB, Ravins M, Anand A, Cheng CY, Biswas D, Tirosh B, Hanski E. Induction of endoplasmic reticulum stress and unfolded protein response constitutes a pathogenic strategy of group A streptococcus. Front Cell Infect Microbiol. 2014;4:105.
3. Birringer M, Pfluger P, Kluth D, Landes N, Brigelius-Flohe R. Identities and differences in the metabolism of tocotrienols and tocopherols in HepG2 cells. J Nutr. 2002;132(10):3113–8.
4. Bolshakova N, Azuaje F, Cunningham P. A knowledge-driven approach to cluster validity assessment. Bioinformatics. 2005;21(10):2546–7.
5. Bravo R, Parra V, Gatica D, Rodriguez AE, Torrealba N, Paredes F, Wang ZV, Zorzano A, Hill JA, Jaimovich E, Quest AF, Lavandero S. Endoplasmic reticulum and the unfolded protein response: dynamics and metabolic integration. Int Rev Cell Mol Biol. 2013;301:215–90.
6. Brigelius-Flohe R. Bioactivity of vitamin E. Nutr Res Rev. 2006;19(2):174–86.
7. Buchakjian MR, Kornbluth S. The engine driving the ship: metabolic steering of cell proliferation and death. Nat Rev Mol Cell Biol. 2010;11(10):715–27.
8. Bulzomi P, Bolli A, Galluzzo P, Acconcia F, Ascenzi P, Marino M. The naringenin-induced proapoptotic effect in breast cancer cell lines holds out against a high bisphenol a background. IUBMB Life. 2012;64(8):690–6.
9. Bustin SA, Benes V, Garson JA, Hellemans J, Huggett J, Kubista M, Mueller R, Nolan T, Pfaffl MW, Shipley GL, Vandesompele J, Wittwer CT. The MIQE guidelines: minimum information for publication of quantitative real-time PCR experiments. Clin Chem. 2009;55(4):611–22.
10. Canali R, Comitato R, Ambra R, Virgili F. Red wine metabolites modulate NF-kappaB, activator protein-1 and cAMP response element-binding proteins in human endothelial cells. Br J Nutr. 2010;103(6):807–14.

11. Chakrabarti A, Chen AW, Varner JD. A review of the mammalian unfolded protein response. Biotechnol Bioeng. 2011;108(12):2777–93.
12. Cho SY, Park PJ, Shin HJ, Kim YK, Shin DW, Shin ES, Lee HH, Lee BG, Baik JH, Lee TR. Catechin suppresses expression of Kruppel-like factor 7 and increases expression and secretion of adiponectin protein in 3T3-L1 cells. Am J Physiol Endocrinol Metab. 2007;292:1166–72.
13. Circu ML, Aw TY. Glutathione and modulation of cell apoptosis. Biochim Biophys Acta. 2012;1823(10):1767–77.
14. Colgan SM, Tang D, Werstuck GH, Austin RC. Endoplasmic reticulum stress causes the activation of sterol regulatory element binding protein-2. Int J Biochem Cell Biol. 2007;39:1843–51.
15. Comitato R, Leoni G, Canali R, Ambra R, Nesaretnam K, Virgili F. Tocotrienols activity in MCF-7 breast cancer cells: involvement of ERbeta signal transduction. Mol Nutr Food Res. 2010;54:669–78.
16. Comitato R, Nesaretnam K, Leoni G, Ambra R, Canali R, Bolli A, Marino M, Virgili F. A novel mechanism of natural vitamin E tocotrienol activity: involvement of ERβ signal transduction. Am J Physiol-Endoc M. 2009;297:427–37.
17. Conte C, Floridi A, Aisa C, Piroddi M, Floridi A, Galli F. Gammatocotrienol metabolism and antiproliferative effect in prostate cancer cells. Ann Ny Acad Sci. 2004;1031:391–4.
18. Dennis Jr G, Sherman BT, Hosack DA, Yang J, Gao W, Lane HC, Lempicki RA. DAVID: Database for Annotation, Visualization, and Integrated Discovery. Genome Biol. 2003;4(5):P3.
19. Fukuda S, Sumii M, Masuda Y, Takahashi M, Koike N, Teishima J, Yasumoto H, Itamoto T, Asahara T, Dohi K, Kamiya K. Murine and human SDF2L1 is an endoplasmic reticulum stress-inducible gene and encodes a new member of the Pmt/rt protein family. Biochem Biophys Res Commun. 2001;280(1):407–14.
20. Gooch JL, Yee D. Strain-specific differences in formation of apoptotic DNA ladders in MCF-7 breast cancer cells. Cancer Lett. 1999;144(1):31–7.
21. Green CD, Olson LK. Modulation of palmitate-induced endoplasmic reticulum stress and apoptosis in pancreatic β-cells by stearoyl-CoA desaturase and Elovl6. Am J Physiol Endocrinol Metab. 2011;300:640–9.
22. Guthrie N, Gapor A, Chambers AF, Carroll KK. Inhibition of proliferation of estrogen receptor-negative MDA-MB-435 and -positive MCF-7 human breast cancer cells by palm oil tocotrienols and tamoxifen, aloneand in combination. J Nutr. 1997;127:544S–8S.
23. Hasson T. Myosin VI: two distinct roles in endocytosis. J Cell Sci. 2003;116(Pt 17):3453–61.
24. Herr I, Debatin KM. Cellular stress response and apoptosis in cancer therapy. Blood. 2001;98(9):2603–14.
25. Ishiwata-Kimata Y, Promlek T, Kohno K, Kimata Y. BiP-bound and nonclustered mode of Ire1 evokes a weak but sustained unfolded protein response. Genes Cells. 2013;18:288–301.
26. Jiang Q. Natural forms of vitamin E: metabolism, antioxidant, and anti-inflammatory activities and their role in disease prevention and therapy. Free Radic Biol Med. 2014;72:76–90.
27. Kannappan R, Gupta SC, Kim JH, Aggarwal BB. Tocotrienols fight cancer by targeting multiple cell signaling pathways. Genes Nutr. 2012;7(1):43–52.
28. Lattka E, Illig T, Koletzko B, Heinrich J. Genetic variants of the FADS1 FADS2 gene cluster as related to essential fatty acid metabolism. Curr Opin Lipidol. 2010;21:64–9.
29. Lee AH, Iwakoshi NN, Glimcher LH. XBP-1 regulates a subset of endoplasmic reticulum resident chaperone genes in the unfolded protein response. Mol Cell Biol. 2003;23(21):7448–59.
30. Lei Z, Dai Y. Assessing protein similarity with Gene Ontology and its use in subnuclear localization prediction. BMC Bioinformatics. 2006;7:491.
31. Li H, Korennykh AV, Behrman SL, Walter P. Mammalian endoplasmic reticulum stress sensor IRE1 signals by dynamic clustering. Proc Natl Acad Sci U S A. 2010;107(37):16113–8.
32. Lopes CT, Franz M, Kazi F, Donaldson SL, Morris Q, Bader GD. Cytoscape Web: an interactive web-based network browser. Bioinformatics. 2010;26(18):2347–8.
33. Magosso E, Ansari MA, Gopalan Y, Shuaib IL, Wong JW, Khan NA, Abu Bakar MR, Ng BH, Yuen KH. Tocotrienols for normalisation of hepatic echogenic response in nonalcoholic fatty liver: a randomised placebo-controlled clinical trial. Nutr J. 2013;12(1):166.
34. McIntyre BS, Briski KP, Tirmenstein MA, Fariss MW, Gapor A, Sylvester PW. Antiproliferative and apoptotic effects of tocopherols and tocotrienols on normal mouse mammary epithelial cells. Lipid. 2000;35:171–80.
35. Meunier L, Usherwood YK, Chung KT, Hendershot LM. A subset of chaperones and folding enzymes form multiprotein complexes in endoplasmic reticulum to bind nascent proteins. Mol Biol Cell. 2002;13(12):4456–69.
36. Mihailidou C, Papavassiliou AG, Kiaris H. A crosstalk between p21 and UPR-induced transcription factor C/EBP homologous protein (CHOP) linked to type 2 diabetes. Biochimie. 2014;99:19–27.
37. Miranda M, Escoté X, Ceperuelo-Mallafré V, Megía A, Caubet E, Näf S, Gómez JM, González-Clemente JM, Vicente V, Vendrell J. Relation between human LPIN1, hypoxia and endoplasmic reticulum stress genes in subcutaneous and visceral adipose tissue. Int J Obes Relat Metab Disord. 2010;34:679–86.
38. Morishima N, Nakanishi K, Takenouchi H, Shibata T, Yasuhiko Y. An endoplasmic reticulum stress-specific caspase cascade in apoptosis. Cytochrome c-independent activation of caspase-9 by caspase-12. J Biol Chem. 2002;277:34287–94.
39. Nakagawa T, Yuan J. Cross-talk between two cysteine protease families. Activation of caspase-12 by calpain in apoptosis. J Cell Biol. 2000;150:887–94.
40. Nesaretnam K, Ambra R, Selvaduray KR, Radhakrishnan A, Canali R, Virgili F. Tocotrienol-rich fraction from palm oil and gene expression in human breast cancer cells. Ann Ny Acad Sci. 2004;1031:143–57.
41. Nesaretnam K, Ambra R, Selvaduray KR, Radhakrishnan A, Reimann K, Razak G, Virgili F. Tocotrienol-rich fraction from palm oil affects gene expression in tumors resulting from MCF-7 cell inoculation in athymic mice. Lipid. 2004; 39:459–67.
42. Nesaretnam K, Selvaduray KR, Abdul Razak G, Veerasenan SD, Gomez PA. Effectiveness of tocotrienol-rich fraction combined with tamoxifen in the management of women with early breast cancer: a pilot clinical trial. Breast Cancer Res. 2010;12(5):R81.
43. Nesaretnam K, Stephen R, Dils R, Darbre PD. Tocotrienols inhibit the growth of human breast cancer cells irrespective of estrogen receptor status. Lipid. 1998;33:461–9.
44. Park SK, Sanders BG, Kline K. Tocotrienols induce apoptosis in breast cancer cell lines via an endoplasmic reticulum stress-dependent increase in extrinsic death receptor signaling. Breast Cancer ResTreat. 2010;124:361–75.
45. Patel V, Rink C, Gordillo GM, Khanna S, Gnyawali U, Roy S, Shneker B, Ganesh K, Phillips G, More JL, Sarkar A, Kirkpatrick R, Elkhammas EA, Klatte E, Miller M, Firstenberg MS, Chiocca EA, Nesaretnam K, Sen CK. Oral tocotrienols are transported to human tissues and delay the progression of the model for end-stage liver disease score in patients. J Nutr. 2012;142(3):513–9.
46. Pfaffl MW. A new mathematical model for relative quantification in real-time RT-PCR. Nucleic Acids Res. 2001;29(9):e45.
47. Rahman MM, Mohamed MR, Kim M, Smallwood S, McFadden G. Co-regulation of NF-kappaB and inflammasome-mediated inflammatory responses by myxoma virus pyrin domain-containing protein M013. PLoS Pathog. 2009;5(10):e1000635.
48. Rasheva VI, Domingos PM. Cellular responses to endoplasmic reticulum stress and apoptosis. Apoptosis. 2009;14:996–1007.
49. Ron D, Walter P. Signal integration in the endoplasmic reticulum unfolded protein response. Nat Rev Mol Cell Biol. 2007;8:519–29.
50. Rong Y, Distelhorst CW. Bcl-2 protein family members: versatile regulators of calcium signaling in cell survival and apoptosis. Ann Rev Physiol. 2008;70:73–91.
51. Rutkowski DT, Kaufman RJ. A trip to the ER: coping with stress. Trends Cell Biol. 2004;14(1):20–8.
52. Srivastava JK, Gupta S. Tocotrienol-rich fraction of palm oil induces cell cycle arrest and apoptosis selectively in human prostate cancer cells. Biochem Biophys Res Commun. 2006;346:447–53.
53. Sundram K, Gapor A. Vitamin E from palm oil. Its extraction and nutritional properties. Lipid Tech. 1992;4:137–41.
54. Sylvester PW, Akl MR, Malaviya A, Parajuli P, Ananthula S, Tiwari RV, Ayoub NM. Potential role of tocotrienols in the treatment and prevention of breast cancer. Biofactors. 2014;40(1):49–58.
55. Sylvester PW, Shah SJ. Mechanisms mediating the antiproliferative and apoptotic effects of vitamin E in mammary cancer cells. Front Biosci. 2005;10:699–709.
56. Szegezdi E, Logue SE, Gorman AM, Samali A. Mediators of endoplasmicreticulum stress-induced apoptosis. EMBO Rep. 2006;7:880–5.
57. Takahashi K, Loo G. Disruption of mitochondria during tocotrienol-induced apoptosis in MDA-MB-231 human breast cancer cells. Biochem Pharmacol. 2004;67(2):315–24.

58. van Harmelen V, Rydén M, Sjölin E, Hoffstedt J. A role of lipin in human obesity and insulin resistance: relation to adipocyte glucose transport and GLUT4 expression. J Lipid Res. 2007;48:201–6.
59. Wada S, Satomi Y, Murakoshi M, Noguchi N, Yoshikawa T, Nishino H. Tumor suppressive effects of tocotrienol in vivo and in vitro. Cancer Lett. 2005;229:181–91.
60. Wali VB, Bachawal SV, Sylvester PW. Endoplasmic reticulum stress mediates gamma-tocotrienol-induced apoptosis in mammary tumor cells. Apoptosis. 2009;14:1366–77.
61. Wu SJ, Ng LT. Tocotrienols inhibited growth and induced apoptosis in human HeLa cells through the cell cycle signaling pathway. Integr Cancer Ther. 2010;9(1):66–72.
62. Xu C, Bailly-Maitre B, Reed JC. Endoplasmic reticulum stress: cell life and death decisions. J Clin Invest. 2005;115:2656–64.
63. Zhang K, Kaufman RJ. Identification and characterization of endoplasmic reticulum stress-induced apoptosis in vivo. Methods Enzymol. 2008;442:395–419.

6

Comparative anti-inflammatory and lipid-normalizing effects of metformin and omega-3 fatty acids through modulation of transcription factors in diabetic rats

Abhijit Ghadge[1], Abhay Harsulkar[1], Manjiri Karandikar[2], Vijaya Pandit[3] and Aniket Kuvalekar[1*]

Abstract

Background: Emerging evidence suggests beneficial effects of omega-3 fatty acids on diabetic complications. The present study compared the progressive effects of metformin and flax/fish oil on lipid metabolism, inflammatory markers, and liver and renal function test markers in streptozotocin-nicotinamide-induced diabetic rats.

Methods: Streptozotocin-induced diabetic rats were randomized into control and four diabetic groups: streptozotocin (STZ), metformin (200 mg/kg body weight (b.w)/day (D)), flax and fish oil (500 mg/kg b.w/D).

Results: Metformin and flax and fish oil exhibited increased expression of transcription factor peroxisome proliferator-activated receptor γ while the treatment downregulated sterol regulatory element-binding protein 1 and nuclear factor kβ as compared to those of the STZ group. Apart from modulation of transcription factor expression, the expression of fatty acid synthase, long chain acyl CoA synthase, and malonyl-CoA-acyl carrier protein transacylase was lowered by flax/fish oil treatment. Serum cholesterol, triglycerides, and VLDL were also significantly reduced in the treatment groups as compared to those in the STZ group. Although pathological abnormalities were seen in the liver and kidneys of rats on metformin, no significant changes in liver/renal function markers were observed at day 15 and day 30 of the treatment groups. Flax/fish oil had protective effects toward pathological abnormalities in the liver and kidney. Flax/fish oil improved lipid profile and alkaline phosphatase at day 30 as compared to that at day 15.

Conclusions: The present study demonstrates potential beneficial effects of metformin and flax/fish oil intervention in improving serum lipid profile by regulating the expression of transcription factors and genes involved in lipid metabolism in diabetic rats. In addition, these interventions also lowered the expression of atherogenic cytokines. The protective effects of flax/fish oil are worth investigating in human subjects on metformin monotherapy.

Keywords: Fish oil, Flax oil, Metformin, Omega-3 fatty acids, Streptozotocin

Background

Omega-3 polyunsaturated fatty acids (n-3 PUFA) constitute a fundamental part of cell membranes and exhibit a diverse range of membrane functions including functioning of transporters, signal transduction pathways, and gene expression (Liu and Ma 2014; Ander et al. 2003). Alpha-linolenic acid (ALA; 18:3 n-3) is a short chain n-3 PUFA obtained from flaxseed (a plant-derived food item) (Dessì et al. 2013; Mozaffarian and Wu 2012; Connor 2000) while eicosapentaenoic acid (EPA) and docosahexaenoic acid (DHA; 22:6 n-3) are the long chain n-3 PUFA derived from a seafood source, fish oil (Swanson et al. 2012). There is strong scientific evidence demonstrating anti-inflammatory, anti-atherogenic, vasodilatory, and lipid-lowering properties of n-3 PUFA (Jangale et al. 2013; Mozaffarian and Wu 2012; Connor 2000) due to which they have been implicated in some chronic diseases like cardiovascular disease (Ander et al. 2003), diabetes (Wu et al. 2012), and autoimmune diseases

* Correspondence: kuaniket@gmail.com
[1]Nutrigenomics and Functional Foods Laboratory, Interactive Research School for Health Affairs (IRSHA), Bharati Vidyapeeth Deemed University, Pune-Satara Road, Pune, Maharashtra 411043, India

(Calder 2007). In view of this, dietary n-3 PUFA are considered as significant nutrients involved in metabolic regulation. There is a recent surge in research on effects of functional foods, like n-3 PUFA for the management of type 2 diabetes mellitus (T2DM).

Diabetes consists of a group of metabolic disorders involving distinct pathogenic mechanisms with hyperglycemia, arising due to impaired metabolism of glucose, lipids, and proteins (Prabhakar et al. 2013). T2DM is frequently associated with abnormal lipid profile (Ozder 2014) with perturbations in the lipid metabolism affected by abnormalities in the expression of hepatic transcription factors and genes (Erejuwa et al. 2012). Moreover, diabetics are more prone to develop chronic complications related to cardiovascular, renal (Forbes and Cooper 2013), and peripheral vascular tissues (King 2008).

Several oral hypoglycemic drugs such as biguanides, sulfonylurea, and thiazolidenediones are commonly used for the treatment of T2DM. Metformin is an old and widely used first-line agent, known for its anti-hyperglycemic properties, and is also reported to improve lipid profile, fat redistribution (Rojas and Gomes 2013), and chronic liver diseases (Zheng et al. 2015) and lower microvascular and macrovascular complications associated with T2DM (Kooy et al. 2009). Though it has rarely been reported to induce hepatocellular and cholestatic hepatic injury (Saadi et al. 2013) and hepatotoxicity (Miralles-Linares et al. 2012), there are very few reports examining its long-term effects for the management of T2DM.

Some investigations have evaluated the individual effects of metformin (Wang et al. 2014) or n-3 PUFA on the regulation of lipid metabolism genes in diabetes (Devarshi et al. 2013). The lipid-lowering actions of n-3 PUFA are attributed to the regulation of key transcription factors like peroxisome proliferator-activated receptors (PPAR) and sterol regulatory element-binding protein (SREBP), that control hepatic lipid metabolism (Di Minno et al. 2012). However, there are some conflicting results stating that supplementation with fish oil does not delay the onset of diabetes in rats at 12 months of age (Cummings et al. 2010) while other reports state that n-3 PUFA slows the progression of T2DM and its complications (Nettleton and Katz 2005). However, there is lack of evidence for these effects of n-3 PUFA in T2DM and the underlying molecular mechanisms have not been well evaluated (Devarshi et al. 2013; Wu et al. 2012). A review by Hendrich points a need to carry out high-quality studies to assess the effects of ALA (Hendrich 2010). The above reports suggest the need for a meticulous evaluation of effects of ALA, EPA, and DHA on lipid metabolism and its underlying mechanism.

It is well known that streptozotocin (STZ) has a selective cytotoxic action on β-cells in the islets of Langerhans whereas nicotinamide has a partial protective role on β-cells against STZ (Szkudelski 2012) and is commonly used for induction of type 2 diabetes mellitus in experimental animals (Devarshi et al. 2013; Pari and Saravanan 2007; Saravanan and Pari 2007; Brenna et al. 2003). Additionally, STZ-nicotinamide is considered as a suitable T2DM model to study the effects of metformin as well as herbal (Maheshwari et al. 2014; Sharma et al. 2012; Mohammadi et al. 2012; Li et al. 2011) and nutritional (Devarshi et al. 2013; Jangale et al. 2013) interventions as indicated by several animal studies. We selected peripheral blood mononuclear cells (PBMCs) to study gene expression profile since the blood is the most accessible tissue in humans, and as the profile of multiple tissues is shared with PBMCs, they reflect important metabolic changes in the liver (Konieczna et al. 2014). However, there are no reports examining the temporal effects of metformin and flax/fish oil diets on the lipid metabolism and biochemical markers in T2DM. Moreover, potential of these treatments to affect duration of the disease is poorly understood.

We hypothesized that metformin and omega-3 fatty acids could improve lipid metabolism and inflammatory cytokines by modulating the expression of transcription factors in STZ-nicotinamide-induced diabetic rats. The objectives of the present study were to examine the comparative effects of metformin and omega-3 fatty acids on serum lipid profile, expression of transcription factors and genes involved in lipid metabolism, and inflammation in STZ-nicotinamide-induced diabetic rats. Additionally, the progressive effects of these treatments on liver/renal function test markers and histological changes in these tissues were evaluated. We also compared the effects of these treatments on the above parameters at post treatment day 15 (D15) and day 30 (D30) to study their effects on the duration of disease.

Methods

Chemicals and reagents

Flax oil (Alvel-500) capsules were purchased from Real World Nutritional Laboratory (Pune, India) that contained 50 % alpha-linolenic acid (ALA), 20 % oleic acid, and 12 % linoleic acid. Fish oil capsules (Maxepa) were purchased from Merck Limited (Goa, India) which contained 60 % EPA and 40 % DHA. Streptozotocin (STZ), nicotinamide (Sigma Life Sciences, USA), and metformin (Glycomet 250 mg; USV Limited) were purchased from a local pharmacy.

Experimental animals

The study was carried out as per the CPCSEA (Committee for the Purpose of Control and Supervision of Experiments on Animals) guidelines after the approval of Institutional Animal Ethics Committee (Ref. No: BVDUMC/189/2014-

2015). The male albino Wistar rats weighing between 150 and 200 g were procured from the institutional animal house and maintained under standard conditions throughout the experimentation (temperature 25 ± 2 °C, 12-h light:12-h dark cycle). Animals were fed with standard pellet diet (Nutrivet life science, Pune, M.S., India), and water was supplied ad libitum.

Diabetes induction

Animals were randomly assigned to five groups ($n = 6$). Diabetes was induced by administration of nicotinamide (110 mg/kg body weight) in saline through intraperitoneal (i.p) injection. After 15 min, STZ was administered (65 mg/kg body weight i.p) in sodium citrate buffer, pH 4.0. The fasting blood glucose levels of the rats were estimated after 48 h and on day 7 of STZ injection. Stable hyperglycemia was confirmed by elevated fasting blood glucose levels on day 7 after STZ injection. Animals with fasting blood glucose levels above 200 mg/dl were considered as diabetic and used for the study. After development of stable hyperglycemia, metformin or flax/fish oil treatment was given for 30 days. The dose of flax and fish oil was based on the earlier study carried out in our laboratory (Chavan et al. 2013). The study protocol is given in Fig. 1. Animals were randomly assigned to one of the following groups: group I: control group ($n = 6$): received feed and water normally throughout the experiment; group II: STZ-induced diabetic group ($n = 6$): administered nicotinamide (110 mg/kg body weight) and STZ (65 mg/kg body weight) i.p single dose; group III: metformin group ($n = 6$): administered metformin (200 mg/kg, body weight/D p.o); group IV: flax oil group ($n = 6$): administered flax oil (500 mg/kg body weight/D, p.o); group V: fish oil group ($n = 6$): administered fish oil (500 mg/kg body weight/D, p.o). After 15 days of treatment, animals were fasted overnight and blood was collected by retro-orbital puncture. Animals were sacrificed after 30 days of treatment. Liver and kidney tissues were excised immediately, washed in saline, weighed, and stored in 10 % neutral buffered formalin for histological analysis. Blood was collected and centrifuged at 2000 rpm for 15 min to collect serum for biochemical estimations.

Blood biochemistry

Serum glucose, total cholesterol, triglyceride, high-density lipoprotein (HDL), low-density lipoprotein (LDL), serum glutamic oxaloacetic transaminase (SGOT), serum glutamic pyruvic transaminase (SGPT) and alkaline phosphatase (ALP), total bilirubin, creatinine, urea, albumin, and total protein were estimated using commercial kits (Coral Clinical Systems, Goa, India). Very low-density lipoprotein cholesterol (VLDL) was estimated by using the formula: (triglyceride/5).

Quantitative real-time reverse transcription-polymerase chain reaction analysis

PBMCs were isolated by density gradient centrifugation by layering the blood sample over Histopaque-1077 (Sigma-Aldrich, Inc., USA). RNA was isolated by TRIzol (Invitrogen Co., Carlsbad, CA, USA) method. Total RNA was quantified using NanoDrop (ND1000, USA). The quality of RNA was analyzed by agarose gel

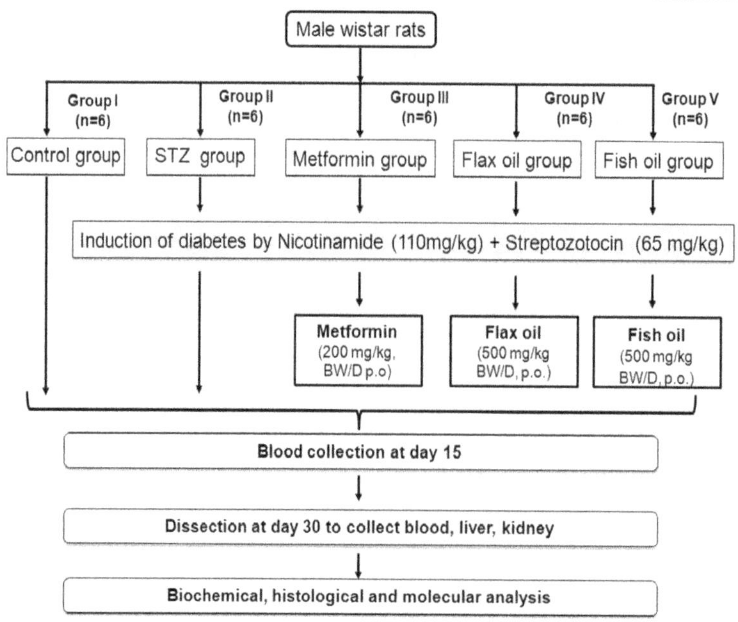

Fig. 1 Study design

electrophoresis. Complementary DNA (cDNA) was prepared by using high-capacity cDNA Reverse Transcription kit (Applied Biosystems). Standard quantitative real-time transcription-polymerase chain reaction (qRT-PCR) was performed with the use of SYBR Green master mix (Applied Biosystems) for the following genes: PPARγ, SREBP1, nuclear factor kappa β (NFκβ), fatty acid synthase (FAS), long chain acyl CoA synthetases (ACSL), malonyl-CoA-acyl carrier protein transacylase (MCAT), tumor necrosis factor α (TNFα). KicqStart Primers (Sigma, USA) were used for gene expression studies and are listed in Table 1. qRT-PCR was performed using the Applied Biosystems 7300 Standard system. The reactions for each gene were performed in duplicate. Relative expression levels of genes were calculated and expressed as $2^{\Delta CT}$ where ΔCT is C_T (GAPDH)–C_T (target gene) and this method is a modification of $2^{-\Delta\Delta C_T}$ method (Gaines et al. 2010).

Histological analysis

Paraffin-embedded liver and kidney tissues were cut at 4 μm and stained with hematoxylin and eosin. The slides were examined under a binocular microscope (Make: Olympus IX71) and photographed by using Image Pro Plus (v5.1.2.59).

Table 1 List of primers used for quantitative real-time PCR

Gene	Primer name	Sequence (5′–3′)
GAPDH	GAPDH F	AGTTCAACGGCACAGTCAAG
	GAPDH R	TACTCAGCACCAGCATCACC
PPARγ	PPARγ F	AAGACAACAGACAAATCACC
	PPARγ R	CAGGGATATTTTTGGCATACTC
SREBP1	SREBP F	AAACCTGAAGTGGTAGAAAC
	SREBP R	TTATCCTCAAAGGCTGGG
NFKB	NFKB F	AAAAACGAGCCTAGAGATTG
	NFKB R	ACATCCTCTTCCTTGTCTTC
FAS	FAS F	AAAAGGAAAGTAGAGTGTGC
	FAS R	GACACATTCTGTTCACTACAG
ACSL	ACSL F	ACATTATGAACGATTGCTCC
	ACSL R	GCATTACACACTCTACAACG
MCAT	MCAT F	AAAACTCTAGGCTCAATCAAC
	MCAT R	GGATGTGTGTATTTATGCCC
TNFα	TNFα F	CTCACACTCAGATCATCTTC
	TNFα R	GAGAACCTGGGAGTAGATAAG

GAPDH glyceraldehyde-3-phosphate dehydrogenase, *PPARγ* peroxisome proliferator-activated receptors γ, *SREBP1* sterol regulatory element-binding protein 1, *NFκβ* nuclear factor kappa β, *FAS* fatty acid synthase, *ACSL* long chain acyl CoA synthetases, *MCAT* malonyl-CoA-acyl carrier protein transacylase, *TNFα* tumor necrosis factor α (Make: Sigma-Aldrich; *F* forward primer sequence, *R* reverse primer sequence)

Statistical analysis

Results are presented as mean ± standard error (SE). All the statistical analyses were performed using SPSS PC+ package (Version 20, Chicago, IL, USA). The data were checked for normal distribution by testing for skewness. Skewed variables were transformed to normality using log to the base 10 transformation. Statistical differences between means in different groups were determined using one-way analysis of variance (ANOVA) test followed by post hoc Bonferonni multiple correction test. Mean values of various parameters from each group at D15 were compared with those at D30 using Student's t test. $P \leq 0.05$ was considered statistically significant.

Results

Food intake, body weights, and organ weights

The food intake of animals from the STZ group was higher at D1 ($p < 0.01$), D15, and D30 ($p < 0.05$) as compared to that from the control. The body weights were lower at D15 ($p < 0.05$) and D30 ($p < 0.01$) when compared with those of the control (Table 2). Liver weights, hepatic index, and kidney weights were comparable while kidney index ($p < 0.01$) was higher in the STZ group as compared to that in the control (Table 2).

Serum glucose levels

Serum glucose levels were significantly higher ($p < 0.01$) in the STZ group than those in the control at D15 and D30 (Table 3).

Comparison of glucose levels at D15 and D30 within the groups

Glucose levels in the control, STZ, metformin, and flax oil groups were comparable at D15 and D30. However, glucose levels in the fish oil group were lower ($p < 0.05$) at D30 as compared to those at D15 (Table 5).

Lipid profile

At D15, the STZ group had higher serum cholesterol ($p < 0.01$), HDL, and LDL levels ($p < 0.01$) than the control group. A higher trend was observed for triglyceride and VLDL ($p = 0.068$) levels in the STZ group than for those in the control group. Animals from the metformin-treated group had lower cholesterol ($p < 0.05$), HDL, and LDL ($p < 0.01$) than those in the STZ group. The fish oil treatment group also lowered HDL and LDL levels ($P < 0.05$) than the STZ group (Table 3).

At D30, higher serum cholesterol ($p < 0.05$), triglyceride, and VLDL levels ($p < 0.01$) were seen in the STZ group than in the control. Metformin group lowered cholesterol, triglyceride, and VLDL ($p < 0.01$) as compared to the STZ group. Flax oil treatment group lowered triglycerides and VLDL levels ($p < 0.01$) than the STZ group. Fish oil treatment group lowered cholesterol,

Table 2 Food intake and body, liver, and kidney weights of animals

	Control ($n = 6$)	STZ ($n = 6$)	Metformin ($n = 6$)	Flax oil ($n = 6$)	Fish oil ($n = 6$)
Food intake (g)					
Day 1	14.66 ± 3.58	30.83 ± 0.21**	33.66 ± 0.58	31.83 ± 2.69	30.00 ± 0.65
Day 15	12.66 ± 2.41	23.33 ± 2.07*	27.00 ± 1.27	28.33 ± 1.80	16.66 ± 2.59
Day 30	16.00 ± 2.22	26.50 ± 3.55*	27.00 ± 1.89	33.66 ± 0.45	31.50 ± 1.93
Body weights (g)					
Day 1	236.50 ± 3.48	235.50 ± 8.54	235.50 ± 13.91	245.83 ± 3.84	243.16 ± 15.15
Day 15	292.16 ± 6.55	232.33 ± 20.28*	201.33 ± 14.02	231.83 ± 12.68	202.50 ± 11.64
Day 30	345.50 ± 10.47	223.33 ± 30.34**	176.50 ± 14.93	211.33 ± 13.90	198.33 ± 11.47
Liver and kidney weights					
Liver weight (g)	9.97 ± 0.60	7.68 ± 0.59	6.60 ± 0.50	7.60 ± 0.51	8.24 ± 0.59
Liver index (%)	2.87 ± 0.12	3.60 ± 0.31	3.78 ± 0.19	3.62 ± 0.20	4.17 ± 0.24
Kidney weight (g)	1.60 ± 0.13	1.89 ± 0.08	1.76 ± 0.12	1.91 ± 0.07	1.84 ± 0.03
Kidney index (%)	0.46 ± 0.03	0.90 ± 0.08**	1.01 ± 0.06	0.91 ± 0.04	0.94 ± 0.05

Data are presented as mean ± SE
*$p < 0.05$, **$p < 0.01$ for comparison between the control and STZ group

triglyceride, and VLDL ($p < 0.01$) as compared to the STZ group (Table 3).

Comparison of lipid profile parameters at D15 and D30 within the groups

In the STZ group, serum HDL and LDL levels were lower ($p < 0.01$) at D30 as compared to those at D15. Serum cholesterol, triglyceride, and VLDL levels were lower ($p < 0.01$) at D30 as compared to those at D15 in the metformin group. In the flax and fish oil group, cholesterol, triglyceride, HDL, LDL, and VLDL levels were lower ($p < 0.01$) at D30 as compared to those at D15 (Table 5).

Expression of genes involved in lipid metabolism

The PPARγ gene expression was lower in the STZ group ($p < 0.05$) as compared to that in the control. The treatment with metformin ($p < 0.05$) and fish oil ($p < 0.01$)

Table 3 Serum glucose level and lipid profile at post treatment days 15 and 30

	Control ($n = 6$)	STZ ($n = 6$)	Metformin ($n = 6$)	Flax oil ($n = 6$)	Fish oil ($n = 6$)
Glucose level (mg/dl)					
At day 15	53.72 ± 3.58	294.11 ± 14.85**	340.98 ± 30.14	280.12 ± 12.62	315.36 ± 10.66
At day 30	54.11 ± 4.89	309.65 ± 33.54**	300.64 ± 6.75	315.18 ± 16.20	269.23 ± 16.96
Lipid profile					
Post treatment day 15					
Cholesterol (mg/dl)	43.37 ± 3.76	98.24 ± 12.83**	58.79 ± 4.47#	87.31 ± 9.03	69.44 ± 3.16
Triglyceride (mg/dl)	72.74 ± 6.15	171.96 ± 39.49	145.58 ± 20.68	114.01 ± 15.45	133.95 ± 23.67
HDL (mg/dl)	10.03 ± 0.83	22.10 ± 2.11**	8.09 ± 1.55##	22.93 ± 1.95	13.80 ± 1.17#
LDL (mg/dl)	17.31 ± 1.44	38.12 ± 3.65**	13.96 ± 2.68##	39.56 ± 3.37	23.82 ± 2.20#
VLDL (mg/dl)	14.54 ± 1.23	34.39 ± 7.89	29.19 ± 4.13	22.80 ± 3.09	26.79 ± 4.73
Post treatment day 30					
Cholesterol (mg/dl)	44.44 ± 2.04	68.22 ± 10.04*	34.35 ± 4.71##	49.25 ± 2.82	34.62 ± 4.75##
Triglyceride (mg/dl)	66.29 ± 5.96	201.33 ± 31.23**	43.14 ± 8.12##	44.81 ± 11.19##	42.03 ± 9.13##
HDL (mg/dl)	10.71 ± 0.70	9.95 ± 1.10	7.97 ± 1.02	13.05 ± 1.06	8.73 ± 0.71
LDL (mg/dl)	18.48 ± 1.21	17.16 ± 1.90	13.75 ± 1.77	22.52 ± 1.83	15.05 ± 1.23
VLDL (mg/dl)	13.25 ± 1.19	40.26 ± 6.24**	8.62 ± 1.62##	8.96 ± 2.23##	8.40 ± 1.82##

Data are presented as mean ± SE
HDL high-density lipoprotein cholesterol, *LDL* low-density lipoprotein cholesterol, *VLDL* very low-density lipoprotein cholesterol
*$p < 0.05$, **$p < 0.01$ for comparison between the control and STZ group and #$p < 0.05$, ##$p < 0.01$ for comparison between the STZ group and treatment groups

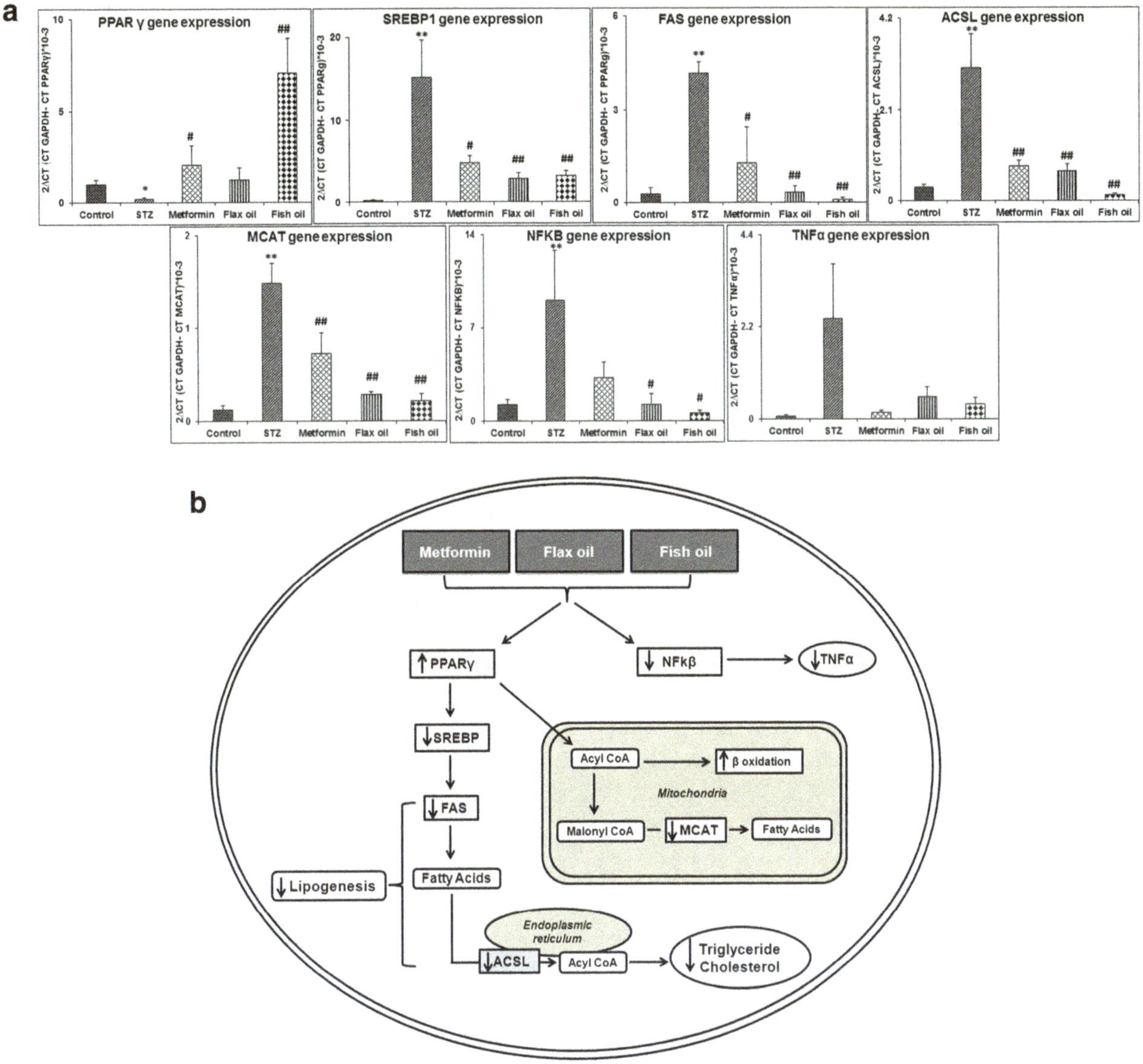

Fig. 2 **a** Expression of genes involved in lipid metabolism and inflammation. Data are presented as mean ± SE. $*p < 0.05$, $**p < 0.01$ for comparison between the control and STZ group and $^{\#}p < 0.05$, $^{\#\#}p < 0.01$ for comparison between the STZ group and treatment groups. *GAPDH* glyceraldehyde-3-phosphate dehydrogenase, *PPARγ* peroxisome proliferator-activated receptors γ, *SREBP1* sterol regulatory element-binding protein, *NFκβ* nuclear factor kappa β, *FAS* fatty acid synthase, *ACSL* long chain acyl CoA synthetases, *MCAT* malonyl-CoA-acyl carrier protein transacylase, *TNFα* tumor necrosis factor α. **b** Diagrammatic representation of the possible mechanism of metformin and flax and fish oil on the lipid metabolism and inflammatory cytokines. *PPARγ* peroxisome proliferator-activated receptors γ, *SREBP* sterol regulatory element-binding protein, *NFκβ* nuclear factor kappa β, *FAS* fatty acid synthase, *ACSL* long chain acyl CoA synthetases, *MCAT* malonyl-CoA-acyl carrier protein transacylase, *TNFα* tumor necrosis factor α, *up arrow* up-regulation, *down arrow* down-regulation

increased PPARγ expression as compared to that in the STZ group (Fig. 2a).

The SREBP1 gene expression was higher in the STZ group ($p < 0.01$) as compared to that in the control while treatment with metformin ($p < 0.05$) and flax and fish oil lowered ($p < 0.01$) the expression as compared to that in the STZ group (Fig. 2a).

The expression of fatty acid synthase (FAS) was higher in the STZ group ($p < 0.01$) as compared to that in the control whereas the expression was lower in metformin ($p < 0.05$) and flax and fish oil groups ($p < 0.01$) when compared to that in the STZ group (Fig. 2a).

The ACSL gene expression was higher in the STZ group ($p < 0.01$) as compared to that in the control. Metformin and flax and fish oil ($p < 0.01$) lowered the expression of ACSL as compared to that in the STZ group (Fig. 2a).

The MCAT gene expression was higher in the STZ group ($p < 0.01$) as compared to that in the control. Metformin and flax and fish oil ($p < 0.01$) lowered the expression as compared to that in the STZ group (Fig. 2a).

Expression of genes involved in inflammation

The NFkβ gene expression was higher in the STZ group ($p < 0.05$) as compared to that in the control. The metformin group did not show any significant difference as compared to the STZ group. Flax and fish oil ($p < 0.05$) lowered the expression as compared to that in the STZ group (Fig. 2a).

The TNFα gene expression did not show a significant difference although it was higher in the STZ group than in the control ($p = 0.123$). Metformin ($p = 0.155$) and flax ($p = 0.404$) and fish ($p = 0.260$) oil groups exhibited decreased expression of TNFα as compared to the STZ group, but the decrease was not statistically significant (Fig. 2a).

Liver function test markers

At D15, serum SGPT and ALP levels were higher ($p < 0.05$) in the STZ group than in the control, but SGOT and bilirubin levels were comparable to those in the control (Table 4).

At D30, serum ALP levels were higher ($p < 0.01$) in the STZ group as compared to those in the control. Metformin and flax and fish oil did not affect liver function test markers at D15 and D30 (Table 4).

Comparison of liver function test markers between D15 and D30 within the groups

In the control group, serum SGPT and ALP levels were lower ($p < 0.05$) at D15 as compared to those at D30. There was no difference in the liver function test markers in STZ and metformin groups. In both flax oil and fish oil groups, ALP levels were lower ($p < 0.05$) at D30 as compared to those at D15 (Table 5).

Liver histology

In the STZ-induced diabetic group, we observed some areas with pathological calcification in the partial triad focal hemorrhages and destruction of some bile ducts. It also showed destruction of hepatocytes, loss of hepatic lobules, and conjunction of the central vein. Surprisingly, the metformin group displayed destruction of some hepatocytes and congestion of the central vein. The flax and fish oil group displayed near-normal liver histology without any histological detectable anomalies (Fig. 3a).

Renal function test markers

At D15, serum urea ($p < 0.01$) levels were higher in the STZ group as compared to those in the control.

Table 4 Liver and renal function test markers at post treatment days 15 and 30

	Control ($n = 6$)	STZ ($n = 6$)	Metformin ($n = 6$)	Flax oil ($n = 6$)	Fish oil ($n = 6$)
Liver function test markers					
Post treatment day 15					
SGOT (U/ml)	104.10 ± 3.97	123.46 ± 6.98	162.11 ± 20.38	133.84 ± 13.60	116.79 ± 8.20
SGPT (U/ml)	113.08 ± 5.56	167.50 ± 15.28*	199.83 ± 20.03	202.16 ± 7.52	220.08 ± 12.47
ALP (KA Unit)	28.15 ± 4.06	113.46 ± 33.45*	103.88 ± 15.53	91.22 ± 11.19	98.98 ± 4.34
Bilirubin (mg/dl)	0.08 ± 0.18	0.11 ± 0.02	0.12 ± 0.04	0.09 ± 0.01	0.10 ± 0.01
Post treatment day 30					
SGOT (U/ml)	113.71 ± 9.81	124.00 ± 8.45	134.48 ± 9.27	120.38 ± 10.69	136.15 ± 6.41
SGPT (U/ml)	87.50 ± 9.10	134.80 ± 24.83	160.33 ± 32.84	150.00 ± 34.53	198.50 ± 22.43
ALP (KA Unit)	15.78 ± 1.59	75.34 ± 6.49**	69.63 ± 9.41	53.80 ± 5.78	58.29 ± 10.88
Bilirubin (mg/dl)	0.08 ± 0.01	0.11 ± 0.03	0.14 ± 0.01	0.06 ± 0.02	0.06 ± 0.02
Renal function test markers					
Post treatment day 15					
Creatinine (mg/dl)	1.44 ± 0.27	2.38 ± 0.23	1.86 ± 0.17	1.49 ± 0.27	1.50 ± 0.28
Urea (mg/dl)	38.37 ± 3.37	56.11 ± 3.57**	56.88 ± 4.24	46.95 ± 2.26	46.33 ± 3.12
Albumin (g/dl)	2.19 ± 0.15	1.83 ± 0.23	1.61 ± 0.26	1.88 ± 0.11	2.15 ± 0.19
Total protein (g/dl)	4.00 ± 0.18	3.68 ± 0.29	3.86 ± 0.68	3.80 ± 0.25	4.07 ± 0.20
Post treatment day 30					
Creatinine (mg/dl)	1.28 ± 0.15	1.69 ± 0.30	1.61 ± 0.33	1.33 ± 0.10	1.22 ± 0.34
Urea (mg/dl)	40.52 ± 4.50	49.38 ± 3.48	50.88 ± 2.29	60.57 ± 2.35	51.22 ± 4.80
Albumin (g/dl)	2.09 ± 0.14	1.70 ± 0.17	1.54 ± 0.10	1.68 ± 0.11	1.80 ± 0.20
Total protein (g/dl)	3.71 ± 0.09	3.42 ± 0.81	3.08 ± 0.19	3.31 ± 0.14	3.23 ± 0.12

Data are presented as mean ± SE

SGOT serum glutamic oxaloacetic transaminase, *SGPT* serum glutamic pyruvic transaminase, *ALP* alkaline phosphatase

*$p < 0.05$, **$p < 0.01$ for comparison between the control and STZ group

Table 5 Comparison of biochemical markers between post treatment days 15 and 30 within the groups

	Glucose	Lipid profile					Liver function test markers				Renal function test markers			
		Cholesterol	Triglyceride	HDL	LDL	VLDL	SGOT	SGPT	ALP	Bilirubin	Creatinine	Urea	Albumin	Total protein
p value														
Control	0.951	0.833	0.469	0.550	0.550	0.469	0.395	*0.037*	*0.017*	1.000	0.612	0.709	0.638	0.192
STZ	0.662	0.108	0.585	*0.001*	*0.001*	0.586	0.961	0.274	0.310	0.966	0.103	0.215	0.673	0.453
Metformin	0.243	*0.004*	*0.001*	0.950	0.950	*0.001*	0.245	0.333	0.088	0.667	0.522	0.242	0.813	0.301
Flax oil	0.118	*0.007*	*0.005*	*0.001*	*0.001*	*0.005*	0.454	0.170	*0.014*	0.425	0.600	*0.001*	0.272	0.123
Fish oil	*0.044*	*0.000*	*0.005*	*0.004*	*0.004*	*0.005*	0.092	0.425	*0.011*	0.186	0.547	0.413	0.233	*0.004*

HDL high-density lipoprotein cholesterol, *LDL* low-density lipoprotein cholesterol, *VLDL* very low-density lipoprotein cholesterol, *SGOT* serum glutamic oxaloacetic transaminase, *SGPT* serum glutamic pyruvic transaminase, *ALP* alkaline phosphatase . The *p* values in italics indicate significant differences in the biochemical markers, within the groups, between post treatment days 15 and 30

However, metformin and flax and fish oil did not show significant differences in renal function test markers at D15 and D30 (Table 4).

Comparison of renal function test markers at D15 and D30 within the groups

There was no difference in the renal function test markers in the control, STZ, and metformin groups. The urea levels were higher ($p < 0.01$) in the flax oil group while total protein levels were lower ($p < 0.05$) in the fish oil group at D30 as compared to those at D15 (Table 5).

Kidney histology

STZ group displayed blood vesicle conjunction, vacuolation of tubular epithelial cells, conjunction of glomerular capillary, cloudy change in many tubular cells, and some degeneration of the glomerulus. The metformin group displayed vacuolation of some tubular epithelial cells and conjunction of glomerular capillary. The flax oil and fish oil groups exhibited near-normal architecture and displayed significant recovery of the damage as compared to the STZ group (Fig. 3b).

Discussion

The general characteristics of STZ-treated diabetic rats include low body weights and elevated blood glucose (Howarth et al. 2005). We observed a significant decrease in body weights and sustained hyperglycemia in nicotinamide-STZ-treated rats indicating successful induction of diabetes. In the present study, both metformin and omega-3 fatty acids could not normalize the glucose levels at D15 which remained higher till D30 of treatment. However, fish oil treatment lowered the glucose levels at D30 as compared to those at D15. It has been reported that metformin alone may not adequately control hyperglycemia (Salama et al. 2013) and omega-3 fatty acids do not directly affect glucose homeostasis (Woodman et al. 2002). However, several studies have reported hypoglycemic- and insulin-sensitizing effects of metformin (Maheshwari et al. 2014; Mohammadi et al. 2012; Erejuwa et al. 2011) and omega-3 fatty acids (Jangale et al. 2013) in the STZ-nicotinamide-induced diabetic rats. Consistent with our findings, metformin treatment at a dose 500 mg/kg for 8 weeks was not able to lower blood glucose in diabetic rats (Alhaider et al. 2011). These differences are probably due to variations in the duration of treatment or dose of metformin/omega-3 fatty acids which needs further investigation.

Effect of n-3 PUFA intervention on lipid profile

Several reports have documented significant lipid abnormalities, like elevated cholesterol, triglyceride, LDL, and VLDL in diabetic rats (Nasrolahi et al. 2012). We observed increase in the serum cholesterol, triglyceride, and VLDL levels in the STZ group indicating adverse effects of elevated glucose on lipid profile. However, long-term metformin treatment for 30 days reduced these levels. The beneficial lipid-lowering effects of metformin have been reported in diabetic rats (Nasrolahi et al. 2012). We have recently reported that long-term use of oral hypoglycemic agents significantly reduce triglyceride levels in diabetic men and LDL and HDL levels in diabetic women (Ghadge et al. 2014).

In the present study, flax oil and fish oil intervention normalized all lipid profile parameters at D30 as compared to those at D15. Several studies have reported triglyceride-lowering effects of dietary fish oil (Bremer et al. 2014; Hartweg et al. 2008) which have been primarily attributed to EPA and DHA (Skulas-Ray et al. 2011; Egert et al. 2009). The present study indicated activation of PPAR and modulation of SREBP1 in the animals treated with n-3 PUFA which are known to be the main mechanisms for a lipid-normalizing action of omega-3 fatty acids (Devarshi et al. 2013).

Modulation of lipid metabolism genes by n-3 PUFA intervention

In the present study, STZ induction markedly reduced the expression of PPAR and increased SREBP1 expression

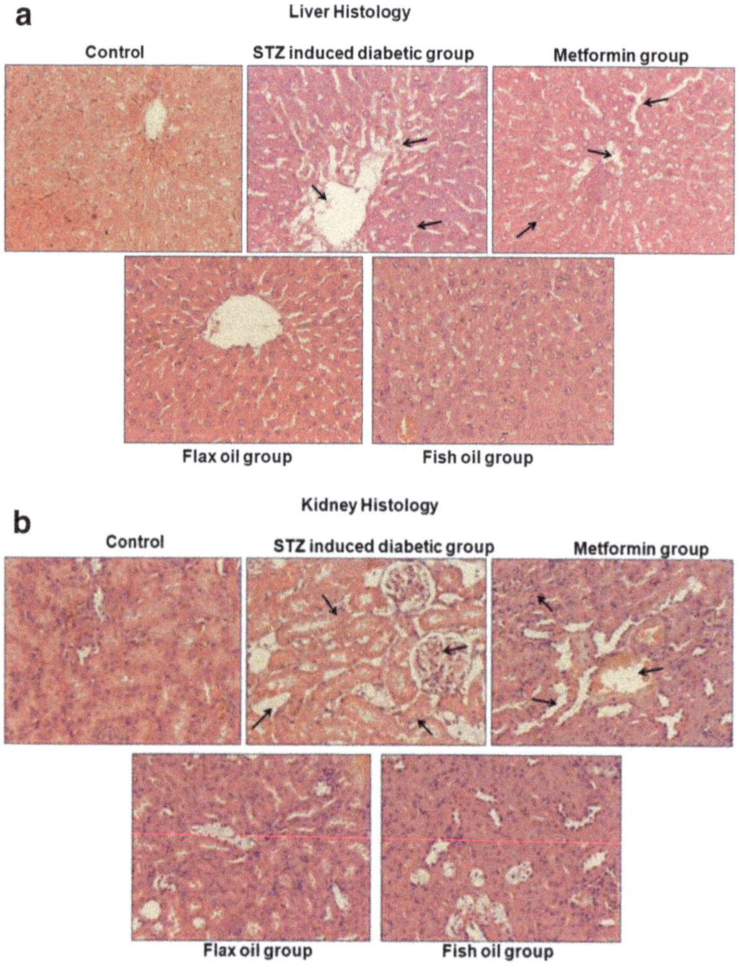

Fig. 3 a Liver histology of control, STZ-induced diabetic, metformin-treated, and flax/fish oil-treated animals. Hematoxylin and eosin-stained cross sections of paraffin-embedded liver tissues of rats from the control and experimental groups (×40). Liver from the control group shows normal architecture. Sections of the liver from the STZ-induced diabetic group show severe destruction of hepatic cells, pathological calcification, hemorrhages, and mild mononuclear cells in the portal tracts. Liver from the metformin-treated group shows some destructive changes and congestion of some central vein. The liver histology of animals treated with flax oil and fish oil shows completely normal liver architecture without any anatomically detectable anomalies. **b** Kidney histology of healthy, STZ-induced diabetic, metformin-treated, and flax/fish oil-treated animals. Hematoxylin and eosin-stained cross sections of paraffin-embedded kidney tissues of rats from the control and experimental groups (×40). Kidney from the control group shows normal kidney architecture. Sections of kidney from the STZ diabetic group showed conjunction of glomerular capillary and blood vesicle. Some tubular epithelial cells show vacuolation and cloudy changes. Kidney from the metformin-treated group shows vacuolation of some tubular epithelial cells and conjunction of glomerular capillary. The liver histology of animals treated with flax and fish oil shows no considerable changes and show normal architecture

which was restored by metformin as well as by fish oil (Fig. 2b). Metformin treatment is known to regulate incretin receptor axis via PPAR-dependent pathway in mice (Maida et al. 2011) and reduce SREBP expression by regulating AMP-activated protein kinase activity in rats (Zhou et al. 2001). Metformin has been shown to reduce fat content by decreasing the expression of SREBP1 and FAS (involved in fatty acid synthesis) in rat kidneys (Wang et al. 2006). A recent study reports reduction in PPAR expression and increase in SREBP expression in diabetic rats which was restored by dietary fish and flax oil supplementation (Devarshi et al. 2013). n-3 PUFA and their metabolites act as natural ligands for PPAR, promoting fatty acid oxidation and suppressing the transcription of lipogenic genes like FAS (Teran-Garcia et al. 2007).

ACSL, catalyzing the thioesterification of fatty acids, is a target of PPAR and is implicated in the pathogenesis of diabetes (Phillips et al. 2010). Recent report suggests that ACSL plays an important role in triglyceride synthesis (Yan et al. 2015). In the present study, STZ-treated animals showed significantly higher ACSL expression with high triglyceride levels. However, metformin and flax and fish oil interventions lowered the expression and consequently had significantly lower triglyceride levels. Metformin has been shown to lower ACSL expression and triglyceride levels in diabetic rats (Forcheron et al. 2009). Besides triglyceride synthesis by ACSL, MCAT, a mitochondrial protein, catalyzes transfer of CoA moiety to free thiol group on the acyl carrier protein in mitochondria, indicating its role in mitochondrial fatty acid synthesis (Zhang et al. 2003). Lower expression of MCAT along with ACSL has beneficial effects in normalizing the fatty acid and triglyceride levels (Li et al. 2009; Zhang et al. 2003). In the present study also, metformin and flax and fish oil showed reduced MCAT expression indicating lower fatty acid synthesis and normal lipid profile (Fig. 2b).

Modulation of inflammatory cytokine genes by n-3 PUFA intervention

T2DM is a chronic inflammatory disease where transcription factor NFkβ activates the transcription of inflammatory cytokines like TNFα increasing the risk of secondary complications owing to their pro-atherogenic nature (Jagannathan-Bogdan et al. 2011). In the present study, NFkβ expression was higher in the STZ group which was significantly lowered by flax and fish oil (Fig. 2b). However, TNFα expression was not significantly altered in the STZ group and treatment groups. Hyperglycemia-induced NFkβ activation in ex vivo isolated PBMCs has been reported in type 1 diabetic patients (Hofmann et al. 1998). Metformin administration has also been shown to downregulate the expression of NFkβ and TNFα and ameliorate β-cell dysfunction (Liu et al. 2014) in diabetes. Recent review highlights the role of n-3 PUFA in reducing TNFα expression (Ellulu et al. 2015).

Effect of n-3 PUFA intervention on liver function test markers

In the present study, SGPT and ALP levels were higher in the STZ group at D15 while ALP remained higher at D30 as compared to that in the control group. There are reports indicating hepatic dysfunction due to higher levels of liver enzymes such as SGPT, SGOT, and ALP in STZ-induced diabetic rats (Sajitha et al. 2012). We have recently reported higher serum SGPT and bilirubin levels in diabetic male subjects and SGPT levels in diabetic female subjects (Ghadge et al. 2015). The biochemical alterations in the hepatic function markers observed in the present study were also associated with destructive changes in hepatocytes and accumulation of lipid droplets.

In this study, metformin treatment did not affect other markers. In contrast, a study in diabetic rats treated with metformin is reported to have elevated bilirubin levels (Nasrolahi et al. 2012). Liver section analysis of these animals displayed destruction of some hepatocytes and congestion of the central vein. A recent study reported mild granular degeneration, mild swelling (narrow sinusoidal capillaries), and normal hepatic architecture in the metformin-treated diabetic rats (Motshakeri et al. 2014). Some case report studies also demonstrated that metformin induces hepatotoxicity in diabetic subjects raising concern about its efficacy and safety profile (Miralles-Linares et al. 2012; Cone et al. 2010).

Hepatoprotective effects of n-3 PUFA in chemically induced hepatotoxicity have been reported earlier from our laboratory (Chavan et al. 2013). In the present study, flax and fish oil intervention showed progressive effects in lowering ALP levels at D30 as compared to D15. Additionally, both of these groups exhibited normal hepatic architecture and displayed significant recovery of destructive changes.

Effect of n-3 PUFA on renal function test markers

Serum urea levels were higher in the STZ group at D15 as compared to those in the control group. Although renal function test markers at D30 were comparable to those of the control group, STZ induction still affected kidney histology and are consistent with other reports (Ahmed et al. 2014; Zafar et al. 2009). The metformin group showed no significant changes in the renal function test markers against the STZ group. However, we observed vacuolation of tubular epithelial cells in some tubules and conjunction of glomerular capillary in metformin-treated group. Similar findings like moderate cellular hydropic degeneration, atrophied renal corpuscle, and mild congestion of glomerular capillaries were reported in metformin-treated diabetic rats (Motshakeri et al. 2014). Further, in the present study, fish oil treatment progressively lowered total protein levels at D30 as compared to those at D15. Flax and fish oil also showed normal kidney histology. Similarly, dietary flax and fish oil have shown to improve renal abnormalities in rats (Hassan et al. 2015; Velasquez et al. 2003).

Conclusion

In conclusion, the treatment with metformin and flax/fish oil intervention in diabetic rats improves serum lipid profile and the expression of transcription factors modulating lipid metabolism such as PPAR-γ and SREBP1 and lowers atherogenic cytokine like NFkβ. In the present study, flax oil and/or fish oil exhibited hepatoprotective and nephroprotective effects under uncontrolled hyperglycemic states. The combination therapy of metformin and n-3 PUFA intervention is worth investigating in T2DM subjects.

Competing interests

The authors have no conflict of interest in connection with the contents of this article.

Authors' contributions

AG performed the experiments, analyzed the data and wrote the manuscript. AH participated in the design and coordination of the study. MK performed histological examinations of the tissue sections and analyzed the histological differences among the study groups. VP participated in the design and coordination of the study. AK conceived, designed and coordinated the study, analyzed the data and wrote the manuscript. All authors read and approved the final manuscript.

Acknowledgements

Authors are thankful to Bharati Vidyapeeth Deemed University for financial support. We gratefully acknowledge Dr. Yogesh Shouche, Microbial Culture Collection (MCC), National Center for Cell Science (NCCS), Pune, for providing the qRT-PCR facility. Authors are also thankful to Prof. Prabhakar Ranjekar, Ex-Director, Interactive Research School for Health Affairs (IRSHA), Bharati Vidyapeeth Deemed University, Pune, for his valuable suggestions.

Author details

[1]Nutrigenomics and Functional Foods Laboratory, Interactive Research School for Health Affairs (IRSHA), Bharati Vidyapeeth Deemed University, Pune-Satara Road, Pune, Maharashtra 411043, India. [2]Department of Pathology, Bharati Vidyapeeth Medical College, Bharati Vidyapeeth Deemed University, Pune-Satara Road, Pune, Maharashtra 411043, India. [3]Department of Pharmacology, Bharati Vidyapeeth Medical College, Bharati Vidyapeeth Deemed University, Pune-Satara Road, Pune, Maharashtra 411043, India.

References

Ahmed D, Kumar V, Verma A, Gupta PS, Kumar H, Dhingra V, Mishra V, Sharma M (2014) Antidiabetic, renal/hepatic/pancreas/cardiac protective and antioxidant potential of methanol/dichloromethane extract of albizzia lebbeck benth. Stem bark (alex) on streptozotocin induced diabetic rats. BMC Complement Altern Med 14:243. doi:10.1186/1472-6882-14-243

Alhaider AA, Korashy HM, Sayed-Ahmed MM, Mobark M, Kfoury H, Mansour MA (2011) Metformin attenuates streptozotocin-induced diabetic nephropathy in rats through modulation of oxidative stress genes expression. Chem Biol Interact 192(3):233–242. doi:10.1016/j.cbi.2011.03.014

Ander BP, Dupasquier CMC, Prociuk MA, Pierce GN (2003) Polyunsaturated fatty acids and their effects on cardiovascular disease. Exp Clin Cardiol 8(4):164–172

Bremer AA, Stanhope KL, Graham JL, Cummings BP, Ampah SB, Saville BR, Havel PJ (2014) Fish oil supplementation ameliorates fructose-induced hyperTG mia and insulin resistance in adult male rhesus macaques. J Nutr 144(1):5–11. doi:10.3945/jn.113.178061

Brenna O, Qvigstad G, Brenna E, Waldum HL (2003) Cytotoxicity of streptozotocin on neuroendocrine cells of the pancreas and the gut. Dig Dis Sci 48(5):906–910. doi:10.1023/A:1023043411483

Calder PC (2007) Immunomodulation by omega-3 fatty acids. Prostaglandins Leukot Essent Fatty Acids 77(5-6):327–335. doi:10.1016/j.plefa.2007.10.015

Chavan T, Khadke S, Harke S, Ghadge A, Karandikar M, Pandit V, Ranjekar P, Kulkarni O, Kuvalekar A (2013) Hepatoprotective effect of polyunsaturated fatty acids against repeated subacute acetaminophen dosing in rats. Int J Pharm Bio Sci 4(2):286–295

Cone CJ, Bachyrycz AM, Murata GH (2010) Hepatotoxicity associated with metformin therapy in treatment of type 2 diabetes mellitus with nonalcoholic fatty liver disease. Ann Pharmacother 44(10):1655–1659. doi:10.1345/aph.1P099

Connor WE (2000) Importance of n-3 fatty acids in health and disease. Am J Clin Nutr 71(1):171–175

Cummings BP, Stanhope KL, Graham JL, Griffen SC, Havel PJ (2010) Supplementation with EPA or fish oil for 11 months lowers circulating lipids, but does not delay the onset of diabetes in UC Davis-type 2 diabetes mellitus rats. Br J Nutr 104(11):1628–1634. doi:10.1017/S0007114510002655

Dessì M, Noce A, Bertucci P, di Villahermosa SM, Zenobi R, Castagnola V, Addessi E, Di Daniele N (2013) Atherosclerosis, dyslipidemia, and inflammation: the significant role of polyunsaturated fatty acids. ISRN Inflamm 2013:191823. doi:10.1155/2013/191823

Devarshi PP, Jangale NM, Ghule AE, Bodhankar SL, Harsulkar AM (2013) Beneficial effects of flaxseed oil and fish oil diet are through modulation of different hepatic genes involved in lipid metabolism in streptozotocin-nicotinamide induced diabetic rats. Genes Nutr 8(3):329–342. doi:10.1007/s12263-012-0326-2

Di Minno MN, Russolillo A, Lupoli R, Ambrosino P, Di Minno A, Tarantino G (2012) Omega-3 fatty acids for the treatment of non-alcoholic fatty liver disease. World J Gastroenterol 18(41):5839–5847. doi:10.3748/wjg.v18.i41.5839

Egert S, Kannenberg F, Somoza V, Erbersdobler HF, Wahrburg U (2009) Dietary alpha-linolenic acid, EPA, and DHA have differential effects on LDL fatty acid composition but similar effects on serum lipid profiles in normolipidemic humans. J Nutr 139(5):861–868. doi:10.3945/jn.108.103861

Ellulu MS, Khaza'ai H, Abed Y, Rahmat A, Ismail P, Ranneh Y (2015) Role of fish oil in human health and possible mechanism to reduce the inflammation. Inflammopharmacology 23(2-3):79–89. doi:10.1007/s10787-015-0228-1

Erejuwa OO, Sulaiman SA, Wahab MS, Sirajudeen KN, Salleh MS, Gurtu S (2011) Glibenclamide or metformin combined with honey improves glycemic control in streptozotocin-induced diabetic rats. Int J Biol Sci 7(2):244–252. doi:10.7150/ijbs.7.244

Erejuwa OO, Sulaiman SA, Wahab MS (2012) Honey- a novel antidiabetic agent. Int J Biol Sci 8(6):913–934. doi:10.7150/ijbs.3697

Forbes JM, Cooper ME (2013) Mechanisms of diabetic complications. Physiol Rev 93(1):137–188. doi:10.1152/physrev.00045.2011

Forcheron F, Basset A, Abdallah P, Del Carmine P, Gadot N, Beylot M (2009) Diabetic cardiomyopathy: effects of fenofibrate and metformin in an experimental model the Zucker diabetic rat. Cardiovasc Diabetol 8:16. doi:10.1186/1475-2840-8-16

Gaines TA, Zhang W, Wang D, Bukun B, Chisholm ST, Shaner DL, Nissen SJ, Patzoldt WL, Tranel PJ, Culpepper AS, Grey TL, Webster TM, Vencill WK, Sammons RD, Jiang J, Preston C, Leach JE, Westra P (2010) Gene amplification confers glyphosate resistance in Amaranthus palmeri. Proc Natl Acad Sci U S A 107(3):1029–1034. doi:10.1073/pnas.0906649107

Ghadge AA, Harke SM, Khadke SP, Diwan AG, Pankaj M, Kulkarni OP, Ranjekar PK, Kuvalekar AA (2014) Circulatory adipocytokines and lipid profile variations in type-2 diabetic subjects: desirable side-effects of antidiabetic drugs. Diabetes Metab Syndr 8(4):230–232. doi:10.1016/j.dsx.2014.09.010

Ghadge A, Harke S, Khadke S, Diwan A, Pankaj M, Kulkarni O, Ranjekar P, Harsulkar A, Kuvalekar AA (2015) Effects of commonly used antidiabetic drugs on antioxidant enzymes and liver function test markers in type 2 diabetes mellitus subjects—pilot study. Exp Clin Endocrinol Diabetes 123(8):500–507. doi:10.1055/s-0035-1554654

Hartweg J, Perera R, Montori V, Dinneen S, Neil HA, Farmer A (2008) Omega-3 polyunsaturated fatty acids (PUFA) for type 2 diabetes mellitus. Cochrane Database Syst Rev 1:Cd003205. doi:10.1002/14651858.CD003205

Hassan HA, Edrees GM, El-Gamel EM, El-Sayed EA (2015) Proanthocyanidin and fish oil potent activity against cisplatin-induced renal cell cycle arrest and apoptosis in rats. Ren Fail 37(8):1356–1362. doi:10.3109/0886022X.2015.1073528

Hendrich S (2010) (n-3) fatty acids: clinical trials in people with type 2 diabetes. Adv Nutr 1(1):3–7. doi:10.3945/an.110.1003

Hofmann MA, Schiekofer S, Kanitz M, Klevesath MS, Joswig M, Lee V, Morcos M, Tritschler H, Ziegler R, Wahl P, Bierhaus A, Nawroth PP (1998) Insufficient glycemic control increases nuclear factor-kappa B binding activity in peripheral blood mononuclear cells isolated from patients with type 1 diabetes. Diabetes Care 21(8):1310–1316. doi:10.2337/diacare.21.8.1310

Howarth FC, Jacobson M, Shafiullah M, Adeghate E (2005) Long-term effects of streptozotocin-induced diabetes on the electrocardiogram, physical activity and body temperature in rats. Exp Physiol 90(6):827–835. doi:10.1113/expphysiol.2005.031252

Jagannathan-Bogdan M, McDonnell ME, Shin H, Rehman Q, Hasturk H, Apovian CM, Nikolajczyk BS (2011) Elevated proinflammatory cytokine production by a skewed T cell compartment requires monocytes and promotes inflammation in type 2 diabetes. J Immunol 186(2):1162–1172. doi:10.4049/jimmunol.1002615

Jangale NM, Devarshi PP, Dubal AA, Ghule AE, Koppikar SJ, Bodhankar SL, Chougale AD, Kulkarni MJ, Harsulkar AM (2013) Dietary flaxseed oil and fish oil modulates expression of antioxidant and inflammatory genes with alleviation of protein glycation status and inflammation in liver of streptozotocin-nicotinamide induced diabetic rats. Food Chem 141(1):187–195. doi:10.1016/j.foodchem.2013.03.001

King GL (2008) The role of inflammatory cytokines in diabetes and its complications. J Periodontol 79(8):1527–1534. doi:10.1902/jop.2008.080246

Konieczna J, Sanchez J, van Schothorst EM, Torrens JM, Bunschoten A, Palou M, Pico C, Keijer J, Palou A (2014) Identification of early transcriptome-based biomarkers related to lipid metabolism in peripheral blood mononuclear cells of rats nutritionally programmed for improved metabolic health. Genes Nutr 9(1):366. doi:10.1007/s12263-013-0366-2

Kooy A, de Jager J, Lehert P, Bets D, Wulffelé MG, Donker AJ, Stehouwer CD (2009) Long-term effects of metformin on metabolism and microvascular and macrovascular disease in patients with type 2 diabetes mellitus. Arch Intern Med 169(6):616–625. doi:10.1001/archinternmed.2009.20

Li LO, Ellis JM, Paich HA, Wang S, Gong N, Altshuller G, Thresher RJ, Koves TR, Watkins M, Muoio DM, Cline GW, Shulman GI, Coleman RA (2009) Liver-specific loss of long chain acyl-CoA synthetase-1 decreases triacylglycerol synthesis and betaoxidation and alters phospholipid fatty acid composition. J Biol Chem 284(41):27816–27826. doi:10.1074/jbc.M109.022467

Li HT, Wu XD, Davey AK, Wang J (2011) Antihyperglycemic effects of baicalin on streptozotocin - nicotinamide induced diabetic rats. Phytother Res 25(2):189–194. doi:10.1002/ptr.3238

Liu J, Ma DWL (2014) The role of n-3 polyunsaturated fatty acids in the prevention and treatment of breast cancer. Nutrients 6(11):5184–5223. doi:10.3390/nu6115184

Liu SN, Liu Q, Sun SJ, Hou SC, Wang Y, Shen ZF (2014) Metformin ameliorates beta-cell dysfunction by regulating inflammation production, ion and hormone homeostasis of pancreas in diabetic KKAy mice. Yao Xue Xue Bao 49(11):1554–1562

Maheshwari RA, Balaraman R, Sen AK, Seth AK (2014) Effect of coenzyme Q10 alone and its combination with metformin on streptozotocin-nicotinamide-induced diabetic nephropathy in rats. Indian J Pharmacol 46(6):627–632. doi:10.4103/0253-7613.144924

Maida A, Lamont BJ, Cao X, Drucker DJ (2011) Metformin regulates the incretin receptor axis via a pathway dependent on peroxisome proliferator-activated receptor-alpha in mice. Diabetologia 54(2):339–349. doi:10.1007/s00125-010-1937-z

Miralles-Linares F, Puerta-Fernandez S, Bernal-Lopez MR, Tinahones FJ, Andrade RJ, Gomez-Huelgas R (2012) Metformin-induced hepatotoxicity. Diabetes Care 35, e21. doi:10.2337/dc11-2306

Mohammadi J, Delaviz H, Malekzadeh JM, Roozbehi A (2012) The effect of hydro alcoholic extract of Juglans regia leaves in streptozotocin-nicotinamide induced diabetic rats. Pak J Pharm Sci 25(2):407–411

Motshakeri M, Ebrahimi M, Goh YM, Othman HH, Hair-Bejo M, Mohamed S (2014) (2014) effects of brown seaweed (sargassum polycystum) extracts on kidney, liver, and pancreas of type 2 diabetic rat model. Evid Based Complement Alternat Med 2014:379407. doi:10.1155/2014/379407

Mozaffarian D, Wu JHY (2012) (n-3) fatty acids and cardiovascular health: are effects of EPA and DHA shared or complementary? J Nutr 142(3):614–625. doi:10.3945/jn.111.149633

Nasrolahi O, Heidari R, Rahmani F, Farokhi F (2012) Effect of natural honey from Ilam and metformin for improving glycemic control in streptozotocin-induced diabetic rats. Avicenna J Phytomed 2(4):212–221

Nettleton JA, Katz R (2005) n-3 long-chain polyunsaturated fatty acids in type 2 diabetes: a review. J Am Diet Assoc 105(3):428–440. doi:10.1016/j.jada.2004.11.029

Ozder A (2014) Lipid profile abnormalities seen in t2dm patients in primary healthcare in turkey: a cross-sectional study. Lipids Health Dis 13:183. doi:10.1186/1476-511x-13-183

Pari L, Saravanan R (2007) Beneficial effect of succinic acid monoethyl ester on erythrocyte membrane bound enzymes and antioxidant status in streptozotocin-nicotinamide induced type 2 diabetes. Chem Biol Interact 169(1):15–24. doi:10.1016/j.cbi.2007.04.010

Phillips CM, Goumidi L, Bertrais S, Field MR, Cupples LA, Ordovas JM, Defoort C, Lovegrove JA, Drevon CA, Gibney MJ, Blaak EE, Kiec-Wilk B, Karlstrom B, Lopez-Miranda J, McManus R, Hercberg S, Lairon D, Planells R, Roche HM (2010) Gene-nutrient interactions with dietary fat modulate the association between genetic variation of the ACSL1 gene and metabolic syndrome. J Lipid Res 51(7):1793–1800. doi:10.1194/jlr.M003046

Prabhakar PK, Prasad R, Ali S, Doble M (2013) Synergistic interaction of ferulic acid with commercial hypoglycemic drugs in streptozotocin induced diabetic rats. Phytomedicine 20(6):488–494. doi:10.1016/j.phymed.2012

Rojas LB, Gomes MB (2013) Metformin: an old but still the best treatment for type 2 diabetes. Diabetol Metab Syndr 5(1):6. doi:10.1186/1758-5996-5-6

Saadi T, Waterman M, Yassin H, Baruch Y (2013) Metformin-induced mixed hepatocellular and cholestatic hepatic injury: case report and literature review. Int J Gen Med 6:703–706. doi:10.2147/IJGM.S49657

Sajitha PC, Punitha D, Danya U, Udhayasankar MR, Baluprakash T, Arumugasamy K (2012) Antidiabetic activity of Anisochillus dysophylloides wall. ex Benth. (lamiaceae) in streptozotocin induced type II diabetes in male wistar albino rats. International Journal of Plant Animal and Environmental Sciences 2(4):40–43

Salama RM, Schaalan MF, Elkoussi AA, Khalifa AE (2013) Potential utility of sodium selenate as an adjunct to metformin in treating type II diabetes mellitus in rats: a perspective on protein tyrosine phosphatase. Biomed Res Int 2013:231378. doi:10.1155/2013/231378

Saravanan R, Pari L (2007) Succinic acid monoethyl ester, a novel insulinotropic agent: effect on lipid composition and lipid peroxidation in streptozotocin-nicotin-amide induced type 2 diabetic rats. Mol Cell Biochem 296(1-2):165–176. doi:10.1007/s11010-006-9312-6

Sharma AK, Sharma A, Kumari R, Kishore K, Sharma D, Srinivasan BP, Sharma A, Singh SK, Gaur S, Jatav VS, Sharma P, Srivastava V, Joshi S, Joshi M, Dhakad PK, Kanawat DS, Mishra A, Sharma A, Singh D, Singh RP, Chawda HS, Singh R, Raikwar SK, Kurmi MK, Khatri P, Agarwal A, Munajjam A (2012) Sitagliptin, sitagliptin and metformin, or sitagliptin and amitriptyline attenuate streptozotocin-nicotinamide induced diabetic neuropathy in rats. J Biomed Res 26(3):200–210. doi:10.7555/JBR.26.20110054

Skulas-Ray AC, Kris-Etherton PM, Harris WS, Vanden Heuvel JP, Wagner PR, West SG (2011) Dose response effects of omega-3 fatty acids on triglycerides, inflammation, and endothelial function in healthy persons with moderate hypertriglyceridemia. Am J Clin Nutr 93(2):243–252. doi:10.3945/ajcn.110.003871

Swanson D, Block R, Mousa SA (2012) Omega-3 fatty acids EPA and DHA: health benefits throughout life. Adv Nutr 3(1):1–7. doi:10.3945/an.111.000893

Szkudelski T (2012) Streptozotocin-nicotinamide-induced diabetes in the rat. Characteristics of the experimental model. Exp Biol Med (Maywood) 237(5):481–490. doi:10.1258/ebm.2012.011372

Teran-Garcia M, Adamson AW, Yu G, Rufo C, Suchankova G, Dreesen TD, Tekle M, Clarke SD, Gettys TW (2007) Polyunsaturated fatty acid suppression of fatty acid synthase (FASN): evidence for dietary modulation of NF-Y binding to the Fasn promoter by SREBP-1c. Biochem J 402(3):591–600. doi:10.1042/BJ20061722

Velasquez T, Bhathena SJ, Ranich T, Schwartz AM, Kardon DE, Ali AA, Haudenschild CC, Hansen CT (2003) Dietary flaxseed meal reduces proteinuria and ameliorates nephropathy in an animal model of type II diabetes mellitus. Kidney Int 64(6):2100–2107. doi:10.1046/j.1523-1755.2003.00329.x

Wang W, Guo XH, Wu HH, Wang NH, Xu XS (2006) Effect of fenofibrate and metformin on lipotoxicity in OLETF rat kidney. Beijing Da Xue Xue Bao 38(2):170–175

Wang C, Liu F, Yuan Y, Wu J, Wang H, Zhang L, Hu P, Li Z, Li Q, Ye J (2014) Metformin suppresses lipid accumulation in skeletal muscle by promoting fatty acid oxidation. Clin Lab 60(6):887–896

Woodman RJ, Mori TA, Burke V, Puddey IB, Watts GF, Beilin LJ (2002) Effects of purified eicosapentaenoic and docosahexaenoic acids on glycemic control, blood pressure, and serum lipids in type 2 diabetic patients with treated hypertension. Am J Clin Nutr 76(5):1007–1015

Wu JH, Micha R, Imamura F, Pan A, Biggs ML, Ajaz O, Djousse L, Hu FB, Mozaffarian D (2012) Omega-3 fatty acids and incident type 2 diabetes: a systematic review and meta-analysis. Br J Nutr 107(2):214–227. doi:10.1017/S0007114512001602

Yan S, Yang XF, Liu HL, Fu N, Ouyang Y, Qing K (2015) Long-chain acyl-CoA synthetase in fatty acid metabolism involved in liver and other diseases: an update. World J Gastroenterol 21(12):3492–3498. doi:10.3748/wjg.v21.i12.3492

Zafar M, Naqvi SN-u-H, Ahmed M, Kaimkhani ZA (2009) Altered kidney morphology and enzymes in streptozotocin induced diabetic rats. Int J Morphol 27(3):783–790

Zhang L, Joshi AK, Smith S (2003) Cloning, expression, characterization, and interaction of two components of a human mitochondrial fatty acid synthase. Malonyltransferase and acyl carrier protein. J Biol Chem 278(41):40067–40074. doi:10.1074/jbc.M306121200

Zheng J, Woo SL, Hu X, Botchlett R, Chen L, Huo Y, Wu C (2015) Metformin and metabolic diseases: a focus on hepatic aspects. Front Med. doi:10.1007/s11684-015-0384-0

Zhou G, Myers R, Li Y, Chen Y, Shen X, Fenyk-Melody J, Wu M, Ventre J, Doebber T, Fujii N, Musi N, Hirshman MF, Goodyear LJ, Moller DE (2001) Role of AMP-activated protein kinase in mechanism of metformin action. J Clin Invest 108(8):1167–1174. doi:10.1172/JCI13505

7

A porcine gluteus medius muscle genome-wide transcriptome analysis: dietary effects of omega-6 and omega-3 fatty acids on biological mechanisms

Magdalena Ogłuszka[1], Agnieszka Szostak[1], Marinus F. W. te Pas[2], Ewa Poławska[1], Paweł Urbański[1], Tadeusz Blicharski[1], Chandra S. Pareek[3], Edyta Juszczuk-Kubiak[1], Jenelle R. Dunkelberger[4], Jarosław O. Horbańczuk[1] and Mariusz Pierzchała[1*]

Abstract

Background: The level of omega-6 and omega-3 polyunsaturated fatty acids can affect many cellular systems and function via nuclear receptors or the bioactive lipid regulation of gene expression. The objective of this study was to investigate changes in the muscle transcriptome and the biological functions regulated by increased consumption of omega-3 and omega-6 fatty acids in the pig gluteus medius muscle.

Results: The transcriptome of the gluteus medius muscle was studied for pigs subjected to either a control diet or a diet supplemented with linseed and rapeseed oil to increase polyunsaturated fatty acid content. Next-generation sequencing (NGS) was used to generate the muscle tissue transcriptome database pointing differentially expressed genes (DEG). Comparative expression analyses identified 749 genes significantly differing at least in the twofold of change between two groups of animals fed with divergent level of omega-3 and omega-6 fatty acids. The expression of 219 genes was upregulated, and the expression of 530 genes was downregulated in the group of pigs supplemented with omega-3 and omega-6 fatty acids in relation to control group pigs. Results of RNA-seq indicated a role of fatty acid in the regulation of the expression of genes which are essential for muscle tissue development and functioning. Functional analysis revealed that the identified genes were important for a number of biological processes including inflammatory response, signaling, lipid metabolism, and homeostasis.

Conclusions: Summarizing, obtained results provide strong evidence that omega-6 and omega-3 fatty acids regulate fundamental metabolic processes in muscle tissue development and functioning.

Keywords: Gluteus medius muscle, Omega-3 fatty acid, Omega-6 fatty acid, Pig, Transcriptome

Background

The expression of animal genes can be modified in response to environmental factors. One such factor is feed, especially the composition of its bioactive dietary components [1]. The newly emerging field of nutrigenomics investigates the relationship between dietary components and genomic expression profiles [2]. Recently, nutrigenomic research has focused much attention on omega-6 and omega-3 fatty acids.

Omega-6 and omega-3 fatty acids are polyunsaturated fatty acids (PUFA), which belong to the essential fatty acid family and must be obtained from food sources [3]. Mammals can, however, metabolize PUFA by utilizing the omega-6 and omega-3 fatty acid conversion pathways to synthesize other omega fatty acids (i.e., arachidonic acid from linoleic acid (LA), as well as eicosapentaenoic acid and docosahexaenoic acid from alpha-linolenic acid (ALA)) [4]. Omega-6 and omega-3 fatty acids modulate gene expression and provide substrates for the production

* Correspondence: m.pierzchala@ighz.pl
[1]Institute of Genetics and Animal Breeding of the Polish Academy of Sciences, Postępu 36A, 05-552 Jastrzębiec, Poland
Full list of author information is available at the end of the article

of signaling molecules or functioning mediators [5]. Additionally, a correct balance of these fatty acids is important for the proper function and development of various cell types [6]. Presence of omega-6 and omega-3 fatty acids and maintaining their optimal ratio in the diet helps to prevent the development of metabolic diseases, such as heart attacks, atherosclerosis, thrombosis, arrhythmia, stroke, immune-inflammatory disorders, asthma, arthritis, cancer proliferation, type II diabetes mellitus, obesity, and psychiatric disorders [7]. Although PUFA are known to have significant biological roles, their mechanisms are not well understood.

Fatty acids are an important cellular component and serve as a source of energy for animals [8]. A major site of fatty acid catabolism in mammals is the skeletal muscle [9]. In fact, it has been suggested that PUFA content can modulate both the function and metabolism of the skeletal muscle. The effect of PUFA on the skeletal muscle also has the potential to substantially impact whole body functioning [10]. PUFA content is important for muscle tissue as well, regulating immunological, hormonal, and metabolic processes [11]. Gluteus medius muscle was selected as the target muscle tissue for this study due to its dynamic energy metabolism and role in independent gait [12]. The gluteus medius muscle contains IIb and IIx fibers as well as IIa (fast oxidative-glycolytic) fibers [13], which can switch between glycolytic and oxidative metabolism in reaction to accessibility of the fatty acids [14]. Although the immune-stimulating effects of PUFA have been studied for decades [15], knowledge of their integrative effects is limited. Therefore, the objective of this study was to investigate changes in the pig gluteus medius muscle transcriptome, including the regulated biological functions as a result of increased omega-3 and omega-6 fatty acid concentration. In our studies, we used pigs, which are one of the best models for studies on effects of omega-6 and omega-3 fatty acids supplementation. Moreover, they are a proven and recognized large animal model due to their anatomical and physiological similarities to humans. We hypothesize that supplementation of omega-6 and omega-3 fatty acids in the diet will modulate the expression of genes essential for muscle homeostasis.

Methods

Animals

Ethical clearance was obtained from the Local Ethics Commission for Experimentation on Animals in Warsaw (No 27/2009). Analyses were conducted on Polish Landrace. The breed was based on improved white German pig and was upgraded using German and Swedish national breeds. Unrelated female pigs ($n = 24$) were bred at a commercial farm and fed with a standard diet until pigs reached approximately 60 kg in body weight (105 ± 2 days of age). Pigs were then divided into two groups and fed with one of two diets until slaughter. Pigs fed with the control diet received a regular feed mixture (Table 1) of 268 mg of LA and 25 mg of ALA/100 g. Pigs fed with the experimental (supplemented) diet received additives of 1% rapeseed oil and 2% linseed oil to the standard diet in the form of 660 mg of LA and 64 mg of ALA/100 g. The fodder mixtures (identical to the fodders used in Szostak et al. [16]) were isocaloric (13 MJ EM per kg of mixture) and balanced according to the amino acid composition. Pigs were delivered to a commercial slaughterhouse at least 24 h prior to slaughter once they reached a body weight of approximately 110 kg (168 ± 2 days of age). Pigs were sacrificed by exsanguination after electrical stunning, reflecting industry standards. Gluteus medius muscle samples were taken immediately after slaughter, frozen in liquid nitrogen, and stored at −80 °C for further analysis.

Gas chromatography determination of the ratio of omega-6 to omega-3 fatty acid

Quantitative data for the ratio of omega-6 to omega-3 fatty acid in all gluteus medius muscle samples were obtained by gas chromatography using flame ionization detection (GC–FID) analysis. For each sample, 1 g of muscle tissue was homogenized and extracted with chloroform-methanol 2:1(*v*/*v*) according to Folch et al. [17]. Fatty acids were analyzed using a GC-7890 Agilent gas chromatograph (Agilent Technologies, Inc., Santa Clara, CA,) equipped with a 60-m capillary column (Hewlett-Packard-88, Agilent J&W GC Columns, Santa Clara, CA) with 0.25-mm inner diameter and coating thickness of 0.20 μm. Helium was used as a carrier gas at a flow rate of 50 mL min^{-1}. The injector and detector were both maintained at 260 °C. Column oven temperature was programmed to increase from 140 °C (held for 5 min) at a rate of 4 °C min^{-1} to 190 °C to 215 °C at a rate of 0.8 °C min^{-1}. Individual fatty acid peaks were identified by comparison with known reference methyl esters (Supelco 37 Component FAME Mix, 47885-U, Sigma-Aldrich Co. Warsaw, Poland) and expressed as a percentage of total fatty acid concentration [18].

Table 1 Composition of pigs diets

	Experimental diet	Control diet
Ingredient %		
Rapeseed meal	7.2	6.0
Soybean meal	9.2	9.0
Wheat	49.6	54.0
Barley	28.5	28.5
Linseed oil	2.0	0
Rapeseed oil	1.0	0
Other	2.5	2.5

RNA isolation

To prepare samples for next-generation sequencing [19], 20 mg of frozen tissue were pulverized with a mortar and pestle precooled with liquid nitrogen. The RNA was isolated using an mRNA extraction kit (RNeasy Fibrous Tissue Mini Kit—Qiagen, Crawley, UK) according to the manufacturer's recommendations. For real-time PCR, 20 mg of frozen tissue was homogenized in 800 μl of TRIzol reagent (Invitrogen, Carlsbad, CA) using tubes with ceramic beads on Magna Lyser (Roche Applied Science, Penzberg, Germany). The extracts of total cellular RNA were isolated from homogenate according to Chomczynski and Sacchi [20]. The concentration and purity of total RNA were checked using a UV-Vis spectrophotometer (Actgene, Piscataway, NJ) at 260 nm. The integrity of ribosomal RNA was evaluated electrophoretically on the Bioanalyser (Agilent Technologies Inc.). Only high-quality RNA isolates, characterized by an RNA integrity number greater than 7, were used for further analysis.

Next-generation sequencing

Equal amounts of total RNA of six randomly selected individuals per group were used to construct libraries for sequencing. The mRNA-Seq library was constructed and sequenced by Genomed (http://www.genomed.pl/, Poland) [21] in accordance with the manufacturer's instructions for the Illumina MiSeq2000 system (Illumina, Inc., San Diego, CA, USA). The TruSeq RNA Sample Pre Kit (Illumina Inc.) was used to construct the libraries. To remove rRNA, bead-based depletion was used. Libraries were synthetized twice from freshly prepared RNA pools (each pool contained material from six pigs) and were sequenced independently on the MiSeq high-throughput sequencing instrument with 150 paired-end sequencing. Obtained sequence reads were aligned to the Sus scrofa 10.2 genome (NCBI GenBank ID GCA_000003025.4). Preprocessing and mapping was performed using the CLC Genomics workbench (CLC bio, Denmark) and DNASTAR Lasergene Genomic Suite (DNASTAR, Inc., Madison, WI). The read mapping was conducted using the RNA-Seq analysis package default settings (mismatch cost 2, insertion cost 3, length fraction 0.8, similarity fraction 0.8, and maximum number of reads 1) within the CLC software. The number of mapped reads was normalized and measured in terms of reads per kilobase per million (RPKM) to determine transcript abundance. For this study, pooled sample was used in order to remove animal-specific differences, allowing for the general reaction mechanism to be highlighted (for comparison, see te Pas et al. [22] and Szostak et al. [16]). As there was a single sample comprised of pooled individuals, in each condition, genes with the highest expression variance were estimated by using the variance across the two conditions. This is known as a "blind" method of dispersion estimate. The analysis assumes that for most genes, there is no true differential expression and that a valid mean-variance relationship can be estimated from treating the two samples as if they were replicates what will lead to emergence of a minority of differentially abundant genes acting as outliers. This method results in overly strict statistical significance testing of differential gene expression [23]. Genes that showed at least a twofold change in expression between control and experimental group and had a t test P value ≤0.05 adjusted for false discovery rate (FDR) were considered for detailed functionally grouped network analysis using DAVID software and Cytoscape 3.2 ClueGO plugin.

Reverse transcription PCR

DNase digestion was performed with RQ1 RNase-free DNase (Promega Corp., Madison, WI) by incubating samples with DNase for 15 min at 20 °C. One microgram of total RNA was reverse transcribed into cDNA using oligo-dT primers and the Transcriptor First Strand cDNA Synthesis Kit (Roche Applied Science) following the manufacturer's recommendations.

Real-time PCR

To validate the NGS data, the expression level of 10 genes was analyzed using two-step quantitative real-time PCR. More pigs were used for validation and were subjected to the same conditions as those involved in NGS analysis: 12 pigs were fed with the experimental fodder and 12 pigs were fed with the control fodder. All samples were analyzed individually. Selected genes were differentially expressed between the two diet treatments. Expression was normalized to the topoisomerase (DNA) II beta (*TOP2B*) gene as an endogenous control, and intron-spanning primers were specifically designed to quantify target mRNA transcripts. Genes and their primers are presented in Table 2. All reactions were performed on the Light Cycler 480 (Roche Applied Science) using the SYBR Green methodology. The standard curve to determine efficiency of the real-time PCR reaction and the appropriate dilution of cDNA template were determined based on a serial dilution of pooled cDNA samples. Cycling conditions were as follows: 95 °C for 5 min followed by 50 cycles (95 °C for 10 s, 58 °C for 10 s, and 72 °C for 10 s). A melting curve was performed from 60 to 95 °C to check the specificity of the amplified product. Real-time PCR was achieved on RNA samples from individual animals. Gene expression levels were calculated using the linear regression method for analyzing real-time PCR data [24]. To determine relative genes expression for independent samples, the bilateral Student t test was used; P value <0.05 was considered as significant.

Table 2 Real-time PCR primer

Gene symbol	Description	Forward primer	Reverse primer	Product length (bp)
TTR	Transthyretin	CTACTGGAAGGCACTTGGCA	AGGGCTGTGGTGGAGTAAGA	132
APOC3	Apolipoprotein C-III	AGGACACCTCCCTTCTGGAC	GTCGGTGAACTTGCCCTTGA	179
RBP4	Retinol-binding protein 4	CGGACTATGACACCTACGCC	GTGACACCCTCCATGTTGCT	245
ADAM19	ADAM metallopeptidase domain 19	AGTTTACGAACCAGACCAAGAA	GCATAATCAGCCACAAGGTAAAG	97
FADS1	Fatty acid desaturase 1	CGTGATTGACCGGAAGGTGT	TAGTCGGTTCAAAGCTGGGC	203
FADS2	Fatty acid desaturase 2	GCGCAGATGCCTACCTTT	TAAATCAAGGTCGCGGTGGAA	198
ADORA1	Adenosine A1 receptor	CCTCTTCCTCTTTGCCCTTAC	GTAGATGAGGATGCTGGACTTG	97
CASQ1	Calsequestrin 1	CCAACAGCGAAGAGGAGATT	TCCTCCCAGGTCTCATACATAC	97
MAPK1	Mitogen-activated protein kinase 1	CCCTCACAAGAGGATTGAAGTAG	GGCTCATCACTTGGGTCATAA	78
FADD	Fas (TNFRSF6)-associated via death domain	GGGCGGGAAGTGTTTGATT	CTCCCTGGCCAATTCTGTTATG	83
CCL4	C-C motif chemokine ligand 4	GCAAGACCATGAAGCTCTGC	AAGCTTCCGCACGGTGTATG	137
TOP2B	Topoisomerase (DNA) II beta	AACTGGATGATGCTAATGATGCT	TGGAAAAACTCCGTATCTGTCTC	464

Functional bioinformatics analysis

DAVID analysis

Differentially expressed genes (DEG) that showed at least a twofold change in expression between control and experimental group and had a *t* test *P* value ≤0.05 adjusted for FDR were selected for DAVID analysis (The Database for Annotation, Visualization, and Integrated Discovery: https://david.ncifcrf.gov/ [25]). DAVID software calculates *P* values for the enrichment of the number of genes in biological mechanisms. These *P* values indicate the importance of the general biological mechanisms active in all animals but do not indicate the inter-individual differences. All DEG were analyzed. The gene list was transferred to NCBI's ENTREZ search engine of cross-database, which recognized 493 unique gene names. Of these 493 genes, 481 of the gene IDs were transferred to human gene IDs, to compensate for poor pig gene annotation. Further analyses were performed using the total human genome as a background. An error rate of 0.05 was assumed significant according to the Benjamini and Hochberg multiple test correction method, and a FDR less than 5% was applied.

Cytoscape analysis

To further elucidate the biological relevance of the DEG, a functional enrichment analysis was performed using ClueGO software, a Cytoscape 3.1.0 plug-in (Institute for Genomics and Bioinformatics, Graz University of Technology, Graz, Austria) [26]. ClueGO facilitates the visualization of functionally related genes by displaying the genes as a clustered network and chart. The statistical test used to determine the enrichment score for terms and groups was based on a right-sided hypergeometric distribution option with a Benjamini-Hochberg correction. A kappa statistic was calculated to determine the strength of the connection between the terms in the network, based on similarity of associated genes [26]. To obtain complex, clear, and readable networks, various kappa scores were applied. The kappa score was preset to 0.9 for analyses covering a complete list of genes. A minimum level of 7 and a maximum level of 15 were set as the GO level interval with a minimum of two genes per category.

Results

Phenotype parameters

There were no significant differences in carcass nor meat quality traits between pigs of the two dietary groups. For animals from the experimental group, we observed a tendency in the reduction of backfat thickness and fodder intake.

The effect of dietary treatment on fatty acid composition in pig gluteus medius muscle is presented in Table 3. The greatest difference between diets was detected for the omega-3 fatty acid level, for which the mean value of the supplemented diet was more than five times that of the control diet (*P* value <0.001). In contrast, there was no evidence of a difference in omega-6 fatty acid level in the muscle of pigs fed with different diets (*P* value >0.05). Pigs fed with the supplemented diet had significantly higher levels of polyunsaturated fatty acids (*P* value <0.05) and decreased levels of monounsaturated fatty acids (*P* value <0.05) compared to pigs fed with the control diet.

Next-generation sequencing

NGS was performed to identify changes induced by omega-6 and omega-3 supplementation in the pig muscle transcriptome. The number of reads per sample obtained from NGS was 25,244,670. Among these reads, 16,040,530 (63.54%) were mapped in pairs and 792,066 (3.14%) in broken pairs and 8,412,074 (33.32%) were unmapped. The number of counted fragments was 8,020,265 (63.54%); among these fragments, 7,475,220 (59.22%) were unique and 545,04 (4,32%) were not specific. The number of uncounted fragments was 4,602,070 (36.46%). The

Table 3 Fatty acid profile [g/100 g FAME] of the muscle of pigs from two examined groups (mean ± SD)

Fatty acid	Supplemented	Control	*P* value
C14:0	1.39 ± 0.18	1.51 ± 0.32	0.42997
C16:0	23.77 ± 1.35	25.17 ± 1.67	0.13779
C18:0	13.96 ± 0.54	13.75 ± 0.57	0.84922
C20:0	0.27 ± 0.13	0.11 ± 0.07	0.66062
C16:1 n-7	2.78 ± 0.34	3.34 ± 0.42	0.02783*
C18:1 n-9	36.23 ± 1.93	38.92 ± 2.02	0.04020*
C18:1 n-7	3.34 ± 0.32	3.92 ± 0.31	0.01022*
C18:2 n-6	9.44 ± 1.49	8.14 ± 2.46	0.29516
C18:3 n-3	4.45 ± 1.09	0.57 ± 0.52	1.37E−5***
C20:4 n-6	1.24 ± 0.24	1.36 ± 0.53	0.62428
Σ saturated FA	41.85 ± 1.30	42.87 ± 1.46	0.23132
Σ monounsaturated FA	42.77 ± 2.41	46.48 ± 2.54	0.02678*
Σ polyunsaturated FA	15.27 ± 2.66	10.19 ± 2.20	0.00476**
Σ n-6 FA	10.69 ± 1.67	9.51 ± 2.79	0.39499
Σ n-3 FA	4.47 ± 1.14	0.89 ± 0.55	0.00035***
n-6/n-3 FA	2.57 ± 1.09	11.57 ± 8.81	0.120

Means and standard deviations of fatty acids and profiles of omega-6/omega-3 fatty acids. Comparisons were made between the muscle tissue of pigs fed with a diet supplemented with fatty acids versus pigs fed with a control diet
*P value <0.05; **P value <0.01;*P value <0.001

sequence reads have been submitted to the NCBI Gene Expression Omnibus under accession series GSE83729. The expression of 14246 genes was registered in the muscle tissue of pigs subjected to NGS. An Additional file 1 shows the heat maps of the transcription levels between control and experimental group. Between genes complying the condition of significance (at least a twofold change in expression between control and experimental group and a t test P value ≤0.05 adjusted for FDR), expression of 219 genes was upregulated and the expression of 530 genes was downregulated.

Real-time PCR verification of NGS data

The reliability of differentially expressed genes detected by NGS was confirmed by real-time PCR analysis for ten selected genes. Results are presented in Figs. 1 and 2. Nine of ten genes were significantly differentially expressed in examined groups. For nine out of ten genes, the direction of change identified by real-time PCR was the same as that detected by NGS.

Functional analysis by DAVID

The DEG in pigs fed with alternative diets were analyzed by DAVID functional clustering analysis. Results identified more than 15 functional clusters (Table 4, Additional file 2). The cluster with the highest enrichment score was related to response to wounding/inflammation. Related clusters included complement and coagulation cascades, acute inflammatory response, and inflammatory response. Decreased expression levels were observed in several genes encoding the chemokines: C-C motif chemokine ligand 2 (*CCL2*), C-C motif chemokine ligand 4 (*CCL4*), C-C motif chemokine ligand 5 (*CCL5*), C-C motif chemokine ligand 16 (*CCL16*), C-C motif chemokine ligand 19 (*CCL19*), and C-C motif chemokine ligand 21 (*CCL21*). Moreover, the expression of complement components (complement component 4 binding protein alpha (C4BPA), complement C5 (C5), complement C7 (C7), complement C8 gamma chain (C8G), and complement C9 (C9)) were observed

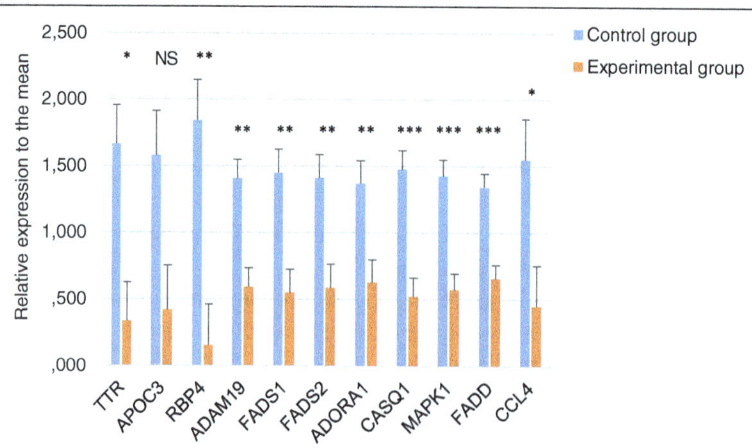

Fig. 1 The validation of NGS results with real-time PCR—comparison of control and experimental group. Mean expression of ten genes: transthyretin (*TTR*), apolipoprotein C-III (*APOC3*), retinol-binding protein 4 (*RBP4*), ADAM metallopeptidase domain 19 (*ADAM19*), fatty acid desaturase 1 (*FADS1*), fatty acid desaturase 2 (*FADS2*), adenosine A1 receptor (*ADORA1*), calsequestrin 1 (*CASQ1*), mitogen-activated protein kinase 1 (*MAPK1*), Fas (*TNFRSF6*)-associated via death domain (*FADD*), and C-C motif chemokine ligand 4 (*CCL4*) determined using real-time PCR for 24 pigs from two diet treatments. Expression was normalized to the topoisomerase (DNA) II beta (TOP2B) gene as an endogenous control. *Error bars* represent standard error.*P value <0.05; **P value <0.01; ***P value <0.001, *ns* not significant

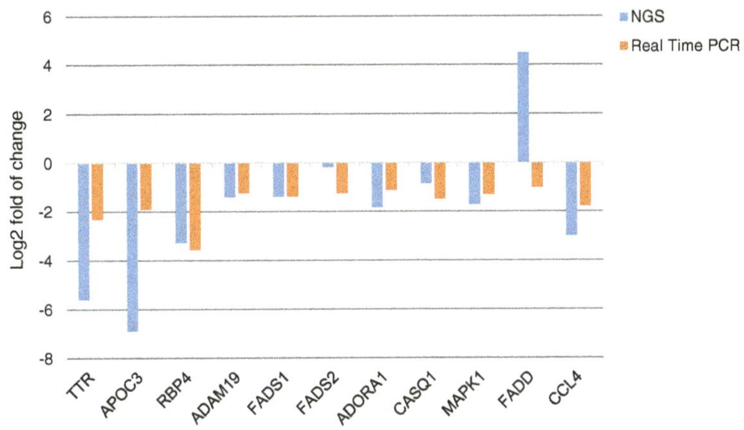

Fig. 2 The validation of NGS results with real-time PCR—comparison of two methods. Log2 fold changes of ten differentially expressed genes measured by NGS (*blue*) versus real-time PCR (*orange*): transthyretin (*TTR*), apolipoprotein C-III (*APOC3*), retinol-binding protein 4 (*RBP4*), ADAM metallopeptidase domain 19 (*ADAM19*), fatty acid desaturase 1 (*FADS1*), fatty acid desaturase 2 (*FADS2*), adenosine A1 receptor (*ADORA1*), calsequestrin 1 (*CASQ1*), mitogen-activated protein kinase 1 (*MAPK1*), Fas (*TNFRSF6*)-associated via death domain (*FADD*), and C-C motif chemokine ligand 4 (*CCL4*)

as downregulated. Finally, we registered changes in the level of two coagulation factors—coagulation factor II, thrombin (F2), and coagulation factor V (F5). Other clusters included processes related to response to endogenous stimulus and organic substance, regulation of response to external stimulus, and negative regulation of response to stimulus. Genes with significantly differential expression were related to retinol and lipid binding, as well as gluconeogenesis, monooxygenase, and microsome. Among the genes related to lipid metabolism, supplementation occurred to decrease expression number of genes coding apolipoproteins, apolipoprotein A1 (*APOA1*), apolipoprotein A2 (*APOA2*), apolipoprotein A4 (*APOA4*), apolipoprotein A5 (*APOA5*), apolipoprotein C3 (*APOC3*), apolipoprotein E (*APOE*), and apolipoprotein N (*APON*). Obtained results of NGS data at the transcriptomic level indicated that omega-6 and omega-3 fatty acid level affected biological processes responsible for keeping homeostasis in muscle tissue.

Functional analysis by Cytoscape

To gain insight into the network interactions of DEG in the muscle tissue of pigs fed with the supplemented diet compared to pigs fed with the control diet, we performed a clustered functional analysis using the Cytoscape software with the ClueGO plug-in. Overall, 34 GO terms were

Table 4 Results of DAVID functional clustering analysis of differentially expressed genes (DEG)

Functional annotation	Enrichment score	Number of DEG	Ontology
Response to wounding/inflammation	7.34	48	Biological processes
Signal/extracellular region	5.32	157	Molecular function
Response to endogenous stimulus and organic substance	4.40	43	Biological processes
Regulation of response to external stimulus	3.70	20	Biological processes
Homeostasis	3.30	44	Biological processes
Complement and coagulation cascades	2.43	19	Biological processes
Retinol binding/vitamin A	2.20	7	Molecular function
Oxidoreductase	2.17	30	Molecular function
Lipid binding	1.90	56	Molecular function
Negative regulation of response to stimulus	1.85	11	Biological processes
Gluconeogenesis	1.83	25	Biological processes
Acute inflammatory response	1.81	38	Biological processes
Inflammatory response	1.77	28	Biological processes
Monooxygenase	1.75	10	Molecular function
Microsome	1.52	10	Cellular component

Analysis of genes identified with differential expression in the muscle of pigs fed with a diet supplemented with fatty acids versus pigs fed a control diet significantly enriched (Figs. 3 and 4, Additional file 3). Among various biological processes, the most affected revealed by functional network analysis were as follows: complement and coagulation cascades, very low-density lipoprotein (VLDL) particle remodeling, negative regulation of fibrinolysis, positive regulation of cholesterol esterification, and intestinal cholesterol absorption (Fig. 3). Several of highlighted terms were related to the same processes: regulation of triglyceride catabolic process and regulation of lipoprotein lipase activity, angiotensin-mediated drinking behavior and positive regulation of gap junction assembly, and vitamin B6 metabolism and pyridoxine biosynthetic process.

Discussion

The objective of this study was to determine the impact of omega-6 and omega-3 fatty acid concentration on the pig muscle transcriptome. Results provide new insight regarding the possible underlying regulatory mechanisms of the muscle tissue's biological response to increased concentration of omega-6 and omega-3 fatty acids.

RNA-seq of muscle tissue identified 759 genes with at least a twofold change in gene expression. The number of downregulated genes in pigs characterized by decreased omega-6 to omega-3 ratio in the muscle (for the supplemented diet) was more than two times greater than the number of upregulated genes in pigs fed with the control diet. Duan et al. [6] reported a dietary ratio of omega-6/omega-3 fatty acids of 1:1 and 5:1, which suppressed gene expression levels of lipid metabolism-related genes and proteins, as well as inflammatory cytokines. The authors concluded that their reported ratio of omega-6 to omega-3 fatty acids is beneficial for lipid metabolism and function of the inflammatory system. However, until now, a few studies have investigated the effect of fatty acid consumption on the muscle transcriptome using high-throughput technology.

Omega-6 and omega-3 fatty acids regulate the inflammatory response by nuclear receptors, which regulate gene expression [27] and synthesize pro- and anti-inflammatory biomarkers. Indeed, the most affected process pointed out both by DAVID and Cytoscape-ClueGo was the response to wounding and inflammation. We observed decreased expression of a number of chemokines: *CCL2, CCL4, CCL5, CCL16, CCL19,* and *CCL21*, recruiting macrophages and monocytes to the site of inflammation. That may

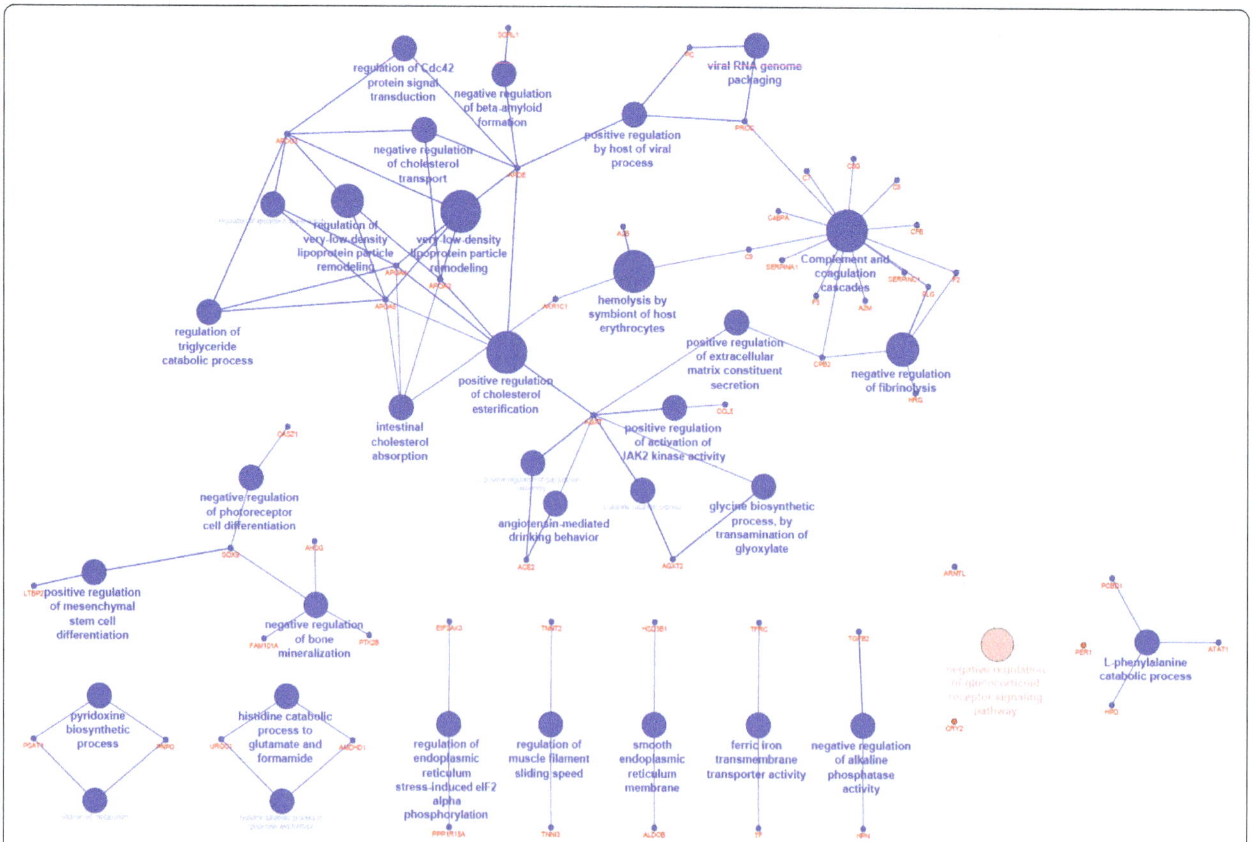

Fig. 3 Cytoscape-ClueGo analysis of differentially expressed genes (DEG). Gene networks of upregulated (*red*) and downregulated (*blue*) genes for the diet supplemented with n-6 and n-3 fatty acids versus the control diet. The edges connecting the nodes are based on the kappa statistic (kappa score of 0.9) that measures the overlap of shared genes between terms

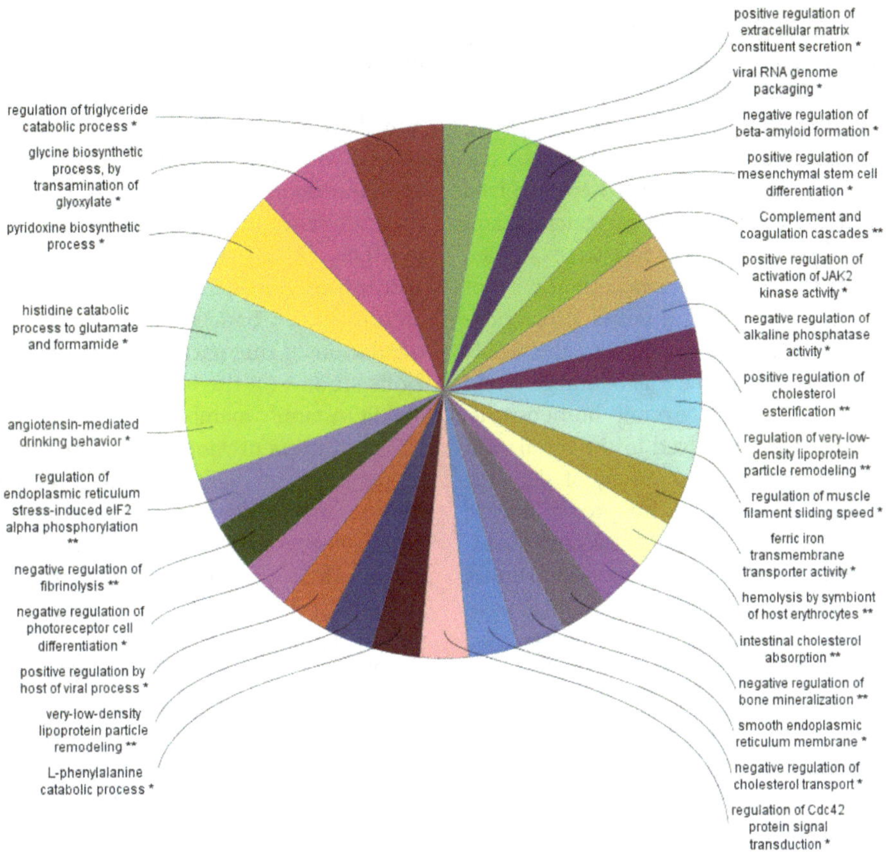

Fig. 4 Cytoscape-ClueGo analysis of functional distribution of differentially expressed genes (DEG). Analysis of genes identified with differential expression in muscle of pigs fed with a diet supplemented with fatty acids versus pigs fed a control diet. Categories of genes were based on GO annotation. Significant terms (Kappa = 0.9) and distribution were determined according to percentage of number of gene association

indicate a diminished activity of macrophages and monocytes themselves. Similar results were obtained by Liang et al. [28], who registered decreased expression of *CCL2* after the administration of omega-3 fatty acid to mice. Further, we observed diminished expression of several complement components, *C4BPA*, *C5*, *C7*, *C8G*, and *C9*, that are components of the complement system, a part of the innate immune system. The usefulness of polyunsaturated fatty acid immunomodulatory activities is well known. Their possible impact on a group of chemokines and complement components explore mechanisms of its acting. That supports their utility in the management of inflammatory and autoimmune diseases.

Among genes with divergent expression that are involved in coagulation, two coagulation factors—*F2* and *F5*—showed reduced expression. These genes encode essential enzymes of the blood coagulation cascade. There are a number of studies on the impact of polyunsaturated fatty acids on coagulation process; however, their results are inconsistent. It is suggested that increased consumption of polyunsaturated fatty acids decreased the blood levels of several coagulation factors and may prevent thrombosis [29–31]. Here, we suggest that the possible mechanism of this phenomenon could be related to diminished levels of *F2* and *F5* due to increased consumption of omega-6 and omega-3 fatty acids.

The significant number of affected genes was related to signal transduction. Long-chain fatty acids can function as lipid second messengers of signaling cascade systems or as modulators and regulators of intracellular signaling pathways. The specific functions depend on the bioavailability of fatty acids (governed by their interaction with soluble proteins capable of binding fatty acids) and the lipid and protein components of biological membranes, including membrane-associated fatty acid-binding proteins [32]. In our studies, affected genes were related to membrane signaling components, such as receptors, ion channels, and membrane glycoproteins. Among them, genes belonging to several families deserve to be highlighted. The differentially expressed genes (DEG) of the ADAM family play an important role in signaling, cell adhesion, and migration. This finding was consistent with results reported by Reiss et al. [33], suggesting that free fatty acids are critical regulators of ADAM family gene function. Another family of genes is signaling membrane proteins. Our results showed that encoded by genes differentially expressed between experimental groups are G protein-coupled receptors and solute carrier proteins. Furthermore, a significant number of DEG were involved in ion transport, especially responsible for calcium and iron which showed different expression between examined groups. The regulation of the free ion concentration is not only important for signaling pathways but is also fundamental in the proper functioning of cells and the whole body. This observation confirmed the role of omega-6 and omega-3 fatty acids in ion and overall homeostasis. Likewise, affected genes were involved in the regulation of Cdc42 protein that is involved in a variety of signaling events and a number of fundamental for proper muscle functioning cellular pathways, determining cell growth, differentiation, and apoptosis. Previous genome-wide studies on pig muscle transcriptome, where compared pigs were divergent in fatty acid composition in the muscle, also pointed out the pathway dedicated to the signaling as one of the most affected [34]. The biological functions of polyunsaturated fatty acids are inter alia, due to their ability to act as secondary messengers or modulators of activities of functionally important proteins. Here, we present that adaptation to omega-6 and omega-3 supplementation is accomplished through signal transduction. Taken together, this finding indicates that the regulatory mechanisms underlying the biological effects of omega-6 and omega-3 fatty acids seem to be strictly connected to signaling pathways.

We have detected differential expression of genes related to the lipid binding between the control and experimental groups. Noteworthy are our observation of the downregulation of many apolipoprotein genes, including *APOA1*, *APOA2, APOA4, APOA5, APOC3, APOE*, and *APON*. Previous studies proved that ALA decreased the level of triacylglycerol, total cholesterol, and low-density lipoprotein (LDL) cholesterol, as well as lipoprotein-A, *APOA1*, and apolipoprotein B (*APOB*) [35]. Likewise, Fox et al. [36] perceived that the supplementation with oils containing higher content of PUFA resulted in longer term effect on decreasing the level of *APOA1* transcript in comparison to oils containing lower levels of PUFA.

Many other observations made by scientists lead to the conclusion that the control of lipoprotein metabolism through proper supplementation with bioactive components is the essential part of metabolic diseases prevention. A number of studies have shown that polyunsaturated fatty acids have a marked hypolipidemic effect. In our studies, we have detected differential expression of genes related to the lipid-binding protein between the groups of pigs. This is consistent with other research made by Canovas et al. [37], where animals showing higher levels of PUFA in the muscle were characterized by decreased level of serum lipids: total cholesterol, high-density lipoprotein (HDL) cholesterol, LDL cholesterol, and triglycerides. The diminished concentration of mentioned lipids could be related with observed in our studies downregulation of apolipoproteins.

APOA1 and *APOA2* are the major proteins constituent of HDLs. While *APOA4* participates in intestinal lipid absorption, *APOA5* regulates VLDLs synthesis and secretion [38]. Changes in their expression may suggest regulation of this particles metabolism. Results of previous studies on the impact of PUFA on the expression of APOA family members are consistent with our findings [35, 39]. It was previously suggested that APOA level can be regulated by PUFA through molecular mechanism or indirect mechanism via changes in plasma lipid or lipoprotein concentration [40]. Nevertheless, additional studies are needed to clarify the mechanism by which omega-6 and omega-3 fatty acids affect APOA expression and further the lipoprotein metabolism.

APOC3 is a component of chylomicrons, both very low and HDLs; inhibits the activity of lipoprotein lipase; and delays very LDLs clearance. The reduction in *APOC3* expression observed in the group supplemented with omega-3 and omega-6 fatty acid may have been a result of a direct effect of omega-3 fatty acids on a reducing *APOC3* production or as an indirect result of synthesis and secretion of fewer very LDL particles. Increased concentrations of *APOC3* are an indicator of a risk factor for coronary heart disease and atherosclerotic lesions [41]. Therefore, it could be hypothesized that reduction in *APOC3* that we observed after omega-6 and omega-3 fatty acids supplementation could have implications for coronary heart disease risk.

In accordance with our results, Canovas et al. [37] observed decreased expression of *APOE* in pigs containing increased levels of PUFA in the muscle. *APOE* removes chylomicron's remnants from circulation through interaction with LDL receptors. It was proven that *APOE* knockout mice exhibit less body fat stores and smaller adipocytes and are more resistant to diet-induced obesity [37]. Possibly, decreased *APOE* expression that is thought to facilitate obesity decreased risk of this disorder.

It became evident that omega-6 and omega-3 fatty acids through regulation of lipoproteins play the essential role in postprandial metabolism. Therefore, they are associated with a lower risk of atherogenesis, heart disease, obesity, and diabetes. Here, we reported that omega-6 and omega-3 fatty acids affect a number of genes related to lipid transport. An important group of regulated genes belongs to apolipoprotein family. Our results highlight the need of further studies that would broaden knowledge about interactions between PUFA, lipoproteins, and metabolic disorders.

Finally, among the pathways overrepresented between both groups of animals was homeostasis. PUFA are powerful endogenous bioregulators, affecting whole body functioning and therefore homeostasis. In fact, they strongly regulate the muscle, an important organ that adjusts systemic metabolic homeostasis. First and foremost, we have observed significant changes in the expression of genes related to ion homeostasis. Homeostatic regulation of ionic gradients is critical for most functions. Here, we reported that omega-6 and omega-3 fatty acids impact expression of a number of genes involved in ion transport, including ion channels, solute carriers, G protein-coupled receptors, and tyrosine kinases. Possibly, through regulation of genes that control calcium, iron sodium and potassium ion concentration which examined fatty acids affect fundamental regulatory system of cellular processes.

Among the strengths of the present study is the scale of NGS analysis that allowed for whole genome sequencing and validation of NGS results with real-time PCR. In addition, pigs as a choice of the model organism are one of the best models for studies on effect of omega-6 and omega-3 fatty acids, which improves studies. However, limitation of lack of biological replicates should be considered in the interpretation of our results.

Conclusions

In our study, we compared the muscle transcriptome of pigs fed with a control diet to that of pigs fed with a diet supplemented with additional fatty acids, causing different muscular fatty acid profiles. Our results showed that the omega-3 and omega-6 fatty acids regulate cellular muscle metabolism at the transcriptome level. This showed that these fatty acids are regulators of fundamental metabolic processes in muscle tissue development and functioning. A total of 749 unique genes were differently expressed between the two diet groups. The expression of 219 genes was upregulated, and the expression of 530 genes was downregulated in the group of pigs supplemented with omega-3 and omega-6 fatty acids in relation to expression in the control group pigs. The roles of these genes were indicated based on their involvement in particular biological functions. Among these biological processes were basic physiological processes such as inflammatory response, signaling pathways and lipid metabolism, leading to a finding that influence of omega-6 and omega-3 fatty on the skeletal muscle substantially impacts the whole body functioning. Obtained results reveal additional information regarding transcriptome-level regulation of biological processes underlying differences in omega-6 and omega-3 fatty acid levels.

Additional files

Additional file 1: Heatmap of global expression levels of mRNA in the muscle of pigs from control group (M-high) and pigs fed with the diet supplemented with omega-6 and omega-3 fatty acids (M-low). The heatmap was clustered by Euclidean distance of expression. It shows gene expression in log 2 cpm (counts per million).

Additional file 2: List of differentially expressed genes (DEG) and results of DAVID analysis for all DEG in the porcine gluteus medius muscle tissue between pigs fed with the diet enriched for omega-6 and omega-3 fatty acids versus pigs fed with the control diet. In file are presented terms fulfilling the criteria of significance (Benjamini <0.05 and FDR <5%).

Additional file 3: Additional information for the Cytoscape-ClueGo networks of differentially expressed genes (DEG) identified between pigs fed with the diet supplemented with omega-6 and omega-3 fatty acids versus pigs fed with the control diet.

Funding

This study was funded by the project "BIOFOOD – innovative, functional products of animal origin" No. POIG.01.01.02-014-090/09 and was co-financed by the European Union from the European Regional Development Fund under Innovative Economy Operational Program 2007–2013.

Authors' contributions

MO participated in the laboratory analysis, analyzed and interpreted the data, and prepared the draft of the manuscript. AS participated in the laboratory analysis and data analysis. MFWTP participated in the data analysis and coordinated the manuscript writing. EP made substantial contributions to the conception and preparation of the manuscript. PU conducted the GC analysis. TB and JOH participated in designing the experiment. CSP and EJK gave comments to the manuscript. JRD participated in the manuscript creation. MP designed and coordinated the experiment and participated in the bioinformatic analyses. All authors read and approved the final manuscript.

Competing interests

The authors declare that they have no competing interests.

Author details

[1]Institute of Genetics and Animal Breeding of the Polish Academy of Sciences, Postępu 36A, 05-552 Jastrzębiec, Poland. [2]Breeding and Genomic Centre, Wageningen UR Livestock Research, 6700 AH Wageningen, The Netherlands. [3]Division of Functional Genomics in Biological and Biomedical Research, Centre for Modern Interdisciplinary Technologies, Nicolaus Copernicus University, 87-100 Torun, Poland. [4]Department of Animal Science, Iowa State University, 2255 Kildee Hall, Ames, IA 50011, USA.

References

1. Pegorier JP, Le May C, Girard J. Control of gene expression by fatty acids. J Nutr. 2004;134:2444S–9.
2. Ouhtit A. Nutrigenomics: from promise to practice. Sultan Qaboos Univ Med J. 2014;14:e1–3.
3. Chondrogianni N, Sakellari M, Lefaki M, Papaevgeniou N, Gonos ES. Proteasome activation delays aging in vitro and in vivo. Free Radic Biol Med. 2014;71:303–20.
4. Liu JJ, Green P, John Mann J, Rapoport SI, Sublette ME. Pathways of polyunsaturated fatty acid utilization: implications for brain function in neuropsychiatric health and disease. Brain Res. 2015;1597:220–46.
5. Kang JX, Liu A. The role of the tissue omega-6/omega-3 fatty acid ratio in regulating tumor angiogenesis. Cancer Metastasis Rev. 2013;32:201–10.
6. Duan Y, Li F, Li L, Fan J, Sun X, Yin Y. n-6:n-3 PUFA ratio is involved in regulating lipid metabolism and inflammation in pigs. Br J Nutr. 2014;111:445–51.
7. Lands B. Consequences of essential fatty acids. Nutrients. 2012;4:1338–57.
8. Zhang W, Zhang J, Cui L, Ma J, Chen C, Ai H, et al. Genetic architecture of fatty acid composition in the longissimus dorsi muscle revealed by genome-wide association studies on diverse pig populations. Genet Sel Evol. 2016;48:5.

9. Jeukendrup AE. Regulation of fat metabolism in skeletal muscle. Ann N Y Acad Sci. 2002;967:217–35.
10. Jeromson S, Gallagher IJ, Galloway SD, Hamilton DL. Omega-3 fatty acids and skeletal muscle health. Mar Drugs. 2015;13:6977–7004.
11. Kohlstadt I. Advancing medicine with food and nutrients. 2nd ed. Boca Raton: CRC Press, Taylor & Francis Group; 2013.
12. Lee SK, Lee SY, Jung JM. Muscle activity of the gluteus medius at different gait speeds. J Phys Ther Sci. 2014;26:1915–7.
13. Bee G, Solomon MB, Czerwinski SM, Long C, Pursel VG. Correlation between histochemically assessed fiber type distribution and isomyosin and myosin heavy chain content in porcine skeletal muscles. J Anim Sci. 1999;77:2104–11.
14. Borer KT. Advanced exercise endocrinology. Champaign: Human Kinetics; 2013.
15. Weylandt KH, Serini S, Chen YQ, Su HM, Lim K, Cittadini A, et al. Omega-3 polyunsaturated fatty acids: the way forward in times of mixed evidence. Biomed Res Int. 2015;2015:143109.
16. Szostak A, Ogluszka M, te Pas MFW, Polawska E, Urbanski P, Juszczuk-Kubiak E, et al. Effect of a diet enriched with omega-6 and omega-3 fatty acids on the pig liver transcriptome. Genes Nutr. 2016;11:9.
17. Folch J, Lees M, Sloane Stanley GH. A simple method for the isolation and purification of total lipides from animal tissues. J Biol Chem. 1957;226:497–509.
18. Polawska E, Horbanczuk JO, Pierzchala M, Strzalkowska N, Jozwik A, Wojcik A, et al. Effect of dietary linseed and rapeseed supplementation on fatty acid profiles in the ostrich. Part 1. Muscles. Anim Sci Paper Rep. 2013;31:239–48.
19. Hicks AA, Pramstaller PP, Johansson A, Vitart V, Rudan I, Ugocsai P, et al. Genetic determinants of circulating sphingolipid concentrations in European populations. PLoS Genet. 2009;5:e1000672.
20. Chomczynski P, Sacchi N. Single-step method of RNA isolation by acid guanidinium thiocyanate-phenol-chloroform extraction. Anal Biochem. 1987;162:156–9.
21. Genomed. http://www.genomed.pl/. Accessed 10 Oct 2016.
22. te Pas MFW, Wijnberg ID, Hoekman AJW, de Graaf-Roelfsema E, Keizer HA, van Breda E, et al. Skeletal muscle transcriptome profiles related to different training intensities and detraining in Standardbred horses: a search for overtraining biomarkers. Vet J. 2013;197:717–23.
23. Anders S, Huber W. Differential expression analysis for sequence count data. Genome Biol. 2010;11:R106.
24. Ramakers C, Ruijter JM, Deprez RH, Moorman AF. Assumption-free analysis of quantitative real-time polymerase chain reaction (PCR) data. Neurosci Lett. 2003;339:62–6.
25. da Huang W, Sherman BT, Stephens R, Baseler MW, Lane HC, Lempicki RA. DAVID gene ID conversion tool. Bioinformation. 2008;2:428–30.
26. Bindea G, Mlecnik B, Hackl H, Charoentong P, Tosolini M, Kirilovsky A, et al. ClueGO: a Cytoscape plug-in to decipher functionally grouped gene ontology and pathway annotation networks. Bioinformatics. 2009;25:1091–3.
27. Siriwardhana N, Kalupahana NS, Fletcher S, Xin WT, Claycombe KJ, Quignard-Boulange A, et al. n-3 and n-6 polyunsaturated fatty acids differentially regulate adipose angiotensinogen and other inflammatory adipokines in part via NF-kappa B-dependent mechanisms. J Nutr Biochem. 2012;23:1661–7.
28. Liang P, Henning SM, Schokrpur S, Wu L, Doan N, Said J, et al. Effect of dietary omega-3 fatty acids on tumor-associated macrophages and prostate cancer progression. Prostate. 2016;76:1293–302.
29. Kristensen SD, Iversen AM, Schmidt EB. n-3 polyunsaturated fatty acids and coronary thrombosis. Lipids. 2001;36 Suppl:S79–82.
30. Shahar E, Folsom AR, Wu KK, Dennis BH, Shimakawa T, Conlan MG, et al. Associations of fish intake and dietary n-3 polyunsaturated fatty acids with a hypocoagulable profile. The Atherosclerosis Risk in Communities (ARIC) Study. Arterioscler Thromb. 1993;13:1205–12.
31. Miller GJ. Effects of diet composition on coagulation pathways. Am J Clin Nutr. 1998;67:542S–5.
32. Glatz JFC, Luiken JJFP. Fatty acids in cell signaling: historical perspective and future outlook. Prostaglandins Leukot Essent Fat Acids. 2015;92:57–62.
33. Reiss K, Cornelsen I, Husmann M, Gimpl G, Bhakdi S. Unsaturated fatty acids drive disintegrin and metalloproteinase (ADAM)-dependent cell adhesion, proliferation, and migration by modulating membrane fluidity. J Biol Chem. 2011;286:26931–42.
34. Corominas J, Ramayo-Caldas Y, Puig-Oliveras A, Estelle J, Castello A, Alves E, et al. Analysis of porcine adipose tissue transcriptome reveals differences in de novo fatty acid synthesis in pigs with divergent muscle fatty acid composition. BMC Genomics. 2013;14:843.
35. Poudyal H, Panchal SK, Diwan V, Brown L. Omega-3 fatty acids and metabolic syndrome: effects and emerging mechanisms of action. Prog Lipid Res. 2011;50:372–87.
36. Fox JC, McGill Jr HC, Carey KD, Getz GS. In vivo regulation of hepatic LDL receptor mRNA in the baboon. Differential effects of saturated and unsaturated fat. J Biol Chem. 1987;262:7014–20.
37. Canovas A, Quintanilla R, Amills M, Pena RN. Muscle transcriptomic profiles in pigs with divergent phenotypes for fatness traits. BMC Genomics. 2010;11:372.
38. Dominiczak MH, Caslake MJ. Apolipoproteins: metabolic role and clinical biochemistry applications. Ann Clin Biochem. 2011;48:498–515.
39. Bloedon LT, Balikai S, Chittams J, Cunnane SC, Berlin JA, Rader DJ, et al. Flaxseed and cardiovascular risk factors: results from a double blind, randomized, controlled clinical trial. J Am Coll Nutr. 2008;27:65–74.
40. Berthou L, Saladin R, Yaqoob P, Branellec D, Calder P, Fruchart JC, et al. Regulation of rat liver apolipoprotein A-I, apolipoprotein A-II and acyl-coenzyme A oxidase gene expression by fibrates and dietary fatty acids. Eur J Biochem. 1995;232:179–87.
41. Davidson MH, Maki KC, Bays H, Carter R, Ballantyne CM. Effects of prescription omega-3-acid ethyl esters on lipoprotein particle concentrations, apolipoproteins AI and CIII, and lipoprotein-associated phospholipase A(2) mass in statin-treated subjects with hypertriglyceridemia. J Clin Lipidol. 2009;3:332–40.

8

Linkage and association analysis of circulating vitamin D and parathyroid hormone identifies novel loci in Alaska Native Yup'ik people

Stella Aslibekyan[1], Laura K. Vaughan[2,4], Howard W. Wiener[1], Bertha A. Hidalgo[1], Dominick J. Lemas[3], Diane M. O'Brien[5], Scarlett E. Hopkins[5], Kimber L. Stanhope[6], Peter J. Havel[6], Kenneth E. Thummel[7], Bert B. Boyer[5] and Hemant K. Tiwari[2*]

Abstract

Background: Vitamin D deficiency is a well-documented public health issue with both genetic and environmental determinants. Populations living at far northern latitudes are vulnerable to vitamin D deficiency and its health sequelae, although consumption of traditional native dietary pattern rich in fish and marine mammals may buffer the effects of reduced sunlight exposure. To date, few studies have investigated the genetics of vitamin D metabolism in circumpolar populations or considered genediet interactions with fish and n-3 fatty acid intake.

Methods: We searched for genomic regions exhibiting linkage and association with circulating levels of vitamin D and parathyroid hormone (PTH) in 982 Yup'ik individuals from the Center for Alaska Native Health Research Study. We also investigated potential interactions between genetic variants and a biomarker of traditional dietary intake, the δ15N value.

Results: We identified several novel regions linked with circulating vitamin D and PTH as well as replicated a previous linkage finding on 2p16.2 for vitamin D. Bioinformatic analysis revealed multiple candidate genes for both PTH and vitamin D, including *CUBN*, *MGAT3*, and *NFKBIA*. Targeted association analysis identified *NEBL* as a candidate gene for vitamin D and *FNDC3B* for PTH. We observed significant associations between a variant in *MXD1* and vitamin D only when an interaction with the δ15N value was included. Finally, we integrated pathway level information to illustrate the biological validity of the proposed candidate genes.

Conclusion: We provide evidence of linkage between several biologically plausible genomic regions and vitamin D metabolism in a circumpolar population. Additionally, these findings suggest that a traditional dietary pattern may modulate genetic effects on circulating vitamin D.

Keywords: Alaska Native, Vitamin D, Linkage, n-3 fatty acids, Parathyroid hormone

Background

Vitamin D, a steroid hormone synthesized in the skin or acquired through diet, and parathyroid hormone (PTH), secreted by parathyroid glands, work synergistically to promote absorption of dietary calcium and phosphates (reviewed by [31]). In addition, vitamin D affects cell cycle, proliferation, differentiation, and apoptosis through vitamin D receptor response elements found on several hundred genes (reviewed by [40]). As a consequence of its physiological importance, a large body of evidence links circulating vitamin D to numerous health outcomes, including skeletal health, cardiovascular disease, type 1 diabetes, type 2 diabetes, metabolic syndrome, autoimmune diseases, multiple sclerosis, and some types of cancer ([22], reviewed by [15, 16]).

The primary form of circulating vitamin D, 25-hydroxy-vitamin D (25(OH)D), is converted to the metabolically active form 1,25-dihydroxy-vitamin D (1,25(OH)$_2$D). The conversion is regulated by PTH as part of a feedback

* Correspondence: htiwari@uab.edu
[2]Department of Biostatistics, University of Alabama at Birmingham, Birmingham, AL, USA
Full list of author information is available at the end of the article

system maintaining calcium and phosphate homeostasis (reviewed by [13, 17, 31]). Concentrations of 25(OH)D in the blood, which aggregately reflect endogenous generation through UVB exposure (D_3), exogenous dietary intake (D_3 from animal sources, D_2 from plant sources), and supplementation, are considered the best indicator of vitamin D status (reviewed by [50]). In addition to the environmental inputs of sunlight and diet, high inter-individual variation in circulating 25(OH)D as well as family studies suggest a role for genetic determinants [1, 14]. Large-scale genome-wide association studies (GWAS) of 25(OH)D have confirmed associations with polymorphisms near cholesterol synthesis, hydroxylation, and vitamin D transport genes in individuals of European descent [1, 46]. Despite the documented importance of ancestry to vitamin D status [42, 46], genetic risk factors for other populations are less established.

Of particular salience is the study of vitamin D in Arctic populations, where exposure to sunlight is greatly reduced for at least half of the year (reviewed in [15]). However, this deficit may be corrected by traditional subsistence diets that are rich in vitamin D due to high intake of fish such as salmon or halibut and marine mammals. Furthermore, there is evidence of physiological adaptations leading to more efficient calcium absorption. For example, in Greenland Inuit people, vitamin D is produced at a lower rate than in Europeans, but the rate of PTH-mediated conversion to $1,25(OH)_2D$ is higher [37]. Another study documented normal serum calcium despite low 25(OH)D and dietary calcium in Canadian Inuit children, postulating that evolutionary pressures have selected for vitamin D receptors that bind more strongly to the vitamin D molecule [10, 41]. For these reasons, investigating genetic determinants of vitamin D and PTH in Arctic populations, as well as gene-diet interactions with the intake of vitamin D-rich fatty fish, is likely to yield unique insights.

To that end, we performed the first genome-wide linkage analysis of both 25(OH)D and PTH in a population of Yup'ik people participating in the Center for Alaska Native Health Research (CANHR) study. We followed up our findings with targeted association and gene-diet interaction analyses and used complementary bioinformatic tools to identify putative genetic contributors to vitamin D and PTH homeostasis in this community.

Methods

The CANHR population and study sample

The CANHR studies genetic, behavioral, and nutritional risk factors for obesity and related cardiometabolic diseases among Yup'ik people in a community-based setting [29]. Recruitment of Yup'ik families was initiated in 2003 and continues in 11 Southwest Alaskan communities, where all residents are invited to participate, resulting in a convenience sample. The present study sample was comprised of 982 non-pregnant Yup'ik individuals (age range, 13[1]–94) and were informative for genetic linkage analysis; of those, 926 passed quality control checks and had either 25(OH)D or PTH measurements or both. All participants signed informed consent documents, and the study protocols were approved by the Institutional Review Boards of the University of Alaska and the National and Alaska Area Indian Health Service Institutional Review Boards, as well as the Yukon Kuskokwim Human Studies Committee.

Laboratory measurements

Blood samples were collected from participants after an overnight fast and were immediately processed in the field, stored at −15 °C for up to a week, and then stored at −80 °C at the University of Alaska Fairbanks [5]. Total 25(OH)D was ascertained through a quantitative chemiluminescent immunoassay (ARUP Laboratories, Salt Lake City, UT). This assay accurately quantifies the sum of $25(OH)D_3$ and $25(OH)D_2$. The intra- and inter-assay coefficients of variation (CVs) were 5.5 and 12.7 %, respectively. ARUP participates in the College of American Pathologists Laboratory Accreditation Program and has CLIA (Clinical Laboratory Improvement Amendments) certification through the Centers of Medicare and Medicaid Services. PTH levels were assayed at the University of California at Davis using the DSL-8000 ACTIVE® Intact PTH IRMA Kit (Diagnostic Systems Laboratories, Inc., Webster, TX). The procedure employs a two-site immuno-radiometric assay principle [28]. The intra- and inter-assay CVs were 4.2 and 10.3 %, respectively. Traditional dietary intake was assessed using red blood cell (RBC) nitrogen stable isotope ratios ($^{15}N/^{14}N$) as previously described [34] and validated [30]. By convention, isotope ratios were expressed in relative abundance using delta values, as follows: $\delta^{15}N = (^{15}N/^{14}N_{sample} - {}^{15}N/^{14}N_{std})/{}^{15}N/^{14}N_{std} \times 1000$ ‰, in which the standard is atmospheric nitrogen ($^{15}N/^{14}N = 0.0036765$). Analytical precision as assessed using reference materials was within 0.2 ‰.

Genotyping and quality control

Detailed descriptions of genotyping procedures, pedigree analyses, and data cleaning have previously been published [3]. Briefly, genotyping at 6090 loci was performed at the Center for Inherited Disease Research at Johns Hopkins University using the Illumina Linkage-IV panel (Illumina, San Diego, CA, USA), spanning the entire genome with an average genetic distance of 0.58 cM. Due to residual kurtosis following trait transformation, all linkage analyses involving vitamin D levels used the *t*-distribution option in Sequential Oligogenic Linkage Analysis Routines (SOLAR) to control type I error rate [2].

The genotypic data was subject to several quality control measures, specifically the removal of single nucleotide polymorphisms (SNPs) exhibiting inconsistencies with Mendelian segregation or Hardy-Weinberg equilibrium, prior to whole-genome linkage analysis as previously described [3]. Variants that passed quality checks were used to ascertain a cryptic population substructure, deriving "community group" as a dichotomous covariate indicating proximity to the coast.

Linkage and association analysis

We estimated the heritability and conducted a whole-genome linkage scan using the variance component approach implemented in the SOLAR program as previously described [3]. All models run in SOLAR included age (quartiles), sex (dichotomous), community group (dichotomous, inland vs. coastal), and $\delta^{15}N$ value quartiles.

We tested all SNPs under the linkage peaks with a LOD score greater than 1.5 for association with the trait using ASSOC from the S.A.G.E. package, which models the full correlation structure of the pedigree [7, 11]. All association models included the same non-genetic covariates that were used for the linkage analysis: sex, age, community, and $\delta^{15}N$ value quartiles. A sensitivity analysis additionally adjusted for the season of blood sample collection as a categorical variable. For each SNP, the following two models were run: one containing non-genetic covariates and the SNP genotype as an additive effect and one containing non-genetic covariates, SNP genotype as an additive effect, and the interaction between SNP effect and $\delta^{15}N$ value quartiles. Likelihood ratio tests were used to compare the models. Corrections for multiple testing were ascertained separately for each linkage peak of interest, calculating the effective number of tested SNPs (i.e., independent SNPs not in linkage disequilibrium (LD)) using spectral decomposition of the correlation matrix [23, 32]. Bonferroni corrections for the effective number of SNPs in each linkage peak were used to determine the number of full model results that met the significance threshold (Additional file 1: Table S1). Full models were defined to include both the additive genotype term and the interactions of that term with n-3 polyunsaturated fatty acids (PUFA) intake.

Bioinformatic analysis

In order to limit the list of potential genes from regions identified by linkage analysis (LOD score >1.5), we used the SIMWALK2 [43] to phase the genotype data. This analysis indicates the positions of recombination events in the haplotypes of the analyzed individuals. We determined the haplotypes for each individual that had no recombination events and included the position of peak evidence for linkage with the trait of interest. The regions thus defined were examined for the full sample, as well as the subsets limited to both the highest and lowest quartile of the trait of interest. Regions in which less than 5 % of the examined sample experienced a recombination event were included in subsequent bioinformatic analysis. This region was very narrow for chromosome 3, so the threshold was relaxed for that region. Within the regions, potential candidate genes were identified using three complementary algorithms: Ingenuity (Qiagen, Redwood City, CA), TOPPGene Suite [6], and ENDEAVOUR [44]. For all three algorithms, training gene lists were based on the keyword "PTH" or "Vitamin D" in the HuGE navigator [49]. Genes were selected if they attained a HuGE score of at least 0.10 and were related to vitamin D and PTH only. Gene names were converted to Ensembl using BioMart Central ID converter as necessary. The settings for all three algorithms were identical to those in a previous analysis by our group [45]. Genes were considered to be putative candidates if the P values for both TOPPGene and ENDEAVOUR were ≤0.005 and if they were shown by Ingenuity to interact with the chosen training genes.

Results

Descriptive characteristics of the Yup'ik study participants are presented in Table 1. All of the P values in this table are based on simple two-sample t tests, without taking the pedigree correlation into account. RBC $\delta^{15}N$ values and circulating PTH were both significantly higher among women, while 25(OH)D levels did not vary by gender. The correlation between serum 25(OH)D and PTH levels was estimated at –0.09. Transformations of both traits reduced residual kurtosis from 9.96 to 0.45 for PTH and from 4.00 to 1.10 for 25(OH)D. Heritability was estimated at 0.43 ± 0.07 for log-transformed PTH (P value = 1.2×10^{-10}) and at 0.54 ± 0.07 for Box-Cox transformed 25(OH)D (P value = 2.3×10^{-18}).

Results for the genome-wide linkage scan are presented in Table 2 and Figs. 1 and 2. Three regions on chromosomes 2, 10, and 22 yielded a LOD score of at least 2 for 25(OH)D. The linkage peak on chromosome 2 exhibited the strongest signal, with the LOD score exceeding 4 for 25(OH)D. Also, three regions on chromosomes 3, 14, and 17 were linked with PTH with LOD scores greater than 2.

After adjusting for multiple testing, two variants on chromosome 2 and one variant on chromosome 10 were significantly associated with 25(OH)D at adjusted α = 0.001 and 0.002, respectively, while only one variant on chromosome 3 was significantly associated with PTH at adjusted $\alpha = 0.001$. However, the two variants on chromosome 2 were in perfect LD. Significant SNPs and the associated genes are presented in Table 3. Significant interactions of variants on chromosome 2 with n-3

Table 1 Descriptive statistics of the study sample ($n = 926$)

	Male	Female	*P* value
N[a]	419 (45)	507 (55)	0.004
Coastal community group[a]	184 (50)	186 (50)	0.92
Inland community group[a]	235 (42)	321 (58)	0.0003
Age, years[b]	36.56 (17.56)	38.07 (17.61)	0.17
δ^{15}N, ‰[b]	8.80 (1.51)	9.13 (1.54)	0.0001
Parathyroid hormone, pg/mL[c]	52.7 (24.21–114.84)	65.60 (27.83–154.61)	<0.0001
25(OH)D, ng/mL[c]	34.57 (11.47–83.32)	33.96 (12.21–77.69)	0.56

The overall study sample consists of 926 individuals after QC; however, two were missing values for 25(OH)D and two different individuals were missing values for parathyroid hormone
[a]*N* = sample size (%), *P* value based on binomial distribution
[b]Mean (SD), *P* value based on two-sample *t* test
[c]Mean (95 % CI), *P* value based on two-sample *t* test

PUFA intake were observed for 25(OH)D, and there was evidence suggestive of similar interactions between a variant on chromosome 3 and circulating PUFA in the PTH models (Additional files 2 and 3: Figures S1 and S2). Additional adjustment for season did not appreciably change the observed genetic associations (data not shown).

Results of the bioinformatic analysis are summarized in Table 4. None of the a priori identified training genes were located under the linkage peaks. All peaks except for the one on chromosome 2 contained candidate genes proposed by all three bioinformatic algorithms.

Discussion

The CANHR Yup'ik study population is ideal for investigation of the genetic determinants of circulating vitamin D and potential gene-diet interactions with n-3 PUFA. Despite low levels of sunlight exposure, mean 25(OH)D levels in our study sample were well within the optimal range currently recommended for the general population [4]. This paradox may be explained by both genetic adaptations as well as the high vitamin D content of the traditional diet of the Yup'ik people, which may buffer the effects of insufficient sunlight at higher latitudes (reviewed by [15, 17]). Indeed, a previous analysis of a CANHR subsample demonstrated that intake of locally harvested foods, namely fatty fish, fish roe, fish liver, and wild game, is correlated with higher levels of 25(OH)D [24]. Yet, another study showed that 25(OH)D mediates PTH levels in our study population [25]. Using genotype data from extended pedigrees, biochemical measurements of 25(OH)D, PTH, and the δ^{15}N value (a marker of traditional diet rich in vitamin D), and established biological pathways, this report further illustrates the complexity of vitamin D metabolism in the Yup'ik people.

Three linkage peaks were identified for 25(OH)D and three for PTH. The peaks for the two traits did not overlap, reflecting distinct genetic contributions underlying the weakly correlated 25(OH)D and PTH levels in our study population as well as others [21, 39]. All were novel findings except for the locus on chromosome 2, which was initially reported as linked to 25(OH)D_3 in Northern European families with asthma [48] and associated with bone mineral density in a large meta-analysis [8]. Few genome-wide linkage studies on 25(OH)D and none on PTH are available to use as a comparison. Interestingly, none of our observed linkage regions contained genes previously reported in genome-wide association studies (GWAS) of 25(OH)D or 1,25(OH)2D, e.g., *GC* on chromosome 4 [1] or *CYP2R1* and *DHCR7* on chromosome 11 [46]. Similarly, the previous GWAS association of loci in the *PTH* gene with circulating PTH

Table 2 Linkage peaks with a LOD score >2

Chromosome bands	Peak LOD score	Start SNP	End SNP	Genomic region
25(OH)D				
2p16.2–2p12	4.25	rs1483869	rs741418	52,906,147–75,363,186
10p13–10p12.1	2.52	rs873849	rs638324	14,509,807–27,730,261
22q13.1–22q13.31	2.17	rs138383	rs929090	38,799,861–44,313,849
Parathyroid hormone				
3q25.32–3q26.32	2.48	rs6799097	rs6443567	158,811,068–178,427,716
14q12–14q22.1	2.93	rs7149108	rs735265	32,962,300–52,120,264
17p13.1–17p11.2	2.15	rs9217	rs1037037	7,363,088–18,765,021

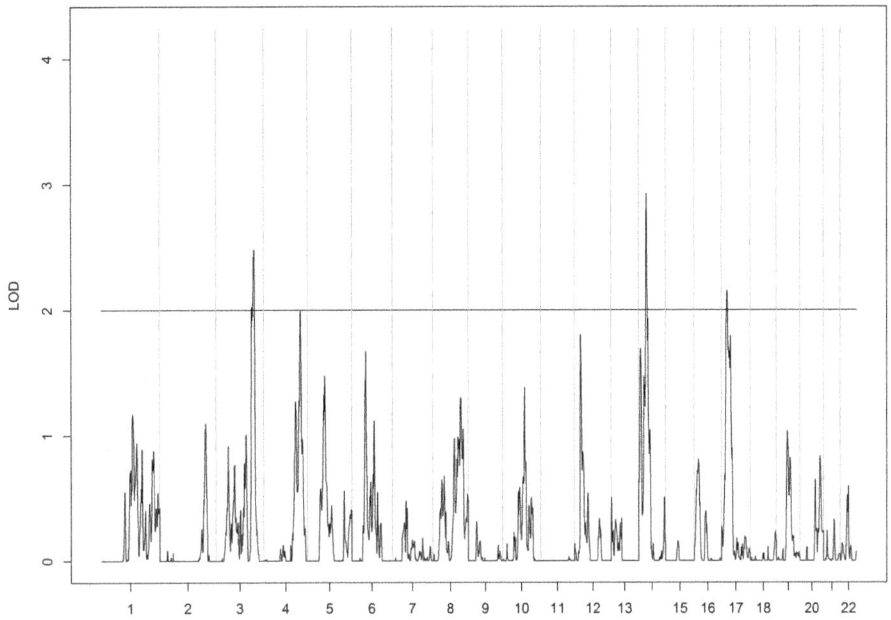

Fig. 1 Linkage results for vitamin D. Whole-genome linkage scan for circulating vitamin D in Yup'ik people ($n = 924$). The *X*-axis shows the chromosomal location, and the *Y*-axis displays the LOD score

was not replicated [27]. The reasons for non-replication may include our genotyping approach, which utilized a linkage-specific panel that was not designed to include all physiologically relevant loci, the uniqueness of our population, and chance. The remaining linkage peaks at 10p13–p12.1 and 22q13.1–13.31 for 25(OH)D and 3q25.32–26.32, 14.12–22.1, and 17p13.1–11.2 for PTH are novel and contain several biologically plausible loci.

Using complementary methods, bioinformatic analysis identified several strong candidate genes located under observed linkage peaks. Of those, the most notable is *CUBN* (cubilin), located on chromosome 10. The

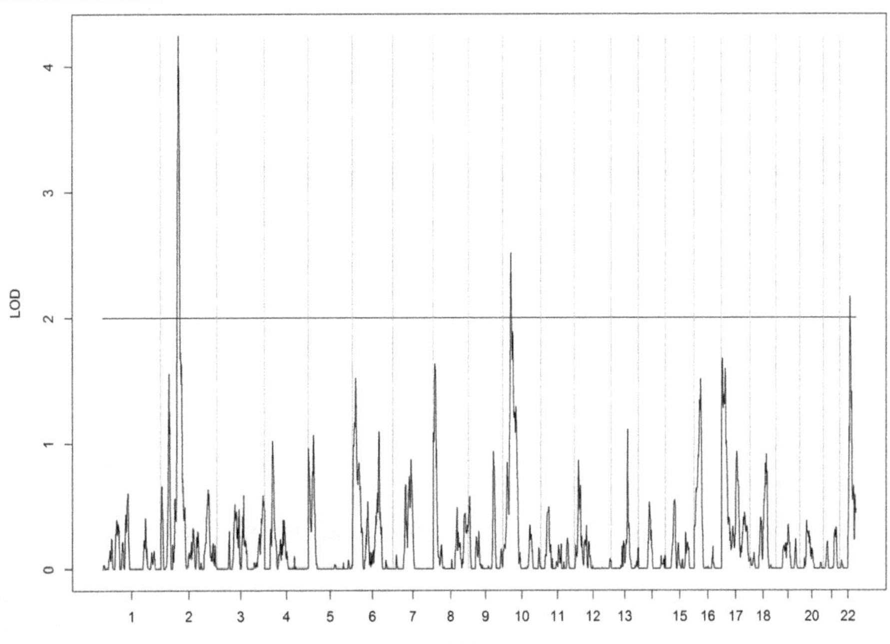

Fig. 2 Linkage results for parathyroid hormone. Whole-genome linkage scan for parathyroid hormone in Yup'ik people ($n = 924$). The *X*-axis shows the chromosomal location, and the *Y*-axis displays the LOD score

Table 3 Significant associations under the linkage peaks

SNP	Chr	Gene	*P* (additive)[a]	*P* (full)[b]	χ^2 (LRT)[c]	*P* (LRT)[c]
25(OH)D						
rs10205487/rs897119[d]	2	*MXD1*	0.22	0.0006	18.15	0.0004
rs10828183	10	*NEBL*	0.0005	0.004	3.18	0.37
Parathyroid hormone						
rs1353894	3	*FNDC3B*	0.03	0.0008	14.21	0.003

[a]*P* value for the model including age, sex, community group, $\delta^{15}N$ quartiles, and additive genotype
[b]*P* value for the model including all of the above plus the interaction term between the additive genotype and $\delta^{15}N$ quartiles
[c]Chi-square statistic and *P* value for the likelihood ratio test comparing the additive model with the full model
[d]rs10205487 and rs897119 were found to be in perfect linkage disequilibrium, with identical estimates of association signal

product of *CUBN*, cubilin, facilitates megalin-mediated delivery of 25(OH)D_3 to kidney epithelial cells, impacting circulating levels of the hormone [33]. In both human and animals, mutations causing cubulin dysfunction are associated with abnormal vitamin D metabolism (e.g., urinary excretion of 25(OH)D_3 in humans) [33]. Another biologically interesting finding from the bioinformatic analysis is *MGAT3* (beta-1,4-mannosyl-glycoprotein 4-beta-N-acetylglucosaminyltransferase), located on chromosome 22. *MGAT3* encodes an enzyme implicated in protein glycosylation and the immune response [20]. Preliminary data illustrate *MGAT3* mRNA as a potential biomarker of response to vitamin D therapy in Alzheimer's disease, hinting at its translational potential; however, these findings remain to be independently validated [9]. Isoforms of two other potential candidate genes, *CACNA1I* (calcium channel, voltage-dependent, *T* type, alpha 1i subunit) and *PDGFB* (plate-derived growth factor beta polypeptide), have been shown to be regulated by the vitamin D receptor, respectively affecting calcium homeostasis [12] and mitosis [36].

Several strong candidate genes for PTH were also identified based on their involvement in relevant physiological pathways. *NFKBIA* (nuclear factor kappa light polypeptide gene enhancer in B cells inhibitor, alpha) is a member of the NFkB inhibitor family that binds with the product of *REL* (v-rel reticuloendotheliosis viral oncogene homolog, regulated by the vitamin D receptor) to inhibit Rel/NFkB complexes. In a previous transcriptome-wide study, the expression of *NFKBIA* in white blood cells was shown to be decreased by vitamin D supplementation, potentially affecting downstream immune response [18]. Reflecting the pleiotropic functions of the vitamin D/PTH axis, other potential candidate genes were also implicated immune/inflammatory processes (*NKX2, PSMA6, SNX6*) as well as cancer (*NKX2*, NKX3, *PAX9*).

Table 4 Potential candidate genes identified by bioinformatic analysis of genes within linkage peaks for 25(OH)D and parathyroid hormone

Chromosome bands	Putative candidate genes
25(OH)D	
10p13–10p12.1	*CUBN, RSU1*
22q13.1–22q13.31	*APOBEC3F, APOBEC3G, ATF4, CACNA1I, CBX7, CBY1, DDX17, DMC1, GTPBP1, MGAT3, PDGFB, RPL3*
Parathyroid hormone	
3q25.32–3q26.32	*NLGN1*
14q12–14q22.1	*CFL2, FOXA1, MYH1, NFKBIA, NKX2-8, PAX9, PSMA6, SFTA3, SNX6*
17p13.1–17p11.2	*GAS7, MIPOL1, MYH2, MYH4, RCVRN*

Extended pedigrees such as those present in the CANHR study provide a powerful framework for targeted association following whole-genome linkage [47]. Targeted association analysis of the observed linkage peaks identified two SNPs in *MXD1* (MAX dimerization protein 1) and one in *NEBL* (nebulette) that were significantly associated with 25(OH)D levels and one in *FNDC3B* (fibronectin type III domain containing 3B) associated with PTH levels. Both *MXD1* and *FNDC3B* are involved in the VDR/RXR activation pathway, the former being regulated by the vitamin D/VDR/RXR complex [38] and the latter suppressing the expression of *RUNX2* [19], which in turn binds to and activates vitamin D/VDR/RXR [35]. On the other hand, *NEBL* has been implicated in calcium homeostasis [26], although a direct link to vitamin D metabolism has not been investigated.

This study presents novel evidence of linkage between several biologically plausible genomic regions and 25(OH)D/PTH in a study population of Yup'ik people with seasonally low exposure to sunlight and high intake of vitamin D-rich foods. These findings are particularly informative in the context of the vitamin D/VDR/RXR pathway, which illustrates the involvement of candidate loci in maintaining the vitamin D/PTH/calcium homeostasis. To our knowledge, this is the first whole-genome linkage study of PTH overall and the first such study of both phenotypes in a circumpolar population. In addition to replicating a previously reported linkage region for 25(OH)D and identifying novel loci for both 25(OH)D and PTH, we present novel evidence of gene-diet interactions with n-3 PUFA intake. Specifically, a variant in *MXD1* was significantly associated with 25(OH)D only after accounting for its interaction with $\delta^{15}N$, a marker of n-3 PUFA intake and traditional lifestyle in Yup'ik people. To the best of our knowledge, no other circumpolar cohorts currently have comparable genotypic and phenotypic measurements, limiting our opportunities for external replication. Future studies in high-latitude populations with unique vitamin D dietary sources and requirements are warranted to establish validity of our findings, laying the groundwork for disease-prevention efforts in Arctic communities.

Conclusions

We provide evidence of linkage between several biologically plausible genomic regions, located on chromosomes 2, 3, 10, 14, 17, and 22, and vitamin D metabolism in a circumpolar population. Additionally, these findings suggest that the traditional dietary pattern of the Yup'ik people, characterized by high intake of n-3 PUFA, may modulate genetic effects on circulating 25(OH)D.

Endnotes

[1]There was only one 13 year old individual, who turned 14 within two weeks of enrollment.

Abbreviations

1,25(OH)$_2$D, 1,25-dihydroxy-vitamin D; 25(OH)D, 25-hydroxy-vitamin D; CANHR, Center for Alaska Native Health Research; CV, coefficient of variation; HWE, Hardy-Weinberg equilibrium; PTH, parathyroid hormone; PUFA, polyunsaturated fatty acids; SNP, single nucleotide polymorphism; SOLAR, Sequential Oligogenic Linkage Analysis Routines

Acknowledgements

We thank the community field research assistants for helping with the study recruitment and data collection and all study participants and their communities for welcoming and teaching our research team so much about the Yup'ik way of life.

Funding

Genotyping services were provided by the Center for Inherited Disease Research (CIDR). CIDR is fully funded through a federal contract from the National Institutes of Health to The Johns Hopkins University, contract HHSN268200782096C. Other funding sources included the National Institutes of Health grants K01DK080188 (LKV), DK074842 (BBB), and RR016430 (BBB). The National Institutes of Health have no influence over the research process, including but not limited to the study design, the data collection/analysis/interpretation, or writing of the manuscript.

Authors' contributions

BBB and HKT designed the study. DMO, SEH, BBB, KLS, and PJH collected the samples and measured the phenotypes and covariates. HWW, BAH, and LKV analyzed the data. SA, BAH, DJL, KT, and LKV wrote the manuscript. SA, BBB, and HKT had primary responsibility for the final content. All authors read and approved the final manuscript.

Competing interests

The authors declare that they have no competing interests.

Financial support

This research was funded by the National Institutes of Health grants and contracts HHSN268200782096C, DK080188, DK074842, RR016430.

Author details

[1]Department of Epidemiology, University of Alabama at Birmingham, Birmingham, AL, USA. [2]Department of Biostatistics, University of Alabama at Birmingham, Birmingham, AL, USA. [3]Department of Health Outcomes and Policy, College of Medicine, University of Florida, Gainesville, FL, USA. [4]Department of Biology, King University, Bristol, TN, USA. [5]Center for Alaska Native Health Research, Institute of Arctic Biology, University of Alaska Fairbanks, Fairbanks, AK, USA. [6]Departments of Molecular Biosciences and Nutrition, University of California at Davis, Davis, CA, USA. [7]Department of Pharmaceutics, University of Washington, Seattle, WA, USA.

References

1. Ahn J, et al. Genome-wide association study of circulating vitamin D levels. Hum Mol Genet. 2010;19(13):2739–45. doi:10.1093/hmg/ddq155.
2. Almasy L, Blangero J. Multipoint quantitative-trait linkage analysis in general pedigrees. Am J Hum Genet. 1998;62(5):1198–211.
3. Aslibekyan S, et al. Evidence for novel genetic loci associated with metabolic traits in Yup'ik people. Am J Hum Biol. 2013;25(5):673–80. doi:10.1002/ajhb.22429.
4. Bischoff-Ferrari HA, et al. Estimation of optimal serum concentrations of 25-hydroxyvitamin D for multiple health outcomes. Am J Clin Nutr. 2006;84(1):18–28.
5. Boyer BB, et al. Building a community-based participatory research center to investigate obesity and diabetes in Alaska Natives. Int J Circumpolar Health. 2005;64(3):281–90.
6. Chen J, et al. ToppGene Suite for gene list enrichment analysis and candidate gene prioritization. Nucleic Acids Res. 2009;37(Web Server issue): W305–11. doi:10.1093/nar/gkp427.
7. Elston RC, et al. The Elston-Stewart algorithm for continuous genotypes and environmental factors. Hum Hered. 1992;42(1):16–27.
8. Estrada K, et al. Genome-wide meta-analysis identifies 56 bone mineral density loci and reveals 14 loci associated with risk of fracture. Nat Genet. 2012;44(5):491–501. doi:10.1038/ng.2249.
9. Fiala M, et al. MGAT3 mRNA: a biomarker for prognosis and therapy of Alzheimer's disease by vitamin D and curcuminoids. J Alzheimers Dis. 2011;25(1):135–44. doi:10.3233/JAD-2011-101950.
10. Frost P. Vitamin D deficiency among northern Native Peoples: a real or apparent problem? Int J Circumpolar Health. 2012;71:18001. doi:10.3402/IJCH.v71i0.18001.
11. George VT, Elston RC. Testing the association between polymorphic markers and quantitative traits in pedigrees. Genet Epidemiol. 1987;4(3):193–201. doi:10.1002/gepi.1370040304.
12. Gezen-Ak D, et al. The effects of vitamin D receptor silencing on the expression of LVSCC-A1C and LVSCC-A1D and the release of NGF in cortical neurons. PLoS One. 2011;6(3):e17553. doi:10.1371/journal.pone.0017553.
13. Heaney RP. The vitamin D requirement in health and disease. J Steroid Biochem Mol Biol. 2005;97(1-2):13–9. doi:10.1016/j.jsbmb.2005.06.020.
14. Hiraki LT, et al. Exploring the genetic architecture of circulating 25-hydroxyvitamin D. Genet Epidemiol. 2013;37(1):92–8. doi:10.1002/gepi.21694.
15. Holick MF. Sunlight and vitamin D for bone health and prevention of autoimmune diseases, cancers, and cardiovascular disease. Am J Clin Nutr. 2004a; 80(6 Suppl): 1678S-88.
16. Holick MF. Vitamin D: importance in the prevention of cancers, type 1 diabetes, heart disease, and osteoporosis. Am J Clin Nutr. 2004b; 79(3): 362-71
17. Holick MF. Vitamin D deficiency. N Engl J Med. 2007;357(3):266–81. doi:10.1056/NEJMra070553.
18. Hossein-Nezhad A, et al. Influence of vitamin D status and vitamin D3 supplementation on genome wide expression of white blood cells: a randomized double-blind clinical trial. PLoS One. 2013;8(3):e58725. doi:10.1371/journal.pone.0058725.
19. Kishimoto K, et al. Fad104, a positive regulator of adipogenesis, negatively regulates osteoblast differentiation. Biochem Biophys Res Commun. 2010;397(2):187–91. doi:10.1016/j.bbrc.2010.05.077.
20. Lauc G, et al. Loci associated with N-glycosylation of human immunoglobulin G show pleiotropy with autoimmune diseases and haematological cancers. PLoS Genet. 2013;9(1):e1003225. doi:10.1371/journal.pgen.1003225.
21. Lee WP, et al. Correlations among serum calcium, vitamin D and parathyroid hormone levels in the elderly in southern Taiwan. J Nurs Res. 2002;10(1):65–72.
22. Levin GP, et al. Genetic variants and associations of 25-hydroxyvitamin D

concentrations with major clinical outcomes. JAMA. 2012;308(18):1898–905. doi:10.1001/jama.2012.17304.
23. Li J, Ji L. Adjusting multiple testing in multilocus analyses using the eigenvalues of a correlation matrix. Heredity (Edinb). 2005;95(3):221–7. doi:10.1038/sj.hdy.6800717.
24. Luick B, et al. Locally harvested foods support serum 25-hydroxyvitamin D sufficiency in an indigenous population of Western Alaska. Int J Circumpolar Health. 2014;73. doi: 10.3402/ijch.v73.22732
25. Luick B, et al. Associations of parathyroid hormone concentration among Alaska Natives of Western Alaska. FASEB J. 2015;29:735(Abstract).
26. Maiellaro-Rafferty K, et al. Altered regional cardiac wall mechanics are associated with differential cardiomyocyte calcium handling due to nebulette mutations in preclinical inherited dilated cardiomyopathy. J Mol Cell Cardiol. 2013;60:151–60. doi:10.1016/j.yjmcc.2013.04.021.
27. Melzer D, et al. A genome-wide association study identifies protein quantitative trait loci (pQTLs). PLoS Genet. 2008;4(5):e1000072. doi:10.1371/journal.pgen.1000072.
28. Miles LE, et al. Measurement of serum ferritin by a 2-site immunoradiometric assay. Anal Biochem. 1974;61(1):209–24.
29. Mohatt GV, et al. The Center for Alaska Native Health Research Study: a community-based participatory research study of obesity and chronic disease-related protective and risk factors. Int J Circumpolar Health. 2007;66(1):8–18.
30. Nash SH, et al. Stable nitrogen and carbon isotope ratios indicate traditional and market food intake in an indigenous circumpolar population. J Nutr. 2012;142(1):84–90.
31. Nussey S, Whitehead S. Endocrinology: an integrated approach. Oxford: BIOS Scientific Publishers, Ltd.; 2001.
32. Nyholt DR. A simple correction for multiple testing for single-nucleotide polymorphisms in linkage disequilibrium with each other. Am J Hum Genet. 2004;74(4):765–9. doi:10.1086/383251.
33. Nykjaer A, et al. Cubilin dysfunction causes abnormal metabolism of the steroid hormone 25(OH) vitamin D(3). Proc Natl Acad Sci U S A. 2001;98(24): 13895–900. doi:10.1073/pnas.241516998.
34. O'Brien DM, et al. Red blood cell delta15N: a novel biomarker of dietary eicosapentaenoic acid and docosahexaenoic acid intake. Am J Clin Nutr. 2009;89(3):913–9. doi:10.3945/ajcn.2008.27054.
35. Paredes R, et al. The Runx2 transcription factor plays a key role in the 1alpha,25-dihydroxy vitamin D3-dependent upregulation of the rat osteocalcin (OC) gene expression in osteoblastic cells. J Steroid Biochem Mol Biol. 2004;89–90(1-5):269–71. doi:10.1016/j.jsbmb.2004.03.076.
36. Pedigo N, et al. A 5'-distal element mediates vitamin D-inducibility of PDGF-A gene transcription. Growth Factors. 2003;21(3-4):151–60.
37. Rejnmark L, et al. Vitamin D insufficiency in Greenlanders on a westernized fare: ethnic differences in calcitropic hormones between Greenlanders and Danes. Calcif Tissue Int. 2004;74(3):255–63. doi:10.1007/s00223-003-0110-9.
38. Salehi-Tabar R, et al. Vitamin D receptor as a master regulator of the c-MYC/MXD1 network. Proc Natl Acad Sci U S A. 2012;109(46):18827–32. doi:10.1073/pnas.1210037109.
39. Saliba W, et al. The relationship between serum 25(OH)D and parathyroid hormone levels. Am J Med. 2011;124(12):1165–70. doi:10.1016/j.amjmed.2011.07.009.
40. Samuel S, Sitrin MD. Vitamin D's role in cell proliferation and differentiation. Nutr Rev. 2008;66(10 Suppl 2):S116–24. doi:10.1111/j.1753-4887.2008.00094.x.
41. Sellers EA, et al. Adaptation of Inuit children to a low-calcium diet. CMAJ. 2003;168(9):1141–3.
42. Signorello LB, et al. Blood vitamin D levels in relation to genetic estimation of African ancestry. Cancer Epidemiol Biomarkers Prev. 2010;19(9):2325–31. doi:10.1158/1055-9965.EPI-10-0482.
43. Sobel E, Lange K. Descent graphs in pedigree analysis: applications to haplotyping, location scores, and marker-sharing statistics. Am J Hum Genet. 1996;58(6):1323–37.
44. Tranchevent LC. ENDEAVOUR update: a web resource for gene prioritization in multiple species. Nucleic Acids Res. 2008;36(Web Server issue):W377–384. doi:10.1093/nar/gkn325.
45. Vaughan LK, et al. Linkage and association analysis of obesity traits reveals novel loci and interactions with dietary n-3 fatty acids in an Alaska Native (Yup'ik) population. Metabolism. 2015;64(6):689–97. doi:10.1016/j.metabol.2015.02.008.
46. Wang TJ, et al. Common genetic determinants of vitamin D insufficiency: a genome-wide association study. Lancet. 2010;376(9736):180–8. doi:10.1016/S0140-6736(10)60588-0.
47. Williams-Blangero S, Blangero J. Collection of pedigree data for genetic analysis in isolate populations. Hum Biol. 2006;78(1):89–101. doi:10.1353/hub.2006.0023.
48. Wjst M, et al. A genome-wide linkage scan for 25-OH-D(3) and 1,25-(OH)2-D3 serum levels in asthma families. J Steroid Biochem Mol Biol. 2007;103(3-5):799–802. doi:10.1016/j.jsbmb.2006.12.053.
49. Yu W, et al. A navigator for human genome epidemiology. Nat Genet. 2008;40(2):124–5. doi:10.1038/ng0208-124.
50. Zerwekh JE. Blood biomarkers of vitamin D status. Am J Clin Nutr. 2008;87(4):1087S–91.

9

Lactase persistence in Tunisia as a result of admixture with other Mediterranean populations

Yosra Ben Halima[1,2], Rym Kefi[1,2*], Marco Sazzini[3], Cristina Giuliani[3], Sara De Fanti[3], Chokri Nouali[1,2], Majdi Nagara[1], Giacomo Mengozzi[3], Sahar Elouej[1], Abdelmajid Abid[1,4], Henda Jamoussi[1,4], Lotfi Chouchane[5], Giovanni Romeo[6], Sonia Abdelhak[1,4] and Donata Luiselli[3]

Abstract

Background: The ability to digest lactose after weaning, namely, lactase persistence (LP), is encoded by polymorphisms in the *MCM6* gene and varies widely in frequency among different human populations. Although, evolution of LP-related genetic variants was investigated in many groups of Sub-Saharan African, Middle Eastern, and European ancestry, only few studies have focused on populations from North Africa and no data are especially available from the Tunisian one. For this reason, there is an urgent need to investigate the frequency patterns at these loci in Tunisia since this adaptive trait is implicated in health.

Methods: Forty SNPs covering the *LCT/MCM6* genes and including the two functional variants – 13,910 C > T and – 22,018 G > A were genotyped in 117 Tunisian individuals using the Sequenom Mass Array technology. The observed nucleotide and haplotype patterns of variation were then compared with those of several African, European, and Mediterranean human groups for which comparable data were publicly available. Admixture analysis on a 5 Mb genomic region surrounding the *LCT/MCM6* loci was also performed by extracting genotypes from a previously generated genome-wide dataset in order to deepen the reconstruction of the evolutionary history of these loci.

Results: We found that lactase non-persistence (LNP)-related alleles and haplotypes were predominantly present in the examined population. A clear differentiation between Tunisian, African, and North European/North Italian samples was found, while the Tunisian population showed more genetic affinity to Central and South Italian groups.

Conclusions: Our study provided a first report of LP-associated alleles and haplotypes in the Tunisian population. We highlighted a gradient followed by LP diffusion from Europe to North Africa. Based on the rich historic background of Tunisia, we suggest that this adaptive trait was introduced in that geographic region by a relatively recent gene flow.

Keywords: Lactase persistence, North Africa, Admixture, Tunisia, Natural selection, *LCT*, *MCM6*

Background

Lactase persistence (LP) or non-persistence (LNP) is a genetically determined trait related to the capacity of maintaining lactase activity till adulthood. LNP or lactase intolerance (LI) represents the ancestral state characterized by the downregulation of lactase activity [1]. Due to the continued expression of the *LCT* gene in some groups of North European descent, pastoralists from Africa, the Arabian Peninsula, and Central Asia [2], it is known that the lactase activity may persist even after weaning [2–7]. In fact, variants at the intronic regions in the neighboring *MCM6* gene were described to regulate transcriptional activity of the *LCT* promoter and to confer therefore LP [4].

Several reports from previous studies emphasized that the worldwide prevalence of the LP phenotype is highly variable between different ethnic groups and is positively correlated with the importance of milk in their diet. LP shows a highly structured global geographic distribution, it is indeed common in Europe, particularly in the

* Correspondence: rym.kefi@pasteur.rns.tn; rym.kefi@yahoo.com
[1]Laboratory of Biomedical Genomics and Oncogenetics, Institut Pasteur de Tunis, BP 74, 13 Place Pasteur, 1002 Tunis, Tunisia
[2]Université de Tunis El Manar, 2092 El Manar I, Tunis, Tunisia
Full list of author information is available at the end of the article

northwestern regions [8], in parts of the Indian subcontinent and in many African and Middle Eastern populations that traditionally practice pastoralism and regularly consume milk [6, 9, 10]. It was thus hypothesized that LP evolved because it confers a selective advantage. For instance, the consumption of fresh milk and other dairy products is supposed to allow efficient caloric intake [11], calcium assimilation even at high latitude [12], and to increase water absorption from milk in arid environments [13].

Different LP-associated variants arose in several populations independently due to convergent evolution. In particular, the – 13,910 T (rs4988235) and – 22,018 A (rs182549) alleles were found to be 100 and 97% associated with LP, respectively, in the Finnish population [8]. Furthermore, the – 13,910 T allele is ~86–98% associated with LP in other European populations [14, 15]. However, in the Middle East and in most regions of Africa three other variants are commonly found in LP individuals (i.e., – 13,915 G, – 13,907 G, and – 14,010 C) [4, 16], as reported for instance for Ethiopian pastoralists [17]. Variation at LP-related loci was recently investigated in other groups from the South of Europe (i.e., Italy) and the Arabian Peninsula [18, 19], but not from the North of Africa. In fact, there are only few studies that reported the frequencies of LP-related alleles in Berber groups from Algeria and Morocco [20, 21].

Several hypotheses were suggested to explain the acquisition of the LP adaptive trait in North Africa. The first one is that the expansion of pastoralists from the Middle East into North Africa would presumably have resulted in the spread of lactose tolerance [11, 22]. The distribution of the – 13,910 T allele may thus provide useful answers concerning the origin of the spread of dairying [23]. Indeed, the age estimate for the – 13,910 T variant ranges from 12,300 to 5000 years ago [4, 20, 21, 24, 25], which broadly coincides with the origins of cattle domestication in North Africa and Levant around 10,000 years ago [26]. Indeed, the origin of the pastoral movement from the East and West of Africa to Tunisia was dated to the trading of gold, salt, and slaves across the Sahara [27]. Genetic studies conducted on populations from this area and performed using mitochondrial DNA (mtDNA) and nuclear markers confirmed also a correlation between genetic and geographic structure and/or distances [28] and a predominantly east-west structure [29]. Another hypothesis suggested by Myles and colleagues is that the – 13,910 T allele was introduced in North Africa from Europe via the Gibraltar Strait [30]. However, several studies showed that the Gibraltar Strait represented a strong boundary for gene flow [31–35]. In addition, archeological evidence indicates that the change to pastoralism in coastal North Africa was abrupt and not developed locally over a long period of time [36].

Tunisia has a geostrategic location since it represents a crossroad between Europe, the Middle East and Sub-Saharan Africa and a stepping-stone for recent human migrations. Therefore, the genetic background of the present Tunisian population may have been influenced by these migrations and the successive invasions of the country [27, 37]. The main focus of this study is thus to explore variation patterns of a large number of single nucleotide polymorphisms (SNPs) located in the *LCT/MCM6* region, potentially related to the LP phenotype. Accordingly, we compared newly generated data with those from worldwide human populations to test whether in Tunisia the same mutations as those found in the other parts of the world are observable and, finally, to determine if the distribution of allele frequencies underlying this trait are due to de novo-mutations or admixture with populations that were already characterized by LP (i.e., gene flow).

Methods

Sample collections and SNPs genotyping

The present study was carried out on 117 subjects collected from three different Tunisian geographic macro-areas: 61 samples from the North of Tunisia (NT), 29 samples from the center of Tunisia (CT), and 27 samples from the south of Tunisia (ST). The collection of blood samples was achieved with the collaboration of the National Institute of Nutrition (Tunis, Tunisia). The study was approved by the Ethics Committee of the Institut Pasteur de Tunis (Tunis, Tunisia-Registration numbers IRB00005445, FWA00010074), and all participants provided written informed consent.

DNA was extracted from blood samples using a salting out method, as described previously [38], and was used to genotype 40 informative SNPs selected over a wide genomic interval encompassing the *LCT/MCM6* loci and covering 3 Mb [18].

The Sequenom's MassARRAY Designer software (Sequenom, Inc., San Diego, CA, USA) was used to design PCR and extension primers for the multiplex-PCR, with the total number of SNPs being divided in two multiplex. The first one was composed of 21 SNPs and the second one of 19 SNPs.

Genotyping was performed using the iPlex Gold Genotyping Assay and Sequenom MassArray DNA analysis [39] with Matrix-assisted laser desorption/ionization time-of-flight (MALDI-TOF) mass spectrometry (Sequenom, Inc., San Diego, CA, USA) at the Centre for Applied Biomedical Research (CRBA) of the Bologna S. Orsola University Hospital.

The obtained data for the Tunisian population (TN, N = 117) were compared with published datasets including 453 healthy Italian subjects [18] from North-Western and Central-Western Italy (NCWI, N = 105), North-Eastern Italy (NEI, N = 139), Central-Eastern and Southern Italy (CESI, N = 159), and from Sardinia (SARD,

N = 47).Then, we merged these data with those for 10 populations of African and European ancestries from the 1000 Genomes Project [40]. Namely, 99 Utah residents, with North and West European ancestry (CEU), 99 Esan in Nigeria (ESN), 99 Finnish in Finland (FIN), 91 British in England and Scotland (GBR), 113 Gambian in Western Division (GWD), 107 Iberian populations in Spain (IBS), 99 Luhya in Webuye, Kenya (LWK), 85 Mende in Sierra Leone (MSL), 107 Tuscany in Italy (TSI), 108 Yoruba in Ibadan, Nigeria (YRI). The final merged dataset contained 38 common SNPs (one SNP was not found in the 1000 genomes data). Further information about the studied populations were reported in Additional file 1.

Data analyses

Summary statistics and allele frequencies analyses

Summary statistics, such as nucleotide (π) and haplotype (H) diversity at the examined genomic regions and the number of haplotypes (k), were calculated for all the studied groups using the Arlequin package v.3.5.2 [41].

Allele frequencies for the common genotyped SNPs were calculated and compared between the examined population samples by applying a Chi-square test with the PLINK software package beta release 1.9 [42], significance level was set at 5%. Bonferroni's correction was applied to the obtained asymptotic p values to account for the adopted multiple testing procedures.

Population structure and differentiation analyses

To test the genetic structure of our samples, we computed principal component analysis (PCA) by using the *adegenet* and *ade4* packages implemented in the R software [http://www.R-project.org/]. For this purpose, SNPs pairs that showed r^2 > 0.2 calculated on sliding window of 5 SNPs were removed from the dataset with PLINK by maintaining only one SNP per pair. After such a LD-pruning, 20 SNPs remained for the Tunisian dataset.

The Arlequin software was also used to calculate genetic diversity and pairwise Fst genetic distances between Tunisian samples and the other studied populations. Generated genetic distances (Fst matrix) were plotted to visualize data in multidimensional scaling (MDS) using the statistical package for the social science (SPSS, version 20.0, Chicago, IL, USA).

Discriminant analysis of principal components (DAPC)

To further corroborate results from population structure analyses, we evaluated the cluster membership probabilities for each subject by applying DAPC to the three identified Tunisian groups using the adegenet R package [43]. This approach allowed to provide assignment of individuals to different groups and to assess relationships between populations.

Admixture analyses

To better understand the genetic background and population structure of the LP-related genomic region, we extracted SNPs data for 5 Mb encompassing the *LCT* and *MCM6* loci and the surrounding genes from a dataset generated by means of the Genome-Wide Human SNP Array 6.0 (Affymetrix, Santa Clara, CA, USA) on 135 Tunisian healthy individuals that were recruited from the middle coast of Tunisia as described previously [44].

The study was conducted according to the declaration of Helsinki principles and approved by the Institutional review board (under the reference PV09/06, IRB#0000000044). These data were merged with the HapMap3 [45] and other publicly available data [46–48] to produce a dataset composed of 1560 variants for 1677 individuals (Additional file 1). The same quality control (QC) procedures used for filtering the Sequenom data (see Results section) were applied also to that dataset, which showed a mean genotyping rate of 77%. To avoid bias due to LD, variants that showed r^2 > 0.8 were filtered by pruning one SNP per five using the sliding windows approach implemented in the PLINK package and as a result 347 SNPs were removed.

Admixture proportions in the *LCT/MCM6* region were inferred for each subject included in the pruned dataset by means of the algorithm implemented in the software ADMIXTURE [49], which provides a maximum likelihood estimation of population structure. Individual genotypes were clustered by running an unsupervised analysis, testing numbers of potential ancestral populations (K) from two to eight, and by performing five iterations for each K.

Linkage disequilibrium and haplotype analyses

Patterns of LD at the genotyped loci were investigated using the software Haploview 4.2 [50]. Haplotypes were statistically inferred by considering all SNPs located within high LD blocks and through the Bayesian algorithm implemented in the PHASE software v.2.1 [51]. Evolutionary relationships of the reconstructed haplotypes were finally visualized by means of a median joining network [52] using the Network package v.4.6.1.1 [http://www.fluxus-engineering.com].

Results

Summary statistics of nucleotide and haplotype variation

Genotyping failed for four of the collected samples and individuals with more than 30% missing genotypes were excluded. One SNP (rs749017) for which experimental problems occurred during PCR reaction was also removed. The remaining 39 multiplexed SNPs showed call rates higher than 99% and minor allele frequencies (MAF) >5%. No loci showed a significant departure from Hardy-Weinberg equilibrium (HWE).

Allele frequencies for the typed functional SNPs −13,910 C/T and −22,018 G/A were calculated for all populations (Tables 1 and 2). The frequencies of reference alleles C and G and LNP associated genotype C/C were high in TN (Tables 1 and 2) and reached almost the same values in TSI, CESI, NEI, and IBS (Tables 1 and 2). The highest values were observed instead in ESN, GWD, LWK, MSL, and YRI (Tables 1 and 2), while the lowest ones were found, as expected, in Northern European populations, such as FIN, GBR, and CEU (Tables 1 and 2).

Since population structure analyses did not show appreciable differentiation patterns within TN (see next section), nucleotide diversity was calculated for the overall Tunisian population showing high values of diversity (0.400 ± 0.211) (Additional file 2: Table S1). We then compared Tunisian patterns of variation at the examined loci with those characterizing African and European populations. The obtained values for the TN population were comparable to those obtained for CESI, GBR, SARD, TSI, and CEU populations (0.399 ± 0.211, 0.392 ± 0.208, 0.390 ± 0.208, 0.366 ± 0.195, and 0.335 ± 0.180, respectively). In combination with the previously published data, Northern Italian groups, such as NEI and NCWI, showed the highest variability (0.472 ± 0.246 and 0.485 ± 0.252, respectively), with values similar to FIN and IBS (0.458 ± 0.239 and 0.489 ± 0.254, respectively). However, lower diversity was observed for ESN, GWD, LWK, YRI, and MSL (0.207 ± 0.119, 0.217 ± 0.124, 0.196 ± 0.114, 0.116 ± 0.075, and 0.167 ± 0.100, respectively). Summary statistics of nucleotide and haplotype variation for each group were reported in Additional file 2: Table S1.

Table 1 Allelic frequencies for functional SNPs in the studied populations

Populations	rs4988235		rs182549	
	C (%)	T (%)	G (%)	A (%)
TN	88.07	11.92	85.89	14.10
NCWI	72.38	27.61	72.38	27.61
NEI	75.53	24.46	73.38	26.61
CESI	89.93	10.06	88.05	11.94
SARD	94.56	5.43	94.68	5.31
CEU	26.26	73.73	26.26	73.73
ESN	100	0	100	0
FIN	40.90	59.09	40.90	59.09
GBR	28.02	71.97	28.02	71.97
GWD	99.11	0.88	99.11	0.88
IBS	54.20	45.79	54.20	45.79
LWK	100	0	100	0
MSL	100	0	100	0
TSI	91.12	8.87	90.65	9.34
YRI	100	0	100	0

Allelic frequencies of functional SNPs in the studied populations are reported in Table 1. Frequencies for both reference and adaptive alleles were represented

Table 2 Genotypic frequencies for functional SNPs in the studied populations

Populations	rs4988235			rs182549		
	C/C (%)	C/T (%)	T/T (%)	G/G (%)	G/A (%)	A/A (%)
TN	77.98	20.18	1.83	73.50	24.78	1.70
NCWI	55.23	34.28	10.47	55.23	34.28	10.47
NEI	58.27	34.53	7.19	54.67	37.41	7.91
CESI	79.87	20.12	0	76.10	23.89	0
SARD	89.13	10.86	0	89.36	10.63	0
CEU	7.07	38.38	54.54	7.07	38.38	54.54
ESN	100	0	0	100	0	0
FIN	14.14	53.53	32.32	14.14	53.53	32.32
GBR	9.89	36.26	53.84	0	0	0
GWD	98.23	1.76	0	98.23	1.76	0
IBS	31.77	44.85	23.36	31.77	44.85	23.36
LWK	100	0	0	100	0	0
MSL	100	0	0	100	0	0
TSI	84.11	14.01	1.86	83.17	14.95	1.86
YRI	100	0	0	100	0	0

Genotypic frequencies of functional SNPs in the studied populations are reported in Table 2. Frequencies of different genotypes (C/C, C/T, and T/T) were represented

Population structure analyses

PCA was applied to the generated Tunisian genotypes and showed no clear genetic clustering of the different examined groups (Additional file 2: Figure S1). In addition, we performed DAPC that confirmed the absence of well-defined population clusters (Additional file 2: Figure S2).

Observed patterns of Tunisian variation were thus compared with those specific to African and European populations using Fst estimates computed for the 15 SNPs spanning the longest identified LD block (see LD block analysis, Additional file 2: Figure S3) and plotted using MDS (Fig. 1). Since PCA and DAPC applied to the Tunisian dataset showed no appreciable internal structure, the overall Tunisian population is considered as a single sample (TN). Accordingly, the first dimension differentiates mainly populations of African and European ancestry. TN was positioned near to the intersection of the axes in close proximity to the Southern European aggregate including CESI, TSI, and SARD, suggesting a higher European influence in TN than in the remaining African samples. African populations then appear to cluster in the lower left quadrant described by the second dimension.

In order to further explore patterns of population differentiation, allele frequencies for both functional SNPs were compared between TN and all populations by applying a Chi-square test (Additional file 2: Table S2). Tunisian

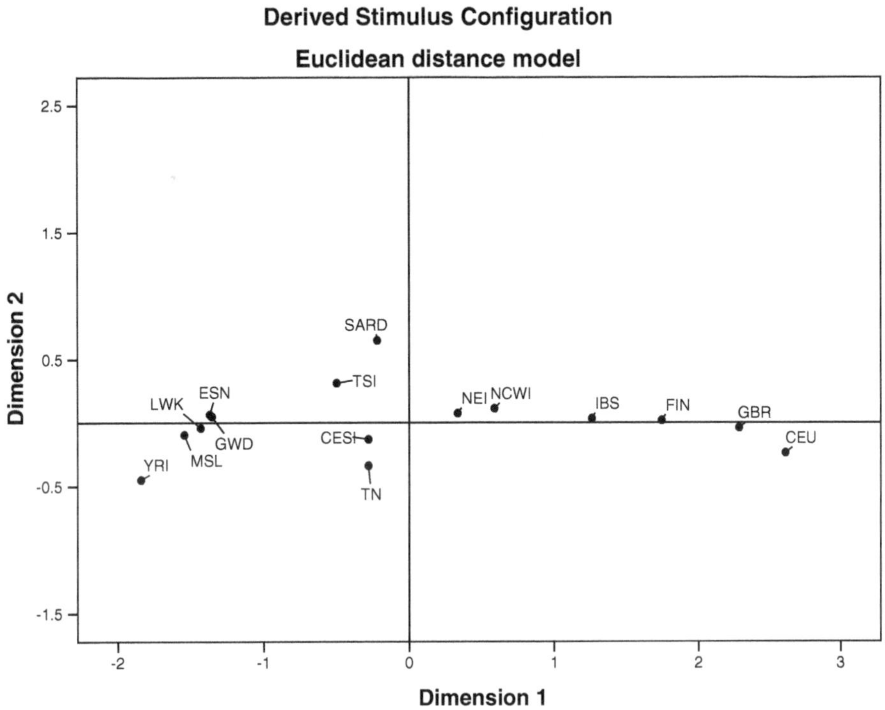

Fig. 1 MDS of Fst estimates based on the LP region for several populations. Non-metric multidimensional scaling analysis of *LCT/MCM6* based on Fst distance showing the relationships among the studied populations. *ESN* Esan in Nigeria, *GWD* Gambian in Western Division, The Gambia, *LWK* Luhya in Webuye, Kenya, *MSL* Mende in Sierra Leone, *YRI* Yoruba in Ibadan, Nigeria, *TSI* Tuscany in Italy, *CESI* Central-Eastern Southern Italy, *NEI* North-Eastern Italy, *NCWI* North Central Western Italy, *SARD* Sardinia, *IBS* Iberian populations in Spain, *FIN* Finnish in Finland, *GBR* British in England and Scotland, *CEU* Utah residents (CEPH) with Northern and Western European ancestry, *TN* Tunisian population

groups were again pooled together since no significant results were obtained when considering the single subgroups. Unadjusted and adjusted differences corresponding to allelic frequencies for the typed SNPs are reported in Additional file 2: Table S2.

The most significant differences were observed mainly between TN and Northern European(i.e. CEU, GBR, and FIN) and Western European populations (i.e., IBS), followed by those compared to the African groups (i.e., GWD, YRI, MSL, ESN, and LWK). In contrast, the lowest differences were observed when we compared TN with Northern Italian samples (i.e., NEI and NCWI).Finally, no significant differences were found when Italian groups with a more Southern European ancestry (i.e., CESI, SARD, and TSI) were considered (Additional file 2: Table S2).

Admixture analysis

We applied the unsupervised ancestry inference algorithm implemented in the ADMIXTURE software on the obtained pruned datasets. As the number of ancestral clusters increased, we observed the emergence of specific population clusters (Fig. 2). At $K = 2$, the ancestry assignment mainly differentiates an African-like (red) and a non-African-like (green) component. $K = 3$ further distinguishes an Asian-like (green) ancestry fraction from a European-like one (blue), while $K = 4$ identifies an additional component (yellow) that is mainly shared among East, Sub-Saharan, and North African clusters. Remarkably, the Tunisian population, and at a lower extent, the Algerian samples appeared to be clearly differentiated from the other African populations. They showed more than 95% contribution from different ancestral populations along different K values. When using the cross validation error, the mean log probability for the successive increase of K levels continues to decrease substantially as K increases. Although, higher values of K reveal additional population-specific ancestries until $K = 4$. For this reason, we focused on $K = 2$ through $K = 4$.

LD block analysis

The analysis of LD patterns that was carried out on the Tunisian dataset showed the existence of a long block of relatively high linkage disequilibrium (266 kb), which includes the two functional variants −13,910 C/T and −22,810 G/A (Additional file 2: Figure S3a). Indeed, the NT group presented a slightly shorter block (157 kb) that contains only six SNPs of the 15 variants observed when the total population was considered (Additional file 2: Figure S3b). However, in CT, the same long haplotype (266 kb) was observed and includes a different SNP

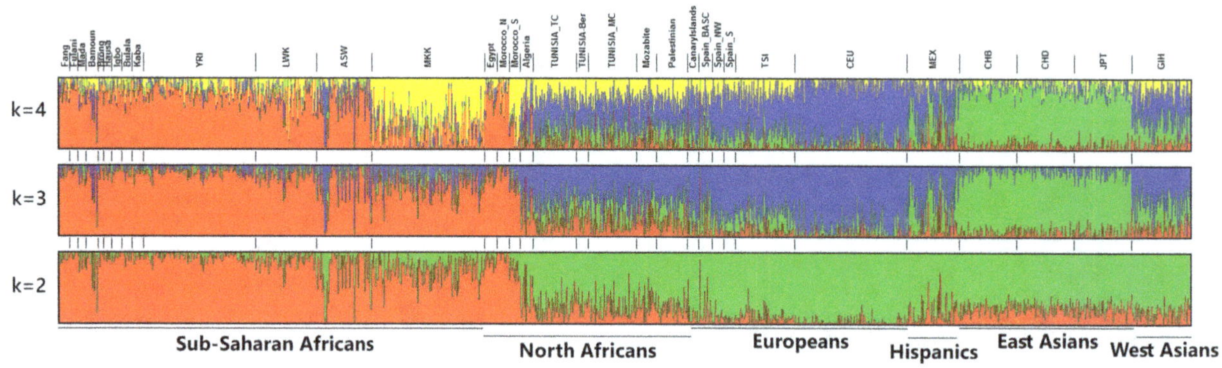

Fig. 2 Ancestry proportions at $K = 2$ to $K = 4$ estimated by means of ADMIXTURE clustering analysis performed on the extended LP-related region. Population structure of worldwide human populations is shown for 1677 individuals from 33 different groups globally distributed (from left to right: 633 Sub-Saharan Africans, 225 North Africans, 399 Europeans, 77 Mexicans, 255 East Asians, 88 Indians)

(rs1438307) (Additional file 2: Figure S3c). Interestingly, this region of high LD appeared to be split into two different blocks spanning respectively (12 kb) and (185 kb) in the ST group (Additional file 2: Figure S3d).

Haplotype reconstruction

We statistically inferred the haplotypes in all the samples that belong to the Tunisian population by considering the 15 SNPs located in the region of overall high LD that is shared among the examined NT, CT, and ST groups. We thus observed a total of 23 different haplotypes, 21 of which carried the − 13,910 C allele and two of them (H19 and H23) showed the functional allele − 13,910 T (Additional file 2: Table S3). The most frequent haplotype (H1) carried the − 13,910 C and the −22,080 G reference alleles, being remarkably represented in NT, CT, and ST groups (0.57, 0.64, and 0.54, respectively). The second most frequent haplotype (H19) carried instead the adaptive alleles, being mainly represented in NT (0.14) and showing instead lower frequencies in CT and ST samples (0.10 and 0.10, respectively).

When we compared the Tunisian population to the other populations, we found that it presented several private haplotypes (e.g., H33, H34, and H35) that carry the reference − 13,910 C and − 22,080 G alleles. The most frequent haplotype (H1) in the merged dataset (Additional file 2: Table S4) carried the − 13,910 C and the − 22,080 G alleles and was represented in all populations. It reaches the highest frequencies in YRI, TN, TSI, MSL, GWD, LWK, CESI, SARD, NEI, ESN, and NCWI, (0.66, 0.58, 0.57, 0.56, 0.56, 0.53, 0.53, 0.51, 0.44, 0.49, and 0.41, respectively). In contrast, the second most common haplotype (H19)which carries the adaptive alleles − 13,910 T and − 22,080 A was highly represented in GBR, CEU, and FIN (0.71,0.70, and 0.55, respectively) and absent in ESN, LWK, MSL, and YRI. The remaining haplotypes finally appeared to be rare and, in some cases, private. Evolutionary relationships among the haplotypes inferred in the studied populations were further explored using a median joining network that highlighted the presence of two clearly distinct groups of allelic combinations separated by several mutational steps. Thus, the haplotype carrying the derived alleles (H19) was segregated into a single cluster and was separated from those carrying the ancestral alleles (H1) (Fig. 3).

Discussion

In the present study, we reported the frequencies and genotypes of the − 13,910 C/T and − 22,810 G/A functional SNPs related to LP [18]. We further described the distribution patterns of *LCT/MCM6* haplotypes in the Tunisian population, and we compared them to those observed in several groups of African and European ancestry that could have intervened in the formation of the Tunisian genetic background as recently hypothesized [48].

The obtained results were discussed in the light of the relatively recent historical relationships between Tunisian and the abovementioned populations [27, 53, 54], in the attempt to clarify the routes followed by LP diffusion and to explore the potential processes of convergent evolution of LP in European and in some non-European populations, such as the Tunisian one.

Investigation of the impact of admixture on a large genomic region related to LP showed that the Tunisian population is highly mixed and displays three major ancestral contributions ascribable to European, African, and Asian ancestry components (Fig. 2). This is in agreement with previous studies that examined uniparental and autosomal markers and showed a multi-ethnic origin of North Africans [27, 37, 46].

Moreover, the study of LP-related genetic diversity revealed that even within the relatively small region represented by Tunisia, a high nucleotide diversity

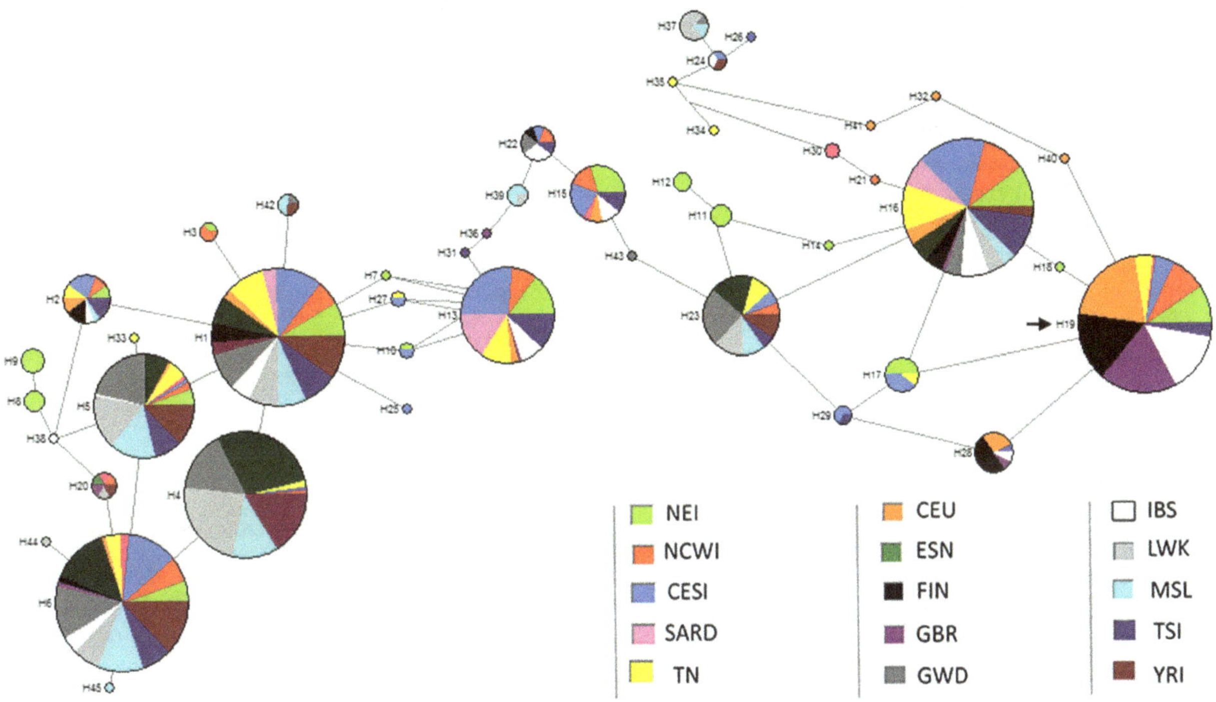

Fig. 3 Median joining network of the inferred haplotypes. Haplotypes proportions were displayed with different colors according to the different examined populations. Adaptive haplotype was indicated by arrow

(0.400 ± 0.212) at *MCM6/LCT* region could be observed (Additional file 2: Table S1). Many studies demonstrated that diversity varied substantially within and between Tunisian and other populations [27, 54]. Furthermore, according to our admixture analysis, the Tunisian population showed higher European proportion compared to other African groups. This was expected if we consider the roots of human migration in Africa. These results corroborate findings from several recent studies [46, 55] and suggest that the TN population has plausibly acquired the LP adaptive variants mainly through admixture with populations of European ancestry.

Our study highlighted an important prevalence of alleles and genotypes related to LI in the Tunisian population, as well as in South European and African groups (Tables 1 and 2). As expected, we found that the North European populations showed the lowest frequencies for these alleles and these findings were consistent with what was found previously [8, 18, 56, 57]. Furthermore, the allele frequencies of the typed SNPs exhibited great variation between Tunisians versus North European and North Italian groups (Additional file 2: Table S2). On the contrary, no differences were detected when we compared different groups from the Mediterranean regions. This distribution of LP-associated − 13,910 T and − 22,018 A alleles is in agreement with the north-south decreasing pattern observed by Anagnostou et al. [58] and De Fanti et al. [18] along the Italian peninsula.

The present study further highlighted the close affinity of the Tunisian population to the South European and Mediterranean populations than to African ones if we consider the LP-related genetic variants. Our data thus support the hypothesis that this adaptive trait was introduced to Tunisia by a relatively recent gene flow and did not evolve locally and independently as occurred for the bulk of Sub-Saharan African groups.

To draw a first picture of the potentially LP-related patterns in the Tunisian population, LD analysis (Additional file 2: Figure S3a, b, c, and d) was also carried out. The presence of a long haplotype block can be interpreted as evidence of a more recent introduction of LP especially in the CT subgroup with respect to those of NT and ST. Our data showed that the − 22,810 A allele was in strong LD with the LP-associated − 13,910 T variant in TN, which is in agreement with prior studies conducted on European populations [8, 18, 24] and to the hypothesis that positive selection at the − 13,910 T allele led to the concomitant rise in frequency of other polymorphisms near to the functional SNP determining the creation of a conserved haplotype block, as observed by Bersaglieri et al. [24].

Finally, we investigated the patterns of Tunisian haplotype variation. We found that the haplotype (H1) carrying the reference LI alleles was the most frequent in all the Tunisian and Italian subgroups, as well as in most African populations. However, the second most frequent haplotype (H19) that carries the adaptive alleles showed the highest frequencies in Northern European populations (i.e., FIN, GBR, and CEU) (Additional file 2: Table S4). Our findings suggest that the distribution of the observed haplotype variation might be due to gene flow that occurred over time from outside or within Africa possibly during key historical events, such as the settlement of the Roman Empire in parts of North Africa. These migration events are also reported in studies based on mtDNA, Y chromosome, and autosomal genetic variation [7, 27, 31, 59, 60]. On the other hand, population structure analyses, such as the MDS plot (Fig. 1), showed that the Tunisian sample was relatively close to the Italian groups. Furthermore, it is differentiated from African populations and especially clustered with samples from Central-Eastern and Southern Italy, supporting the occurrence of appreciable gene flow from Southern Europe to North Africa.

Accordingly, the present study provided a very first view of the genetic structure of the Tunisian population considering the genomic region that modulates the LP phenotype by analyzing subpopulations distributed geographically along the Tunisian territory. Moreover, the investigation of diversity at a wide genomic interval surrounding the *LCT* gene could potentially help to detect genetic variants that may contribute to the development of certain diseases [61]. Indeed, LP was previously shown to be able to confer susceptibility to certain diseases, such as obesity or metabolic disorders [62]. The LP alleles may thus contribute to the complexity of the currently novel and obesogenic environment also in Tunisia.

Conclusions

Our study was the first to report the distribution of LP-associated alleles and haplotypes in the Tunisian population. We thus described the gradient followed by LP diffusion from Europe to Northern Africa. Based on the rich history of gene flow documented for this population, we support the hypothesis of introgression of the LP-associated alleles from outside the region. For this reason, we suppose that the current patterns of diversity observed at this locus in Tunisia may be the result of the interaction of a large number of evolutionary factors, such as genetic drift, demographic processes, people migrations, and admixture.

Further molecular investigation and dissection of the underlying evolutionary forces are needed to fully understand this phenomenon. It could be possible in the future to identify other loci than those on the *LCT/MCM6* that have undergone recent positive selection and that contributed to the modulation of the LP phenotype, thus leading to new insights into human evolution.

Additional files

Additional file 1: Supplementary information about the studied populations.

Additional file 2: Figure S1. Principal component analysis (PCA) plot of genetic variation in Tunisian groups. Distribution of northern, central, and southern samples in the space of two first component of LP-related genotypes. **Figure S2.** Discriminant analysis of principal component (DAPC) in Tunisian groups. DAPC analysis confirmed results of PCA. **Figure S3.** Linkage disequilibrium patterns (LD) of the investigated genomic region in Tunisian population. Each number in squares indicates the r^2 index of LD between the corresponding SNPs. **a** Tunisian population. b Northern Tunisian group. c Central Tunisian group. d Southern Tunisian group. **Table S1.** Summary statistics for the studied populations. Table includes number of chromosome, nucleotide diversity, number of haplotypes, and haplotype diversity. **Table S2.** Results of allelic frequencies comparison between Tunisia and African and European populations. A chi-square test was used to test allelic differences; to reduce the false discovery rate of multiple testing, Bonferroni's multiple comparison adjustment was performed. The statistical significance reached a *p* value less or equal to 5%. **Table S3.** Haplotype list in Tunisian population. A list of 23 different haplotypes generated by PHASE software, distributed between Northern, Central, and Southern Tunisian subgroups. **Table S4.** Haplotype list in the merged dataset. A list of 45 different haplotypes generated when comparing our data with other populations.

Acknowledgements
We thank the Centre for Applied Biomedical Research (CRBA) of the Bologna S. Orsola University Hospital and in particular Dr. Vilma Mantovani and Dr. Elena Marasco for their technical support.

Funding
This work was supported in part by Italian National Grant PRIN 2010EL8TXP_006 to DL, the Tunisian Ministry of Public Health, the Ministry of Higher Education and Scientific Research (LR11IPT05) and the E.C. Grant agreement no. 295097 for FP7 project GM-NCD-Inco (www.genomedika.org).

Authors' contributions
RK, SA, and DL conceived the study. YBH performed the statistical analysis and drafted the manuscript. AA and HJ contributed to the collection of biological material during their consultations. SE assisted to the collection of biological material and extraction of DNA. SDF performed the design of primers. CG, GM, and YBH performed the genotyping analysis. MS, CN, and MN assisted with the statistical analysis. RK, SA, and DL controlled the work progress. RK, MS, GR, SA, and DL critically reviewed the manuscript. All authors approved the final version of the manuscript.

Competing interests
The authors declare that they have no competing interests.

Author details
[1]Laboratory of Biomedical Genomics and Oncogenetics, Institut Pasteur de Tunis, BP 74, 13 Place Pasteur, 1002 Tunis, Tunisia. [2]Université de Tunis El Manar, 2092 El Manar I, Tunis, Tunisia. [3]Laboratory of Molecular Anthropology and Centre for Genome Biology, Department of Biological, Geological and Environmental Sciences (BiGeA), University of Bologna, 40126 Bologna, Italy. [4]Department of external consultation, National Institute of Nutrition and Food Technology, Tunis, Tunisia. [5]Laboratory of Genetic Medicine and Immunology, Weill Cornell Medical College in Qatar, Qatar Foundation, Doha, Qatar. [6]Medical Genetics Unit, Department of Medical and Surgical Sciences, Polyclinic S. Orsola-Malpighi, University of Bologna, Bologna, Italy.

References

1. Hollox E. Evolutionary genetics: genetics of lactase persistence—fresh lessons in the history of milk drinking. Eur J Hum Genet. 2005;13(3):267–9.
2. Swallow DM. Genetics of lactase persistence and lactose intolerance. Annu Rev Genet. 2003;37:197–219.
3. Mulcare CA, et al. The T allele of a single-nucleotide polymorphism 13.9 kb upstream of the lactase gene (LCT) (C-13.9kbT) does not predict or cause the lactase-persistence phenotype in Africans. Am J Hum Genet. 2004;74(6): 1102–10.
4. Tishkoff SA, et al. Convergent adaptation of human lactase persistence in Africa and Europe. Nat Genet. 2007;39(1):31–40.
5. Hollox EJ, et al. Lactase haplotype diversity in the old world. Am J Hum Genet. 2001;68(1):160–72.
6. Itan Y, et al. A worldwide correlation of lactase persistence phenotype and genotypes. BMC Evol Biol. 2010;10:36.
7. Imtiaz F, et al. The T/G 13915 variant upstream of the lactase gene (LCT) is the founder allele of lactase persistence in an urban Saudi population. J Med Genet. 2007;44(10):e89.
8. Enattah NS, et al. Identification of a variant associated with adult-type hypolactasia. Nat Genet. 2002;30(2):233–7.
9. Holden C, Mace R. Phylogenetic analysis of the evolution of lactose digestion in adults. Hum Biol. 1997;69(5):605–28.
10. Gallego Romero I, et al. Herders of Indian and European cattle share their predominant allele for lactase persistence. Mol Biol Evol. 2012;29(1):249–60.
11. Simoons FJ. Primary adult lactose intolerance and the milking habit: a problem in biologic and cultural interrelations. II. A culture historical hypothesis. Am J Dig Dis. 1970;15(8):695–710.
12. Flatz G, Rotthauwe HW. Lactose nutrition and natural selection. Lancet. 1973;2(7820):76–7.
13. Cook GC. Did persistence of intestinal lactase into adult life originate on the Arabian peninsula? Man. 1978;13:418–27.
14. Poulter M, et al. The causal element for the lactase persistence/non-persistence polymorphism is located in a 1 Mb region of linkage disequilibrium in Europeans. Ann Hum Genet. 2003;67(Pt 4):298–311.
15. Ridefelt P, Hakansson LD. Lactose intolerance: lactose tolerance test versus genotyping. Scand J Gastroenterol. 2005;40(7):822–6.
16. Ingram CJ, et al. A novel polymorphism associated with lactose tolerance in Africa: multiple causes for lactase persistence? Hum Genet. 2007;120(6):779–88.
17. Ingram CJ, et al. Multiple rare variants as a cause of a common phenotype: several different lactase persistence associated alleles in a single ethnic group. J Mol Evol. 2009;69(6):579–88.
18. De Fanti S, et al. Inferring the genetic history of lactase persistence along the Italian peninsula from a large genomic interval surrounding the LCT gene. Am J Phys Anthropol. 2015;158(4):708–18.
19. Bayoumi R, et al. Positive selection of lactase persistence among people of southern Arabia. Am J Phys Anthropol. 2016;161(4):676–84.
20. Enattah NS, et al. Evidence of still-ongoing convergence evolution of the lactase persistence T-13910 alleles in humans. Am J Hum Genet. 2007;81(3):615–25.
21. Enattah NS, et al. Independent introduction of two lactase-persistence alleles into human populations reflects different history of adaptation to milk culture. Am J Hum Genet. 2008;82(1):57–72.
22. McCracken RD. Lactase deficiency: an example of dietary evolution. Curr Anthropol. 1971;12:497–517.
23. Barker G. Transitions to farming and pastoralism in North Africa. In: Bellwood P, Renfrew C, editors. Examining the farming/language dispersal hypothesis. Cambridge: McDonald Institute for Archaeological Research; 2003. p. 151–61.
24. Bersaglieri T, et al. Genetic signatures of strong recent positive selection at the lactase gene. Am J Hum Genet. 2004;74(6):1111–20.
25. Coelho M, et al. Microsatellite variation and evolution of human lactase persistence. Hum Genet. 2005;117(4):329–39.
26. Hanotte O, et al. African pastoralism: genetic imprints of origins and migrations. Science. 2002;296(5566):336–9.
27. Kefi R, et al. Phylogeny and genetic structure of Tunisians and their position within Mediterranean populations. Mitochondrial DNA. 2015;26(4):593–604.
28. Cavalli-Sforza LL, Menozzi P, Piazza A. The history and geography of human genes. Princeton: Princeton Univ Press; 1994.
29. Bosch E, et al. Population history of north Africa: evidence from classical genetic markers. Hum Biol. 1997;69(3):295–311.
30. Myles S, et al. Genetic evidence in support of a shared Eurasian-North African dairying origin. Hum Genet. 2005;117(1):34–42.
31. Arredi B, et al. A predominantly neolithic origin for Y-chromosomal DNA variation in North Africa. Am J Hum Genet. 2004;75(2):338–45.
32. Bosch E, et al. Variation in short tandem repeats is deeply structured by genetic background on the human Y chromosome. Am J Hum Genet. 1999; 65(6):1623–38.
33. Bosch E, et al. High-resolution analysis of human Y-chromosome variation shows a sharp discontinuity and limited gene flow between northwestern Africa and the Iberian peninsula. Am J Hum Genet. 2001;68(4):1019–29.
34. Bosch E, et al. Genetic structure of north-west Africa revealed by STR analysis. Eur J Hum Genet. 2000;8(5):360–6.
35. Simoni L, et al. Patterns of gene flow inferred from genetic distances in the Mediterranean region. Hum Biol. 1999;71(3):399–415.
36. Holl AFC. The dawn of African pastoralisms: an introductory note. J AnthropolArchaeol. 1998;17:81–96.
37. Fadhlaoui-Zid K, et al. Genetic structure of Tunisian ethnic groups revealed by paternal lineages. Am J Phys Anthropol. 2011;146(2):271–80.
38. Miller SA, Dykes DD, Polesky HF. A simple salting out procedure for extracting DNA from human nucleated cells. Nucleic Acids Res. 1988;16(3): 1215.
39. Jurinke C, et al. The use of MassARRAY technology for high throughput genotyping. Adv Biochem Eng Biotechnol. 2002;77:57–74.
40. Abecasis GR, et al. A map of human genome variation from population-scale sequencing. Nature. 2010;467(7319):1061–73.
41. Excoffier L, Laval G, Schneider S. Arlequin (version 3.0): an integrated software package for population genetics data analysis. Evol Bioinformatics Online. 2005;1:47–50.
42. Purcell S, et al. PLINK: a tool set for whole-genome association and population-based linkage analyses. Am J Hum Genet. 2007;81(3):559–75.
43. Jombart T, Devillard S, Balloux F. Discriminant analysis of principal components: a new method for the analysis of genetically structured populations. BMC Genet. 2010;11:94.
44. Shan J, et al. Genome scan study of prostate cancer in Arabs: identification of three genomic regions with multiple prostate cancer susceptibility loci in Tunisians. J Transl Med. 2013;11:121.
45. International HapMap Consortium. The International HapMap Project. Nature. 2003;426(6968):789-96.
46. Henn BM, et al. Genomic ancestry of North Africans supports back-to-Africa migrations. PLoS Genet. 2012;8(1):e1002397.
47. Haber M, et al. Genome-wide diversity in the levant reveals recent structuring by culture. PLoS Genet. 2013;9(2):e1003316.
48. Botigue LR, et al. Gene flow from North Africa contributes to differential human genetic diversity in southern Europe. Proc Natl Acad Sci U S A. 2013; 110(29):11791–6.
49. Alexander DH, Novembre J, Lange K. Fast model-based estimation of ancestry in unrelated individuals. Genome Res. 2009;19(9):1655–64.
50. Wall JD, Pritchard JK. Haplotype blocks and linkage disequilibrium in the human genome. Nat Rev Genet. 2003;4(8):587–97.
51. Stephens M, Donnelly P. A comparison of Bayesian methods for haplotype reconstruction from population genotype data. Am J Hum Genet. 2003;73(5):1162–9.
52. Bandelt HJ, Forster P, Rohl A. Median-joining networks for inferring intraspecific phylogenies. Mol Biol Evol. 1999;16(1):37–48.
53. Arauna LR, et al. Recent historical migrations have shaped the gene pool of Arabs and Berbers in North Africa. Mol Biol Evol. 2017;34(2):318–29.
54. Cherni L, et al. Genetic variation in Tunisia in the context of human diversity worldwide. Am J Phys Anthropol. 2016;161(1):62–71.
55. Bekada A, et al. Genetic heterogeneity in Algerian human populations. PLoS One. 2015;10(9):e0138453.
56. Sahi T. Genetics and epidemiology of adult-type hypolactasia. Scand J Gastroenterol Suppl. 1994;202:7–20.
57. Kuokkanen M, et al. Lactase persistence and ovarian carcinoma risk in Finland, Poland and Sweden. Int J Cancer. 2005;117(1):90–4.
58. Anagnostou P, et al. Tracing the distribution and evolution of lactase persistence in southern Europe through the study of the T(−13910) variant. Am J Hum Biol. 2009;21(2):217–9.
59. Tishkoff SA, et al. The genetic structure and history of Africans and African Americans. Science. 2009;324(5930):1035–44.
60. Hassan HY, et al. Y-chromosome variation among Sudanese: restricted gene flow, concordance with language, geography, and history. Am J Phys Anthropol. 2008;137(3):316–23.
61. Ronald J, Akey JM. Genome-wide scans for loci under selection in humans. Hum Genomics. 2005;2(2):113–25.

10

Several type 2 diabetes-associated variants in genes annotated to WNT signaling interact with dietary fiber in relation to incidence of type 2 diabetes

George Hindy*, Inês G. Mollet, Gull Rukh, Ulrika Ericson and Marju Orho-Melander

Abstract

Background: TCF7L2 is a central transcription factor in the canonical wingless-type MMTV integration site (WNT) signaling pathway, and genetic variants in *TCF7L2* have been found to interact with dietary fiber intake on type 2 diabetes risk. Here, we investigate whether other type 2 diabetes genes could be involved in the WNT signaling pathway and whether variants in such genes might interact with dietary fiber on type 2 diabetes incidence.

Results: We included 26,905 individuals without diabetes from the Malmö Diet and Cancer Study cohort. Diet data was collected at baseline using a food frequency questionnaire, a 7-day food record, and an interview. Altogether, 51 gene loci were analyzed for putative links to WNT signaling. Over a mean follow-up period of 14.7 years, 3132 incident cases of type 2 diabetes were recorded. Seven genes (nine single nucleotide polymorphisms (SNPs)) were annotated as involved in WNT signaling including *TCF7L2* (rs7903146 and rs12255372), *HHEX* (rs1111875), *HNF1A* (rs7957197), *NOTCH2* (rs10923931), *TLE4* (rs13292136), *ZBED3* (rs4457053), and *PPARG* (rs1801282 and rs13081389). SNPs in *TCF7L2*, *NOTCH2*, and *ZBED3* showed significant interactions with fiber intake on type 2 diabetes incidence ($P_{interaction}$ = 0.034, 0.005, 0.017, and 0.002, respectively). The magnitude of the association between the *TCF7L2* risk allele and incident type 2 diabetes increased from the lowest to the highest quintiles of fiber intake. Higher fiber associated with lower type 2 diabetes risk only among risk allele carriers of the *NOTCH2* variant and homozygotes of the risk allele of the *ZBED3* variant.

Conclusions: Our results suggest that several type 2 diabetes susceptibility SNPs in genes involved in WNT signaling may interact with dietary fiber intake on type 2 diabetes incidence.

Keywords: Gene-diet interactions, TCF7L2, WNT signaling, Type 2 diabetes, Dietary fiber

Background

Type 2 diabetes is a multifactorial disease, and both genetic and environmental factors, and their complex interactions, are thought to contribute to the disease development. Recently, more than 80 type 2 diabetes associated genetic variants have been discovered mainly through genome-wide association studies (GWAS) [24, 28]. Of these, the transcription factor 7-like 2 gene (*TCF7L2*) variant rs7903146 shows the strongest association with type 2 diabetes [12].

TCF7L2 is a principal transcription factor in the canonical wingless-type MMTV integration site (WNT) signaling pathway [29]. This highlights the importance of the canonical WNT pathway in the pathogenesis of type 2 diabetes. Many studies have demonstrated an essential role for the WNT signaling pathway in pancreatic islet beta cell genesis and proliferation [33]. Glucagon-like peptide-1 (GLP-1)-mediated proliferation of rat beta cell line (INS-1) has been shown to occur through activation of the WNT pathway [19]. In addition, WNT signaling has been reported to mediate the expression of the pro-glucagon gene in intestinal L cells and thus the synthesis of GLP-1 [43]. Moreover,

* Correspondence: george.hindy@med.lu.se
Department of Clinical Sciences in Malmö, Lund University, Skåne University Hospital, Jan Waldenströms gata 35, SE-205 02 Malmö, Sweden

activation of the WNT pathway has been observed to prevent pre-adipocyte differentiation [32].

Several studies have reported a protective association between higher dietary fiber intake and type 2 diabetes [25, 39]. This inverse relationship seems to be likely driven by the cereal fiber component. In a meta-analysis of prospective studies, cereal fiber but not vegetable/fruit fiber intake has been shown to associate with lower risk of type 2 diabetes [34]. Short chain fatty acids (SCFA), the by-products of colonic fermentation of dietary fiber, have been reported to hyper-activate WNT signaling in a colorectal cell line [5]. Fiber intake could thus exert its protective effect at least partially by modifying WNT activity through SCFAs. SCFAs have previously been associated with increased insulin secretion [27], promotion of adipocyte differentiation [44], and induction of GLP-1 secretion via the free fatty acid receptor 2 (FFAR2) [36]. Biological interactions could conceivably occur between fiber intake through SFCAs and the WNT pathway on type 2 diabetes risk at the level of pancreatic beta cells, intestinal L cells, or adipocytes.

We have previously reported that the protective associated effect of higher fiber intake may be restricted to the non-risk CC genotype carriers of *TCF7L2* rs7903146 [14]. Similar results were also reported in the EPIC-Potsdam case-control study showing a protective association between higher whole grain intake and type 2 diabetes only among the non-risk allele carriers [9]. In line with these results, lower risk of type 2 diabetes by higher whole grain and cereal fiber intake was restricted to the non-risk allele carriers in a subgroup of men in the Stockholm Diabetes Prevention Program [42]. Further, another lifestyle intervention demonstrated a greater weight loss by higher fiber intake after a 9-month intervention among individuals carrying the non-risk CC genotype compared to risk allele carriers [13].

As association between *TCF7L2* and type 2 diabetes has highlighted an important role for WNT signaling in type 2 diabetes pathogenesis, we therefore used pathway analysis tools to evaluate whether other type 2 diabetes associated loci might be connected to this pathway. As several studies have indicated that dietary fiber or whole grain intake might modify the association between *TCF7L2* variants and type 2 diabetes or weight loss, we hypothesized that additional type 2 diabetes susceptibility genes in the WNT pathway may interact with fiber intake on type 2 diabetes incidence.

Results

Association between fiber intake and type 2 diabetes incidence and related quantitative traits

Association between fiber intake and type 2 diabetes incidence and related quantitative traits in the Malmö Diet and Cancer Study (MDCS) are shown in Table 1. A total of 3132 incident cases of type 2 diabetes were recorded after a mean follow-up time of 14.7 years. Higher fiber intake was observed to strongly associate ($P < 0.001$) with reduced baseline fasting plasma glucose (FPG), fasting plasma insulin (FPI), homeostasis model for assessment of insulin resistance (HOMA-IR), and glycated hemoglobin (HbA_{1C}) (Table 1).

Table 1 Association between fiber intake and type 2 diabetes and related traits in MDCS

		Quintiles of fiber intake						
	Total	Q1	Q2	Q3	Q4	Q5	Beta (SE) or HR (CI)	*P* value[a]
N	26,905	5381	5381	5381	5381	5381		
Sex (% males)	10,429 (39 %)	3039 (57 %)	2426 (45 %)	2062 (38 %)	1635 (30 %)	1267 (24 %)		
Age (years)	58.0 ± 7.6	57.4 ± 7.5	57.7 ± 7.7	58.2 ± 7.7	58.3 ± 7.7	58.3 ± 7.5		
Incident type 2 diabetes	3132 (10.6 %)	666 (11.3 %)	650 (11.0 %)	670 (11.4 %)	564 (9.56 %)	582 (10.9 %)	0.98 (0.96–1.01)	0.17
BMI (kg/m^2)	25.6 ± 3.9	25.5 ± 3.9	25.6 ± 3.8	25.8 ± 3.9	25.7 ± 3.9	25.5 ± 4.0	0.02 (0.02)	0.22
FPG (mmol/L)[b]	5.64 ± 0.82	5.81 ± 1.04	5.68 ± 0.78	5.63 ± 0.79	5.58 ± 0.73	5.54 ± 0.72	−0.03 (0.008)	0.0001
FPI (pmol/L)[b]	46.5 ± 46.2	50.7 ± 43.5	46.2 ± 33.6	47.5 ± 50.5	45.1 ± 59.3	43.9 ± 38.9	−0.95 (0.48)	6×10^{-07}
HOMA-IR[b]	1.60 ± 1.22	1.75 ± 1.32	1.64 ± 1.06	1.65 ± 1.62	1.53 ± 1.04	1.48 ± 1.00	−0.06 (0.01)	6×10^{-09}
HbA_{1C} (%)[b]	4.81 ± 0.49	4.89 ± 0.58	4.82 ± 0.45	4.82 ± 0.53	4.80 ± 0.43	4.76 ± 0.47	−0.02 (0.005)	0.00002
HbA_{1C} (mmol/mol)[b]	39.7 ± 5.00	40.5 ± 5.88	39.8 ± 4.56	39.8 ± 5.36	39.5 ± 4.38	39.2 ± 4.75	−0.22 (0.05)	0.00002
Fiber (g/1000 Kcal)	9.03 ± 2.72	5.77 ± 0.81	7.47 ± 0.36	8.69 ± 0.36	10.09 ± 0.48	13.13 ± 2.19		

Data are means ± SD unless otherwise stated. Number of individuals included in MDCS cohort, $n = 26{,}905$

HR hazard ratio, *BMI* body mass index, *FPG* fasting plasma glucose, *FPI* fasting plasma insulin, *HOMA-IR* homeostatic model assessment for insulin resistance, HbA_{1C} glycated hemoglobin

[a]Adjusted for age, sex, BMI, total energy intake, dietary assessment method, season, leisure-time physical activity, smoking, alcohol intake, and education where appropriate

[b]Data available only for the MDC-CC, $n = 5499$

Annotation of type 2 diabetes associated genes to the WNT pathway

A total of nine type 2 diabetes associated genes were annotated to the WNT signaling pathway, and of these, seven genes (nine single nucleotide polymorphisms (SNPs)) were annotated and selected for further analyses. We included SNPs mapping to genes with roles upstream of TCF7L2 in the WNT signaling pathway. Functional positioning of these genes within the WNT pathway is detailed in the Additional file 1: Figure S1. These included *TCF7L2* (rs7903146 and rs12255372), *HHEX* (rs1111875), *HNF1A* (rs7957197), *NOTCH2* (rs10923931), *TLE4* (rs13292136), *ZBED3* (rs4457053), and *PPARG* (rs1801282 and rs13081389).

Association between WNT-annotated gene variants and type 2 diabetes and related traits

Both *TCF7L2* variants (rs7903146 and rs12255372), *HHEX* rs1111875, and *HNF1A* rs7957197 were associated with increased risk of type 2 diabetes (Table 2). In addition, the *TCF7L2* variants and the *HNF1A* variant associated with elevated baseline FPG. The *HHEX* variant associated with lower baseline FPI, and the *TCF7L2* variants and the *ZBED3* variant associated with elevated baseline HbA_{1C} (Table 2).

Interaction between WNT-annotated gene variants and fiber intake on incidence of type 2 diabetes

The *TCF7L2* rs7903146 variant interacted with quintiles of fiber intake on type 2 diabetes incidence ($P_{interaction}$ = 0.034). Additionally, another *TCF7L2* variant, rs12255372, showed a somewhat stronger interaction with fiber intake on type 2 diabetes incidence ($P_{interaction}$ = 0.005) (Table 3). The magnitude of the associated effect of the *TCF7L2* risk allele on type 2 diabetes incidence was higher among individuals in the higher fiber intake quintiles as compared to individuals in the lower quintiles. Moreover, individuals in the lowest fiber quintile did not show any increased risk of type 2 diabetes by the risk (T) allele of rs12255372 (Table 4). Higher fiber intake showed a tendency for association with lower risk of type 2 diabetes among non-risk GG genotype carriers of rs12255372 (hazard ratio (HR) 0.96; 95 % confidence interval (CI) 0.92–1.00; $P = 0.06$) but not among GT and TT genotype carriers.

Of the WNT-annotated SNPs (in genes upstream of TCF7L2), we found, in addition to *TCF7L2*, the SNPs in *NOTCH2* and *ZBED3* loci (Table 4) to significantly interact with fiber intake on type 2 diabetes incidence. The *NOTCH2* locus was observed to interact with fiber intake on type 2 diabetes incidence ($P_{interaction}$ = 0.017). Higher fiber intake was observed to associate with lower risk of type 2 diabetes only among carriers of the risk (T) allele; GT (HR 0.93; CI 0.87–0.996; $P = 0.038$); and TT (HR 0.63; CI 0.44–0.90; $P = 0.01$). The *NOTCH2* risk allele did not associate with type 2 diabetes incidence in the whole population (HR 0.99; CI 0.91–1.09; $P = 0.90$); however, it was associated significantly with decreased risk of type 2 diabetes in the fourth fiber intake quintile (HR 0.75; CI 0.60–0.95; $P = 0.015$) (Table 4). Another interaction was observed between quintiles of fiber intake and *ZBED3* rs4457053 on type 2 diabetes incidence ($P_{interaction}$ = 0.002). Higher fiber intake was observed to associate with lower risk of type 2 diabetes only among homozygotes for the risk (G) allele (HR 0.85; CI 0.76–0.95; $P = 0.003$) (Table 4).

Discussion

In this prospective study, we observe interactions between dietary fiber intake and variants in three genes annotated to the canonical WNT signaling pathway influencing the risk of type 2 diabetes in a large population-based cohort over a 15-year follow-up period. This indicates a putative role of the WNT pathway in the pathogenesis of type 2

Table 2 Association between SNPs in WNT-associated genes and type 2 diabetes and related traits in MDCS

	Incident type 2 diabetes[a]		FPG (mmol/L)[b]		FPI (pmol/L)[b]		HbA_{1C} (%)[b]	
	HR (95 % CI)	*P* value	Beta (SE)	*P* value	Beta (SE)	*P* value	Beta (SE)	*P* value
TCF7L2 rs7903146	1.33 (1.25–1.40)	1×10^{-23}	0.04 (0.02)	0.03	0.16 (1.05)	0.82	0.02 (0.01)	0.04
TCF7L2 rs12255372	1.24 (1.17–1.31)	9×10^{-14}	0.03 (0.02)	0.15	−0.73 (1.07)	0.79	0.02 (0.01)	0.07
HHEX rs1111875	1.06 (1.01–1.12)	0.03	−0.02 (0.02)	0.20	−3.07 (0.99)	0.016	0.01 (0.01)	0.31
HNF1A rs7957197	1.12 (1.05–1.20)	0.001	0.04 (0.02)	0.04	1.11 (1.23)	0.54	0.01 (0.01)	0.30
NOTCH2 rs10923931	0.99 (0.91–1.09)	0.90	0.04 (0.03)	0.19	−0.14 (1.73)	0.69	0.02 (0.02)	0.35
TLE4 rs13292136	1.03 (0.94–1.12)	0.60	-7×10^{-05} (0.03)	1.00	1.71 (1.72)	0.40	0.02 (0.02)	0.30
ZBED3 rs4457053	1.01 (0.96–1.08)	0.64	0.01 (0.02)	0.44	−1.41 (1.14)	0.22	0.02 (0.01)	0.04
PPARG rs1801282	1.08 (1.00–1.16)	0.051	0.03 (0.02)	0.24	1.16 (1.38)	0.42	−0.002 (0.01)	0.88
PPARG rs13081389	1.00 (0.91–1.11)	0.97	0.03 (0.03)	0.35	1.67 (1.79)	0.33	0.01 (0.02)	0.68

HR hazard ratio, *FPG* fasting plasma glucose, *FPI* fasting plasma insulin, HbA_{1C} glycated hemoglobin
[a]Adjusted for age and sex, $N = 26{,}905$
[b]Adjusted for age and sex; data available only for the MDC-CC, $N = 5499$

Table 3 Interaction between variants in WNT-associated genes and quintiles of fiber intake on type 2 diabetes incidence

	Alleles	Risk allele	Genotype			HR[b, c, d, e]	95 % CI	p[b, c, d, e]
			XX	XR[a]	RR			
TCF7L2 rs7903146	C/T	T	13,475	9414	1720	1.20[c]	1.05–1.36	0.006
Fiber						0.96[d]	0.93–0.998	0.037
TCF7L2 rs7903146 × Fiber						1.04[e]	1.003–1.09	0.034
TCF7L2 rs12255372	G/T	T	13,517	9689	1785	1.06	0.93–1.21	0.36
Fiber						0.95	0.91–0.98	0.003
TCF7L2 rs12255372 × Fiber						1.06	1.02–1.10	0.005
HHEX rs1111875	A/G	G	4329	12,518	8816	0.99	0.88–1.11	0.83
Fiber						0.95	0.90–1.00	0.05
HHEX rs1111875 × Fiber						1.03	0.99–1.07	0.14
HNF1A rs7957197	A/T	T	1067	8549	16,401	1.15	0.99–1.34	0.06
Fiber						1.00	0.92–1.08	0.92
HNF1A rs7957197 × Fiber						0.99	0.95–1.04	0.75
NOTCH2 rs10923931	G/T	T	20,612	4372	228	1.24	1.02–1.51	0.035
Fiber						1.00	0.97–1.03	0.97
NOTCH2 rs10923931 × Fiber						0.93	0.87–0.99	0.017
TLE4 rs13292136	C/T	C	186	3928	21,962	0.99	0.81–1.23	0.96
Fiber						0.97	0.86–1.10	0.66
TLE4 rs13292136 × Fiber						1.01	0.94–1.07	0.88
ZBED3 rs4457053	A/G	G	13,455	9362	1642	1.22	1.06–1.39	0.004
Fiber						1.02	0.98–1.05	0.38
ZBED3 rs4457053 × Fiber						0.94	0.90–0.98	0.002
PPARG rs1801282	G/C	C	548	6263	19,038	1.18	0.99–1.40	0.06
Fiber						1.01	0.92–1.12	0.77
PPARG rs1801282 × Fiber						0.98	0.93–1.04	0.52
PPARG rs13081389	A/G	A	165	3256	21,423	0.97	0.77–1.21	0.77
Fiber						0.93	0.81–1.07	0.30
PPARG rs13081389 × Fiber						1.03	0.96–1.10	0.46

HR hazard ratio
[a]X designates the non-risk allele and R designates the risk allele
[b]Adjusted for age, sex, BMI, total energy intake, dietary assessment method, season, leisure-time physical activity, smoking, alcohol intake, and education
[c]Main effect per risk allele from the multivariable model including the interaction term
[d]Main effect per quintile of fiber intake from the multivariable model including the interaction term
[e]Interaction effect

diabetes and a potential modulating role of dietary fiber through this pathway.

Annotation of the 51 gene loci corresponding to 58 SNPs associated with type 2 diabetes resulted in identification of seven genes having known connections with WNT signaling. We could replicate our previous finding of interaction between *TCF7L2* variants and fiber intake in relation to the risk of developing type 2 diabetes over time [14]. In addition, novel interactions between dietary fiber intake and two type 2 diabetes-associated variants in the *NOTCH2* and *ZBED3* loci were observed. Higher fiber intake was observed to associate with lower incidence of type 2 diabetes only among risk allele carriers of the *NOTCH2* variant and homozygotes for the risk allele of the *ZBED3* variant.

The WNT pathway may play a central role in the pathogenesis of type 2 diabetes. Pancreatic beta cell genesis and GLP-1-mediated proliferation have been shown to be mediated through activation of the WNT pathway [19, 33]. In addition to effects on beta cells, the WNT pathway mediates pro-glucagon gene expression in intestinal L cells and thus the synthesis of GLP-1 [43]. Activation of the WNT pathway has been shown to keep pre-adipocytes in their undifferentiated state and could eventually result in ectopic fat accumulation and insulin resistance [32]. Recently, a liver-specific knock out of *tcf7l2* in mice was linked to reduced hepatic glucose production [4]. WNT transcriptional activity has been reported to be hyper-activated by butyrate which is one of

Table 4 HR of incident type 2 diabetes by genotype and quintiles of fiber intake

		Genotype					
		XX	XR[a]	RR	HR per R allele	P^{b}_{trend}	$P^{c}_{interaction}$
TCF7L2 rs7903146							
	Q1	1.16 (0.98–1.39)	1.58 (1.32–1.89)	1.56 (1.14–2.15)	1.24 (1.09–1.40)	0.001	0.034
	Q2	1.13 (0.95–1.35)	1.52 (1.27–1.82)	1.92 (1.43–2.60)	1.26 (1.11–1.42)	0.0002	
	Q3	1.15 (0.97–1.37)	1.62 (1.36–1.93)	2.10 (1.60–2.77)	1.37 (1.22–1.55)	1×10^{-7}	
	Q4	1.02 (0.85–1.22)	1.35 (1.12–1.62)	1.93 (1.48–2.58)	1.31 (1.15–1.49)	5×10^{-5}	
	Q5	1 (ref)	1.70 (1.42–2.03)	2.00 (1.49–2.70)	1.47 (1.30–1.66)	2×10^{-9}	
	HR per Q	0.97 (0.93–1.01)	0.99 (0.95–1.03)	1.05 (0.95–1.15)			
	P^{c}_{trend}	0.19	0.64	0.37			
TCF7L2 rs12255372							
	Q1	1.22 (1.03–1.45)	1.44 (1.20–1.73)	1.27 (0.90–1.78)	1.08 (0.95–1.22)	0.26	0.005
	Q2	1.16 (0.98–1.38)	1.32 (1.10–1.58)	1.74 (1.31–2.32)	1.16 (1.02–1.31)	0.02	
	Q3	1.07 (0.90–1.28)	1.53 (1.29–1.82)	1.89 (1.44–2.47)	1.36 (1.21–1.53)	3×10^{-7}	
	Q4	1.02 (0.86–1.22)	1.27 (1.05–1.52)	1.68 (1.25–2.26)	1.23 (1.08–1.40)	0.002	
	Q5	1 (ref)	1.41 (1.18–1.68)	1.99 (1.48–2.67)	1.40 (1.23–1.59)	4×10^{-7}	
	HR per Q	0.96 (0.92–1.00)	0.98 (0.94–1.02)	1.05 (0.96–1.16)			
	P_{trend}	0.060	0.37	0.28			
NOTCH2 rs10923931							
	Q1	1.00 (0.87–1.14)	1.14 (0.92–1.42)	1.66 (0.86–3.23)	1.12 (0.93–1.34)	0.24	0.017
	Q2	1.00 (0.88–1.14)	1.04 (0.85–1.28)	0.76 (0.28–2.04)	1.06 (0.88–1.28)	0.51	
	Q3	1.03 (0.91–1.18)	1.10 (0.90–1.35)	1.05 (0.47–2.34)	1.08 (0.90–1.30)	0.41	
	Q4	0.97 (0.85–1.11)	0.70 (0.55–0.90)	0.75 (0.28–2.00)	0.75 (0.60–0.95)	0.015	
	Q5	1 (ref)	1.00 (0.80–1.25)	0.25 (0.04–1.80)	0.93 (0.75–1.15)	0.50	
	HR per Q	1.00 (0.97–1.03)	0.93 (0.87–0.996)	0.63 (0.44–0.90)			
	P_{trend}	0.89	0.038	0.010			
ZBED3 rs4457053							
	Q1	0.96 (0.81–1.13)	1.03 (0.86–1.23)	1.51 (1.14–2.01)	1.16 (1.02–1.31)	0.06	0.002
	Q2	0.96 (0.81–1.12)	1.00 (0.84–1.20)	1.04 (0.74–1.46)	1.03 (0.90–1.17)	0.36	
	Q3	1.04 (0.89–1.21)	1.04 (0.88–1.24)	0.85 (0.59–1.22)	0.99 (0.87–1.12)	0.97	
	Q4	0.93 (0.79–1.09)	0.93 (0.78–1.12)	0.67 (0.46–0.99)	0.95 (0.83–1.10)	0.55	
	Q5	1 (ref)	0.98 (0.82–1.17)	0.72 (0.50–1.04)	0.94 (0.81–1.07)	0.25	
	HR per Q	1.01 (0.97–1.05)	0.98 (0.94–1.03)	0.85 (0.76–0.95)			
	P_{trend}	0.69	0.40	0.003			

HR hazard ratio, *Q* quintile
[a]X designates the non-risk allele and R designates the risk allele
[b]Adjusted for age and sex
[c]Adjusted for age, sex, BMI, total energy intake, dietary assessment method, season, leisure-time physical activity, smoking, alcohol intake, and education

the SCFAs produced by microfloral fermentation of dietary fiber leading to apoptosis of colorectal cancer cells [5, 17]. Fiber intake is mainly linked to elevated luminal concentrations of SCFAs in the intestines. In addition, it has been linked to elevated SCFAs in plasma after 1 year of high-fiber intervention [10]. Fiber intake could thus at least partially exert its systemic anti-diabetogenic effects through modulation of the WNT signaling pathway by SCFAs.

In line with our previous report, we observed an interaction between *TCF7L2* rs7903146 and fiber intake on type 2 diabetes incidence. However, our present study included 3132 type 2 diabetes cases instead of 1649 cases in our previous study [14]. Another *TCF7L2* SNP (rs12255372) showed a somewhat stronger interaction with fiber. However, the two SNPs are in linkage disequilibrium ($r^2 = 0.70$ and $D' = 0.91$) and are thus very likely reflecting the same interaction. In this study, we observe that the direction of the interaction effects was in opposite direction with variants in *NOTCH2* and *ZBED3* as compared to the *TCF7L2* variants. Reports from colon cancer research show that the WNT pathway should not be viewed as having an additive effect but rather as a continuum since both high and low WNT activity has been shown to promote colorectal cancer cell apoptosis [5, 17]. The dual role played by TCF7L2 adds to this complexity where it can act as a transcriptional activator in the presence of beta catenin or as a repressor in the absence of beta catenin [3, 31]. This highlights the complexity by which WNT signaling may operate in the pathogenesis of type 2 diabetes and could explain the directional discrepancies observed in the interactions with fiber. Both *NOTCH2* and *ZBED3* variants showed no association with type 2 diabetes risk in MDCS with HRs close to null. Although this could be partly because of power limitations due to the smaller sample size compared to large-scale GWASs, the results of our interaction analyses may indicate that environmental factors such as higher fiber intake may in fact attenuate and possibly reverse the risk associated with these genetic variants.

The *TCF7L2* rs7903146 shows the strongest association with type 2 diabetes, as compared to more than 65 other loci identified to date among Europeans, with each risk allele of rs7903146 associating with around 40 % elevated risk of type 2 diabetes [28]. Most of the studies so far have reported beta cell dysfunction and an attenuated incretin effect associated with the risk allele [21,37]. A 1-year high-fiber intervention was linked to elevated plasma SCFAs and GLP-1 in hyperinsulinemic subjects [10]. Furthermore, SCFAs have been shown to induce GLP-1 secretion via the FFAR2 in mice [36]. Therefore, the carriers of the *TCF7L2* risk allele may suffer from beta cell incretin resistance and thus could be less prone to the beneficial associated effects of higher fiber intake through increased GLP-1 secretion. SCFAs, and particularly butyrate, are potent histone deacetylase inhibitors (HDACi), and this is particularly important as the *TCF7L2* variant has been linked to an islet-specific open chromatin state which could be exacerbated by higher fiber intake [11]. ZBED3 has been recently identified as an axin-binding protein that modulates the WNT signaling pathway [8]. Binding of the ZBED3 to axin prevents the formation of the destruction complex that normally phosphorylates beta catenin and targets it for proteasomal degradation. *ZBED3* risk allele has been shown to be associated with increased ZBED3 expression in adipose tissue, and this could translate to elevated WNT activity [38]. The *NOTCH2* gene encodes a transmembrane protein which physically associates with active beta catenin and decreases its levels leading to lower WNT activity in both stem and colon cancer cells [16]. However, whether the *NOTCH2* variant associates with NOTCH2 expression is not yet known.

The high relative validity of our dietary assessment method, the combination of a diet diary with a questionnaire, the large sample size, and the prospective design with a long follow-up period are the major strengths of our study. In addition, the detailed and extensive ascertainment of type 2 diabetes cases from more than six registers is another strength that decreases error and improves the power of our study. However, our study has several limitations that need to be discussed. First of all, the T2D gene loci used for annotation were obtained from the GWASs which in most cases are based on proximity to the SNPs and are not necessarily the causal genes. Further, although our study population is large, it still has a limited power for detecting interactions which could result in many false negative outcomes. Therefore, replication of our results in other studies with reasonable power and good quality of diet data is important. We did not correct for multiple testing as our study is hypothesis driven, and we believe that the selected WNT-associated genes are biologically dependent and the interactions with the *NOTCH2* and *ZBED3* variants may reflect essentially the interactions with *TCF7L2*. Finally, our diet data was collected at baseline and may fail to detect the effect of the changes in dietary habits over the follow-up period.

Conclusions

Our results indicate that several type 2 diabetes susceptibility SNPs in genes involved in WNT signaling may interact with dietary fiber intake on type 2 diabetes incidence. The putative mechanisms by which fiber intake could modify WNT signaling through these variants in type 2 diabetes pathogenesis include effects on beta cell survival, adipogenesis and adipocyte proliferation, and/or GLP-1 production in intestinal L cells. In addition, functional studies are needed to better understand the putative role played by dietary fiber in type 2 diabetes through the WNT signaling pathway.

Methods

Study population

The MDCS is a population-based prospective cohort in the city of Malmö in Sweden. The source population (74,138 individuals) was defined in 1991 to include all individuals living in Malmö and born between the years 1926 and 1945. In 1995, this definition was modified to include all men born between 1923 and 1945 and women born between 1923 and 1950 [2, 22]. Study participants were recruited through public advertisements or personal letters. Individuals with mental disability and limited Swedish language skills were excluded. Study participants visited the screening center twice during the baseline examination period between March 1991 and October 1996. During the first visit, participants received instructions on recording their meals in the menu book and on filling in the diet questionnaire and the extensive questionnaire covering socioeconomic and lifestyle factors. Approximately 10 days later, subjects returned for a diet history interview. By the end of the baseline examination period, complete dietary, anthropometric and lifestyle data, was collected for 28,098 participants. Details of the recruitment procedures are described elsewhere [23].

After exclusion of prevalent type 2 diabetes patients, identified as individuals with a self-reported diabetes diagnosis or on a self-reported anti-diabetic regimen, we were left with 26,905 individuals for our prospective analyses. From the MDCS, 6103 individuals were randomly selected to participate in a cardiovascular sub-cohort (Malmö Diet and Cancer Study Cardiovascular Cohort (MDC-CC)). Additional measurements were obtained for these individuals, including analysis of FPG, FPI, and HbA_{1C} levels. After excluding prevalent cases of diabetes and individuals with no diet data, this sub-cohort consisted of 5499 individuals.

The MDCS was approved by the Ethical Committee at Lund University (LU 51-90). All participants provided written informed consent.

Incident type 2 diabetes

Incident cases of type 2 diabetes were identified using the nationwide Swedish National Diabetes Register [7], the regional Diabetes 2000 register of the Scania region [18], or the Swedish National Patient Register, which is a principal source of data for numerous research projects and which covers more than 99 % of all somatic and psychiatric hospital discharges and Swedish hospital-based outpatient care [20]. Individuals could also be classified as diabetes cases if their cause of death was registered as diabetes in the Swedish Cause-of-Death Register, which comprises all deaths in Swedish residents occurring in Sweden or abroad [15], if they had been prescribed anti-diabetic medication according to the Swedish Prescribed Drug Register [40], or if they had at least two HbA_{1C} recordings ≥6.0 % using the Swedish Mono-S standardization system (corresponding to 7.0 % according to the US National Glycohemoglobin Standardization Program (NGSP) and 52 mmol/mol using International Federation of Clinical Chemistry and Laboratory Medicine units) in the Malmö HbA_{1C} register, which analyzed and cataloged all HbA_{1C} samples at the Department of Clinical Chemistry taken in institutional and non-institutional care in the greater Malmö area from 1988 onwards.

In addition, diabetes cases at the baseline examination of MDC-CC were identified based on self-reports of a physician diagnosis or the use of diabetes medication in a baseline questionnaire, or fasting whole blood glucose of ≥6.1 mmol/L (corresponding to FPG concentration of ≥7.0 mmol/L). Furthermore, a diabetes diagnosis could be determined at the MDC-CC reinvestigation between the years 2007 and 2012 based on self-reports of a physician diagnosis or the use of diabetes medication based on a questionnaire or FPG of ≥7.0 mmol/L or a 120-min value post-OGTT plasma glucose of >11.0 mmol/L. A total of 3132 incident cases of type 2 diabetes were identified during the mean follow-up period of 14.7 years until December 2010.

Dietary assessment

A modified dietary history method specifically designed for the MDCS was used consisting of a 7-day menu book, a dietary 168-item questionnaire, and an interview. In the menu book, participants were asked to record lunch and dinner meals, cold beverages including alcohol, medicinal drugs, natural remedies, and nutrient supplements. The 168-item questionnaire was used to assess meal patterns, consumption frequencies, and portion sizes of regularly consumed foods. A 48-page booklet was used to help participants at home estimate the portion sizes for the questionnaire. During the interview, a more extensive book with photographs was used to estimate portion sizes and dishes in the menu book. Participants were also asked about their meal pattern, cooking methods, and food choices.

The average daily intake of foods was calculated using data from the menu book and diet questionnaire. The MDC Food and Nutrient Database, which was derived from PC KOST2-93 of the Swedish National Food Administration, was used to convert the average daily food intake to energy and nutrient intakes [6, 41].

A slight alteration of the coding routines for dietary data was introduced in September 1994 [41]. A method variable, classifying data collected before and after September 1994, along with a four-category season variable (i.e., winter, spring, summer, and autumn) was created and used as covariate to adjust for variation in data collection over time.

Dietary variables used in our analysis included total energy intake and dietary fiber. Fiber intake was adjusted for total energy intake by expressing it as grams per 1000 kcal. The relative validity of the dietary assessment method in MDCS has previously been evaluated in a sample of 50- to 69-year-old Malmö residents, 105 women, and 101 men. The reference method used was 18 days' weighed food records (3 days every second month) collected over 1 year. Energy-adjusted Pearson correlation coefficients for fiber intake was 0.69 for women and 0.74 for men [30].

Other variables used as potential confounders

An extensive lifestyle questionnaire adapted from the Minnesota Leisure Time Physical Activity Questionnaire was used to assess leisure-time physical activity. Participants had to estimate the number of minutes per week for each season they spent performing each of 17 different physical activities. The duration was multiplied by an intensity factor to create a physical activity score that was divided into tertiles. Alcohol intake was classified into four categories based on grams of alcohol consumed per day: zero-consumers, low (<15 g/day in women or <20 g/day in men), medium (15–30 g/day in women or 20–40 g/day in men), and high consumers (>30 g/day in women or >40 g/day in men). Participants were classified as current smokers, ex-smokers, and never-smokers. The education variable was created by classifying participants according to their highest educational level (≤8 years, 9–10 years, and 11–13 years at school and university degree).

Genotyping

A total of 58 previously reported type 2 diabetes-associated single nucleotide polymorphisms were selected for genotyping in the MDCS (Additional file 1: Table S1) [24, 28]. Genotyping was performed by MassARRAY iPLEX (Sequenom, San Diego, CA, USA) or Taqman 5′ nuclease (Applied Biosystems, Foster City, CA, USA) assays according to the manufacturers' instructions. The concordance rate was >99 % in 5500 samples which were genotyped using Human Omni Express Exome Bead Chip Kit (Illumina, San Diego, CA, USA). Genotyping success rate ranged between 96 and 99 %. All genotypes were in the Hardy-Weinberg equilibrium ($P > 0.0009$).

Gene annotation

A list of 51 unique gene loci, corresponding to 58 SNPs (MDCS) associated with type 2 diabetes, were analyzed for links to WNT signaling (Additional file 1: Table S2) using a combination of annotation from the Gene Ontology [1], the Kyoto Encyclopedia of Genes and Genomes (http://www.kegg.jp/kegg/, accessed on the 15th of March 2013), Biocarta pathways (http://cgap.nci.nih.gov/Pathways/BioCarta_Pathways, accessed on the 15th of March 2013), Panther pathways [26, 35], and Literature integrated within the DAVID Annotation Bioinformatics Resource (http://david.abcc.ncifcrf.gov, accessed on the 15th of March 2013).

Statistical analysis

Assuming an additive model, Cox proportional hazards regression was used to calculate the HR of incident type 2 diabetes associated with each risk allele in the MDCS adjusting for age and sex. After stratification to quintiles of relative intakes of fiber (g/1000 kcal), interactions between the SNP genotypes and quintiles of fiber intakes on type 2 diabetes incidence were analyzed by introducing a multiplicative factor of the genotype and dietary quintiles as continuous variables in addition to these variables to the equation. Interactions were analyzed adjusting for age, sex, BMI, total energy intake, dietary assessment method, season leisure-time physical activity, alcohol intake, smoking habits, and level of education. In the MDC-CC sub-cohort, we performed cross-sectional analysis using linear regression to calculate the effect sizes of each WNT-annotated risk allele on baseline FPG, FPI, HOMA-IR, and HbA_{1C} adjusting for age and sex.

We used IBM SPSS Statistics, version 19 (IBM Corporation, Armonk, NY, USA), for the analyses. Two-sided P values of <0.05 were considered significant.

Compliance with ethics guidelines

All procedures followed were in accordance with the ethical standards of the responsible committee on human experimentation (Ethical Committee at Lund University LU 51-90) and with the Helsinki Declaration of 1975, as revised in 2000. Informed consent was obtained from all participants for being included in the study.

Abbreviations

CI: confidence interval; FFAR2: free fatty acid receptor 2; FPG: fasting plasma glucose; FPI: fasting plasma insulin; GLP-1: glucagon-like peptide-1; GWAS: genome-wide association study; HbA_{1C}: glycated hemoglobin; HOMA-IR: homeostasis model for assessment of insulin resistance; HR: hazard ratio; MDC-CC: Malmö Diet and Cancer Study Cardiovascular Cohort; MDCS: Malmö Diet and Cancer Study; SCFA: short chain fatty acid; SNP: single nucleotide polymorphism; TCF7L2: transcription factor 7-like 2 gene; WNT: wingless-type MMTV integration site.

Competing interests

All authors declare that they have no competing interests.

Authors' contributions

GH and MOM contributed to the study concept and design, data analysis, and drafting of the manuscript. IGM, GR, and UE contributed to the acquisition and/or analysis of the data. All authors critically revised or reviewed the manuscript for important intellectual content.

Acknowledgements

We would like to thank Mrs. Malin Svensson and Mrs. Widet Tas for their excellent technical assistance. We would also like to thank the staff and participants of the Malmö Diet and Cancer Study.

Funding

This study was supported by grants from the Swedish Research Council, the Swedish Heart and Lung Foundation, the Novo Nordisk Foundation, the Swedish Diabetes Foundation, and the Påhlsson Foundation and by equipment grants from the Knut and Alice Wallenberg Foundation, the Skåne University Hospital, and the Linneus Foundation for the Lund University Diabetes Center.

The funders had no role in the design of the study and collection, analysis, and interpretation of the data and in writing the manuscript.

References

1. Ashburner M et al. Gene ontology: tool for the unification of biology. The gene ontology consortium. Nat Genet. 2000;25:25–9. doi:10.1038/75556.
2. Berglund G, Elmstahl S, Janzon L, Larsson SA. The Malmo Diet and Cancer Study. Design and feasibility. J Intern Med. 1993;233:45–51.
3. Bienz M. TCF: transcriptional activator or repressor? Curr Opin Cell Biol. 1998;10:366–72.
4. Boj SF et al. Diabetes risk gene and Wnt effector Tcf7l2/TCF4 controls hepatic response to perinatal and adult metabolic demand. Cell. 2012;151: 1595–607. doi:10.1016/j.cell.2012.10.053.
5. Bordonaro M, Lazarova DL, Sartorelli AC. The activation of beta-catenin by Wnt signaling mediates the effects of histone deacetylase inhibitors. Exp Cell Res. 2007;313:1652–66. doi:10.1016/j.yexcr.2007.02.008.
6. Callmer E, Riboli E, Saracci R, Akesson B, Lindgarde F. Dietary assessment methods evaluated in the Malmo food study. J Intern Med. 1993;233:53–7.
7. Cederholm J, Eeg-Olofsson K, Eliasson B, Zethelius B, Nilsson PM, Gudbjornsdottir S, et al. Risk prediction of cardiovascular disease in type 2 diabetes: a risk equation from the Swedish National Diabetes Register. Diabetes Care. 2008;31:2038–43. doi:10.2337/dc08-0662.
8. Chen T et al. Identification of zinc-finger BED domain-containing 3 (Zbed3) as a novel Axin-interacting protein that activates Wnt/beta-catenin signaling. J Biol Chem. 2009;284:6683–9. doi:10.1074/jbc.M807753200.
9. Fisher E, Boeing H, Fritsche A, Doering F, Joost HG, Schulze MB. Whole-grain consumption and transcription factor-7-like 2 (TCF7L2) rs7903146: gene-diet interaction in modulating type 2 diabetes risk. Br J Nutr. 2009;101:478–81. doi:10.1017/S0007114508020369.
10. Freeland KR, Wilson C, Wolever TM. Adaptation of colonic fermentation and glucagon-like peptide-1 secretion with increased wheat fibre intake for 1 year in hyperinsulinaemic human subjects. Br J Nutr. 2010;103:82–90. doi:10.1017/S0007114509991462.
11. Gaulton KJ et al. A map of open chromatin in human pancreatic islets. Nat Genet. 2010;42:255–9. doi:10.1038/ng.530.
12. Grant SF et al. Variant of transcription factor 7-like 2 (TCF7L2) gene confers risk of type 2 diabetes. Nat Genet. 2006;38:320–3. doi:10.1038/ng1732.
13. Heni M, Herzberg-Schafer S, Machicao F, Haring HU, Fritsche A. Dietary fiber intake modulates the association between variants in TCF7L2 and weight loss during a lifestyle intervention. Diabetes Care. 2012;35:e24. doi:10.2337/dc11-2012.
14. Hindy G et al. Role of TCF7L2 risk variant and dietary fibre intake on incident type 2 diabetes. Diabetologia. 2012;55:2646–54. doi:10.1007/s00125-012-2634-x.
15. Johansson LA, Westerling R. Comparing Swedish hospital discharge records with death certificates: implications for mortality statistics. Int J Epidemiol. 2000;29:495–502.
16. Kwon C, Cheng P, King IN, Andersen P, Shenje L, Nigam V, et al. Notch post-translationally regulates beta-catenin protein in stem and progenitor cells. Nat Cell Biol. 2011;13:1244–51. doi:10.1038/ncb2313.
17. Lazarova DL, Bordonaro M, Carbone R, Sartorelli AC. Linear relationship between Wnt activity levels and apoptosis in colorectal carcinoma cells exposed to butyrate. Int J Cancer. 2004;110:523–31. doi:10.1002/ijc.20152.
18. Lindholm E, Agardh E, Tuomi T, Groop L, Agardh CD. Classifying diabetes according to the new WHO clinical stages. Eur J Epidemiol. 2001;17:983–9.
19. Liu Z, Habener JF. Glucagon-like peptide-1 activation of TCF7L2-dependent Wnt signaling enhances pancreatic beta cell proliferation. J Biol Chem. 2008;283:8723–35. doi:10.1074/jbc.M706105200.
20. Ludvigsson JF et al. External review and validation of the Swedish national inpatient register. BMC Public Health. 2011;11:450. doi:10.1186/1471-2458-11-450.
21. Lyssenko V et al. Mechanisms by which common variants in the TCF7L2 gene increase risk of type 2 diabetes. J Clin Invest. 2007;117:2155–63. doi:10.1172/JCI30706.
22. Manjer J, Elmstahl S, Janzon L, Berglund G. Invitation to a population-based cohort study: differences between subjects recruited using various strategies. Scand J Public Health. 2002;30:103–12. doi:10.1080/14034940210133771.
23. Manjer J et al. The Malmo diet and cancer study: representativity, cancer incidence and mortality in participants and non-participants. Eur J Cancer Prev. 2001;10:489–99.
24. McCarthy MI. Genomics, type 2 diabetes, and obesity. N Engl J Med. 2010; 363:2339–50. doi:10.1056/NEJMra0906948.
25. Meyer KA, Kushi LH, Jacobs Jr DR, Slavin J, Sellers TA, Folsom AR. Carbohydrates, dietary fiber, and incident type 2 diabetes in older women. A J Clin Nutr. 2000;71:921–30.
26. Mi H et al. The PANTHER database of protein families, subfamilies, functions and pathways. Nucleic Acids Res. 2005;33:D284–8. doi:10.1093/nar/gki078.
27. Montague W, Taylor KW. Regulation of insulin secretion by short chain fatty acids. Nature. 1968;217:853.
28. Morris AP et al. Large-scale association analysis provides insights into the genetic architecture and pathophysiology of type 2 diabetes. Nat Genet. 2012;44:981–90. doi:10.1038/ng.2383.
29. Prunier C, Hocevar BA, Howe PH. Wnt signaling: physiology and pathology. Growth Factors. 2004;22:141–50.
30. Riboli E, Elmstahl S, Saracci R, Gullberg B, Lindgarde F. The Malmo food study: validity of two dietary assessment methods for measuring nutrient intake. Int J Epidemiol. 1997;26 Suppl 1:S161–73.
31. Roose J, Clevers H. TCF transcription factors: molecular switches in carcinogenesis. Biochim Biophys Acta. 1999;1424:M23–37.
32. Ross SE, Hemati N, Longo KA, Bennett CN, Lucas PC, Erickson RL, et al. Inhibition of adipogenesis by Wnt signaling. Science. 2000;289:950–3.
33. Rulifson IC et al. Wnt signaling regulates pancreatic beta cell proliferation. Proc Natl Acad Sci U S A. 2007;104:6247–52. doi:10.1073/pnas.0701509104.
34. Schulze MB, Schulz M, Heidemann C, Schienkiewitz A, Hoffmann K, Boeing H. Fiber and magnesium intake and incidence of type 2 diabetes: a prospective study and meta-analysis. Arch Intern Med. 2007;167:956–65. doi:10.1001/archinte.167.9.956.
35. Thomas PD et al. PANTHER: a library of protein families and subfamilies indexed by function. Genome Res. 2003;13:2129–41. doi:10.1101/gr.772403.
36. Tolhurst G et al. Short-chain fatty acids stimulate glucagon-like peptide-1 secretion via the G-protein-coupled receptor FFAR2. Diabetes. 2012;61:364–71. doi:10.2337/db11-1019.
37. Villareal DT, Robertson H, Bell GI, Patterson BW, Tran H, Wice B, Polonsky KS. TCF7L2 variant rs7903146 affects the risk of type 2 diabetes by modulating incretin action. Diabetes 59:479-485. doi:db09-1169 [pii]10.2337/db09-1169.
38. Voight BF et al. Twelve type 2 diabetes susceptibility loci identified through large-scale association analysis. Nat Genet. 2010;42:579–89. doi:10.1038/ng.609.
39. Wannamethee SG, Whincup PH, Thomas MC, Sattar N. Associations between dietary fiber and inflammation, hepatic function, and risk of type 2 diabetes in older men: potential mechanisms for the benefits of fiber on diabetes risk. Diabetes Care. 2009;32:1823–5. doi:10.2337/dc09-0477.
40. Wettermark B et al. The new Swedish prescribed drug register—opportunities for pharmacoepidemiological research and experience from the first six months. Pharmacoepidemiol Drug Saf. 2007;16:726–35. doi:10.1002/pds.1294.
41. Wirfalt E, Mattisson I, Johansson U, Gullberg B, Wallstrom P, Berglund G. A methodological report from the Malmo diet and cancer study: development and evaluation of altered routines in dietary data processing. Nutr J. 2002;1:3.
42. Wirstrom T, Hilding A, Gu HF, Ostenson CG, Bjorklund A. Consumption of whole grain reduces risk of deteriorating glucose tolerance, including progression to prediabetes. Am J Clin Nutr. 2013;97:179–87. doi:10.3945/ajcn.112.045583.
43. Yi F, Brubaker PL, Jin T. TCF-4 mediates cell type-specific regulation of proglucagon gene expression by beta-catenin and glycogen synthase kinase-3beta. J Biol Chem. 2005;280:1457–64. doi:10.1074/jbc.M411487200.
44. Yoo EJ, Chung JJ, Choe SS, Kim KH, Kim JB. Down-regulation of histone deacetylases stimulates adipocyte differentiation. J Biol Chem. 2006;281: 6608–15. doi:10.1074/jbc.M508982200.

11

Effect of a diet enriched with omega-6 and omega-3 fatty acids on the pig liver transcriptome

Agnieszka Szostak[1], Magdalena Ogłuszka[1], Marinus F. W. te Pas[2], Ewa Poławska[1], Paweł Urbański[1], Edyta Juszczuk-Kubiak[1], Tadeusz Blicharski[1], Chandra Shekhar Pareek[3], Jenelle R. Dunkelberger[4], Jarosław O. Horbańczuk[1] and Mariusz Pierzchała[1*]

Abstract

The optimal ratio of omega-6 to omega-3 polyunsaturated fatty acids (PUFAs) is important for keeping the homeostasis of biological processes and metabolism, yet the underlying biological mechanism is poorly understood. The objective of this study was to identify changes in the pig liver transcriptome induced by a diet enriched with omega-6 and omega-3 fatty acids and to characterize the biological mechanisms related to PUFA metabolism.

Polish Landrace pigs ($n = 12$) were fed diet enriched with linoleic acid (LA, omega-6) and α-linolenic acid (ALA, omega-3) or standard diet as a control. The fatty acid profiling was assayed in order to verify how feeding influenced the fatty acid content in the liver, and subsequently next-generation sequencing (NGS) was used to identify differentially expressed genes (DEG) between transcriptomes between dietary groups. The biological mechanisms and pathway interaction networks were identified using DAVID and Cytoscape tools. Fatty acid profile analysis indicated a higher contribution of PUFAs in the liver for LA- and ALA-enriched diet group, particularly for the omega-3 fatty acid family, but not omega-6. Next-generation sequencing identified 3565 DEG, 1484 of which were induced and 2081 were suppressed by PUFA supplementation. A low ratio of omega-6/omega-3 fatty acids resulted in the modulation of fatty acid metabolism pathways and over-representation of genes involved in energy metabolism, signal transduction, and immune response pathways.

In conclusion, a diet enriched with omega-6 and omega-3 fatty acids altered the transcriptomic profile of the pig liver and would influence animal health status.

Keywords: Fatty acid profile, Transcriptome, Omega-3 fatty acids, Omega-6 fatty acids, Liver, Pig

Introduction

A balanced ratio of omega-6 to omega-3 polyunsaturated fatty acids (PUFAs) plays an essential role in multiple biological processes and maintains the metabolic homeostasis. It is widely accepted that long-chain PUFAs are considered as a bioactive molecules, which serve beneficial outcomes to health. However, the mechanism responsible for a health-promoting effect as a result of fatty acid consumption is still not fully clarified.

Polyunsaturated fatty acids, particularly omega-6 or omega-3 family, counteract cardiovascular (Stanley et al. 2013) and metabolic disorders (Warensjo et al. 2006). Efficacy of omega-3-rich diet for reducing blood cholesterol levels and decreasing risk of cardiovascular disease, arthritis, neurodegenerative diseases (Lands 2012), and risk of progression to psychotic disorders (Amminger et al. 2015) is unambiguous. Omega-3 PUFAs derivatives can act as signaling molecules, modulating the anti-inflammatory response, and controlling cellular processes involved in programmed cell death (apoptosis), lymphocyte proliferation, suppression of inflammatory cytokines, and phagocytosis (de Pablo and Alvarez de Cienfuegos 2000; Kruger et al. 2010; Wymann and Schneiter 2008). Since omega-6 PUFAs are involved in the regulation of eicosanoid synthesis, they control the activity of the immune system. They are also associated with a reduced risk of cardiovascular diseases.

* Correspondence: m.pierzchala@ighz.pl

[1]Institute of Genetics and Animal Breeding, Polish Academy of Science, Jastrzębiec, Poland

Full list of author information is available at the end of the article

Many recent studies have investigated fish oils and plant oils (for instance linseed and rapeseed oils) rich in omega-3 fatty acids, indicating the protective actions against the development of cardiovascular and metabolic diseases such as obesity, type II diabetes, and metabolic syndrome (Hanke et al. 2013; Lionetti et al. 2014; Morine et al. 2011). Especially, a low omega-6/omega-3 ratio decreases the risk of metabolic diseases (Jump 2011).

In regard to plant oils, diet can provide short-chain linoleic acid (LA) and α-linolenic acid (ALA), which are the main precursors of omega-6 and omega-3 fatty acids, respectively, and are considered as essential fatty acids for humans and other mammals. They can be stored in tissues or converted into long-chain fatty acids such as arachidonic acid (AA), eicosapentaenoic acid (EPA), and docosahexaenoic acid (DHA), which are subsequently involved in the synthesis of hormones such as prostaglandins, prostacyclins, thromboxanes, or leukotrienes (Aro 2003; Harris et al. 2006). There is now significant evidence that one of the mechanisms by which omega-6 and omega-3 fatty acids exert their protective role is interaction with nuclear receptors. They are the natural ligands that influence gene expression and regulate the activity of numerous transcription factors, including sterol regulatory element-binding protein (SREBP), peroxisome proliferator-activated receptor (PPAR), liver X receptor (LXR), farnesoid X receptor (FXR), and retinoid X receptor (RXR) (Getek et al. 2013; Gormaz et al. 2010; Vallim and Salter 2010).

In our studies, we have chosen the pig as an animal model for humans. Such a model has additional advantage because of the relatively similar anatomy, body morphology, physiological and metabolic processes to humans as well as high sequence homology, and a similar chromosomal structure to the human genome, compared to other domestic animal species (Lunney 2007). Therefore, processes revealed in the pig transcriptome are more likely to be similar to those in humans. For these reasons, the pig is considered to be a good animal model for nutrigenomic and metabolic research.

Since the liver is an organ which plays a major role in the regulation of the availability of lipids for other tissues by modulating the uptake and synthesis of lipids and the secretion of lipoproteins, it is adequate to study the fatty acid metabolism dysregulations (Nguyen et al. 2008). Besides adipose tissue, the liver is one of the main locations of synthesis for both cholesterol and triglyceride fatty acids (Bergen and Mersmann 2005). The synthesis of triglycerides depends largely on the availability of fatty acids, which are derived from de novo synthesis, received from diet, or released from tissues (Vallim and Salter 2010). Fatty acid oxidation occurs in hepatic mitochondria and peroxisomes. Dietary fatty acids affect de novo lipogenesis in the liver by controlling the expression of the key enzymes of fatty acid synthesis, particularly acetyl-CoA carboxylase (ACC) and fatty acid synthase (FAS) by PUFA (Guillevic et al. 2009) or stearoyl-CoA desaturase (SCD) by monounsaturated fatty acids (MUFA) (Ntambi 1999).

Nowadays, high-throughput technology, such as next-generation sequencing (NGS), becomes increasingly popular, providing identification of changes in the transcriptome in nutrigenomics investigations (Chen et al. 2011; Li et al. 2011), further validated by standard quantitative real-time PCR (qRT-PCR) (Nygard et al. 2007; Shi and Chiang 2005). The objective of this study was the use of the RNA-Seq approach to identify changes in the pig liver transcriptome induced by a diet enriched with LA (omega-6 family) and ALA (omega-3) fatty acids and to indicate the general biological mechanisms underlying the effects related to PUFA metabolism.

Materials and methods

Animals and treatments

The experiment was carried out on Polish Landrace pigs ($n = 12$) housed at a commercial farm (Wronie, Poland) in two separate pens under standard conditions. The first stage of feeding was composed of standard diet appropriate for age group and included all of the pigs, which were fed until reaching 60 kg in body weight (BW) (see scheme in Fig. 1). In the second fattening period, the pigs were divided into two feeding groups (six pigs per group) and fed diets differing in omega-6 and omega-3 fatty acid content based on linseed and rapeseed oil supplementation. In the control group (C, $n = 6$), feed contained 268 mg LA/100 g (linoleic acid—omega-6) and 25 mg ALA/100 g (α-linolenic acid—omega-3 family). The experimental diet (E, $n = 6$) was enriched with LA and ALA and contained 660 mg and 64 mg/100 g diet, respectively. The feeding experiment was performed on an equal number of pigs from each treatment group, and all experiment included gilts. Diets were provided ad libitum with a constant access to water.

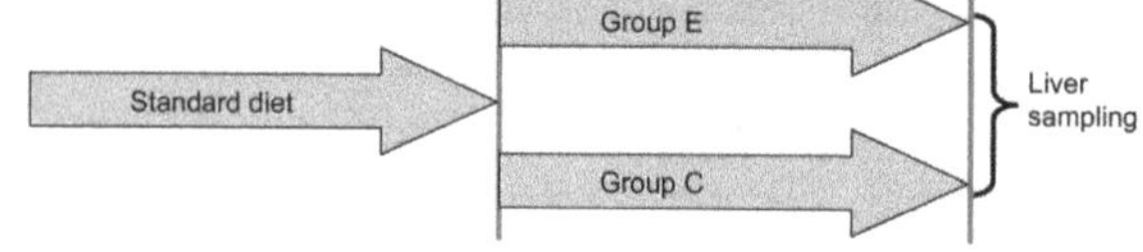

Fig. 1 Experimental design. The first stage of feeding was composed of a standard diet until the pigs reached 60 kg in body weight. In the second stage, the pigs were divided into two groups (six pigs per group): the experimental (E) group—fed a diet enriched with LA and ALA, which contained 660 mg and 64 mg/100 g diet, respectively; and the control (C) group—fed a standard diet which contained 268 mg LA/100 g and 25 mg ALA/100 g

The fodder mixtures were isoenergetic (13 MJ EM per kg of mixture) and isoprotein balanced (15.5 % crude protein), while differing in fat content ranging from 1.78 % (C group) to 4.72 % (E group). Diets were composed of the same components, except linseed and rapeseed oils, which were provided as a polyunsaturated fatty acid source (Table 1). The feed was administered for approximately 4 months until slaughter at the average BW of 110 kg. All animals were characterized by aligned age and body weight. Pigs were sacrificed by electrical stunning and exsanguination, according to industry standards. After slaughter, liver samples were excised and immediately frozen in liquid nitrogen and further stored at −80 °C. Slaughter procedure was carried out with the required permits and according to Minister of Agriculture and Rural Development dated April 2, 2004.

Fatty acid profiling

The fatty acid composition in the liver was assayed in order to verify how feeding influenced the fatty acid content in tissues. Subsequently, the ratio of omega-6/omega-3 fatty acids in the liver was calculated for both dietary groups and used as the basis for further investigation. For *p*-value determination, unpaired Student's test was used.

The fatty acid profile analysis was performed using the chloroform-methanol (2:1 *v*/*v*) method (Folch et al. 1957) on 1 g of liver sample. Fatty acid methyl esters were determined by gas chromatography (GC-FID) on the Agilent 7890 Series GC system equipment with a Hewlett-Packard-88 capillary column (60 m × 0.25 mm × 0.20 μm) (Agilent, J&W GC Columns, USA) with helium as a carrier gas. The details of the analysis are described in Polawska et al. (2013). Fatty acids were identified by comparison with fatty acid standards (Supelco 37 Component FAME mix, 47885-U—10 mg/ml in methylene chloride, analytical standard, Sigma-Aldrich Co.) and expressed in g/100 g fatty acid methyl esters (FAME).

Table 1 Raw material composition of mixtures (%)

Ingredients	Diets	
	C	E
Rapeseed meal	6	7.2
Soybean meal	9	9.2
Wheat	54	49.6
Barley	28.5	28.5
Linseed oil	–	2
Rapeseed oil	–	1
Other	2.5	2.5
Total	100	100

Gene expression analysis

Next-generation sequencing

The total RNA for sequencing were purified from 20 mg of tissue sample of 12 pigs (6 animals in control group and 6 animals in PUFA treatment group) using the messenger RNA (mRNA) extraction kit RNeasy Fibrous Tissue Mini Kit (Qiagen, Hilden, Germany) following the manufacturer's recommendations. The concentration and purity of total RNA were checked using the UV/Vis spectrophotometer (Actgene, New Jersey, USA) at 260 nm, and the integrity was evaluated using a microfluidic assay on Bioanalyzer (Agilent Technologies, Inc., Santa Clara, CA, USA). Only high quality RNA extracts (RNA integrity number (RIN) ≥8) were used for pooling within each treatment group using equal amounts of RNA per animal.

Next-generation sequencing data were obtained from pooled RNA samples within each group to ensure the most robust transcriptome. Construction of complementary DNA (cDNA) libraries for RNA sequencing was prepared using the TruSeq RNA Sample Prep Kit v2 (Illumina, San Diego, CA, USA). RNA-Seq analysis was performed for identification of transcriptional changes using MiSeq instrument (Illumina) according to the manufacturer's recommendations at the laboratory of Genomed (http://www.genomed.pl/) using paired-end libraries. Two replicates of each pool independent for library synthesis and sequencing were done. The number of reads equivalent to mapped reads (reads per kilobase per million (RPKM)) was used to normalize the expression of each gene. Benjamini and Hochberg test (an error rate 0.05) and false discovery rate correction test (FDR < 0.05) were used for adjusting the *p*-value. In this study, a minimum twofold change (FC ≥ 2) difference in gene expression between treatment groups was used as the inclusion criteria for a gene. Reads were mapped to the *Sus scrofa* v. 10.2 genome as a reference genome. The quality of obtained data was checked in regard to the presence and abundance of contaminating sequences, average read length, and GC content. The NGS experiment conformed to the MIAME guidelines (Brazma et al. 2001) except for the microarray design. The RNA-Seq raw data were deposited in NCBI GEO (Gene Expression Omnibus) (Barrett et al. 2013) under accession number GSE72123.

Quantitative real-time PCR

Total cellular RNA was extracted according to the Chomczyński protocol (Chomczynski and Sacchi 1987; Chomczynski and Sacchi 2006). The samples of liver tissue (20 mg) were lysed with TRIzol reagent (Invitrogen, Carlsbad, CA, USA) and homogenized on MagNA Lyser (Roche Diagnostics, Mannheim, Germany). The concentration and purity of the RNA extracts were measured using UVS-99 micro-volume UV/Vis spectrophotometer

(ACTgene, Piscataway, NJ, USA) at 260 nm. Integrity was checked using the Agilent 2100 Bioanalyzer (Agilent Technologies Inc., Santa Clara, CA, USA) based on the RNA integrity number (RIN) parameter. The RIN values for all samples were higher than 7.5. Genomic DNA was removed from RNA extracts by incubation with RQ1 RNase-free DNase (Promega, Madison, WI, USA) for 15 min at 25 °C. The RNA extracts were stored in RNase-free water at −80 °C. The reverse transcription reaction was performed using the Transcriptor First Strand cDNA Synthesis Kit (Roche Applied Science, Penzberg, Germany) from 1.5 μg of total RNA in a final volume of 20 μl using the oligo-dT primers.

Quantitative real-time PCR was performed on 30 individual samples (biological replicates—15 samples for each dietary group) to validate the reliability of RNA-Seq gene expression data. For confirmation, we have chosen the differentially expressed genes EXTL1, APOA4, APOA5, ACSL1, ELOVL6, FASN, COL1A1, DGAT2, FADS1, FADS2, and MMP2. Most of the selected genes are involved in lipid metabolism. Gene expression was normalized by the use of topoisomerase (DNA) II beta (TOP2B) (Nygard et al. 2007; Pierzchala et al. 2011) as a most stable gene revealed by NormFinder algorithm, which was used to determine the optimal normalization gene among a set of candidates (GAPDH, TBP, TOP2B). The primer sets for real-time PCR were designed using Primer-BLAST tool (Ye et al. 2012) (www.ncbi.nlm.nih.gov/tools/primer-blast/) and Primer Premier 5.0 software (PREMIER Biosoft, Palo Alto, CA, USA). The sequences of the primers and their annealing temperatures are described in Table 2.

The reaction mixture for real-time PCR consisted of 4.5 μl of cDNA template (1/20 dilution), 5 pmol reaction primers, and 5 μl SYBR Green I in a final volume of 10 μl. All PCR reactions were performed in duplicate. For each gene, negative controls without the cDNA template were included. The reactions were performed in a 96-well optical plate on the Light Cycler 96 instrument (Roche Applied Science, Germany). Cycling conditions

Table 2 Oligonucleotide primer sequences used for quantitative real-time PCR experiments

Gene	Sequences (5′–3′)	Amplicon size (bp)	Annealing temperature (°C)	GenBank accession no.
DGAT2	For. GACCCTCATAGCTGCCTACTC	136	59	NM_001160080.1
	Rev. CAGCACGGAGATGACCTGTA			
ELOVL6	For. GAACACGTAGCGACTCCGAA	178	59	XM_003357048.2
	Rev. ATGCCGACCGCCAAAGATAA			
EXTL1	For. TGGGATGGGCACTGTGAGC	78	59	XM_003356212.1
	Rev. GCAGAAGGTGGCATTGGGTA			
MMP2	For. CGGACAAAGAGTTGGCTGTG	158	59	NM_214192
	Rev. CATGGTCTCGATGGTGCTCT			
COL1A1	For. TTCAGCTTTGTGGACCTCCG	136	59	XM_005668927
	Rev. CGTTCTGTACGCAGGTGACT			
ACSL1	For. TCAGAAGGTTGCCAGTGAAG	115	59	NM_001167629
	Rev. CTGGAGGAGAGGATCAGAGAATA			
APOA4	For. CAGCAGCTCAACACTCTCTT	142	59	NM_214388
	Rev. GAATCTCCTCCTTCAGCTTCTC			
APOA5	For. GGAAGAGAAGGGAAGAAGGAAG	83	59	NM_001159308
	Rev. CATCGGCCAACAGGGATATT			
FADS1	For. GGGCCTTGTGAGGAAGTATATG	104	59	NM_001113041
	Rev. GGAACTCATCTGTCAGCTCTTT			
FADS2	For. CCTTACAACCACCAGCATGA	118	59	NM_001171750
	Rev. CCAAGTCCACCCAGTCTTTAC			
FASN	For. CTTGTCCTGGGAAGAGTGTAAG	83	59	NM_001099930
	Rev. AGATGGTCACCGTGTCTTTG			
TOP2B	For. AACTGGATGATGCTAATGATGCT	137	59	NM_001258386.1
	Rev. TGGAAAAACTCCGTATCTGTCTC			

were as follows: pre-incubation at 95 °C for 5 min followed by 45 amplification cycles of 95 °C (10 s), 59 °C (10 s), and 72 °C (10 s). After each experiment, the qRT-PCR products were verified for specific amplification by melting curve analysis: 95 °C (5 s), 70 °C (1 min), heating to 95 °C, and cooling step to 37 °C for 30 s. Additionally, PCR product quality and specificity with regard to the applied primer pairs were checked using gel electrophoresis.

The gene expression levels were calculated using the LinRegPCR analysis program according to the baseline estimation method (Ramakers et al. 2003; Ruijter et al. 2013; Ruijter et al. 2009). In order to evaluate the relative gene expressions for independent samples, bilateral Student's test was used and p-value <0.05 was considered significant. The quantitative real-time PCR was performed according to the MIQE guidelines (Bustin et al. 2013).

Bioinformatics analysis

For transcriptome assembling and dispersion evaluation, the CLC Genomics workbench v. 6.0. was used. Since pooled samples were used in the NGS experiment, the expression variance for each gene was estimated by using the variance across the four sequencing for that gene. This "blind" method of dispersion estimate is used in the absence of biological replicates, even though it can overly conservative statistical significance testing of differential gene expression (Anders and Huber 2010).

All data processing steps were performed using Lasergene Genomic Suite v. 5 software package (DNASTAR, Madison, WI, USA) for differential gene expression evaluation. The first step included selection of the genes that showed high variation for all identified gene transcripts. Only genes that demonstrated more than a two-fold change in differential expression between dietary groups with a p-value ≤0.05 for the T test were selected for further analysis. Additionally, genes that demonstrated dietary group-specific expression (and remained below the detection level in the opposite dietary group) were investigated separately.

Biological mechanisms underlying DEGs were investigated using the DAVID v. 6.7 software (the Database for Annotation, Visualization, and Integrated Discovery) (http://david.abcc.ncifcrf.gov/) (Huang et al. 2009a; Huang et al. 2009b). The sets of genes were uploaded using ENTREZ gene IDs. To obtain maximal annotation results, the pig gene IDs were converted to the homologues human gene IDs. The p-values of the enrichment of the number of genes in biological mechanisms were evaluated by Benjamini correction, and values less than 0.05 were considered significant. The data were analyzed for the following situations: (1) all DEGs, (2) DEGs with expression levels below the detection level in the C group, and (3) DEGs with expression levels below the detection level in the E group. The analysis performed using the DAVID software allowed to derive the comprehensive information about the genes' participation in biological pathways from the Kyoto Encyclopedia of Genes and Genomes (KEGG) database (http://www.genome.jp/kegg/) (Kanehisa and Goto 2000; Kanehisa et al. 2014). The p-values calculated in the DAVID software indicate the importance of the general biological mechanisms revealed in all animals but do not distinguish the inter-individual differences. For this purpose, we examined the alterations in the pig transcriptome in pooled liver samples per treatment group in order to clear out the bias caused by variation in a heterogeneous group of individuals derived from the general population. Apart from RNA-Seq, qRT-PCR was performed for individual samples, and indeed, high variation between individual animals was observed. The physiological effects of dietary omega-6 and omega-3 fatty acid intake were measured in the individual animals which are the consequence of the interactions between the animals' genotype and the omega-6/omega-3 ratio. Therefore, it was expected that animal-specific mechanisms were observed, which were not intended for our study. In a pooled sample experiment, the contribution of these individual-specific reactions is diluted, while the general mechanisms active in all animals remain emphasized.

Finally, the molecular interaction networks of DEGs were investigated using the Cytoscape v. 3.1.0 software (http://www.cytoscape.org/) (Saito et al. 2012) as a complementary and more comprehensive approach for the identification of central hub genes. The networks of gene relationships were based on the *Homo sapiens* gene annotation databases. Results were visualized using the ClueGO v. 2.1.1. app. of the Cytoscape software to create clusters of functionally related genes, using the gene ontology databases: KEGG, Wiki Pathways, REACTOME, GO Immune System Process, GO Molecular Function, GO Cellular Component, and GO Biological Process.

The probability value was calculated using Enrichment/Depletion (a two-sided hypergeometric test) with Bonferroni correction. The networks of genes were created for the following situations: (1) all DEGs, (2) DEGs expressed only in the E group and were below the detection level for the C group, (3) DEGs expressed only in the C group and were below the detection level in the E group, (4) DEGs expressed only in the C or E group when combined in one network. The parameters "number of genes per node" and "minimum percentage of genes per node" were chosen empirically for different analyses.

Results

Animals and fatty acid profiles

There were no significant differences in growth performance and carcass characteristics between the pigs in the two treatment groups (data not shown). However, a tendency toward a lower daily gain and a lower backfat thickness in the experimental group was observed, but it was statistically insignificant. No interaction was observed between addition of PUFA and slaughter weight.

The analysis of the fatty acid profile showed a higher level of PUFAs in the liver of the experimental group (p-value = 0.0026), as a consequence of the increased content of PUFAs in the diet. Supplementation of the diet with PUFAs was associated with a higher content of most omega-3 fatty acids in the liver and unchanged or lower omega-6 fatty acid content, hence, pronounced reduction of the omega-6/omega-3 fatty acid ratio (Table 3). Particularly, contents of eicosapentaenoic acid (EPA) (p-value = 0.0006) and docosahexaenoic acid (DHA) (p-value = 0.0006) of the omega-3 family were higher, while that of arachidonic acid (AA)—omega-6 was lower in the E group in comparison to the C group (p-value = 0.0055). Interestingly, the mean value of the omega-6/omega-3 fatty acid ratio was approximately 30 in standard diet group (C group) and approximately 4 for the group with increased content of PUFAs.

We did not observe any statistically significant differences in regard to the content of saturated fatty acids (SFA). We observed a lower content of MUFA in the liver of the E group compared to the C group (p-value = 0.07).

Next-generation sequencing

Next-generation sequencing using RNA-Seq approach was performed to characterize the pig liver transcriptome. The number of reads per sample obtained from the NGS was 13,509,248 sequences using paired-end libraries (PE). Among these, 9,812,246 (72.63 %) reads were mapped in pairs, 381,668 (2.83 %) were mapped in broken pairs, and 3,315,334 (24.54 %) reads were not mapped. The average read was 151 base-pair lengths.

In regard to the fragment counting, the total number of fragments was 6,754,624, in which 1,848,501 (27.37 %) remained uncounted. Among 4,906,123 counted fragments (72.63 % of total fragments), 4,401,376 (65.16 %) were unique and 504,747 (7.47 %) were non-specific. An intact pair was counted as one, and broken pairs were ignored.

In total, 20,325 transcripts were annotated to genes revealed by the RNA-Seq technology for the pig liver

Table 3 Fatty acid content (g/100 g FAME) in liver samples from two dietary groups. Data are presented as averages

Fatty acids		C diet group		E diet group		p-value (T test)
		Mean	SD	Mean	SD	
Σ SFA		43.18	9.12	42.35	5.09	0.7041
	C12:0	3.21	2.44	2.31	1.90	0.1754
	C14:0	0.62	0.28	0.58	0.27	0.6893
	C16:0	17.93	4.61	6.17	2.48	0.1114
	C18:0	21.77	5.8	23.42	4.64	0.2824
Σ MUFA		22.96	7.2	19.65	5.38	0.0792
	C16:1 n-7	3.47	4.62	1.85	0.75	0.1094
	C18:1 n-9	17.56	5.42	16.30	4.67	0.3918
	C18:1 n-7	1.93	0.42	1.64	0.23	0.0058**
Σ PUFA		27.23	8.05	33.9	6.28	0.0026*
	C18:2 n-6 (LA)	13.7	3.4	15.61	2.27	0.0284*
	C18:3 n-3 (ALA)	0.82	1.17	3.32	1.17	0.0000**
	C20:3 n-6	3.02	6.09	1.57	2.61	0.5676
	C20:4 n-6 (AA)	12.66	4.18	9.41	2.87	0.0055**
	C20:5 n-3 (EPA)	0.87	0.74	3.16	0.92	0.0006**
	C22:6 n-3 (DHA)	1.88	1.08	3.38	1.02	0.0006**
	Σ Omega-6[a]	25.63	7.72	25.69	4.13	0.9763
	Σ Omega-3[b]	2.16	1.83	8.22	3.50	10^{-9}**
Omega-6/omega-3 ratio		32.73	62.02	4.25	3.93	0.0769
Other[c]		6.63		4.1		

SFA saturated fatty acids, *MUFA* monounsaturated fatty acids, *PUFA* polyunsaturated fatty acids

[a]LA + ETA + AA

[b]ALA + EPA + DHA

[c]FA not identified according to the used standard

*P < 0.05

**P < 0.01

samples (Table 4). Analysis identified 3565 DEGs between the two dietary groups, 1484 of which were up-regulated and 2081 of which were down-regulated in the E group compared to the C group. The differentially expressed genes identified in the both dietary groups included 2098 annotated transcripts. Results also indicated that expression of certain genes in the liver were unique to a particular dietary group. For instance, 809 genes were unique to the E group while the expression of these genes in the opposite group was below our detection level and 658 genes were unique to the C group.

The mean value of the absolute expression level was 67.95 for all reads in both dietary groups. However, high-throughput sequencing results also identified genes that were characterized by an extreme high absolute value of expression level (RPKM ≥1000). Among the 3565 DEGs, 30 genes in the E group and 41 genes in the C group had an extreme high absolute value of expression, 27 of which were common to both dietary groups.

Fold change (FC) for highly expressed genes (RPKM ≥1000) ranged mainly from 2.0 to 5.0. Two genes had higher FC—retinol saturase (RETSAT, FC = 9.1) and serine dehydratase (SDS, FC = 27.3). Among the up-regulated genes characterized by the highest value of absolute expression were as follows: APOA4, APOA5, HMGCS2, ACSL1, and CYP2C49, while highly expressed down-regulated genes were COX1, SULT2A1, HPD, FMO1, and CPS. These genes are mainly related to fatty acid activation, fatty acid β-oxidation, lipid binding, and lipid transport activity (up-regulated) or were enzymes involved in prostaglandin biosynthesis or peroxidase activity (down-regulated).

Table 4 Summary of RNA sequencing analysis data of pig liver tissues fed a control (C) diet or the experimental (E) diet consisting of additional omega-6 and omega-3 fatty acids

	Number of DEGs	
Total number of DEGs	3565	
Genes up-regulated among all DEGs	1484 UP[a]	
Genes down-regulated among all DEGs	2081 DOWN[b]	
Expression in both groups	2098	
Highly expressed genes common to both groups	27	
	C diet	E diet
Expression in one group only	658	809
Highly expressed genes (RPKM ≥1000)	41	30

DEGs differentially expressed genes
[a]Up-regulated genes—the expression level higher in E diet group than in C diet group
[b]Down-regulated genes—the expression level lower in E diet group than in C diet group

The mean FC value of all DEGs was 9.4. The next-generation sequencing analysis also revealed genes characterized by a high FC value caused by a low level of expression for genes within one dietary group.

Quantitative real-time PCR

Differentially expressed genes selected from RNA-Seq generated data were validated using quantitative real-time PCR. Almost all genes chosen for validation were regulated in the same direction in both approaches excluding EXTL1 and FASN. The differences in Log2-fold of change between both methods were observed as shown in Fig. 2a. The differences in mean relative expression between control and experimental groups were observed (Fig 2b) in agreement with RNA-Seq data using RPKM expression values for almost all genes excluding EXTL1 (opposite results) FASN and FADS2 (statistically insignificant). High variability between the particular individuals among groups was visible.

Functional categorization of DEGs and pathway analysis

Fatty acid metabolism

The different ratio of omega-6/omega-3 fatty acids in the liver was reflected in altered fatty acid metabolism pathways revealed by the Cytoscape-ClueGo software. The visualization of potential networks for selected genes was consistent with previous observations of the most highly expressed genes and revealed the major biological mechanisms related to fatty acid metabolism: triglyceride metabolic process, lipid homeostasis, the PPAR signaling pathway, and fat digestion and absorption (Fig. 3 and Additional file 1).

All DEG

To further investigate the biological importance of DEG, we performed gene category analysis in DAVID software. Among gene sets comprising all DEGs, 1623 records were assigned to gene identifiers recognized by the DAVID tool. Table 5 shows 12 significant functional annotation clusters (for more details see Additional file 2). The created clusters represented genes involved in cell membrane-related processes and signal transduction. The cluster with the highest enrichment score (8.6) included 363 genes related to the plasma membrane. The functional clusters that demonstrated the highest number of involved genes were transmembrane proteins in the cellular component category, signal peptide and glycoproteins in the biological processes category, and ion binding for the molecular function category. Taken together, major functions within this group appeared to be related to plasma membrane proteins, extracellular matrix, and cell transport and signaling. Functional classification in the DAVID tool adjusted DEG to terms in the

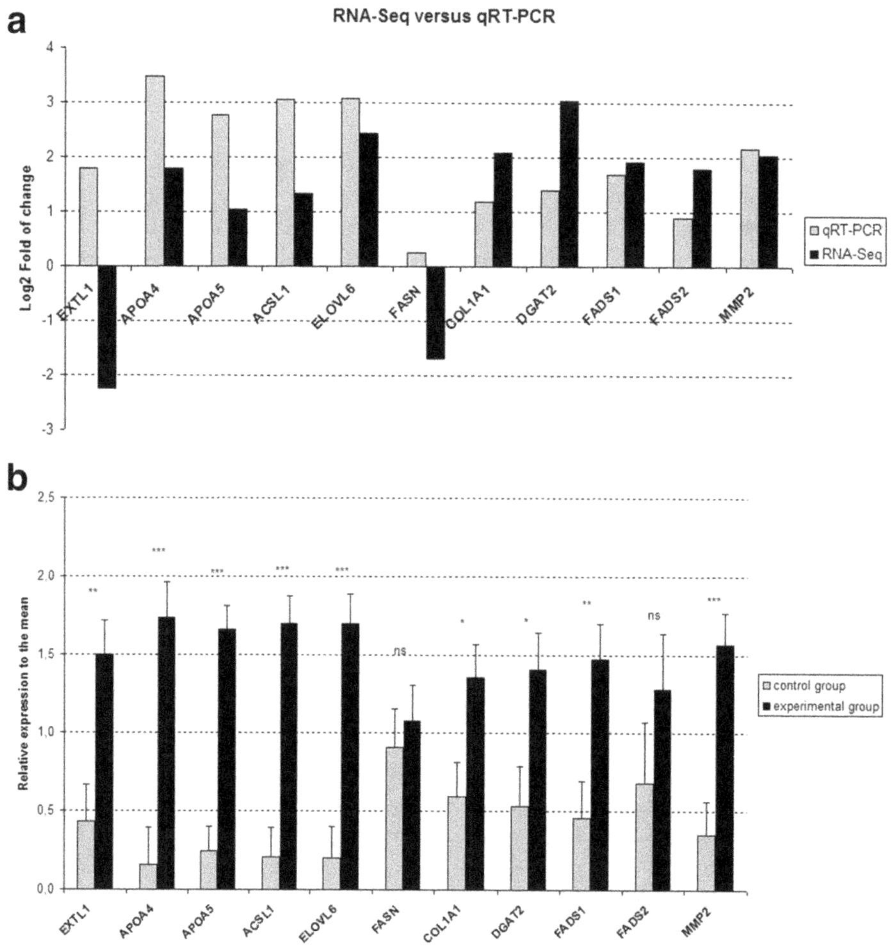

Fig. 2 Validation of differentially expressed genes (DEGs) by qRT-PCR. **a** comparison of the RNA-Seq (6 animals per group) and qRT-PCR (15 animals per group), Log2-fold of change between experimental and control groups, **b** individual variability of validated differentially expressed genes in qRT-PCR. For qRT-PCR, fold change was assessed on the basis of mean values of gene expression for 2 dietary groups with 15 individual samples per group. All Ct values were normalized to the topoisomerase (DNA) II beta (TOP2B) gene. Error bars represent standard error of variability among individual samples. *p-value <0,05; **p-value <0,01; ***p-value <0,001, *ns* not significant

KEGG database and showed the importance of 3 KEGG pathways—cytokine-cytokine receptor interactions (42 genes), focal adhesion (34 genes), and dilated cardiomyopathy (21 genes).

Cytoscape bioinformatics analysis of potential interactions between proteins for all DEGs was performed on 729 genes (Additional file 3). The major biological functions revealed by Cytoscape-ClueGo software were as follows: positive regulation of the JAK-STAT cascade, muscle cell development, dilated cardiomyopathy, growth of symbiont in the host, positive regulation of leukocyte proliferation, regulation of intracellular protein transport, positive regulation of inflammatory response, response to molecules of bacterial origin, and cerebellum development (Fig. 4). Several of these pathways were grouped around biological themes, such as inflammatory/pathogen response (10 pathways), signaling pathways (4), brain/nerve development (3), carbohydrate/lipid metabolism (3), and muscle development and function (2). The JAK-STAT pathways (on the right, near the immune response pathways) and the pathogen response pathway (in the lower right) were grouped relatively close to the inflammatory response pathways (Fig. 4). Muscle development was located near the top of the figure, above and close to the cardio-related pathways. The main groups representing the brain development pathways are in the upper left, separated from the other pathways. The carbohydrate/lipid metabolism pathway is on the bottom left. The regulation of the intracellular protein transport pathway is located in the center. All signaling-related pathways were dispersed throughout the network. Overall, the processes, which were grouped together, were more related to each other than they were to the others. The distribution of

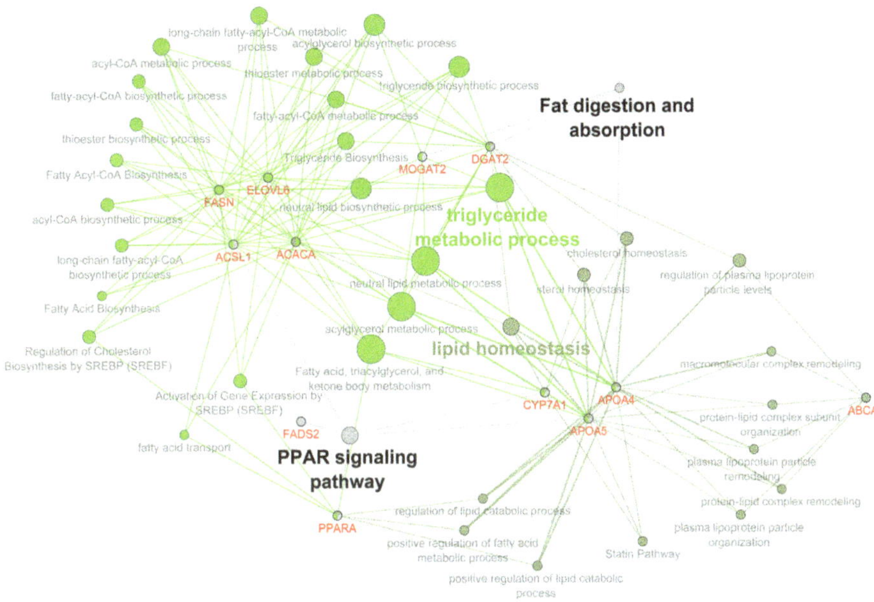

Fig. 3 The gene network pathways related to fatty acid metabolism. Visualization generated by Cytoscape-ClueGo software after selection criteria: at least three genes per one pathway node and 4 % of the associated genes from all genes in one node

pathways for all DEGs as specific clusters is presented in Fig. 5.

Genes expressed only in the experimental group

The analysis in DAVID, which comprised set of genes specific to the E group, recognized and analyzed 359 gene IDs. The results for this subset of genes are presented in Table 6 (more details are listed in the Additional file 4). The cluster with the highest enrichment score was the glycoprotein/transmembrane cluster. The signal peptide and ion transport clusters belong to the functional mechanisms in this category. No pathways were revealed from the KEGG database for the set of genes expressed exclusively in the E dietary group.

Visualization of the molecular interaction networks in Cytoscape for DEGs detected only in the E group was performed for 59 genes (Additional file 5). Selected genes were involved mainly in the regulation of steroid hormone biosynthesis (Fig. 6). Other affected pathways involved muscle contraction, nervous system, signaling, immune response, and ion channels. The results also included a number of small networks that were separated from the main network.

Table 5 Functional clusters created for all DEGs

Functional cluster analysis			
Biological function	Enrichment score	Number of involved genes	Ontology
Plasma membrane	8.6	363	CC
Glycoprotein/signal peptide	7.6	487	CC/BP
Transmembrane protein	6.4	646	CC
Extracellular matrix	4.5	115	CC
Ossification	4.0	44	BP
Fibronectin type 3	3.9	36	MF
Protein kinases	3.7	98	BP
Calmodulin binding	3.6	24	MF
Angiogenesis	3.4	39	BP
Ion binding	3.2	414	MF
Cell motion	3.0	63	BP
Cardio-related	3.0	26	BP

Clustering was performed using DAVID software
CC cellular component, *BP* biological process, *MF* molecular function

Genes expressed only in the control group

In total, 275 DEGs were converted to the DAVID-recognized gene IDs, but no functional cluster was assigned in this group (Additional file 6). The KEGG pathway analysis in DAVID software revealed two molecular interaction networks: cytokine-cytokine receptor interaction (12 genes) and type I diabetes mellitus (5 genes).

Cytoscape classification of DEGs specific for the C group was conducted on 31 genes (Additional file 7). Adjusted pathways included chemokine biosynthetic process, inflammatory response, and regulation of calcidiol 1-monooxygenase activity involved in vitamin D biosynthesis (Fig. 7). Besides the main network, other functions located outside of this network included

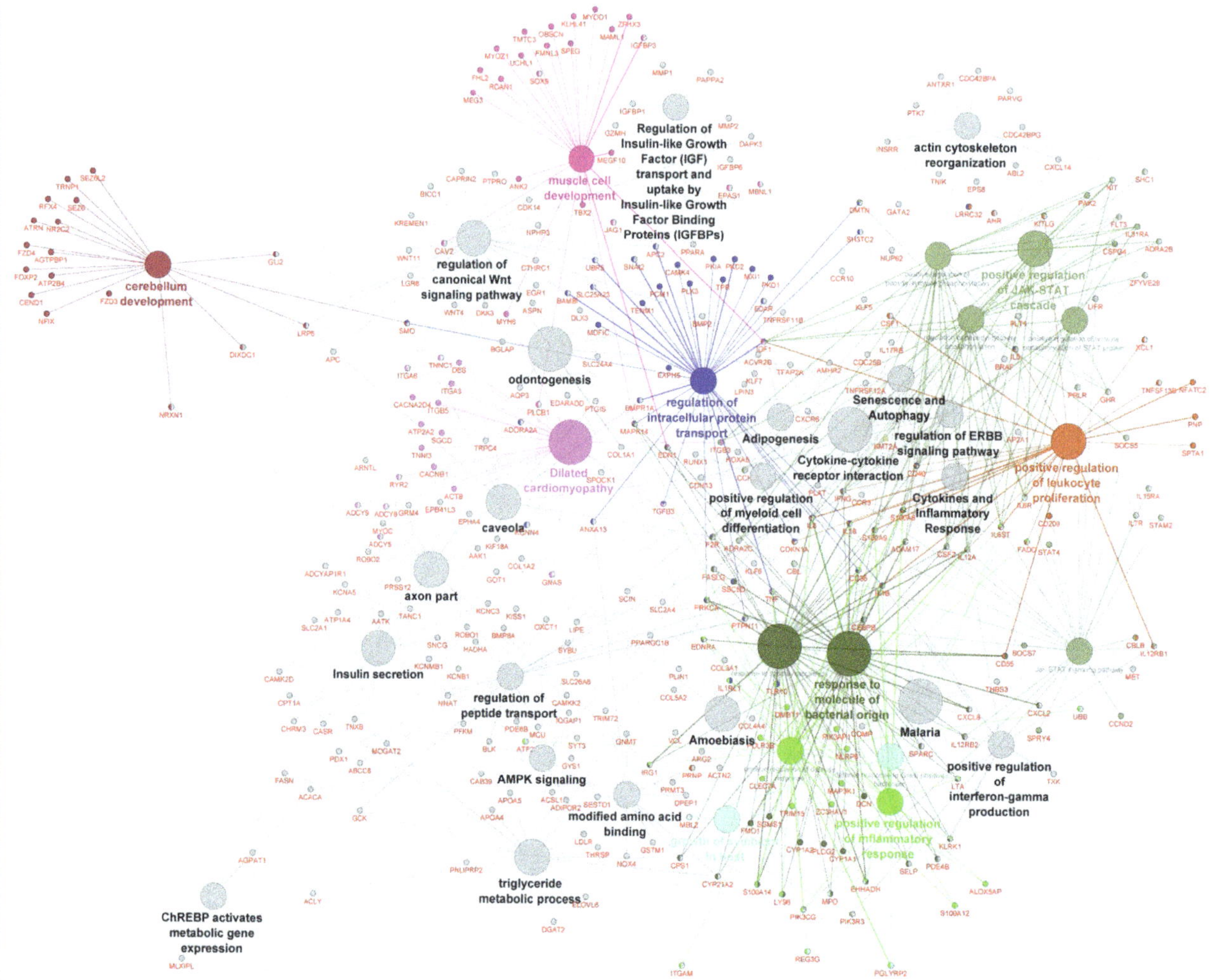

Fig. 4 The gene network and biological processes for all DEGs. Figure generated by Cytoscape-ClueGo. The *red* and *green* dots represent the up-regulated and down-regulated genes in the E group compared to the C group, respectively. The *lines* represent interactions among genes. The processes marked in *grey* are processes without direct connections to any of the other processes. The selection criteria for this network were to have at least two genes per node with a minimum of 5 % of the associated genes from all loaded genes in one node. The group percentage was 50 % with a kappa score threshold of 0.4

potassium-transporting ATPase activity, cGMP biosynthetic processes, and syncytium formation.

Genes exclusively expressed in both groups

Cytoscape analysis preformed on DEGs identified exclusively in the E or C group but not in both of the groups showed that the most of the pathways were related to neurological system processes (5 pathways), immunity response (2), and cation transport (2) (Fig. 8). Two specific clusters were assigned in the interaction network processes: regulation of neurological process and regulation of alcohol biosynthetic process.

Discussion

In our study, the RNA-Seq analysis showed modulatory effects of dietary omega-6 and omega-3 fatty acids on mRNA expression in pig liver. Liver transcriptomes of pigs fed a diet with increased LA and ALA content (the precursors for the synthesis of long-chain PUFA) were compared to those of pigs fed the standard diet. The scope of our study was to investigate the general biological mechanisms underlying the physiological effects of increased dietary intake of PUFA.

Increase of omega-3 PUFA contribution in fatty acid profile

As we expected, our data indicated specific differences between dietary groups in regard to the fatty acid profile. Results showed a higher contribution of PUFAs among all analyzed series of fatty acids in liver for pigs fed the LA and ALA-enriched diet compared to the standard diet, particularly for the omega-3 fatty acids EPA and

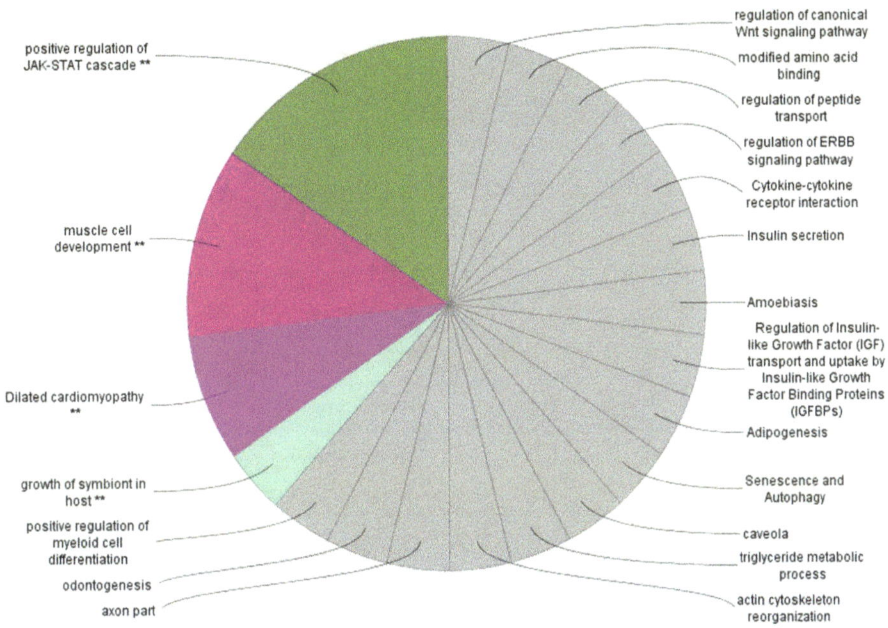

Fig. 5 The pathway distribution of the specific clusters for all DEGs. Analysis performed in Cytoscape-ClueGo. The selection criteria for this network were to have at least two genes per node with a minimum of 5 % of the associated genes from all loaded genes in one node. The group percentage was 50 % with a kappa score threshold of 0.4

DHA, but not omega-6. These results are consistent with those reported for previous gene expression studies in pigs (Corominas et al. 2013) and also rats (Hanke et al. 2013). This finding indicates higher absorption, transport and storage, or lower degradation of unsaturated fatty acids, which suggests inhibition of lipogenesis, but not for the omega-3 pathway. Substantial differences in the omega-6/omega-3 ratio in the liver, lowered ratio in the tissue after PUFA supplementation, outlined that the diet presumably affected body composition, which was the basis for further investigation on the transcriptome level. We can suppose that in the group characterized by increased content of LA and ALA in the diet, appeared specifically increased absorption of omega-3 fatty acids, not omega-6, on the base of fatty acid profile. Even though we consider that the conversion of ALA to EPA and DHA in vivo is less than 2 % (Brenna et al. 2009; Burdge and Calder 2005), the effect on omega-3 pathway was clear.

Table 6 Functional clusters for genes expressed only in E diet group

Functional cluster analysis			
Biological function	Enrichment score	Number of involved genes	Ontology
Glycoprotein/transmembrane	5.4	166	CC
Signal peptide	5.2	129	BP
Plasma membrane	3.8	98	CC
Fibronectin type 3	2.3	13	MF
Ion transport	2.3	41	MF

CC cellular component, *BP* biological process, *MF* molecular function

Enhancement of fatty acid β-oxidation in liver through induction of the PPAR signaling pathway

Among the most highly DEGs (FC ≥ 8), we identified genes involved in lipid metabolism, which play a key role in the synthesis of fatty acids. We observed lower expression of those genes in the liver of pigs with increased omega-3 fatty acids contribution in the liver, suggesting a major down-regulation of lipid metabolism and increase of β-oxidation. This is thought to relate to the omega-3 and omega-6 fatty acids (Jump 2011). One of the identified genes characterized by significantly reduced expression in our study was CYP7A1, which was shown to be important for the PPAR signaling pathway and is one of the target genes of LXR. The liver X receptor plays a major role in the PPAR signaling pathway and is a key regulator of fatty acid synthesis by regulation of lipogenic gene transcription and induction of SREBP-1c gene expression (Afman and Muller 2012). The effects of omega-3 fatty acids on changes in the expression of LXR's target genes agreed with the findings of a recent study in pigs (Ramayo-Caldas et al. 2012).

Additionally, the expression of another transcription factor, PPARα, was affected. The peroxisome proliferator-activated receptor is a liver-specific gene and plays a central role in fatty acid β-oxidation in hepatocytes. It is thought to be the main indicator of the fatty acid oxidation-metabolic state (Gormaz et al. 2010). A

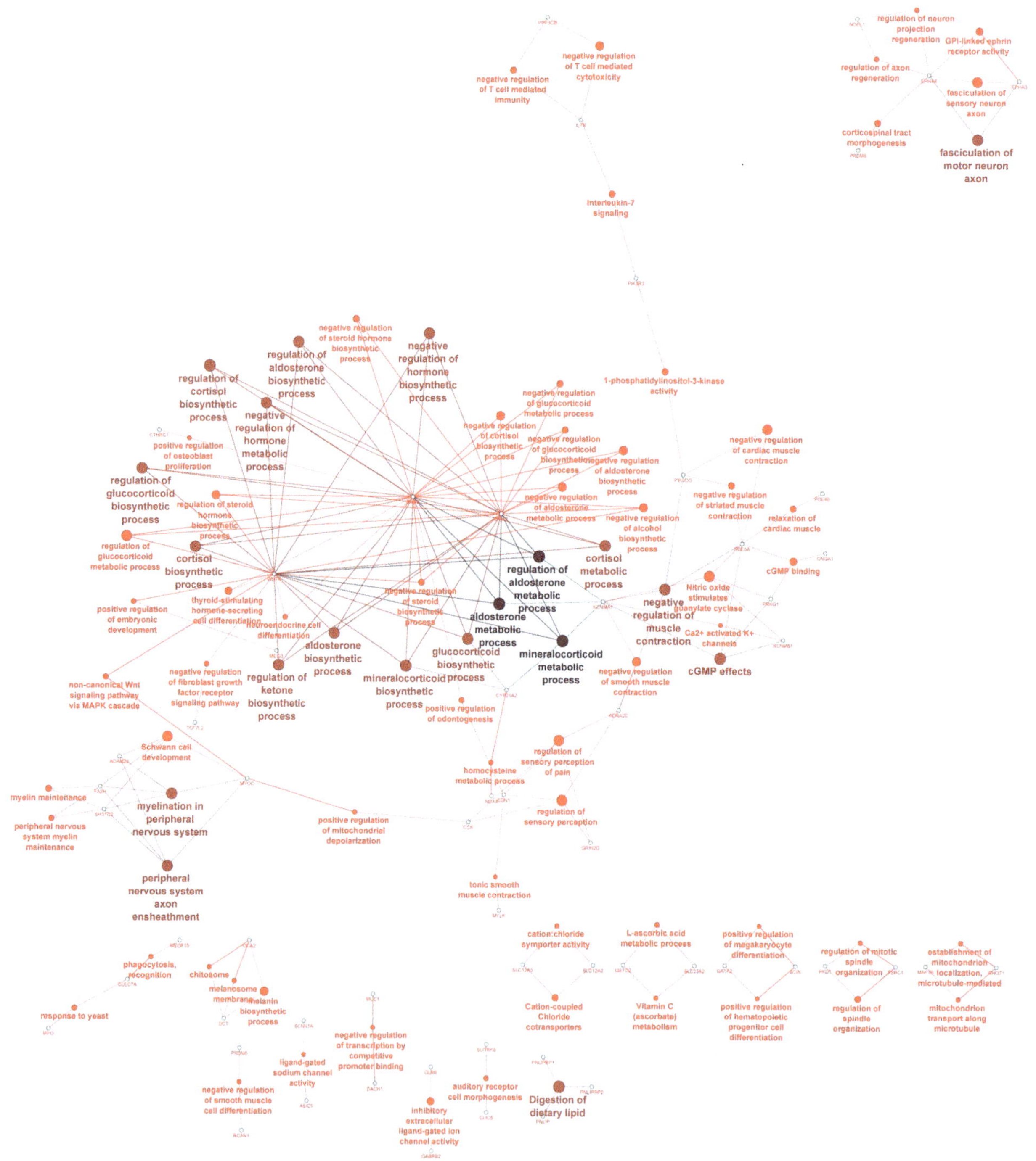

Fig. 6 The gene network and biological processes for genes specific to experimental (E) group. Analysis performed in Cytoscape-ClueGo. The selection criteria for this network were to have at least two genes per node with 15 % of the associated genes from all loaded genes in one node. The kappa score threshold was 0.51

higher content of omega-6 and omega-3 fatty acids in our study resulted in higher expression of the PPARα gene in the liver. Ramayo-Caldas et al. (2012) reported a similar effect on nuclear factors where the influence on the liver transcriptome of a PUFA-rich diet was compared to monounsaturated fatty acid (MUFA)- and saturated fatty acid (SFA)-enriched diet. Here, we pointed out how different contents of omega-6 and omega-3 PUFAs in the diet resulted in a different ratio of these two fatty acid families in the liver and how these alterations are reflected in the transcriptome. In our study, it is proposed that an omega-6 and omega-3

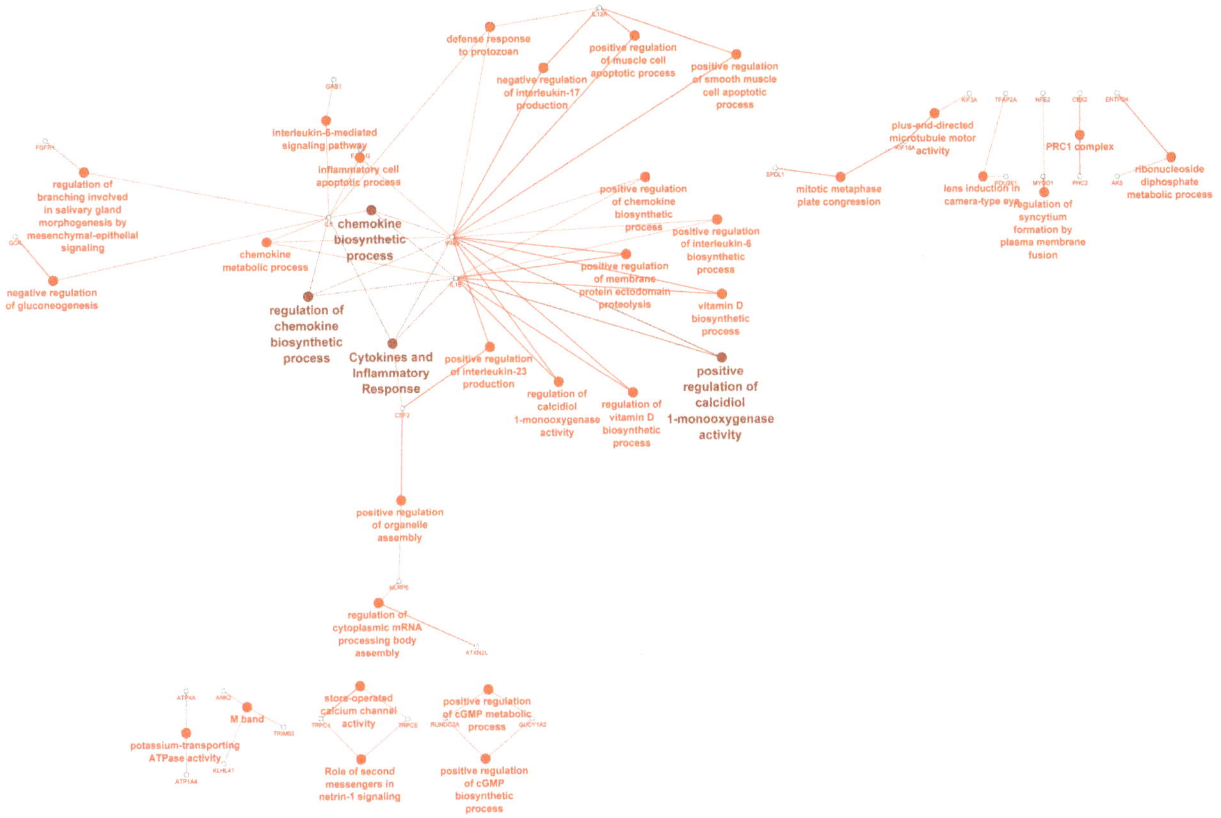

Fig. 7 The genes network and biological processes for genes specific to control (C) group. Analysis performed in Cytoscape-ClueGo. The selection criteria for this network were to have at least two genes per node with 15 % of associated genes from all loaded genes in one node. The kappa score threshold was 0.51

PUFA-enriched diet induced β-oxidation on the transcriptomic level in comparison to the influence of standard diet. It is generally accepted that omega-3 fatty acids induce hepatic fatty acid oxidation, possibly via PPARα activation, and suppress hepatic fatty acid synthesis through SREBP-1c (for reviews see El-Badry et al. (2007). However, some investigators have reported contrary results. Hanke et al. (2013) showed that omega-3-rich diets had no apparent effect on molecular markers of fatty acid oxidation on protein level. In particular, PPAR and ACOX were not affected nor were markers of fatty acid synthesis (SREBP-1c and ACC1) for livers of rats with diet-induced obesity.

Lastly, we found that up-regulated genes of the genes with the highest value of absolute expression registered by RNA-Seq analysis were involved in fatty acid activation, fatty acid β-oxidation, lipid binding, and lipid transport activity. To summarize, the direction of the expression level for major transcription factors responsible for fatty acid homeostasis, such as PPARα, LXR, or SREBP-1c, showed that omega-6 and omega-3-enriched diets influenced transcription of fatty acid β-oxidation genes and had significant impact on their molecular status what highlight their role as bioactive components of a diet. The higher PPARα expression in the liver suggested the biological modulatory effect of the LA- and ALA-enriched diet at the molecular level.

Increase of conversion intensity for omega-3 PUFA pathways in the liver

In our study, the FADS2 and FADS1 genes, which are responsible for coding enzymes delta-6-desaturase and delta-5-desaturase, respectively, where up-regulated in the RNA-Seq analysis (validated by qRT-PCR, statistically significant for FADS1). They are common for the conversion of fatty acids on three different pathways of omega fatty acid metabolism, being involved in introducing additional double bonds to dietary PUFAs, linoleic (omega-6) and α-linolenic acid (omega-3), and also to oleic acid (omega-9 MUFA) derived from de novo synthesis or the diet (Ratnayake and Galli (2009).

On the base of transcriptomic analysis, we cannot unambiguously confirm to which pathway delta-6-desaturase and delta-5-desaturase are directed. However, we can hypothesize a potential mechanism from the contributions of the derivatives of omega-6 and omega-3 fatty acid precursors in the fatty acid profile in the liver. Increased content of EPA and DHA (omega-3) and decreased AA

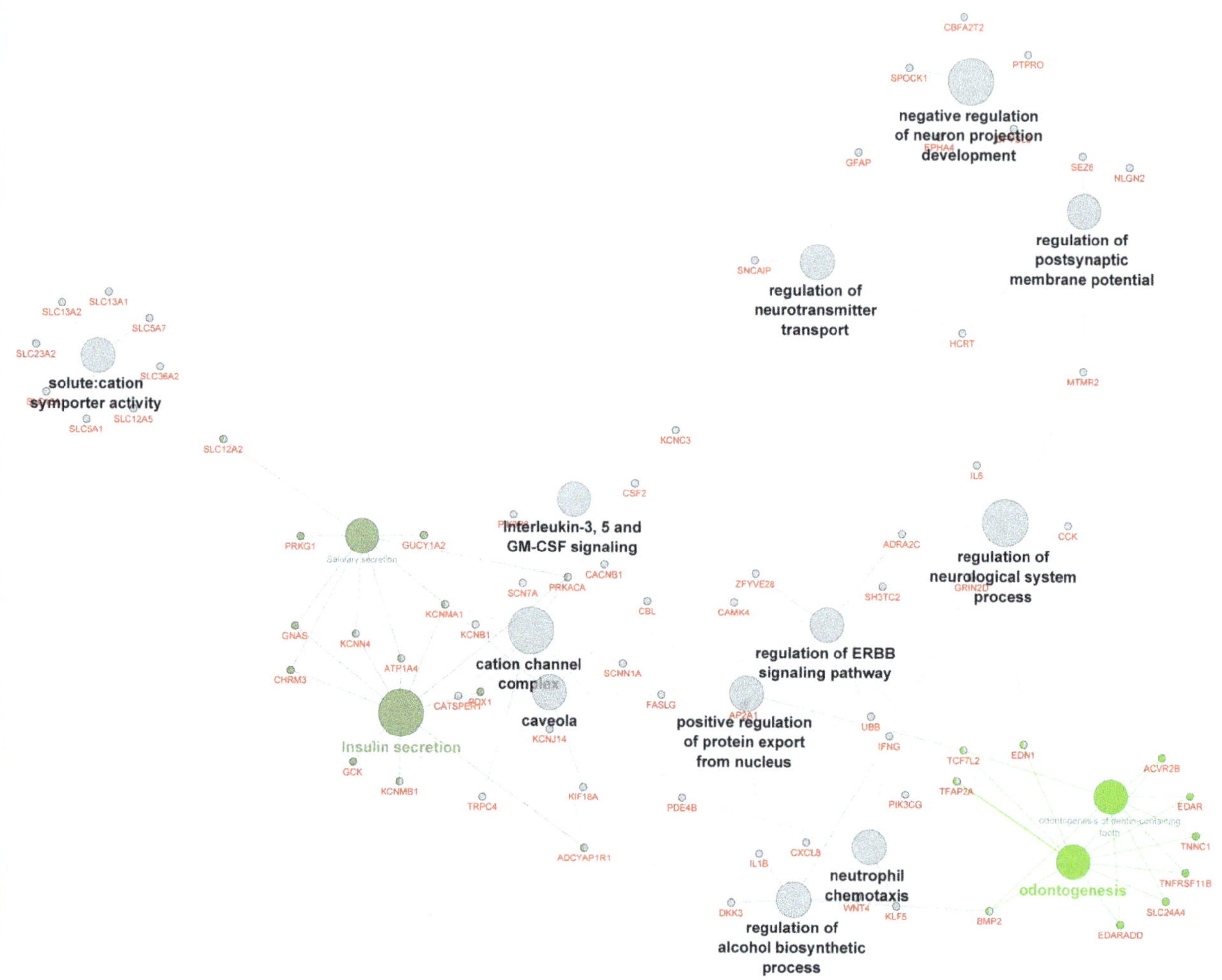

Fig. 8 The genes network for genes expressed above detection only in one of the groups merged in one network. Analysis performed in Cytoscape-ClueGo. The data sets of genes expressed only in one of groups were combined together in one analysis to create one figure. The selection criteria for this network were to have at least two genes per node with a minimum of 4 % of the associated genes from all loaded genes in one node. The group percentage was 50 % with a kappa score threshold of 0.4

(omega-6) suggest that ALA is converted into EPA and further to DHA, but conversion of LA to AA seems to be suppressed. Therefore, we suggest an increased intensity of conversion for omega-3 PUFA in the liver and suppose that FADS2 and FADS1 act mainly in the omega-3 metabolic pathway.

Furthermore, we observed a decreased expression of lipogenic gene coding for acetyl-CoA carboxylase-1 (ACACA). This suggests that the synthesis of short-chain fatty acids was decreased as a consequence of influence of the diet on these lipogenic genes. However, one of another lipogenic gene fatty acid synthase (FASN) was not confirmed by qRT-PCR. Conversely, enhanced activity of the conversion occurs to the long-chain fatty acids related to increased expression of ELOVL6 gene coding elongase (confirmed by qRT-PCR), which convert SFA-palmitic acid to stearic acid and is limiting enzyme for conversion between SFA and MUFA.

The production of acetyl-CoA derived from fatty acid degradation processes does not impact the Krebs cycle independently from the PUFAs content in the diet.

The main difference between the dietary groups in our studies was increased omega-3 intake from the diet and consequently higher conversion of omega-3 in the fatty acid pathway metabolism. Increased contents of omega-6 and omega-3 fatty acids in the diet resulted in altered metabolic pathways in the liver in a specific manner. The main biochemical pathways of unsaturated fatty acid metabolism seem to be directed to the omega-3 pathway, but not omega-6.

Further considerations in our future studies will concern identification of genes participating in the regulation of enzymes involved in lipid metabolism, which are common for different pathways of fatty acid metabolism.

Activation of pathways related to signal transduction, membrane composition, and mitigation of inflammation state

Analysis in DAVID demonstrated that most of the differentially expressed genes identified among two treatment groups affected by increased omega-3 fatty acid conversion were involved in signal transduction and plasma membrane-related proteins (Table 5). The biological function of signaling pathways is to forward information from the extracellular region via receptors on the plasma membrane and ion channels to support their transfer to the cytoplasm, what is supposed to be influenced by a low ratio of omega-6/omega-3 PUFA in our study and highlighted by the DAVID analysis. For example, extracellular fibronectins, one of the functional clusters revealed by DAVID, are ligands for the integrins located on the plasma membrane surface (Huveneers et al. 2008). An interaction network of reactions mediate between the transmission of various extracellular signals to the nucleus and is responsible for positive regulation of molecular function. All biological functions listed in the functional annotation clustering from DAVID are related to the processes taking place between cell membrane and the extracellular matrix such as ion transport or kinases activation. Polyunsaturated fatty acids are important components of the cell membranes and influence membrane fluidity as well as the action of membrane-bound enzymes and receptors. Thus, it is not surprising that oral administration of omega-6 and omega-3 fatty acids in pigs resulted in alterations emphasizing major functions of fatty acids in organisms—signal transduction and building of membrane, revealed in DAVID and Cytoscape-ClueGo analysis.

DAVID analysis concatenated with the KEGG database further support findings mentioned above and revealed focal adhesion molecules as a significant pathway, which is responsible for signal transduction, functionality of cell membranes, kinases activity, and ion transport. This pathway was related to the PUFA supplemented group, for which the omega-3 fatty acid content was increased.

Additionally, processes specific to pigs fed the supplemental diet (E group) were analyzed, and we observed results consistent with our findings mentioned above concerning the directions of alterations in lipid metabolism. We observed that the regulation of steroid hormone biosynthesis was the most affected pathway of the up-regulated genes, which were expressed only in the group characterized by increased intensity of conversions on omega-3 pathway. Steroid hormones are breakdown products of the EPA and DHA conversion pathways, and these metabolites were influenced by the administration of excess omega-3 fatty acid precursors in the diet.

Conversely, down-regulated genes, expressed only in the standard diet group, represent signaling molecules assigned as a cytokine-cytokine receptor interaction pathway identified by the KEGG database in the DAVID, (see also below) what reflects the anti-inflammatory properties of a high content of omega-3 fatty acids or low ratio of omega-6/omega-3 fatty acids in the liver. The expression of pro-inflammatory cytokines, which occurs in the control group of pigs under a normal physiological condition, is not observed in the PUFA supplemented group, what can hint at mitigation of the inflammation state. Our findings are consistent with studies on omega-3 fatty acid interventions against inflammatory status (Liu et al. 2015). Omega-3 fatty acids have been shown to inhibit expression of cytokine mRNAs, which are stimulated via omega-6 fatty acids (Kruger et al. 2010; Roy et al. 2007). Omega-3 fatty acids disturb the action of omega-6 fatty acid excess. Thus, our results suggest that the diet enriched with omega-3 fatty acids can modulate the immune response and could possibly improve the health of animals.

When we analyzed the processes specific to pigs fed the standard diet, we also observed perturbations of health-related pathways. Under a normal, physiological state, in the standard diet group of pigs, cytokine interaction was the most prominent pathway for genes expressed above detection level registered only in this group, while in the group with increased conversion of omega-3 fatty acids, expression of these genes were either not expressed or were down-regulated. Therefore, we can assume that increased conversion of omega-3 fatty acids revealed anti-inflammatory effect. This is in agreement with a recent study that investigated the effects of different omega-6/omega-3 ratios in pigs (Duan et al. 2014). Duan et al. (2014) revealed that inhibition of immune stimulation in pigs was characterized by a low ratio of omega-6/omega-3 fatty acids. Similarly, Papadopoulos et al. (2009) observed inflammation modulation in sows after administration of high doses of omega-3 fatty acids during the perinatal period. The up-regulation of TNFα in our study, which is an indicator of the inflammatory state, and additionally KEGG pathway and Cytoscape results further support this observation.

Additionally, calcidiol 1-monooxygenase activity, which is involved in vitamin D synthesis, was down-regulated. Vitamin D is known to promote vascular regeneration and possesses anti-proliferative and pro-apoptotic functions. Deficiency of vitamin D was associated with the inflammatory state (Wong et al. 2014). Presence of pro-inflammatory cytokines (such as TNFα and IL-6) might impair activation of vitamin D, which plays a pivotal role in the regulation of the prostaglandin pathway, thereby affecting both PGE2 synthesis by inhibition of COX2 expression (down-regulated in our studies), as well as its degradation by stimulation of 15-PGDH expression (Hummel et al. 2014). Thus, it could be proposed that a higher conversion of omega-3 fatty acids in the liver, caused by increased dietary intake of LA resulted in inhibition of inflammation in vascular tissue possibly via activation of the vitamin D system.

In summary, the presented work utilized high-throughput sequencing to identify the biological and metabolic processes of the pig liver transcriptome most affected by different omega-6 and omega-3 fatty acid content in the diet. A low ratio of omega-6/omega-3 fatty acids in the liver, caused by increased intake of omega-3 fatty acids from the diet, modulated gene expression and affected a set of genes related mainly to energy metabolism, signaling pathways, and the inflammatory response.

Additional files

Additional file 1: The list of genes related to fatty acid metabolism from Cytoscape-ClueGo.

Additional file 2: The list of significantly differentially expressed genes (DEGs). Significant annotation clusters were listed based on the analysis of functional ontologies using the DAVID tools including all DEGs.

Additional file 3: Cytoscape-ClueGo analysis including all DEGs.

Additional file 4: The list of DEGs specific to experimental (E) group. A list of significant annotation clusters based on the analysis of functional ontologies using the DAVID tools including DEGs above detection level only in the E diet group.

Additional file 5: Cytoscape-ClueGo analysis, including genes with detectable gene expression found only in the E diet group.

Additional file 6: The list of DEGs specific to control (C) group. A list of significant annotation clusters based on the analysis of functional ontologies using the DAVID tools including DEGs detected only in the C diet group.

Additional file 7: Cytoscape-ClueGo analysis of genes with detectable gene expression found only in the C diet group.

Competing interests
The authors declare that they have no competing interests.

Authors' contributions
AS wrote the manuscript. AS and MO performed the gene expression experiments. AS, MO and MP analyzed the NGS data and performed the functional ontology and pathways analysis. MP designed the experiment. MP and MFWP supervised the experiment and helped in writing the manuscript. EP had significant participation in study design, edited the manuscript and performed fatty acids analysis. PU participated in carry out gas chromatography analysis. EJK, JOH and TB participated in the design of the study. All authors read and approved the final manuscript.

Acknowledgements
The research was realized within the project "BIOFOOD—innovative, functional products of animal origin" no. POIG.01.01.02-014-090/09 co-financed by the European Union from the European Regional Development Fund within the Innovative Economy Operational Programme 2007 – 2013, and this work was supported by The National Science Centre, grant no. 2014/13/N/NZ9/00906. We would like to thank Genomed for performing next-generation sequencing analysis and for data production.

Author details
[1]Institute of Genetics and Animal Breeding, Polish Academy of Science, Jastrzębiec, Poland. [2]Animal Breeding and Genetics Centre, Wageningen UR Livestock Research, Lelystad, The Netherlands. [3]Functional Genomics Laboratory, Faculty of Biology and Environment Protection, Nicolaus Copernicus University, Toruń, Poland. [4]Department of Animal Science, Iowa State University, Ames, IA, USA.

References
Afman LA, Muller M (2012) Human nutrigenomics of gene regulation by dietary fatty acids. Prog Lipid Res 51:63–70
Amminger GP, Schafer MR, Schlogelhofer M, Klier CM, McGorry PD (2015) Longer-term outcome in the prevention of psychotic disorders by the Vienna omega-3 study. Nat Commun 6:7934
Anders S, Huber W (2010) Differential expression analysis for sequence count data. Genome Biol 11:R106
Aro A (2003) Fatty acid composition of serum lipids: is this marker of fat intake still relevant for identifying metabolic and cardiovascular disorders? Nutr Metab Cardiovasc Dis 13:253–255
Barrett T, Wilhite SE, Ledoux P, Evangelista C, Kim IF, Tomashevsky M, Marshall KA, Phillippy KH, Sherman PM, Holko M, Yefanov A, Lee H, Zhang N, Robertson CL, Serova N, Davis S, Soboleva A (2013) NCBI GEO: archive for functional genomics data sets—update. Nucleic Acids Res 41:D991–D995
Bergen WG, Mersmann HJ (2005) Comparative aspects of lipid metabolism: impact on contemporary research and use of animal models. J Nutr 135: 2499–2502
Brazma A, Hingamp P, Quackenbush J, Sherlock G, Spellman P, Stoeckert C, Aach J, Ansorge W, Ball CA, Causton HC, Gaasterland T, Glenisson P, Holstege FCP, Kim IF, Markowitz V, Matese JC, Parkinson H, Robinson A, Sarkans U, Schulze-Kremer S, Stewart J, Taylor R, Vilo J, Vingron M (2001) Minimum information about a microarray experiment (MIAME)—toward standards for microarray data. Nat Genet 29:365–371
Brenna JT, Salem N Jr, Sinclair AJ, Cunnane SC, International Society for the Study of Fatty A, Lipids I (2009) alpha-Linolenic acid supplementation and conversion to n-3 long-chain polyunsaturated fatty acids in humans. Prostaglandins Leukot Essent Fatty Acids 80:85–91
Burdge GC, Calder PC (2005) Conversion of alpha-linolenic acid to longer-chain polyunsaturated fatty acids in human adults. Reprod Nutr Dev 45:581–597
Bustin SA, Benes V, Garson J, Hellemans J, Huggett J, Kubista M, Mueller R, Nolan T, Pfaffl MW, Shipley G, Wittwer CT, Schjerling P, Day PJ, Abreu M, Aguado B, Beaulieu JF, Beckers A, Bogaert S, Browne JA, Carrasco-Ramiro F, Ceelen L, Ciborowski K, Cornillie P, Coulon S, Cuypers A, De Brouwer S, De Ceuninck L, De Craene J, De Naeyer H, De Spiegelaere W, Deckers K, Dheedene A, Durinck K, Ferreira-Teixeira M, Fieuw A, Gallup JM, Gonzalo-Flores S, Goossens K, Heindryckx F, Herring E, Hoenicka H, Icardi L, Jaggi R, Javad F, Karampelias M, Kibenge F, Kibenge M, Kumps C, Lambertz I, Lammens T, Markey A, Messiaen P, Mets E, Morais S, Mudarra-Rubio A, Nakiwala J, Nelis H, Olsvik PA, Perez-Novo C, Plusquin M, Remans T, Rihani A, Rodrigues-Santos P, Rondou P, Sanders R, Schmidt-Bleek K, Skovgaard K, Smeets K, Tabera L, Toegel S, Van Acker T, Van den Broeck W, Van der Meulen J, Van Gele M, Van Peer G, Van Poucke M, Van Roy N, Vergult S, Wauman J, Tshuikina-Wiklander M, Willems E, Zaccara S, Zeka F, Vandesompele J (2013) The need for transparency and good practices in the qPCR literature. Nat Methods 10:1063–1067
Chen C, Ai H, Ren J, Li W, Li P, Qiao R, Ouyang J, Yang M, Ma J, Huang L (2011) A global view of porcine transcriptome in three tissues from a full-sib pair with extreme phenotypes in growth and fat deposition by paired-end RNA sequencing. BMC Genomics 12:448
Chomczynski P, Sacchi N (1987) Single-step method of RNA isolation by acid guanidinium thiocyanate-phenol-chloroform extraction. Anal Biochem 162:156–159
Chomczynski P, Sacchi N (2006) The single-step method of RNA isolation by acid guanidinium thiocyanate–phenol–chloroform extraction: twenty-something years on. Nat Protoc 1:581–585
Corominas J, Ramayo-Caldas Y, Puig-Oliveras A, Estelle J, Castello A, Alves E, Pena RN, Ballester M, Folch JM (2013) Analysis of porcine adipose tissue

transcriptome reveals differences in de novo fatty acid synthesis in pigs with divergent muscle fatty acid composition. BMC Genomics 14:843

de Pablo MA, Alvarez de Cienfuegos G (2000) Modulatory effects of dietary lipids on immune system functions. Immunol Cell Biol 78:31–39

Duan Y, Li F, Li L, Fan J, Sun X, Yin Y (2014) n-6:n-3 PUFA ratio is involved in regulating lipid metabolism and inflammation in pigs. Br J Nutr 111:445–451

El-Badry AM, Graf R, Clavien PA (2007) Omega 3 - omega 6: what is right for the liver? J Hepatol 47:718–725

Folch J, Lees M, Sloane Stanley GH (1957) A simple method for the isolation and purification of total lipides from animal tissues. J Biol Chem 226:497–509

Getek M, Czech N, Fizia K, Bialek-Dratwa A, Muc-Wierzgon M, Kokot T, Nowakowska-Zajdel E (2013) Nutrigenomics—bioactive dietary components. Postepy Hig Med Dosw 67:255–260

Gormaz JG, Rodrigo R, Videla LA, Beems M (2010) Biosynthesis and bioavailability of long-chain polyunsaturated fatty acids in non-alcoholic fatty liver disease. Prog Lipid Res 49:407–419

Guillevic M, Kouba M, Mourot J (2009) Effect of a linseed diet on lipid composition, lipid peroxidation and consumer evaluation of French fresh and cooked pork meats. Meat Sci 81:612–618

Hanke D, Zahradka P, Mohankumar SK, Clark JL, Taylor CG (2013) A diet high in alpha-linolenic acid and monounsaturated fatty acids attenuates hepatic steatosis and alters hepatic phospholipid fatty acid profile in diet-induced obese rats. Prostaglandins Leukot Essent Fatty Acids 89:391–401

Harris WS, Assaad B, Poston WC (2006) Tissue omega-6/omega-3 fatty acid ratio and risk for coronary artery disease. Am J Cardiol 98:19i–26i

Huang DW, Sherman BT, Lempicki RA (2009a) Bioinformatics enrichment tools: paths toward the comprehensive functional analysis of large gene lists. Nucleic Acids Res 37:1–13

Huang DW, Sherman BT, Lempicki RA (2009b) Systematic and integrative analysis of large gene lists using DAVID bioinformatics resources. Nat Protoc 4:44–57

Hummel DM, Fetahu IS, Groschel C, Manhardt T, Kallay E (2014) Role of proinflammatory cytokines on expression of vitamin D metabolism and target genes in colon cancer cells. J Steroid Biochem Mol Biol 144(Pt A):91–95

Huveneers S, Truong H, Fassler R, Sonnenberg A, Danen EH (2008) Binding of soluble fibronectin to integrin alpha5 beta1—link to focal adhesion redistribution and contractile shape. J Cell Sci 121:2452–2462

Jump DB (2011) Fatty acid regulation of hepatic lipid metabolism. Curr Opin Clin Nutr Metab Care 14:115–120

Kanehisa M, Goto S (2000) KEGG: Kyoto encyclopedia of genes and genomes. Nucleic Acids Res 28:27–30

Kanehisa M, Goto S, Sato Y, Kawashima M, Furumichi M, Tanabe M (2014) Data, information, knowledge and principle: back to metabolism in KEGG. Nucleic Acids Res 42:D199–D205

Kruger MC, Coetzee M, Haag M, Weiler H (2010) Long-chain polyunsaturated fatty acids: selected mechanisms of action on bone. Prog Lipid Res 49:438–449

Lands B (2012) Consequences of essential fatty acids. Nutrients 4:1338–1357

Li H, Xi Q, Xiong Y, Cheng X, Qi Q, Yang L, Shu G, Wang S, Wang L, Gao P, Zhu X, Jiang Q, Zhang Y, Yuan L (2011) A comprehensive expression profile of microRNAs in porcine pituitary. PLoS ONE 6:e24883

Lionetti L, Mollica MP, Sica R, Donizzetti I, Gifuni G, Pignalosa A, Cavaliere G, Putti R (2014) Differential effects of high-fish oil and high-lard diets on cells and cytokines involved in the inflammatory process in rat insulin-sensitive tissues. Int J Mol Sci 15:3040–3063

Liu Y-H, Li X-Y, Chen C-Y, Zhang H-M, Kang JX (2015) Omega-3 fatty acid intervention suppresses lipopolysaccharide-induced inflammation and weight loss in mice. Mar Drugs 13:1026–1036

Lunney JK (2007) Advances in swine biomedical model genomics. Int J Biol Sci 3:179–184

Morine MJ, Tierney AC, van Ommen B, Daniel H, Toomey S, Gjelstad IM, Gormley IC, Perez-Martinez P, Drevon CA, Lopez-Miranda J, Roche HM (2011) Transcriptomic coordination in the human metabolic network reveals links between n-3 fat intake, adipose tissue gene expression and metabolic health. PLoS Comput Biol 7:e1002223

Nguyen P, Leray V, Diez M, Serisier S, Le Bloc'h J, Siliart B, Dumon H (2008) Liver lipid metabolism. J Anim Physiol Anim Nutr (Berl) 92:272–283

Ntambi JM (1999) Regulation of stearoyl-CoA desaturase by polyunsaturated fatty acids and cholesterol. J Lipid Res 40:1549–1558

Nygard AB, Jorgensen CB, Cirera S, Fredholm M (2007) Selection of reference genes for gene expression studies in pig tissues using SYBR green qPCR. BMC Mol Biol 8:67

Papadopoulos GA, Maes DG, Van Weyenberg S, van Kempen TA, Buyse J, Janssens GP (2009) Peripartal feeding strategy with different n-6: n-3 ratios in sows: effects on sows' performance, inflammatory and periparturient metabolic parameters. Br J Nutr 101:348–357

Pierzchala M, Pareek CS, Urbanski P, Goluch D, Kamyczek M, Rozycki M, Kuryl J (2011) Selection of reference genes for gene expression studies in porcine hepatic tissue using quantitative real-time polymerase chain reaction. Anim Sci Pap Rep 29:53–63

Polawska E, Horbanczuk JO, Pierzchala M, Strzalkowska N, Jozwik A, Wojcik A, Pomianowski J, Gutkowska K, Wierzbicka A, Hoffman LC (2013) Effect of dietary linseed and rapeseed supplementation on fatty acid profiles in the ostrich. Part 1. Muscles. Anim Sci Pap Rep 31:239–248

Ramakers C, Ruijter JM, Deprez RH, Moorman AF (2003) Assumption-free analysis of quantitative real-time polymerase chain reaction (PCR) data. Neurosci Lett 339:62–66

Ramayo-Caldas Y, Mach N, Esteve-Codina A, Corominas J, Castello A, Ballester M, Estelle J, Ibanez-Escriche N, Fernandez AI, Perez-Enciso M, Folch JM (2012) Liver transcriptome profile in pigs with extreme phenotypes of intramuscular fatty acid composition. BMC Genomics 13:547

Ratnayake WM, Galli C (2009) Fat and fatty acid terminology, methods of analysis and fat digestion and metabolism: a background review paper. Ann Nutr Metab 55:8–43

Roy N, Barnett M, Knoch B, Dommels Y, McNabb W (2007) Nutrigenomics applied to an animal model of inflammatory bowel diseases: transcriptomic analysis of the effects of eicosapentaenoic acid- and arachidonic acid-enriched diets. Mutat Res 622:103–116

Ruijter JM, Ramakers C, Hoogaars WM, Karlen Y, Bakker O, van den Hoff MJ, Moorman AF (2009) Amplification efficiency: linking baseline and bias in the analysis of quantitative PCR data. Nucleic Acids Res 37:e45

Ruijter JM, Pfaffl MW, Zhao S, Spiess AN, Boggy G, Blom J, Rutledge RG, Sisti D, Lievens A, De Preter K, Derveaux S, Hellemans J, Vandesompele J (2013) Evaluation of qPCR curve analysis methods for reliable biomarker discovery: bias, resolution, precision, and implications. Methods 59:32–46

Saito R, Smoot ME, Ono K, Ruscheinski J, Wang PL, Lotia S, Pico AR, Bader GD, Ideker T (2012) A travel guide to Cytoscape plugins. Nat Methods 9:1069–1076

Shi R, Chiang VL (2005) Facile means for quantifying microRNA expression by real-time PCR. Biotechniques 39:519–525

Stanley WC, Cox JW, Asemu G, O'Connell KA, Dabkowski ER, Xu W, Ribeiro RF Jr, Shekar KC, Hoag SW, Rastogi S, Sabbah HN, Daneault C, des Rosiers C (2013) Evaluation of docosahexaenoic acid in a dog model of hypertension induced left ventricular hypertrophy. J Cardiovasc Transl Res 6:1000–1010

Vallim T, Salter AM (2010) Regulation of hepatic gene expression by saturated fatty acids. Prostaglandins Leukot Essent Fatty Acids 82:211–218

Warensjo E, Sundstrom J, Lind L, Vessby B (2006) Factor analysis of fatty acids in serum lipids as a measure of dietary fat quality in relation to the metabolic syndrome in men. Am J Clin Nutr 84:442–448

Wong MS, Leisegang MS, Kruse C, Vogel J, Schurmann C, Dehne N, Weigert A, Herrmann E, Brune B, Shah AM, Steinhilber D, Offermanns S, Carmeliet G, Badenhoop K, Schroder K, Brandes RP (2014) Vitamin d promotes vascular regeneration. Circulation 130:976–986

Wymann MP, Schneiter R (2008) Lipid signalling in disease. Nat Rev Mol Cell Biol 9:162–176

Ye J, Coulouris G, Zaretskaya I, Cutcutache I, Rozen S, Madden TL (2012) Primer-BLAST: a tool to design target-specific primers for polymerase chain reaction. BMC bioinformatic 13:134

12

Synbiotic effects of β-glucans from cauliflower mushroom and *Lactobacillus fermentum* on metabolic changes and gut microbiome in estrogen-deficient rats

Seong-Yeop Jeong[1], Suna Kang[2], Cao Shi Hua[2], Zhang Ting[2] and Sunmin Park[2*]

Abstract

Background: We investigated whether the long-term consumption of a symbiotic formulation with *Lactobacillus fermentum* (probiotic) and β-glucan from cauliflower mushroom (prebiotic) would delay the progression of post-menopausal symptoms in ovariectomized (OVX) rats and explored their mechanisms of action, including changes in gut microbiota.

Methods: OVX rats were fed with high-fat diets containing 1% dextrin (control), 1% lyophilized cauliflower mushroom extract (CFM), 0.1% *L. fermentum* JS (LFE), 1% CFM plus 0.1% LFE (CFLF), or 30 μg 17β-estradiol/kg body weight (positive-control) for 8 weeks.

Results: CFM contained 95.8% β-glucans. OVX increased the ratio of *Firmicutes* and *Bacteroidetes* in the large intestines. Only CFLF lowered tail skin temperature without increasing serum 17β-estradiol and uterine index. Visceral fat mass was lower in CFLF and positive-control groups by increasing daily energy expenditure and fat oxidation. Dyslipidemia induced by OVX was improved by CFM and CFLF as much as in the positive-control group. Homeostasis model assessment estimate of insulin resistance was lower in CFLF than in the positive-control. Hepatic insulin signaling (pAkt→GSK-3β) was potentiated in the ascending order of the control, LFE, CFM, CFLF, and positive-control. AMPK phosphorylation showed similar patterns of hepatic insulin signaling but LFE increased it more than CFM. The changes in gut microbiota were prevented by CFLF in OVX rats, and the ratio of *Firmicutes* and *Bacteroidetes* in the CFLF was similar to the positive-control group.

Conclusion: OVX changed gut microbiota and was associated with menopausal symptoms; however, the synbiotics, CFM and LFE, prevented menopausal symptoms and improved the gut microbiota in estrogen-deficient rats.

Keywords: Cauliflower mushroom, β-Glucan, *Lactobacillus fermentum*, Gut microbiota, Ovariectomy, Synbiotics

Background

Estrogen deficiency causes disturbances of energy, lipid, glucose, and bone metabolism and induces vasomotor symptoms such as daytime hot flushes, night sweats, sleep and mood disorder, and difficulty in concentration. These menopausal symptoms result in a lower quality of life and increase the incidence of metabolic disease. Although hormone replacement therapy ultimately prevents menopausal symptoms and improves quality of life, hormone replacement therapy is often not recommended due to its risk of adverse side-effects [1]. Alternative therapies with less adverse effects have been suggested for the treatment of menopausal symptoms.

Firmicutes among the gut microbiota is associated with obesity and its progression towards metabolic disease [2], and dietary interventions to modulate the gut microbiota can alleviate metabolic diseases [3]. Sex hormones including estrogen and testosterone have been reported to modulate microbial communities [4], and gut microbiota influence systemic levels of sex hormones [5, 6]. Intestinal tissues mainly contain estrogen receptor (ER)-β. ER-β affects the composition of gut microbiota

* Correspondence: smpark@hoseo.edu
[2]Department of Food & Nutrition, Obesity/Diabetes Center, Hoseo University, 165 Sechul-Ri, BaeBang-Yup, Asan-Si, ChungNam-Do 336-795, South Korea
Full list of author information is available at the end of the article

in female mice [7]. Cox-York et al. [8] have demonstrated that ovariectomized (OVX) rats with higher aerobic capacity increase microbial diversity and the number of the *Bacteroidetes phylum* in the gut. In addition, equol production in the gut produces the beneficial effects of soy and isoflavones on menopausal symptoms and gut microbiota is associated with equol production in the gut from soy-isoflavone concentrates in post-menopausal women [9]. Thus, the changes of gut microbiota composition can prevent the menopausal symptoms.

Diets including prebiotics and probiotics can modulate gut microbiota [7, 10]. Probiotics consumption seems to be a feasible approach to modulate the intestinal microbiota and to maintain or restore human health [11]. *Bifidobacterium* and *Lactobacillus*, natural components of the colon microbiota, are the most commonly used probiotics in many functional foods and dietary supplements. Various *Lactobacillus* species such as *Lactobacillus fermentum, Lactobacillus plantarium*, and *Lactobacillus reuteri* are naturally present in fermented foods and milk products [12] and especially, *L. fermentum*, which was isolated from human milk, can inhibit pathogens, decrease cholesterol synthesis, and change gut microbiota [13, 14]. Dietary supplementation with prebiotics, including lactulose, galacto-oligosaccharides, and fructo-oligosaccharides, increases the contents and proportion of bifidobacteria in the intestines [15] and improves nutrient absorption, prevents gut inflammation, and stimulates energy and glucose metabolism [16, 17]. Synbiotics, a combination of probiotics and prebiotics, may have better efficacy for changing gut microbiota and to improving metabolic symptoms [17]. However, there are still some debates about consumption of prebiotics and probiotics, gut microbiota, and metabolic efficacy.

Cauliflower mushroom (*Sparassis crispa* Wulf.:Fr.) contains about 40% of six-branched 1,3-beta-glucan that can change gut microbiota [18, 19]. However, β-glucan is known to improve inflammation and to alleviate inflammatory bowel diseases, cancer, atopic dermatitis, and arthritis. In addition, β-glucan potentiates glucagon-like peptide-1 secretion in L cells in the intestines to improve glucose metabolism. Thus, cauliflower mushroom may prevent the energy, glucose, lipid, and bone metabolism disturbances that occur in estrogen-deficient animals while modulating the gut microbiota.

We hypothesized that the long-term consumption of *L. fermentum* (probiotics) and cauliflower mushroom (prebiotics) would prevent and/or delay the progression of post-menopausal symptoms in estrogen-deficient animals with diet-induced obesity. The present study tested this hypothesis and explored their mechanisms of action in OVX rats fed a high-fat diet supplemented with *L. fermentum* and cauliflower mushroom.

Methods

Water extract of cauliflower mushroom and β-glucan contents

Cauliflower mushroom was purchased from Haemaru Biotechnology (Asan, Korea). Dried cauliflower mushroom was powdered, and the powder was extracted with water at 90 °C for 4 h in an extractor. The extract was concentrated by 50% with a rotary evaporator and centrifuged at 8000×*g* for 30 min. The concentrates were then freeze dried, and the yield of the mushroom was 28.8%.

To calculate the β-glucan contents, cauliflower mushroom extract was sequentially degraded with digestive enzymes by incubating in a shaking incubate with specific pH and temperature for 2 h. The enzymes used to digest the cauliflower mushroom were amylase (20 units, pH 6.9) at 20 °C, cellulase (50 units, pH 5.0) at 37 °C, protease (10 units, pH 7.5) at 37 °C, and amyloglucosidase (70 units, pH 4.8) at 60 °C. After digesting the cauliflower mushroom with enzymes, 95% ethanol was added into the digested mixture and the mixture was left at 4 °C for 12 h. The mixture was centrifuged at 10,000 rpm for 10 min, and the precipitates were mixed with water. The mixture was homogenized and diluted with distilled water, and then sulfuric acid was added (1:5). The mixture was left at room temperature for 20 min, and the optical density was measured at 470 nm. Glucose solution was used as a standard.

Ovariectomy operation

Female Sprague–Dawley rats (weighing 271 ± 9 g) were housed individually in cages in a controlled environment (23 °C, with a 12-h light/dark cycle). Animal care and surgery were conducted according to the NIH Guide for the Care and Use of Laboratory Animals. The Sprague–Dawley rats from DBL (Yeumsung-Kun, Korea) had an acclimation for 1 week in our animal facility. The rats had an ovariectomy (OVX) operation under anesthesia by a subcutaneous injection of a mixture of ketamine and xylazine (100 and 10 mg/kg body weight, respectively) [20]. A mid-ventral incision was made, and both ovaries were dissected after each ovary was separated by the ligation of the most proximal portion. The OVX rats were randomly assigned into five groups of 10 each.

L. fermentum JS is an acid and bile salt-resistant lactic acid bacteria [21]. *L. fermentum* JS (KCCM 10499) has been registered as a probiotic for improving intestinal health and immunity [22, 23] in Korea Food & Drug Administration. *L. fermentum* JS KCCM 10499 was routinely grown in Difco MRS broth or agar (BD, NJ, USA) and incubated in shaking incubator (Daihan Science, Wonjoo, Korea) with aerobic condition at 37 °C for 24 h. After incubation, the media was centrifuged at 900×*g* and the precipitates were lyophilized. The freeze-dried powder contained 1×10^8–1×10^{10} CFU *L. fermentum* JS/g.

Diet preparation

High-fat diets were used in the study since they are known to exacerbate the progression of menopausal symptoms compared with a low fat diet [24–26]. Water extracts of cauliflower mushroom and *L. fermentum* JS KCCM 10499 were purchased from Haemaru-Biotech (Cheonan, Korea) and Well-being LS (Gang Reung, Korea), respectively, and were supplemented into high-fat diets. The high-fat diet was a semi-purified modified AIN-93 formulation containing 37 energy percent (En%) from carbohydrates, 20 En% from protein, and 43 En% from fats [27]. The sources of carbohydrate, protein, and fat were starch plus sugar, casein (milk protein), and lard (CJ Co., Seoul, Korea), respectively. CFM included 1% lyophilized water extracts of cauliflower mushroom plus 0.1% casein; LFE contained 0.1% *L. fermentum* (1×10^8–1×10^{10} CFU/g) plus 1% dextrin; CFLF included 1% CFM plus 0.1% LFE; control contained 1% dextrin plus 0.1% casein; or positive-control contained 30 μg/kg body weight 17β-estradiol plus1% dextrin and 0.1% casein. The CFM and LFE powders were homogeneously mixed with the vitamin and mineral mixture and sugar components of the diet. The mixture was sifted to remove the lumps. Each mixture was blended with the appropriate amounts of starch, casein, and lard, sifted again, and stored at 4 °C. The nutrient composition of the diets was the same. The amounts of each supplement consumed were calculated from daily food intake.

Experimental design

Sixty OVX rats were randomly assigned to the following groups: (1) CFM, (2) LFE, (3) CFLF, (4) positive-control (30 μg/kg body weight 17β-estradiol), or (5) OVX-control (dextrin; placebo). The OVX rats had free access to water and their respective diets for 8 weeks. After an overnight-fast, the serum glucose levels, food intake, and body weights were measured every Tuesday at 10 am.

Tail skin temperature

The tail skin temperature was measured during the dark-period every week of the experimental period using an infrared thermometer for small rodents (BIO-152-IRB, Bioseb, Chaville, France) [26]. Three measurements were made 10 min apart each time, and the average value was used as a single data point.

Body composition measurement

At the seventh week of the experimental period, the body composition of the rats was measured in a dual-energy X-ray absorptiometer (DEXA; Norland pDEXA Sabre; Norland Medical Systems Inc., Fort Atkinson, WI, USA) after calibrating it with a phantom supplied by the manufacturer. After anesthetization with ketamine and xylazine (100 and 10 mg/kg bw, respectively), bone mineral density (BMD) and lean body mass were assessed in the leg and hip using the DEXA instrument equipped with the appropriate software for small animals [26]. Fat mass was measured in the leg and abdominal areas using the DEXA equipment.

Energy expenditure analysis by indirect calorimetry

At 2 days after the DEXA analysis, energy expenditure was assessed at the beginning of the dark-phase of the light/dark cycle after removing foods for 6 h. The rats were acclimated into the metabolic chambers (airflow = 800 mL/min) for 30 min, and then the chambers were connected with a computer-controlled O_2 and CO_2 measurement system (BIOPAC Systems, Inc., Goleta, CA). Oxygen consumption (VO_2) and carbon dioxide production (VCO_2) were measured over 1 min intervals and integrated over periods of 30 min. The VO_2 and VCO_2 values were corrected for the animals' metabolic body size ($kg^{0.75}$). The respiratory quotient and resting energy expenditure were calculated using reported equations [20, 26]. Carbohydrate and fat oxidation were calculated from non-protein oxygen consumption according to their relative oxidative proportions. They were reported as the amount of oxygen consumed per gram of substrate oxidized [24, 26].

Glucose homeostasis, lipid profiles, and sample collection at the end of experiment

An oral glucose tolerance test (OGTT) was performed on overnight-fasted animals at the eighth week. Blood samples were taken by tail bleeding at 0, 10, 20, 30, 40, 50, 60, 70, 80, 90, and 120 min after orally giving 2 g of glucose/kg body weight. The serum glucose levels were measured with a Glucose Analyzer II (Beckman, Palo Alto, CA). The serum insulin levels were determined at 0, 20, 40, 90, and 120 min using a radioimmunoassay kit (Linco Research, Billerica, MA). The areas under the curves (AUC) of the first (0–40 min) and second (40–120 min) parts for the serum glucose and insulin levels were calculated using the trapezoidal rule.

Three days after the OGTT, food was removed for 6 h and an intraperitoneal insulin tolerance test (IPITT) was conducted. The serum glucose levels were measured every 15 min for 90 mins after an intraperitoneal injection of insulin (0.75 U/kg body weight). At 2 days after the IPITT, the rats were anesthetized with ketamine and xylazine (100 and 10 mg/kg body weight, respectively) and human insulin (5 U/kg body weight) was injected through the inferior vena cava after collecting blood by abdominal cardiac puncture. The epididymal and retroperitoneal fat mass and uteri were then collected and weighed. The uterus index was calculated as the uterus weight divided by the body weight. Feces in the large intestine were collected from the large intestine of all rats in each group. Feces from two of samples were pooled to make five fece samples of each group. The pooled contents were mixed, and the gut microbiomes were measured. Serum, tissue, and large intestine specimen were stored at − 70 °C for biochemical analysis.

Insulin resistance and insulin secretion capacity were estimated using the homeostasis model assessment estimate (HOMA) of insulin resistance (HOMA-IR) and insulin secretion (HOMA-B). HOMA-IR and HOMA-B were calculated as previously described [26, 28]. Serum 17β-estradiol levels were assessed by ELISA kits (Enzo Life Sciences, NY, USA). The levels of serum tumor necrosis factor (TNF)-α and monocyte chemoattractant protein-1 (MCP-1) were measured with ELISA kits (R & D Systems, Minneapolis, MN). Total cholesterol, HDL cholesterol, and triglycerides levels in the circulation were assessed by using colorimetry kits for (Asan Pharmaceutical, Seoul, Korea). Serum LDL cholesterol was calculated with the Friedewald equation [29].

Gut microbiome

Gut microbiome was measured from five fece samples from each group by Microgen (Seoul, Korea) by analyzing metagenome sequencing using next-generating sequencing. Bacterial DNA was extracted from each sample by Power water DNA Isolation Kit (MoBio, Carlsbad, CA) according to the manufacturer's instructions. Each library was prepared using PCR products according to the GS FLX plus library prep guide. Libraries were quantified using Picogreen assay (Victor 3). The emPCR, corresponding to clonal amplification of the purified library, was carried out using the GS-FLX plus emPCR Kit (454 Life Sciences, Branford, CT). Briefly, libraries were immobilized onto DNA capture beads. The library beads were added to amplification mix and oil, and the mixture was vigorously shaken on a Tissue Lyser II (Qiagen, Valencia, CA) to create "micro-reactors" containing both amplification mix and a single bead. Emulsion was dispensed into a 96-well plate and the PCR amplification program was run according to the manufacturer's recommendations. The 16S universal primers, 27F (5′ GAGTTTGATCMTGGCTCAG 3′) and 518R (5′ WTTACCGCGGCTGCTGG 3′), were used for the amplification of 16 s rRNA genes by PCR. PCR was conducted in the FastStart High Fidelity PCR System (Roche, Basel, Switzerland) under the following conditions: 94 °C for 3 min followed by 35 cycles of 94 °C for 15 s, 55 °C for 45 s and 72 °C for 1 min, and a final elongation step at 72 °C for 8 min. After the PCR procedure, we purified the products using AMPure beads (Beckman coulter, Brea, CA).

Next-generation sequencing using Roche 454 GS-FLX plus

Sequencing was performed by the Macrogen Ltd. (Seoul, Korea). Following PCR amplification, the emulsion was chemically broken and the beads carrying the amplified DNA library were recovered and washed by filtration. Positive beads were purified using the biotinylated primer A (complementary to adaptor A), which binds to streptavidin-coated magnetic beads. The DNA library beads were then separated from the magnetic beads by melting the double-stranded amplification products, leaving a population of bead-bound single-stranded template DNA fragments. The sequencing primer was then annealed to the amplified single-stranded DNA. Lastly, beads carrying amplified single-stranded DNA were counted with a Particle Counter (Beckman Coulter). Sequencing was performed on a Genome Sequencer FLX plus (454 Life Sciences), and each sample was loaded in one region of a 70–75-mm PicoTiter plate (454 Life Sciences) fitted with an eight-lane gasket.

Immunoblot analysis

The liver was lysed with a 20 mM Tris buffer (pH 7.4) containing 2 mM EGTA, 137 mM NaCl, 1% NP40, 10% glycerol, and 12 mM α-glycerol phosphate and protease inhibitors. Lysates containing equal amounts of protein (30–50 μg) were used for immunoblotting with specific antibodies against protein kinase B (PKB/Akt), glycogen synthase (GSK)-3β, AMP kinase (AMPK), phosphoenolpyruvate carboxykinase (PEPCK), and β-actin, and phosphorylated forms of PKB^{ser473}, GSK-3β ^{ser9}, and $AMPK^{the172}$ (Cell Signaling, Danvers, MA), as previously described [24]. The intensity of protein expression was determined using Imagequant TL (Amersham Biosciences, Piscataway, NJ).

Statistical analysis

Statistical analysis was performed using SAS software version 7 (SAS Institute). Sample size was calculated using a G power program (power = 0.90), and sample size of each group was 10. Results were expressed as means ± standard deviation (SD) when the normal distribution was checked using Proc univariate. The variables that were measured over multiple time points were tested with two-way repeated measure ANOVA, with time and group as the independent variables and an interaction term between time and groups. One-way ANOVA was used to determine the metabolic effects of the OVX-control, CFM, LFE, CFLF, and 17β-estradiol (a positive-control) groups at a single time point, when the results were measured once at the end of the experiment. Significant differences in the main effects among the groups were identified by Tukey's test at $p < 0.05$.

Results

β-Glucan contents of CFM and *L. fermentum* in LFE

The β-glucan contents were 33.4 ± 2.2 g/100 g cauliflower mushroom. The water extracts mainly contained β-glucans (about 95.8%). The yield of its water extracts was 28.8% because some β-glucan was lost during the water extraction process. Rats in the CFM group

Table 1 Serum 17β-estradiol levels, uterine index, and skin tail temperature

	Control	CFM	LFE	CFLF	Positive-control
Serum 17β-estradiol levels (pg/mL)	1.6 ± 0.6^{b}	1.9 ± 0.7^{b}	1.7 ± 0.5^{b}	2.0 ± 0.7^{b}	7.3 ± 1.1^{a}
Uterine index	0.49 ± 0.10^{b}	0.52 ± 0.11^{b}	0.50 ± 0.12^{b}	0.56 ± 0.10^{b}	1.80 ± 0.29^{a}
Tail skin temperature (°C)	29.6 ± 0.17^{a}	28.8 ± 0.17^{ab}	29.3 ± 0.15^{a}	28.2 ± 0.14^{b}	27.9 ± 0.15^{b}
Serum TNF-α (pg/mL)	52.1 ± 4.6^{a}	46.2 ± 4.5^{b}	48.5 ± 4.4^{ab}	41.1 ± 4.2^{c}	42.5 ± 4.3^{bc}
Serum MCP-1 (pg/mL)	60.5 ± 6.4^{a}	50.4 ± 5.7^{b}	55.3 ± 5.6^{b}	43.7 ± 4.9^{c}	44.5 ± 4.7^{c}

Values represented means ± standard deviation (n = 10)
Different letters represent a significant difference in Tukey test at $p < 0.05$
CFM 1% water extract of cauliflower mushroom, *LFE* 0.1% *L. fermentum*, *CFLF* 1% water extract of cauliflower mushroom +0.1% *L. fermentum*, *positive-control* 30 μg/kg body weight 17β-estradiol, *TNF-α* tumor necrosis factor-a, *MCP-1* monocyte chemoattractant protein-1

consumed 0.15–0.2 g β-glucan and those in the LFE group had 1–2 × 10^7 CFU on a daily basis. Rats in the CFLF group consumed 0.15–0.2 g β-glucan plus 1–2 × 10^7 *L. fermentum* daily.

Serum 17β-estradiol levels, uterine index, tail skin temperature and inflammation index

Serum 17β-estradiol levels were much lower in the OVX-control group than the positive-control group and the levels were slightly higher in CFLF, but it was not significantly different (Table 1). Uterine index was also much lower in the OVX-control group than the positive-control group, and none of the treatments changed the index. Due to the estrogen deficiency, tail skin temperature was higher in OVX-control group than the positive-control (Table 1). Only CFLF lowered skin temperature.

Serum TNF-α and MCP-1 levels, inflammation indexes, were higher in the control group than the positive-control group. They were lower in both CFM and LFE than the control group, and CFLF synergistically decreased then to similar levels as the positive-control group (Table 1).

Energy metabolism

The OVX-control group had higher body weights than the positive-control group and CFLF prevented its increase in OVX rats (Table 2). As a result, final body weight was greater in the OVX-control group than the positive-control group but CFLF also lowered final body weight but it was not significantly different from the OVX-control or positive-control groups (Table 2). Peri-uterine fat and retroperitoneum fat mass, the visceral fat mass, was much greater in OVX-control group than the positive-control group. CFLF lowered the visceral fat mass to less than the OVX-control, but the visceral fat mass in the CFLF was greater than that in the positive-control group (Table 2). The body weight gain and visceral fat mass are associated with the balance of food intake and energy expenditure. Food intake was not significantly different among any of the groups (Table 2). However, OVX-control rats exhibited a decrease in daily energy expenditure compared to the positive-control and CFLE prevented its decrease in OVX rats. Carbohydrate oxidation as an energy fuel was not significantly different among all the groups. However, fat oxidation was much lower in the OVX-control group than the

Table 2 Body composition and energy metabolism at the end of experimental periods

	Control	CFM	LFE	CFLF	Positive-control
Final weight (g)	416 ± 29^{a}	407 ± 38^{a}	414 ± 42^{a}	395 ± 19^{ab}	373 ± 32^{b}
Weight gain (g)	145 ± 19^{a}	134 ± 30^{ab}	145 ± 22^{a}	123 ± 17^{b}	101 ± 27^{c}
Peri-uterine fat (g)	15.5 ± 2.2^{a}	13.6 ± 1.5^{ab}	16.0 ± 1.9^{a}	12.1 ± 1.7^{b}	9.9 ± 1.8^{c}
Retroperitoneum fat (g)	11.3 ± 1.6^{a}	9.7 ± 1.1^{b}	11.7 ± 1.6^{a}	8.2 ± 0.9^{c}	6.0 ± 0.8^{d}
Visceral fat mass (g)	26.8 ± 3.1^{a}	23.3 ± 2.9^{b}	27.7 ± 2.9^{a}	20.4 ± 2.6^{c}	15.9 ± 2.3^{d}
Food intake (g/day)	13.9 ± 1.7	14.2 ± 1.7	14.5 ± 1.8	14.0 ± 1.3	13.2 ± 1.6
Energy expenditure (kcal/kg$^{0.75}$/day)	89.4 ± 10.2^{b}	94.0 ± 10.7^{b}	88.6 ± 9.6^{b}	105.5 ± 11.5^{a}	110.1 ± 12.7^{a}
Carbohydrate oxidation (mg/kg$^{0.75}$/min)	5.1 ± 0.7	5.3 ± 0.7	5.0 ± 0.7	4.9 ± 0.7	5.3 ± 0.8
Fat oxidation (mg/kg$^{0.75}$/min)	4.4 ± 0.6^{b}	4.7 ± 0.6^{b}	4.4 ± 0.7^{b}	6.3 ± 0.7^{a}	6.4 ± 0.8^{a}

Visceral fat was the sum of epididymal fat pads and inguinal fat. Values represented means ± standard deviation (n = 10)
Different letters represent a significant difference in Tukey test at $p < 0.05$
CFM 1% water extract of cauliflower mushroom, *LFE* 0.1% *L. fermentum*, *CFLF* 1% water extract of cauliflower mushroom +0.1% *L. fermentum*, *positive-control* 30 μg/kg body weight 17β-estradiol

positive-control group and CFLF protected its decrease in OVX rats (Table 2).

Body composition

BMD in the lumber spine and femur was much lower in the OVX-control group than the positive-control group (Fig. 1a). CFLF prevented the decrease in BMD in the lumber spine and femur as much as the positive-control although neither CMF nor LFE prevented it (Fig. 1a). LBM in the hip and leg was also lower in the OVX-control group than the normal-control group, and CFLF exhibited a similar LBM as the positive-control group

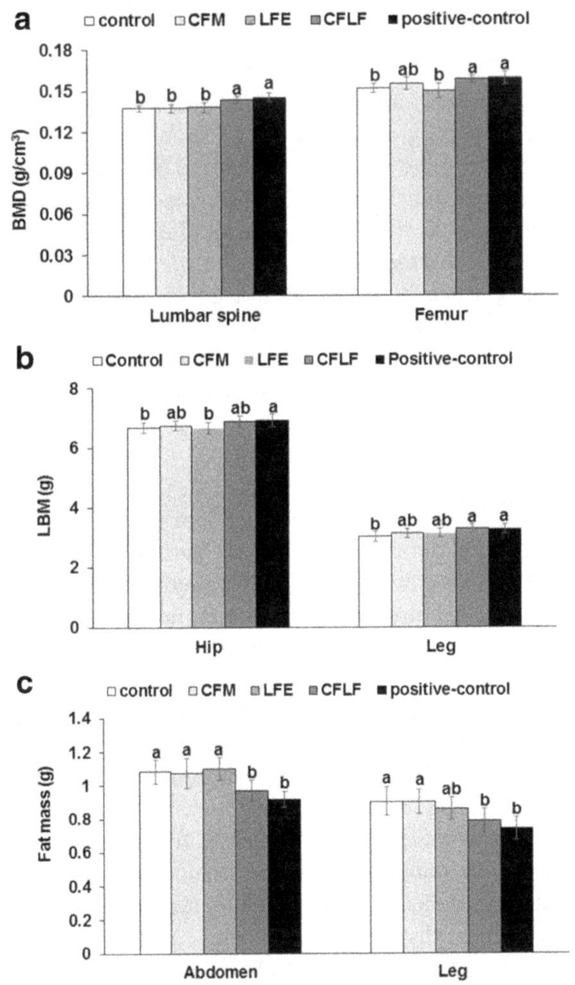

Fig. 1 Body composition including bone mineral density (BMD), lean mass (LM), and fat mass (FM) measured by DEXA. Control, OVX rats fed a high-fat diet (HFD) with 1% dextrin; CFM, OVX rats fed an HFD with 1% lyophilized cauliflower mushroom; LFE, OVX rats fed an HFD with 0.1% *L. fermentum* plus 1% dextrin; CFLF, OVX rats fed an HFD with 1% CFM plus 0.1% *L. fermentum*; positive-control, OVX rats fed an HFD with 1% dextrin plus 30 μg/kg body weight 17β-estradiol. At the end of the experimental period, BMD (**a**) in the lumbar spine and femur and LM (**b**) and FM (**c**) in the abdominal and leg regions were measured by DEXA. Values are expressed as means ± SD ($n = 12$). Different letters represent a significant difference in Tukey test at $p < 0.05$

(Fig. 1b). In contrast to the LBM, fat mass in the abdomen and leg was much higher in the OVX-control group than the positive-control (Fig. 1c). CFLF lowered fat mass in the abdomen and leg as much as the positive-control group.

Lipid metabolism

OVX-control rats exhibited dyslipidemia including elevated serum total cholesterol, LDL cholesterol, and triglyceride concentrations and lower serum HDL cholesterol concentrations in overnight-fasted states in comparison to the normal-control rats (Table 3). CFM prevented the decrease of serum HDL cholesterol and triglyceride concentrations but not total and LDL cholesterol concentrations in the circulation (Table 3). CFLF protected against the development of dyslipidemia in OVX rats, and lipid profiles in the blood were similar to the positive-control group.

Glucose metabolism

Serum glucose concentrations in overnight-fasted states were higher in the OVX-control rats than the normal-control rats, and CFLF lowered it to concentrations as low as the positive-control rats. Serum insulin concentrations were much higher in the OVX-control group than the positive-control group (Table 3). Serum insulin concentrations were lower in the descending order of OVX-control, CFM, positive-control, LFE, and CFLF. Consistent with serum insulin concentrations, HOMA-IR, an index of insulin resistance, was much higher in OVX-control rats than the positive-control. HOMA-IR was lower in CFM and LFE than in OVX-control, and it was lowest in CFLF among all the groups (Table 3).

OVX-control rats had higher serum glucose concentrations that continued to increase until 60 min after glucose challenge, and then slowly decreased in comparison to the positive-control rats, indicating that the OVX-control rats had increased insulin resistance (Fig. 2a). CFM and LFE rats had peak of serum glucose concentrations at about 40 min, and the concentrations at 40 min were similar in the OVX-control (Fig. 2a). However, serum glucose in CFM and LFM quickly decreased after the peak levels in comparison to the OVX-control group. The peak concentrations in the CFLF and positive-control rats were lower than the OVX-control group, and the levels quickly declined Fig. 2a). Since glucose concentration of most rats peaked at 40 min, the AUC of serum glucose levels was divided into two parts at 40 min after glucose loading. The first part of AUC represented the glucose metabolism by insulin secretion capacity and insulin sensitivity at hyperglycemia whereas the second part of AUC was mainly explained by insulin sensitivity (Fig. 2b). Serum insulin concentrations during OGTT were much higher in control rats than in positive-control

Table 3 Glucose and lipid metabolism in overnight-fasted states

	Control	CFM	LFE	CFLF	Positive-control
Total cholesterol (mg/dL)	146.4 ± 16.4[a]	149.1 ± 15.2[a]	147.4 ± 15.2[a]	126.3 ± 13.0[b]	123.2 ± 12.5[b]
HDL cholesterol (mg/dL)	17.7 ± 1.8[c]	24.8 ± 2.6[a]	19.9 ± 2.2[c]	24.1 ± 2.5[a]	20.9 ± 2.2[b]
LDL cholesterol (mg/dL)	106.9 ± 11.0[a]	107.3 ± 12.0[a]	106.1 ± 11.0[a]	84.8 ± 8.8[b]	86.4 ± 9.1[b]
Triglyceride (mg/dL)	108.8 ± 12.2[a]	85.4 ± 8.9[bc]	107.1 ± 12.0[a]	87.1 ± 9.1[b]	79.4 ± 8.3[c]
Serum glucose (mg/dL)	122.2 ± 10.7[a]	115.8 ± 8.4[ab]	116.6 ± 7.7[ab]	113.7 ± 8.6[b]	112.9 ± 9.1[b]
Serum insulin (ng/mL)	2.87 ± 0.42[a]	2.05 ± 0.31[b]	1.81 ± 0.34[c]	1.77 ± 0.26[c]	1.96 ± 0.34[bc]
HOMA-IR	8.4 ± 1.2[a]	5.9 ± 0.9[b]	5.2 ± 0.8[b]	4.5 ± 0.6[c]	5.5 ± 0.7[b]
HOMA-B	367 ± 44[a]	280 ± 40[b]	256 ± 31[b]	227 ± 28[c]	283 ± 32[b]

Values represented means ± standard deviation ($n = 10$)
Different letters represent a significant difference in Tukey test at $p < 0.05$
CFM 1% water extract of cauliflower mushroom, *LFE* 0.1% *L. fermentum*, *CFLF* 1% water extract of cauliflower mushroom +0.1% *L. fermentum*, *positive-control* 30 μg/kg body weight 17β-estradiol

rats whereas the levels were lower in CFM, LFE, and CFLF than the control (Fig. 2c). However, the decrease by the treatments was not as great as the positive-control. The AUC of serum insulin levels was much higher in the control group than in the positive-control group, whereas it was lower in descending order of the control (630 ± 93 ng/mL min), CFM (443 ± 64 ng/mL min), CFLF (344 ± 49 ng/mL min), LFE (316 ± 43 ng/mL min), and positive-control (227 ± 34 ng/mL min).

In IPITT, serum glucose levels markedly decreased until 30–45 min, and then began to rebound from 60 min in all rats after an intraperitoneal injection of insulin (Fig. 3a). After no food for 6 h, serum glucose levels were higher in OVX-control rats than in the positive-control rats and CFLF also lowered the serum glucose levels in OVX rats (Fig 3a). AUC of serum glucose concentrations during the first part and second part was higher in OVX-control group than in positive-control group whereas CFM and CFLF lowered the AUC as much as the positive-control group (Fig. 3b). OVX-control rats had lower insulin sensitivity and 17β-estradiol, but CFM and CFLF improved the insulin sensitivity.

Hepatic insulin signaling

The phosphorylation of Akt and GSK-3β were much lower in the control group than in the positive-control, and it increased in the ascending order of control, CFM, LFE, CFLF, and positive-control (Fig. 4). PEPCK expression was higher in the control than in the positive-control and CFM, LFE and CFLF decreased its expression. The phosphorylation of AMPK was much lower in the control than in the positive-control, and CFM and CFLF prevented the decrease (Fig. 4). The phosphorylation of AMPK was higher in CFLF than in the positive-control.

Gut microbiome

OVX rats exhibited different proportions of taxonomic assignment (Fig. 5). OVX increased the ratio of *Firmicutes* to *Bacteroidetes*, and the changes were reversed in the positive-control group (Table 4). CFM and LFE prevented the increase in the ratio of *Firmicutes* to *Bacteroidetes*, but it was not as much as CFLF. CFLF lowered the ratio to similar values as the positive-control (Table 4). The number of proteobacteria was reduced in the CFM and CFLF groups, compared to the control group, but it was not significantly different between the control and positive-control groups (Table 4). The growth of proteobacteria was not affected by estrogen deficiency, but it was modulated by β-gluten.

Discussion

Gut microbiota has a profound influence on metabolism, immunity, and protection against pathogens. The gut microbiota also influences obesity and BMD [17, 30], and probiotics, prebiotics, and synbiotics may attenuate menopausal symptoms by modulating gut microbiota in estrogen-deficient animals. However, the efficacy of probiotics, prebiotics, and synbiotics for improving gut microbiota still remains controversial. The present study suggested that OVX changes gut microbiota and the changes are associated with menopausal symptoms, but that the synbiotics, CFM and LFE, can prevent many of the gut microbiota changes and menopausal symptoms in estrogen-deficient animals. CFM itself also alleviated the metabolic disturbances of energy, glucose, lipid, and bone metabolism in OVX rats but it was not as much as CFLF. LFE itself had the least effect. Thus, the synbiotics might be effective for alleviating menopausal symptoms.

Cauliflower mushrooms mainly contain six-branched 1,3-β-glucan (about 40% of the mushroom weight) and small amounts of the flavor components including 3-octanone, DL-3-octanol, and 1-octen-3-ol and vitamin D_2 [31]. Oat β-glucans have been mainly known to lower blood glucose and cholesterol levels in animals and humans [32, 33]. However, cauliflower mushroom has been shown to possess anti-bacterial

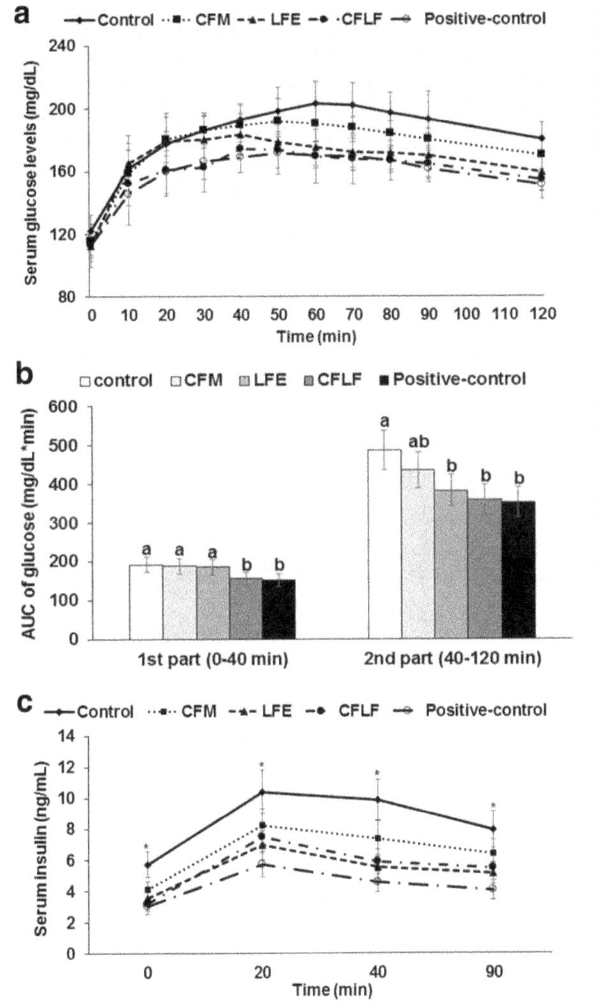

Fig. 2 Serum glucose concentrations and area under the curve of glucose and insulin during oral glucose tolerance test (OGTT). Control, OVX rats fed a high-fat diet (HFD) with 1% dextrin; CFM, OVX rats fed an HFD with 1% lyophilized cauliflower mushroom; LFE, OVX rats fed an HFD with 0.1% *L. fermentum* plus 1% dextrin; CFLF, OVX rats fed an HFD with 1% CFM plus 0.1% *L. fermentum*; positive-control, OVX rats fed an HFD with 1% dextrin plus 30 μg/kg body weight 17β-estradiol. Changes of serum glucose concentration were measured during OGTT (**a**) and the average of the area under the curve (AUC) of glucose during the first part (0–40 min) and second part (40–120 min) of OGTT (**b**) was given. The changes of serum insulin levels were shown (**c**). Each dot and bar represents the mean ± SD ($n = 12$). Asterisk indicates significantly different among the treatments of OVX rats at $p < 0.05$. Different letters represent a significant difference in Tukey test at $p < 0.05$

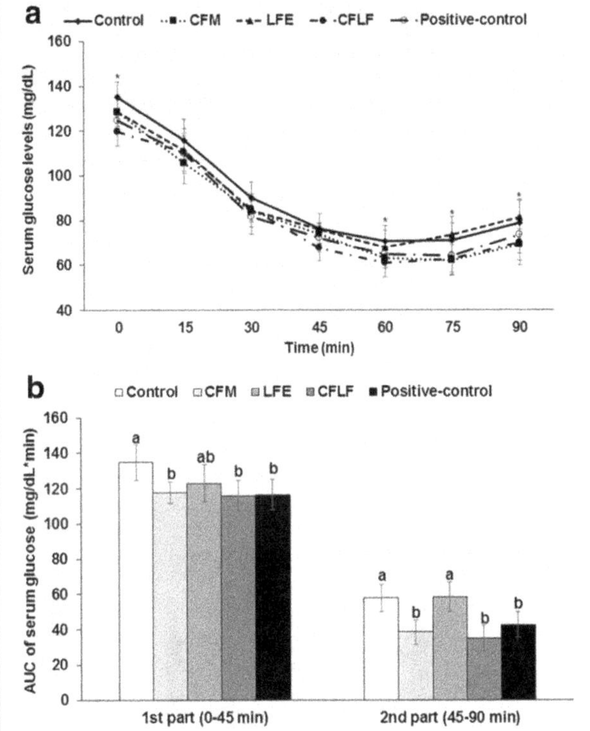

Fig. 3 Changes in serum glucose concentrations during the insulin tolerance test (ITT). Control, OVX rats fed a high-fat diet (HFD) with 1% dextrin; CFM, OVX rats fed an HFD with 1% lyophilized cauliflower mushroom; LFE, OVX rats fed an HFD with 0.1% *L. fermentum* plus 1% dextrin; CFLF, OVX rats fed an HFD with 1% CFM plus 0.1% *L. fermentum*; positive-control, OVX rats fed an HFD with 1% dextrin plus 30 μg/kg body weight 17β-estradiol. ITT was conducted with intraperitoneal injection of 0.75 IU insulin/kg body weight and measured serum glucose concentrations in blood collected from the tail every 15 min for 90 min. Changes of serum glucose concentrations were shown during ITT (**a**). The average of the area under the curve (AUC) of glucose during the first part (0–45 min) and second part (45–90 min) of ITT (**b**) was given. Each dot and bar represents the mean ± SD ($n = 12$). Asterisk indicates significantly different among the treatments of OVX rats at $p < 0.05$. Different letters represent a significant difference in Tukey test at $p < 0.05$

and anti-fungal, anti-inflammatory hypocholesterolemic, and immunomodulatory activities [18, 29, 31]. Thus, β-glucans of different origins might have similar or different activities against metabolic disturbances. β-Glucans in cauliflower mushroom, six-branched 1,3-beta-glucan, are different from β-glucans in oats and barleys. However, no studies have investigated CFM effects on menopausal symptoms. The present study showed some beneficial synbiotic effects of CFM and LFE in an estrogen-deficient animal model.

Probiotics and prebiotics can change gut microbiota, but neither of them consistently changes gut microbiota efficiently and synbiotics, a mixture of probiotics and prebiotics, may be more effective for making beneficial changes to the gut microbiota [34]. Probiotics, prebiotics, and synbiotics have mainly been reported to improve bowel-related diseases such as irritable bowel syndrome and colon cancer [35]. In addition, a "leaky gut" may deliver toxins, antigens, or bacteria into the liver and may play a pathogenic role in liver damage [36]. In this aspect, gut microbiota may play an important role by improving intestinal barriers. Recently, gut microbiota have been associated with obesity and its related diseases such as type 2 diabetes and dyslipidemia.

Lactobacillus species have a common characteristic of producing lactic acid or alcohol from sugars. *Lactobacillus* species have probiotic activities, but different species have

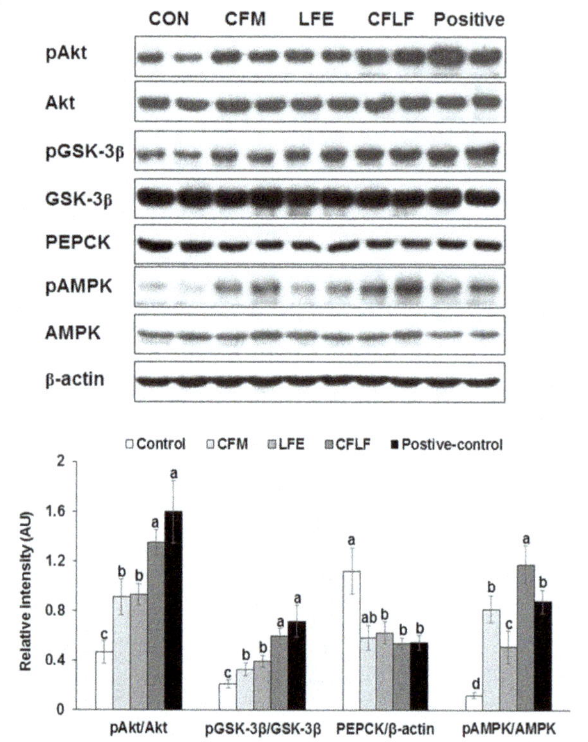

Fig. 4 Hepatic insulin signaling. Control, OVX rats fed a high-fat diet (HFD) with 1% dextrin; CFM, OVX rats fed an HFD with 1% lyophilized cauliflower mushroom; LFE, OVX rats fed an HFD with 0.1% *L. fermentum* plus 1% dextrin; CFLF, OVX rats fed an HFD with 1% CFM plus 0.1% *L. fermentum*; positive-control, OVX rats fed an HFD with 1% dextrin plus 30 μg/kg body weight 17β-estradiol. Hepatic insulin signaling was determined by immunoblotting assays. Each bar represents the mean ± SD ($n = 4$). Different letters represent a significant difference in Tukey test at $p < 0.05$

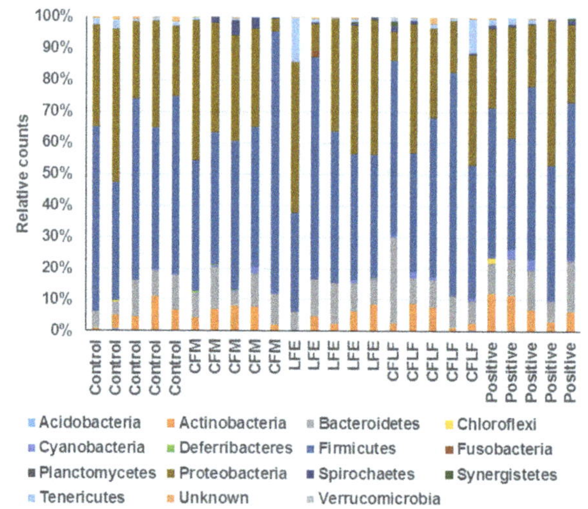

Fig. 5 Proportion of taxonomic assignments [Phylum] for gut microbiomes. Control, OVX rats fed a high-fat diet (HFD) with 1% dextrin; CFM, OVX rats fed an HFD with 1% lyophilized cauliflower mushroom; LFE, OVX rats fed an HFD with 0.1% *L. fermentum* plus 1% dextrin; CFLF, OVX rats fed an HFD with 1% CFM plus 0.1% *L. fermentum*; positive-control, OVX rats fed an HFD with 1% dextrin plus 30 μg/kg body weight 17β-estradiol

specific activities. *L. fermentum* produces lactic acid from sugars, and it is found in sourdough. Since *L. fermentum* tolerates acid environments and 3 g/L of bile salts, it is found to survive in the intestines and it can act as a probiotic, although *L. fermentum* does not use dietary fiber [37]. *L. fermentum* is safe up to a level of 10^{10} CFU/kg body weight/day during 2–4 weeks of treatment in animals, and it has also been shown to be safe in infant formulas in 1–6-month old infants [38, 39]. It enables harmful intestinal bacterial enzymes to be inhibited, decreases pathogenic bacterial populations, and increases beneficial bacterial populations [38]. Interestingly, *L. fermentum* was first isolated from healthy elderly Koreans [40] and it has the strongest binding to intestinal epithelial cells and has potent immune-enhancing, anti-inflammatory, anti-oxidative, and anti-dyslipidemia activities and reverses alcohol-induced liver diseases [14, 41, 42]. These studies suggest that *L. fermentum* is a beneficial probiotic in humans. However, it has not been studied for alleviating menopausal symptoms. Previous studies have demonstrated that *L. reuteri* and *Bifidobacterium longum* increased BMD in OVX rats [30, 43] whereas in the present study, LFE itself did not change BMD, but CFM + LFE elevated BMD to densities as high as the positive-control group. LFE improved glucose tolerance and insulin resistance compared to the control group. In other menopausal symptoms, LFE itself had limited capacity for improving menopausal symptoms in OVX rats, but LFE plus CFM prevented menopausal symptoms as much as 17β-estradiol treatment in the present study. These results suggested that LFE itself did not improve menopausal symptoms as much as CFLF and positive-control groups, but it was associated with the changes of gut microbiota flora. Thus, symbiotic treatment of CFLF may be beneficial for post-menopausal women.

CFM has been reported to have immunomodulatory, anti-tumor, and hypocholesterolemic activities in animals [18, 29, 31], and also β-glucans, the major components of CFM, have hypoglycemic activity [44]. *Bacteroidetes* are well-known bacteria that use dietary fibers as an energy source, and their growth may be increased with CFM [45]. Thus, *Bacteroidetes* can be increased in the intestines when CFM is provided to the animals. CFM may improve the estrogen deficiency-linked disturbances of energy, glucose, lipid, and bone metabolism by modulating gut microbiota. The present study showed that CFM reduced visceral fat mass, serum triglyceride levels, and insulin resistance. CFM partly reduced the ratio of *Firmicutes* and *Bacteroidetes* in comparison to the control group. However, CFLF improved menopausal symptoms much better than CFM. Therefore, CFLF, but not CFM, was sufficient for protecting against menopausal symptoms.

Early studies of the gut microbiomes concentrated on selectively stimulating the growth of a limited number of

Table 4 Gut microbiomes (unit: counts)

	Control	CFM	LFE	CFLF	Positive-control
Actinobacteria	199 ± 31[b]	209 ± 36[b]	142 ± 29[c]	161 ± 28[c]	295 ± 42[a]
Firmicutes	1837 ± 241[a]	1548 ± 224[b]	1427 ± 251[b]	1593 ± 232[b]	1549 ± 236[b]
Proteobacteria	1323 ± 186[a]	960 ± 167[b]	1232 ± 184[a]	928 ± 142[b]	1365 ± 192[a]
Bacteroidetes	268 ± 44[c]	275 ± 36[c]	295 ± 42[c]	368 ± 48[b]	421 ± 51[a]
Cyanobacteria	5.8 ± 1.1[d]	19.4 ± 4.7[c]	7.2 ± 1.7[d]	28.8 ± 6.6[b]	54.6 ± 12.2[a]
Ratio of F/B[1]	6.85 ± 1.01[a]	5.64 ± 0.87[b]	4.84 ± 0.79[bc]	4.33 ± 0.64[c]	3.68 ± 0.61[c]

Values represented means ± standard deviation ($n = 5$)
Different letters represent a significant difference in Tukey test at $p < 0.05$
CFM 1% water extract of cauliflower mushroom, *LFE* 0.1% *L. fermentum*, *CFLF* 1% water extract of cauliflower mushroom +0.1% *L. fermentum*, *positive-control* 30 μg/kg body weight 17β-estradiol
[1]The ratio of Firmicutes and Bacteroidetes

health-promoting bacteria; the application of prebiotics was focused on improving host welfare [10]. However, the applications of synbiotics have recently progressed to the alleviation of metabolic diseases [34]. Some studies have reported that synbiotics have beneficial effects on obesity and metabolic syndrome in human clinical studies [46] and synbiotics are somewhat better than individual effects on conditions such as obesity, ethanol-induced hepatic steatosis, and inflammation-related diseases [34, 47]. The present study also definitively demonstrated that synbiotics had much better efficacy for improving menopausal symptoms than either CFM or LFE alone. CFLF prevented the disturbance of energy, glucose, and lipid metabolism in OVX rats and also it reduced fat mass and increased BMD. In parallel with the alleviation of menopausal symptoms, the gut microbiota in the CFLF group showed similar patterns as the positive-control group: CFLF reduced the ratio of *Firmicutes* and *Bacteroidetes* and increased total counts of bacteria in the gut.

Conclusions

Estrogen deficiency causes menopausal symptoms including higher tail skin temperature, increasing visceral fat mass, dyslipidemia, glucose intolerance, and BMD loss. Additionally, estrogen-deficient rats had higher ratios of *Firmicutes* to *Bacteroidetes* and lower total bacterial counts. CFM containing mainly β-glucans partly prevented the disturbance of glucose and lipid metabolism while potentiating hepatic insulin signaling without changing serum 17β-estradiol levels. Although LFE itself did not protect against the metabolic disturbance caused by estrogen deficiency, CFLF synergistically improved energy, glucose, lipid, and bone metabolism as much as the positive-control group. The improvement of metabolism was associated with the prevention of gut microbiota patterns. Therefore, the synbiotics, CFM and LFE, can be a potential therapeutic agent for menopausal symptoms in post-menopausal women.

Abbreviations

AMPK: AMP kinase; AUCG: Area under the curve of glucose; AUCI: Area under the curve of insulin; BMD: Bone mineral density; CFLF: 1% CFM plus 0.1% LFE; CFM: Cauliflower mushroom plus 0.1% casein; DEXA: Dual-energy X-ray absorptiometer; En%: Energy percent; ER: Estrogen receptor; GSK-3β: Glycogen synthase-3β; HOMA-IR: Homeostasis model assessment estimate of insulin resistance; IL-1β: Interleukin-1β; IPITT: Intraperitoneal insulin tolerance test; LFE: 0.1% *L. fermentum* plus 1% dextrin; MCP-1: Monocyte chemoattractant protein-1; OGTT: Oral glucose tolerance test; OVX: Ovariectomy; PEPCK: Phosphoenol-pyruvate carboxykinase; PKB/Akt: Protein kinase B; TNF-α: Tumor necrosis factor-α; VCO_2: Average carbon dioxide production; VO_2: Average oxygen consumption

Funding

This study was supported by a grant from Traditional Culture Convergence Research Program through the National Research Foundation of Korea(NRF) funded by the Ministry of Science and ICT (NRF- 2016M3C1B5907152) and the Business for Cooperative R&D between Industry, Academy, and Research Institute funded Korea Small and Medium Business Administration.

Authors' contributions

SP and SYJ participated in the experimental design; SK and NRL conducted the animal studies; SYJ performed biochemical studies. SP and SYJ wrote the manuscript. All authors participated in analysis of the data and review of the manuscript. All authors read and approved the final manuscript.

Competing interests

The authors declare that they have no competing interests.

Author details

[1]Department of R&D, Microbial Institute for Fermentation Industry, Sunchang, South Korea. [2]Department of Food & Nutrition, Obesity/Diabetes Center, Hoseo University, 165 Sechul-Ri, BaeBang-Yup, Asan-Si, ChungNam-Do 336-795, South Korea.

References

1. Stevenson JC, Panay N, Pexman-Fieth C. Oral estradiol and dydrogesterone combination therapy in postmenopausal women: review of efficacy and safety. Maturitas. 2013;76:10–21.
2. Patterson E, Ryan PM, Cryan JF, Dinan TG, Ross RP, Fitzgerald GF, et al. Gut microbiota, obesity and diabetes. Postgrad Med J. 2016;92:286–300.
3. Brahe LK, Le Chatelier E, Prifti E, Pons N, Kennedy S, Blaedel T, et al. Dietary modulation of the gut microbiota—a randomized controlled trial in obese postmenopausal women. Br J Nutr. 2015;114:406–17.
4. Markle JG, Frank DN, Mortin-Toth S, Robertson CE, Feazel LM, Rolle-Kampczyk U, et al. Sex differences in the gut microbiome drive hormone-dependent regulation of autoimmunity. Science. 2013;339:1084–8.
5. Plottel CS, Blaser MJ. Microbiome and malignancy. Cell Host Microbe. 2011; 10:324–35.

6. Flores R, Shi J, Fuhrman B, Xu X, Veenstra TD, Gail MH, et al. Fecal microbial determinants of fecal and systemic estrogens and estrogen metabolites: a cross-sectional study. J Transl Med. 2012;10:253.
7. Menon R, Watson SE, Thomas LN, Allred CD, Dabney A, Azcarate-Peril MA, et al. Diet complexity and estrogen receptor beta status affect the composition of the murine intestinal microbiota. Appl Environ Microbiol. 2013;79:5763–73.
8. Cox-York KA, Sheflin AM, Foster MT, Gentile CL, Kahl A, Koch LG, et al. Ovariectomy results in differential shifts in gut microbiota in low versus high aerobic capacity rats. Physiol Rep. 2015;3:e12488–502.
9. Guadamuro L, Delgado S, Redruello B, Florez AB, Suarez A, Martinez-Camblor P, et al. Equol status and changes in fecal microbiota in menopausal women receiving long-term treatment for menopause symptoms with a soy-isoflavone concentrate. Front Microbiol. 2015;6:777–87.
10. Gibson GR, Roberfroid MB. Dietary modulation of the human colonic microbiota: introducing the concept of prebiotics. J Nutr. 1995;125:1401–12.
11. Reid G, Jass J, Sebulsky MT, McCormick JK. Potential uses of probiotics in clinical practice. Clin Microbiol Rev. 2003;16:658–72.
12. Swain MR, Anandharaj M, Ray RC, Parveen RR. Fermented fruits and vegetables of Asia: a potential source of probiotics. Biotechnol Res Int. 2014; 2014:250424–35.
13. Russo M, Fabersani E, Abeijon-Mukdsi MC, Ross R, Fontana C, Benitez-Paez A, et al. *Lactobacillus fermentum* CRL1446 ameliorates oxidative and metabolic parameters by increasing intestinal feruloyl esterase activity and modulating microbiota in caloric-restricted mice. Nutrients. 2016;8:415–29
14. Tomaro-Duchesneau C, Saha S, Malhotra M, Jones ML, Rodes L, Prakash S. *Lactobacillus fermentum* NCIMB 5221 and NCIMB 2797 as cholesterol-lowering probiotic biotherapeutics: in vitro analysis. Benef Microbes. 2015;6:861–9.
15. Gibson GR. Dietary modulation of the human gut microflora using the prebiotics oligofructose and inulin. J Nutr. 1999;129:1438s–41s.
16. Goetze O, Fruehauf H, Pohl D, Giarre M, Rochat F, Ornstein K, et al. Effect of a prebiotic mixture on intestinal comfort and general wellbeing in health. Br J Nutr. 2008;100:1077–85.
17. Vitali B, Ndagijimana M, Cruciani F, Carnevali P, Candela M, Guerzoni ME, et al. Impact of a synbiotic food on the gut microbial ecology and metabolic profiles. BMC Microbiol. 2010;10:4–14.
18. Hida TH, Kawaminami H, Ishibashi K, Miura NN, Adachi Y, Ohno N. Oral administration of soluble beta-glucan preparation from the cauliflower mushroom, *Sparassis crispa* (Higher Basidiomycetes) modulated cytokine production in mice. Int J Med Mushrooms. 2013;15:525–38.
19. Ferrario C, Statello R, Carnevali L, Mancabelli L, Milani C, Mangifesta M, et al. How to feed the mammalian gut microbiota: bacterial and metabolic modulation by dietary fibers. Front Microbiol. 2017;8:1749.
20. Ko BS, Lee HW, Kim DS, Kang S, Ryuk JA, Park S. Supplementing with *Opuntia ficus-indica* Mill and *Dioscorea nipponica* Makino extracts synergistically attenuates menopausal symptoms in estrogen-deficient rats. J Ethnopharmacol. 2014;155:267–76.
21. Choi JS. Acid-resistant microorganism *Lactobacillus fermentum* JS, and composition containing the same microorganism. KR100435168B1. 2003.
22. Bai SP, AM W, Ding XM, Lei Y, Bai J, Zhang KY, et al. Effects of probiotic-supplemented diets on growth performance and intestinal immune characteristics of broiler chickens. Poult Sci. 2013;92:663–70.
23. Lee DS. Compositions containing green tea and lactic-acid bacteria. KR20070056153A. 2009.
24. Kim MJ, Park JH, Kwon DY, Yang HJ, Kim DS, Kang S, et al. The supplementation of Korean mistletoe water extracts reduces hot flushes, dyslipidemia, hepatic steatosis, and muscle loss in ovariectomized rats. Exp Biol Med. 2015;240:477–87.
25. Litwak SA, Wilson JL, Chen W, Garcia-Rudaz C, Khaksari M, Cowley MA, et al. Estradiol prevents fat accumulation and overcomes leptin resistance in female high-fat diet mice. Endocrinology. 2014;155:4447–60.
26. Park S, Kang S, Jeong DY, Jeong SY, Park JJ, Yun HS. Cyanidin and malvidin in aqueous extracts of black carrots fermented with Aspergillus oryzae prevent the impairment of energy, lipid and glucose metabolism in estrogen-deficient rats by AMPK activation. Genes Nutr. 2015;10:455–69.
27. Reeves PG, Nielsen FH, Fahey GC Jr. AIN-93 purified diets for laboratory rodents: final report of the American Institute of Nutrition ad hoc writing committee on the reformulation of the AIN-76A rodent diet. J Nutr. 1993; 123:1939–51.
28. Hermans MP, Ahn SA, Mahadeb YP, Rousseau MF. Sleep apnoea syndrome and 10-year cardiovascular risk in females with type 2 diabetes: relationship with insulin secretion and insulin resistance. Diabetes Metab Res Rev. 2013; 29:227–34.
29. Hong KB, Hong SY, Joung EY, Kim BH, Bae SH, Park Y, et al. Hypocholesterolemic effects of the cauliflower culinary-medicinal mushroom, *Sparassis crispa* (higher Basidiomycetes), in diet-induced hypercholesterolemic rats. Int J Med Mushrooms. 2015;17:965–75.
30. Britton RA, Irwin R, Quach D, Schaefer L, Zhang J, Lee T, et al. Probiotic L. reuteri treatment prevents bone loss in a menopausal ovariectomized mouse model. J Cell Physiol. 2014;229:1822–30.
31. Kimura T. Natural products and biological activity of the pharmacologically active cauliflower mushroom *Sparassis crispa*. Biomed Res Int. 2013;2013: 982317–26.
32. Charlton KE, Tapsell LC, Batterham MJ, O'Shea J, Thorne R, Beck E, et al. Effect of 6 weeks' consumption of beta-glucan-rich oat products on cholesterol levels in mildly hypercholesterolaemic overweight adults. Brit J Nutr. 2012;107:1037–47.
33. Wang Q, Ellis PR. Oat beta-glucan: physico-chemical characteristics in relation to its blood-glucose and cholesterol-lowering properties. Brit J Nutr. 2014;112(Suppl 2):S4–s13.
34. Kolida S, Gibson GR. Synbiotics in health and disease. Annu Rev Food Sci Technol. 2011;2:373–93.
35. Wasilewski A, Zielinska M, Storr M, Fichna J. Beneficial effects of probiotics, prebiotics, synbiotics, and psychobiotics in inflammatory bowel disease. Inflamm Bowel Dis. 2015;21:1674–82.
36. Fukui H. Gut-liver axis in liver cirrhosis: how to manage leaky gut and endotoxemia. World J Hepatol. 2015;7:425–42.
37. Pan DD, Zeng XQ, Yan YT. Characterisation of *Lactobacillus fermentum* SM-7 isolated from koumiss, a potential probiotic bacterium with cholesterol-lowering effects. J Sci Food Agric. 2011;91:512–8.
38. Shokryazdan P, Faseleh Jahromi M, Liang JB, Kalavathy R, Sieo CC, Ho YW. Safety assessment of two new *Lactobacillus* strains as probiotic for human using a rat model. PLoS One. 2016;11:e0159851–60.
39. Maldonado-Lobon JA, Gil-Campos M, Maldonado J, Lopez-Huertas E, Flores-Rojas K, Valero AD, et al. Long-term safety of early consumption of *Lactobacillus fermentum* CECT5716: a 3-year follow-up of a randomized controlled trial. Pharmacol Res. 2015;95-96:12–9.
40. Park JS, Shin E, Hong H, Shin HJ, Cho YH, Ahn KH, et al. Characterization of *Lactobacillus fermentum* PL9988 isolated from healthy elderly Korean in a longevity village. J Microbiol Biotechnol. 2015;25:1510–8.
41. Archer AC, Muthukumar SP, Halami PM. Anti-inflammatory potential of probiotic *Lactobacillus* spp. on carrageenan induced paw edema in Wistar rats. Int J Biol Macromol. 2015;81:530–7.
42. Barone R, Rappa F, Macaluso F, Caruso Bavisotto C, Sangiorgi C, Di Paola G, et al. Alcoholic liver disease: a mouse model reveals protection by *Lactobacillus fermentum*. Clin Transl Gastroenterol. 2016;7:e138–51.
43. Parvaneh K, Ebrahimi M, Sabran MR, Karimi G, Hwei AN, Abdul-Majeed S, et al. Probiotics (Bifidobacterium longum) increase bone mass density and upregulate SPARC and BMP-2 genes in rats with bone loss resulting from ovariectomy. Biomed Res Int. 2015;2015:897639-48.
44. Shen XL, Zhao T, Zhou Y, Shi X, Zou Y, Zhao G. Effect of oat beta-glucan intake on glycaemic control and insulin sensitivity of diabetic patients: a meta-analysis of randomized controlled trials. Nutrients. 2016;8:39–49.
45. Reeves AR, Wang GR, Salyers AA. Characterization of four outer membrane proteins that play a role in utilization of starch by *Bacteroides thetaiotaomicron*. J Bacteriol. 1997;179:643–9.
46. Saez-Lara MJ, Robles-Sanchez C, Ruiz-Ojeda FJ, Plaza-Diaz J, Gil A. Effects of probiotics and synbiotics on obesity, insulin resistance syndrome, type 2 diabetes and non-alcoholic fatty liver disease: a review of human clinical trials. Int J Mol Sci. 2016;17:928–43.
47. Chiu WC, Huang YL, Chen YL, Peng HC, Liao WH, Chuang HL, et al. Synbiotics reduce ethanol-induced hepatic steatosis and inflammation by improving intestinal permeability and microbiota in rats. Food Funct. 2015;6:1692–700.

13

Circulating microRNAs are deregulated in overweight/obese children

Giuseppe Iacomino[1*], Paola Russo[1], Ilaria Stillitano[1], Fabio Lauria[1], Pasquale Marena[1], Wolfgang Ahrens[2,3], Pasquale De Luca[4] and Alfonso Siani[1]

Abstract

Background: MicroRNAs (miRNAs) are small non-coding RNAs involved in the modulation of gene expression and in the control of numerous cell functions. Alterations of miRNA patterns frequently occur in cancer and metabolic disorders, including obesity. Recent studies showed remarkable stability of miRNAs in both plasma and serum making them suitable as potential circulating biomarkers for a variety of diseases and conditions.
The aim of this study was to assess the profile of circulating miRNAs expressed in plasma samples of overweight or obese (OW/Ob) and normal weight (NW) prepubertal children from a European cohort (www.ifamilystudy.eu). The project, aimed to assess the determinants of eating behavior in children and adolescents of eight European countries, is built on the IDEFICS cohort (www.ideficsstudy.eu), established in 2006. Among the participants of the I.Family Italian Cohort, ten OW/Ob (age 10.7 ± 1.5 years, BMI 31.6 ± 4.3 kg/m^2) and ten NW (age 10.5 ± 2.7 years, BMI 16.4 ± 1.7 kg/m^2) children were selected for the study. Gene arrays were employed to differentially screen the expression of 372 miRNAs in pooled plasma samples. Deregulated miRNAs ($p < 0.05$) were further validated in the individual samples using a real-time PCR (RT-qPCR) approach.

Results: Using a significance threshold of $p < 0.05$ and a fold-change threshold of ± 4.0, we preliminarily identified in the pooled samples eight miRNAs that differed between the OW/Ob and NW groups. The validation by RT-qPCR in the individual plasma samples showed a twofold upregulation of miR-31-5p, a threefold upregulation of miR-2355-5p, and a 0.5-fold downregulation of miR-206 in OW/Ob as compared with NW. The molecular functions of these differentially expressed plasma miRNAs as well as their expected mRNA targets were predicted by bioinformatics tools.

Conclusions: This pilot study shows that three circulating miRNAs are differentially regulated in OW/Ob as compared with NW children. Although causal pathways cannot be firmly inferred by these results, that deserve confirmation in larger samples, it is conceivable that circulating miRNAs may be novel biomarkers of obesity and related metabolic disturbances.

Keywords: Circulating miRNAs, Childhood obesity, Metabolic disorders, Biomarker

Background

The obesity epidemic represents a major health challenge worldwide since it is associated with severe adverse consequences for human health [1–3]. Excess energy intake and lack of physical activity are the main factors that drive the development of obesity. Individual traits, such as the genetic profile, likewise contribute to obesity. A quantity of studies has found a number of genes associated with obesity and obesity-related phenotypes [4–6].

Adipose tissue, the storage site of triglycerides, acts as an endocrine organ contributing to regulate energy homeostasis [7, 8]. Anomalous fat accumulation in obesity increases the risk of severe diseases such as metabolic syndrome, type 2 diabetes, atherosclerosis, and cancer [9]. Evidence suggests that in obesity, adipose tissues stay in a state of subclinical chronic inflammation [10]

* Correspondence: piacomino@isa.cnr.it
[1]Institute of Food Sciences, CNR, Via Roma, 64, 83100 Avellino, Italy
Full list of author information is available at the end of the article

mainly prompted by the massive recruitment of macrophages into adipose tissues [11]. Adipogenesis is tightly controlled by a mixture regulatory signals including endocellular transcription factors and circulating hormones [12]. Additional regulators of adipogenesis also include microRNAs (miRNAs) [13–17]. These small non-coding RNAs, which have a length of only 20–24 nucleotides, are involved in the modulation of gene expression and, consequently, in the control of numerous cell functions [18–20]. At present, more than 2.000 different miRNAs have been described in humans and their number is still increasing (miRBase) (http://www.mirbase.org). miRNAs are important elements of the cell epigenetic machinery that, opposing to the other known players of epigenetic regulation (DNA methylation and post-translational histone modifications), can affect gene expression by binding to the 3′ untranslated sequence of a target messenger RNA (mRNA) [21]. Each miRNA can target many transcripts, and transcription levels of a gene may be regulated by multiple miRNAs [21, 22]. Computational and experimental analyses indicate that endogenous miRNAs regulate the expression of up to 30 % of mouse and human genes [23]. miRNAs have been shown to be involved in fundamental cellular processes including proliferation, differentiation, DNA repair, apoptosis, and metabolism [24, 25].

As a consequence, remarkable evidence indicates that dysregulation of miRNAs is causative and/or indicator of a number of disease processes including cancer [26]. Altered circulating miRNA profiles have been linked to numerous cardiometabolic diseases, including hypertension (let-7e), type 2 diabetes (miR-126), hepatic injury (miR-122), and atherosclerosis (miR-223) [14].

The presence of extracellular circulating miRNAs in blood and other biological fluids is well established [27, 28], but the reason for the nuclease resistance of miRNAs outside the cell remained unclear for a long period [29]. The discovery that cell-free miRNAs are detectable in serum and plasma and that their expression varies as a result of disease offers great potential for the discovery of novel health/disease biomarkers and candidate therapeutic targets [30].

Various miRNAs have been recognized to play a role in adipogenesis [31]. Preliminary evidence showed that some circulating miRNAs are associated with obesity and related metabolic disturbances in adults as well as in children (see [16, 32] for review).

The primary aim of our study was to identify circulating miRNAs potentially associated to early obesity via an integrated study comprising miRNA signatures and bioinformatic analyses in children participating to the I.Family survey. Here, we present the results of a pilot study on a relatively small sample of children belonging to the Italian cohort of the I.Family survey.

Results and discussion

Distinct miRNA expression in plasma of OW/Ob and NW children

The present study was aimed to identify new insights into the pathogenesis of childhood obesity according to the experimental scheme reported in Fig. 1. The main characteristics of the participants are described in Table 1. As time saving and efficiency strategy, samples from ten overweight or obese (OW/Ob) and ten normal weight (NW) were analyzed as pools in triplicate by PCR arrays.

The geometric mean Ct value of multiple selected housekeeping genes was 26.13 for NW and 26.38 for OW/Ob. Reverse transcription control average C_t (RTC) was 20.68 for NW and 20.75 for OW/Ob. Absent calls were 1.82 % for NW and 2.34 % for OW/Ob.

Using a significance threshold of $p < 0.05$ and a fold-change threshold of ±4.0, we identified in the pooled samples eight out of 372 total screened miRNAs that differed between the OW/Ob and NW groups (Table 2). A scatter plot (Fig. 2) shows the relative expression levels of miRNAs in OW/Ob vs. NW pooled plasma samples.

The eight miRNAs found to be differentially expressed in the pooled analysis were subsequently validated in real-time PCR (RT-qPCR) as distinct assays performed in triplicate in the 20 individual plasma samples. PCR reference gene included the endogenous spike-in *C.el*-miR-39-3p. As reported in Table 3, the differential expression of three miRNAs was statistically confirmed (*p* value <0.05): a twofold upregulation of miR-31-5p, a threefold upregulation of miR-2355-5p, and a 0.5-fold downregulation of miR-206 were observed in OW/Ob as compared with NW.

miRNAs target prediction, KEGG pathway analysis

The specialized algorithm miRPath v2.0 [33] was used to understand the molecular functions of deregulated miRNAs and to predict their putative mRNA targets. To recognize biologically relevant molecular networks and pathways, we further explored miRNA targets by analyzing molecular interactions on the comprehensive knowledge base including the Kyoto Encyclopedia of Genes and Genomes (KEGG) [34] and Ingenuity Pathways Analysis. Both IPA and KEGG technologies provided hints for the functions of miRNAs.

Top pathways predicted to be actively regulated by miRNAs were classified according to the KEGG functional annotation (Table 4).

Results of mir-31-5p MiRPath analysis on experimentally validated miRNA interactions (derived from DIANA-TarBase v6.0) or predicted targets (provided by the DIANA-microT-CDS algorithm) are reported in Table 5.

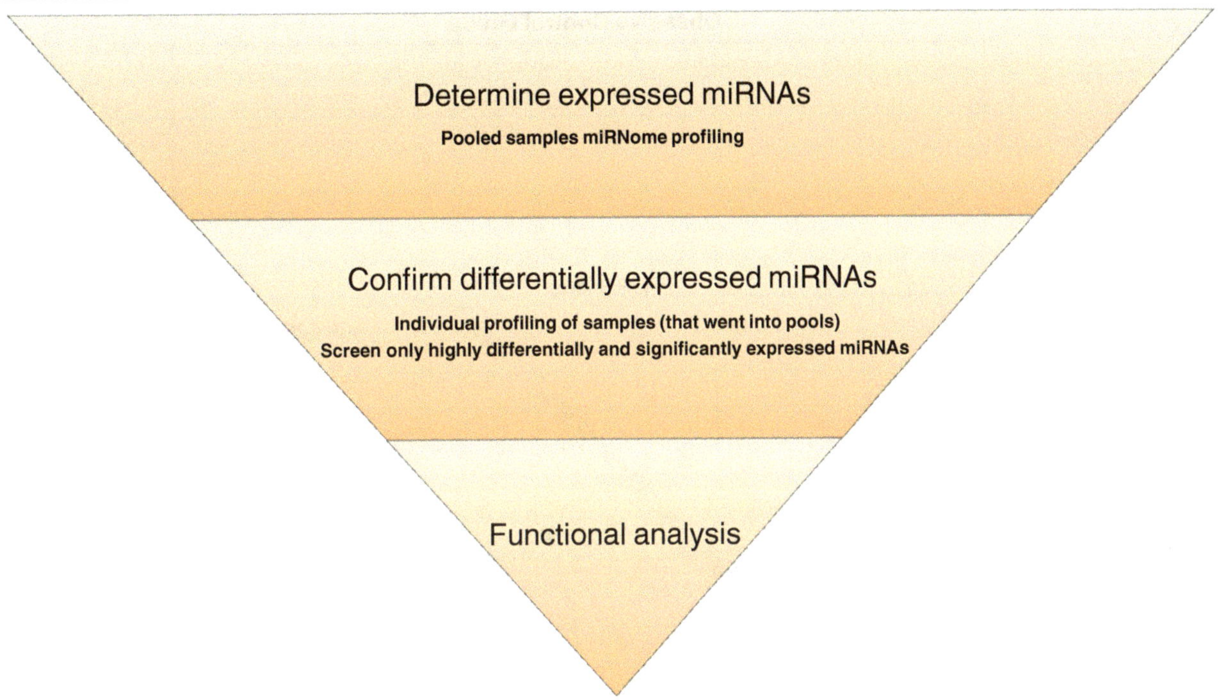

Fig. 1 Experimental scheme

Computational prediction of miR-31 identified the following targets in the "fatty acid degradation" pathway: (a) the enoyl-CoA hydratase, a key enzyme in the breakdown of fatty acids essential to metabolizing fatty acids to produce both acetyl CoA and energy, and (b) the alcohol dehydrogenase 1A (Additional file 1: Figure S1).

Among the top predicted targets of miR-31-5p, we also identify the CCAAT-enhancer-binding protein-α (C/EBPα), a main modulator of the expression of genes involved in cell cycle regulation as well as adipocyte functions during adipogenesis (Fig. 2).

As relevant miR-206 targets, we recognized the "insulin signaling," the "pentose phosphate" pathways, and the liver X receptor-α (LXRα), a ligand-dependent transcription factor playing a relevant role in the metabolism and homeostasis of lipids, cholesterol, bile acids, and steroid hormones with a preeminent expression in the liver.

Further, we identified the oleoyl-ACP hydrolase, a medium-chain acyl-[acyl-carrier-protein] hydrolase in the "fatty acid biosynthesis" pathway as a target of miR-2355 ($p = 0.005$).

Finally, the target prediction of concurrently deregulated miRNAs gave evidence for the "Notch" signaling ($p = 0.0008$) (Additional file 2: Figure S2) and the

Table 1 Anthropometric and metabolic variables of the individuals included in this study

	Normal weight	Overweight/Obese	*p*
Sex (M/F)	5/5	6/4	
Age (years)	10.50 ± 2.76	10.70 ± 1.57	n.s
BMI (kg/cm^2)	16.45 ± 1.71	31.68 ± 4.32	<0.001
Trg (mg/dL)	53.80 ± 22.08	84.20 ± 30.01	0.02
TC (mg/dL)	146.80 ± 24.10	163.40 ± 33.87	n.s
HDL (mg/dL)	62.30 ± 12.33	52.10 ± 12.37	n.s
LDL (mg/dL)	77.60 ± 22.51	100.70 ± 30.57	n.s
Glu (mg/dL)	91 ± 6.16	94.6 ± 3.53	n.s

Value are mean ± standard deviation
n.s = not significant

Table 2 Differential miRNA expression profile determined by gene-arrays screening

miRNA	Fold regulation	
miR-26b-5p	25.3723	↑
miR-31-5p	4.9499	↑
miR-2355-5p	6.5216	↑
miR-1231	−8.7217	↓
miR-361-3p	−4.8918	↓
miR-136-5p	−4.8356	↓
miR-320a	−9.9692	↓
miR-206	−6.0515	↓

miRNAs showing significant differences in expression levels between the compared groups are reported. Analyses were generated setting the threshold at ±4 and *p* value <0.05
up arrow = upregulated; down arrow = downregulated

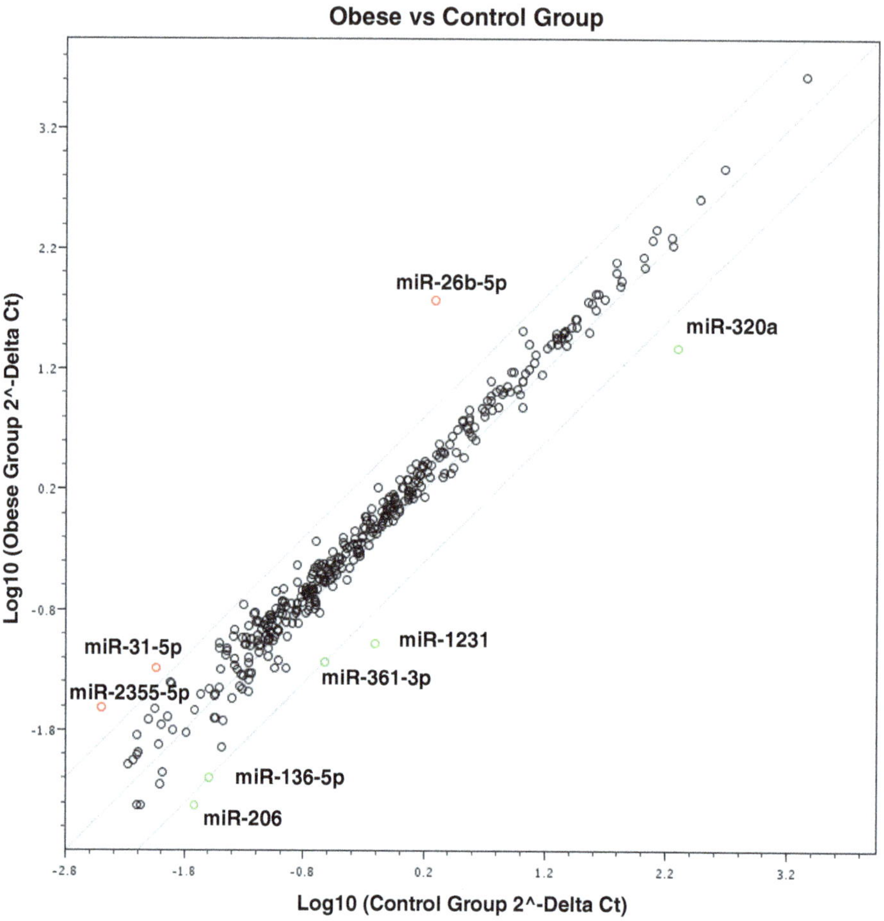

Fig. 2 Differential expression of circulating miRNAs in plasma. Comparisons of OW/Ob vs. NW circulating miRNA profiles. The expression levels were queried by qPCR arrays. Means of each data point are presented as a scatter plot ($n = 3$ in each group). Selection threshold is ±4.0. Upregulated miRNAs are marked *red* whereas downregulated miRNAs are marked *green*

"Arrhythmogenic right ventricular cardiomyopathy" pathways ($p = 2.905898 \times 10^{-05}$) (Additional file 3: Figure S3).

Discussion

We identified three circulating miRNAs differentially expressed in plasma samples of OW/Ob children. Bioinformatic exploratory analysis predicted their involvement in critical pathways including lipid metabolism and adipocyte differentiation.

Table 3 Differential miRNA profile confirmed by RT-qPCR

miRNA	OW/Ob	NW	Fold regulation	*p*	
miR-31-5p	3.60 (3.42–3.97)	1.86 (0.47–2.40)	1.92	0.0003	↑
miR-2355-5p	3.65 (2.52–5.35)	1.23 (0.21–1.78)	2.93	0.0166	↑
miR-206	1.28 (0.63–1.83)	2.45 (1.29–4.92)	0.52	0.0461	↓

Differential miRNAs were confirmed by RT-qPCR. Reported values are mean (minimum-maximum). Fold regulation was expressed as fold change with respect to non-obese controls. Reference included the endogenous spike-in *C.el*-miR-39-3p
up arrow = upregulated; down arrow = downregulated

Table 4 MiRPath analysis

KEGG pathway	*p* value
Gap junction	1.13E-13
Arrhythmogenic right ventricular cardiomyopathy (ARVC)	2.90E-05
Notch signaling pathway	0.0003
Regulation of actin cytoskeleton	0.0005
Dorso-ventral axis formation	0.0008
Bacterial invasion of epithelial cells	0.0009
Axon guidance	0.0026
Shigellosis	0.0200
Endocrine and other factor-regulated calcium reabsorption	0.0397
Glycosaminoglycan biosynthesis—heparan sulfate/heparin	0.0483
Pathways in cancer	0.0490
Thyroid cancer	0.0500

Target genes were classified according to KEGG functional annotations to identify top pathways that were actively regulated by miRNAs. Merged *p* value is extracted by combining calculated significance levels using Fisher's meta-analysis method

Table 5 miRPath analysis of Hsa-mir-31-5p interactions

(A) KEGG-predicted pathway derived from DIANA-microT-CDS database	*p* value	genes
Metabolism of xenobiotics by cytochrome P450	1.46E-07	3
Inositol phosphate metabolism	0.00442	4
Fatty acid metabolism	0.02773	2
(B) KEGG-predicted targets provided by the DIANA-TarBase v6.0 database	*p* value	genes
Regulation of actin cytoskeleton	6.24E-06	5
Bacterial invasion of epithelial cells	1.79E-05	3
Axon guidance	8.85E-05	3
Shigellosis	0.00062	2
Pathogenic *Escherichia coli* infection	0.00276	2
Chemokine signaling pathway	0.00653	3
Pertussis	0.00746	2
Hypertrophic cardiomyopathy (HCM)	0.00979	2
Dilated cardiomyopathy	0.01157	2
T cell receptor signaling pathway	0.01604	2
Leukocyte transendothelial migration	0.01604	2
Arrhythmogenic right ventricular cardiomyopathy (ARVC)	0.01604	2
Dorso-ventral axis formation	0.03214	1

miRPath analysis of miR-31-5p (A) of predicted targets provided by the DIANA-microT-CDS algorithm or (B) of experimentally validated miRNA interactions derived from the DIANA-TarBase v6.0. Target pathways were classified according to KEGG functional annotations

Adipose tissue is involved in pathophysiological processes because it influences metabolism. In adipogenesis, pluripotent adipose-derived mesenchymal stem cells differentiate into adipocytes. This process is finely regulated by both hormones and transcription factors in a complex signaling network. A number of miRNAs and their targets were recently identified to play regulatory roles in adipocyte differentiation [35–37]. To date, up to 221 miRNAs have been found to be expressed or dysregulated in adipose tissue or adipocytes in mammals [16].

Differentiation from pre-adipocytes into mature adipocytes is orchestrated by several transcription factors such as peroxisome proliferator-activated receptor-γ (PPARγ) and C/EBPs (C/EBPs). C/EBPβ and C/EBPδ are induced by adipogenic stimuli and represent primary regulators of adipogenesis. Targets of C/EBPβ and C/EBPδ are the promoters of the genes encoding crucial adipogenic factors as C/EBPα and PPARγ as well as the sterol regulatory element-binding protein (SREBP1), the key regulator of lipogenic genes. The protein encoded by the C/EBPα intronless gene is a leucine zipper transcription factor which can bind to specific promoters and enhancers as a homodimer or it can form heterodimers with the related proteins C/EBPβ and C/EBPγ (Fig. 3). The C/EBPα has been shown to bind to the promoter and to also modify the expression of the leptin gene that plays a central role in body weight homeostasis. C/EBPα is sufficient to trigger differentiation of pre-adipocytes into mature adipocytes [38]. Peculiarly, PPARγ directly triggers endogenous C/EBPα transcription. In turn, C/EBPα activates the PPARγ gene through a positive feedback loop and thereby promotes adipogenesis [12]. Concurrently, PPARγ and C/EBPα induce the expression of genes that are involved in insulin sensitivity, lipogenesis, and lipolysis and, ultimately, in terminal differentiation and mature functions of adipocytes.

miR-31 directly targets C/EBPα transcript whose levels are in vivo downregulated by miR-31 [37]. Notably, miR-31 expression is inversely correlated with adipogenic differentiation status [39], and consequently, it has a decisive anti-adipogenic function.

We found that miR-31 was significantly upregulated in plasma of OW/Ob children identifying C/EBPα as a privileged target of miR-31. miR-31 upregulation may be considered as an apparent contradiction, but it probably reflects the well-established role of circulating miRNAs as "endocrine signals." The concept that miRNAs may be transferred from donor to recipient cells is now well established with the relevant implication that miRNAs could affect gene expression distally, so acting as paracrine or endocrine signaling molecules. Accordingly, a panel of "endocrine miRNAs" released from fat cells that may be used as a marker of disturbed adipose tissue function has been characterized [16]. The idea that miR-31 acts as an obesity controlling signal seems to be supported by the literature. Actually, in analyzing the expression of miRNAs in the livers of leptin-deficient obese (ob/ob) mice compared to normal C57BL/6 mice, Li et al. found that ob/ob mice exhibited an upregulation of miR-31 [40], despite its well-established anti-adipogenic role.

Computational prediction of miR-31 recognized several targets in the "fatty acid degradation" pathway ($p = 0.027$) (Additional file 1: Figure S1). Whether miR-31 deregulation plays a causative role or is merely an epiphenomenon in the etiology of obesity still remains to be determined.

In this study, we also observed that miR-206 was significantly downregulated in plasma of OW/Ob children. miR-206 belongs to the cluster of the so-called myomiRs and represents one of the most studied tissue-specific miRNAs involved in skeletal muscle differentiation. Several studies indicate that miR-206 plays a key role in the growth and development of skeletal muscle, promoting myogenic differentiation [41]. Moreover, it has been well established that it is related to the pathogenesis of numerous diseases including heart failure, chronic obstructive pulmonary disease, and Alzheimer's disease

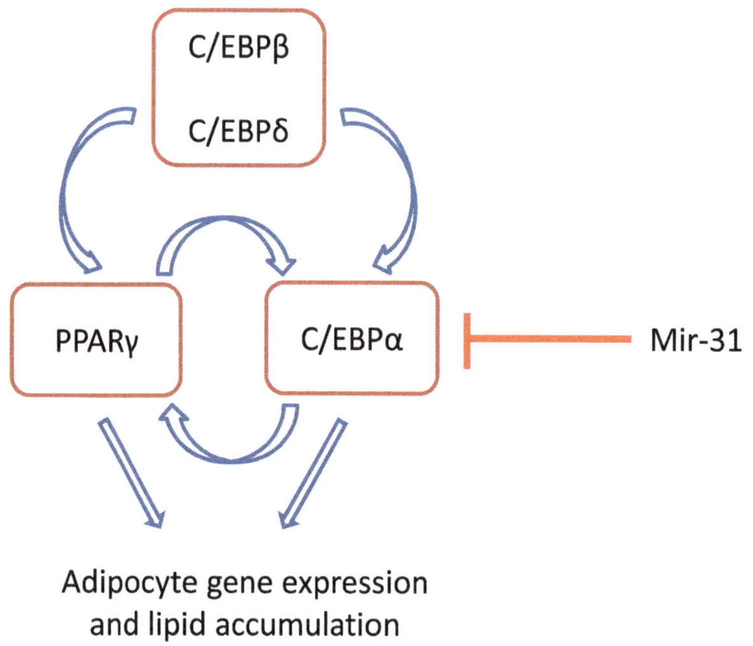

Fig. 3 C/EBPα, a key target. The C/EBPα intronless gene encodes a transcription factor containing a basic leucine zipper domain. The protein acts in homodimers or heterodimers that recognize the CCAAT motifs in the promoters of target genes. Complexes modulate the expression of genes involved in cell cycle regulation as well as adipocyte functions: during adipogenesis highly induced genes are synergistically controlled by both PPARγ and C/EBPα

and in numerous kinds of cancers. Interestingly, in most of these diseases, miR-206 levels are downregulated, which leads to the recognition of miRNA as a "disease-avoiding" molecule. Moreover, miR-206 expression is abundant in brown adipocytes but missing in white adipocytes [42]. Remarkably, it has been shown that miR-206 suppresses liver LXRα, a gene target of PPAR, consequently inhibiting lipogenesis and controlling lipid metabolism [43]. The insulin signaling pathway ($p = 0.01$, 11 target genes) and the pentose phosphate pathway ($p = 0.01$, 4 target genes) were also identified as candidate targets of miR-206. Therefore, the reduced level of circulating miR-206 in OW/Ob children may be either representative of a functional decreased synthesis [42] or an epiphenomenon reflecting the reduced relative skeletal muscle mass in the OW/Ob group.

Among the top pathways that were predicted to be targeted by the three differentially expressed miRNAs, "Notch" signaling appears relevant ($p = 0.0008$, 5 target genes, Additional file 2: Figure S2). Notch signaling represents a basic biological pathway primarily related to cell communication and development with extensive integration and crosstalk with other signaling pathways. Perturbations in this pathway have been linked to many genetic disorders and cancers. Accordingly, the direct involvement of Notch signaling has recently been demonstrated in obesity and type 2 diabetes [44]: through transcriptional binding partners FoxO1 and Rbpj, Notch activation enhances pathologic glucose output and fatty liver in obese, in combination with a reduced Akt activation by insulin. Activation of the Notch pathway in obesity results in heightened diabetes and fatty liver production, as a consequence of an augmented lipogenesis that is not blocked despite the reduced insulin signaling. Notably, blocking Notch signaling in mice caused white fat cells to transform into beige fat consequently reducing the risk of obesity and related health problems [44].

While we recognize the limitations and the relative reliability of our target prediction analyses, this hypothesis-generating exercise suggested the involvement of the detected miRNAs in metabolic relevant pathways, to be obviously confirmed by larger and ad hoc designed studies.

Our results confirm those of recent papers indicating that circulating miRNAs are deregulated in obese children [45] and are associated with obesity and lipid abnormalities in adolescents [46]. However, differentially detected miRNA signals in refs. 46 and 47 are not consistent with those identified in our study. Of note, all these miRNAs are present in the 372 miRNA arrays we used in our study but did not pass the threshold we set to consider them as differentially expressed. A solid explanation of these discrepancies is not at hand. Considering the rapidly changing scenario in this field, the interpretation and discussion of the inconsistent findings regarding the association of circulating miRNAs with obesity in children [45, 46] is far beyond the objective of this study. However, recent reviews extensively summarized potentiality, but also uncertainties, of the role of extracellular miRNAs as potential regulators and/or biomarkers of obesity and metabolic diseases [16, 32]. In particular, the inconsistencies of the findings may be ascribed to inter-population differences, but even, and perhaps most likely, to methodological differences in sampling, RNA isolation, detection, and normalization [32]. The need for consistent analysis strategies and quality control has been recently discussed [47].

Conclusions

This pilot study showed that three circulating miRNAs are differentially regulated in OW/Ob as compared with NW children. Although causal pathways cannot be firmly inferred—but only suggested—by these preliminary results, that deserve confirmation in other populations, it is conceivable that circulating miRNAs may be novel biomarkers of obesity and related metabolic disturbances.

The planned completion of the miRNA studies in the much larger sample of children from the eight European countries participating to the I.Family project will certainly contribute to the ongoing debate whether circulating miRNAs play a role in disease pathogenesis, are (early) indicators of a metabolic dysfunction, or both.

Methods

Study cohort

The I.Family project aimed to assess the determinants of eating behavior in children and adolescents of eight European countries and related health outcomes was built on the IDEFICS cohort (http://www.ideficsstudy.eu), established in 2006. We selected our sample among OW/Ob and NW participants of the Italian cohort of the project. The weight status of children was defined according to age- and sex-specific BMI categories [48]. Ten OW/Ob (four females and six males, age 10.7 ± 1.5 years, BMI 31.7 ± 4.3 kg/m^2) and ten NW (five females and five males, age 10.5 ± 2.7 years, BMI 16.4 ± 1.7 kg/m^2) children were included in the study.

The study protocol was approved by the local Ethics Committee of the local Health Authority (ASL Avellino) and informed written parental consent was obtained for each participant.

Sample processing

Whole blood was collected according to the standard operating procedures in BD Vacutainer® blood collection tubes. The optimal approach for miRNA purification from whole blood necessitates collecting fresh blood and processes the sample as quickly as possible. Accordingly, plasma was isolated by centrifugation at 1900×*g* for 10 min at 4 °C in an Eppendorf benchtop centrifuge (Eppendorf, Germany), aliquoted into 1.5 mL Eppendorf tubes, and promptly stored at −80 °C, in the absence of freeze-thaw cycles, until processing.

miRNA extraction, reverse transcription, and pre-screening

Prior to miRNA extraction, spectrophotometry was carried out on plasma samples to test for hemolysis by measuring the absorbance of free hemoglobin at 414 nm; samples with OD_{414} greater than 0.2 were excluded from the study. RNA was extracted from both plasma pooled samples and from individual plasma samples using the commercial column-based system miRNeasy serum/plasma Kit (Qiagen, Germany) according to the manufacturer's instructions with minor modifications. Plasma was thawed on ice and spun for 10 min at 13,000×*g* at 4 °C in an Eppendorf benchtop centrifuge (Eppendorf, Germany) to pellet any debris. An aliquot of 200 μL of plasma was transferred to a new microcentrifuge tube and 800 μL of a Qiazol (Qiagen) mixture, containing 1.25 μg/mL of MS2 bacteriophage RNA (Roche Applied Science), was added to the sample. *Caenorhabditis elegans* miR-39 (*C.el*-miR-39) was spiked into the sample (5.6×10^8 molecules) before the extraction process to assess RNA recovery. A rinse step (500 μL Qiagen RPE buffer) was repeated two times. Total RNA was eluted by adding 14 μL of RNase-free water to the membrane of the column and incubating for 1 min before centrifugation at 13,000×*g* for 1 min at room temperature. The obtained RNA was stored at −80 °C.

Complementary DNA (cDNA) was generated by means of the miScript RTII kit (Qiagen), in HiSpec Buffer with miRNA-specific stem-looped RT primers. Nine microliters of isolated RNA were reverse transcribed in 20-μL reactions according to the manufacturer's recommendations. The obtained cDNA was diluted 1:5.5 in RNase-free water. This procedure was repeated three times. To identify hemolyzed samples, the levels of miR-451, highly abundant in RBCs, were preliminarily assessed in cDNA samples by qPCR. Hemolyzed samples were excluded from the analysis.

Circulating miRNA profiling

Selected samples from ten OW/Ob and ten NW children (Table 1) were pooled, and miRNAs were extracted as described above. miRNA profiling was performed by using the Serum and Plasma 384HC miScript miRNA PCR Arrays (SABiosciences, Qiagen) to assess the expression of 372 miRNAs typically detectable in serum and plasma. The SYBR green-based qPCR assay was performed with cDNA (dil. 1:225) in 10-uL reaction volume using a 7900HT fast Real-Time PCR System instrument (Applied Biosystems). Reaction conditions were as follows: 15 min at 95 °C and 40 cycles of 15 s at 94 °C, 30 s at 60 °C, and 30 s at 72 °C with a set of technical controls on each plate which included the spike-in control and small non-coding RNAs (SNORDs) as reference genes. References for data normalization included the spike-in *C.el*-miR-39-3p, SNORD61, SNORD68, SNORD72, SNORD95, and SNORD96A, which have been verified to hold relatively stable expression levels across tissues and cell types. Normalization of expression was done using the geometric mean of the endogenous controls. All assays were inspected for distinct melting curves, and the Tm was checked. The amplification efficiency was also calculated. Ct values >35 were considered as negative amplification. Data that did not pass these criteria were omitted from further analysis. The efficiency of reverse transcription was assessed with miRTC.

Statistically significant deregulated miRNAs with a fold-change ≥4.0 were selected and further validated by individual microRNA assays (SABiosciences, Qiagen) performed on the individual plasma samples of ten OW/Ob and ten NW children, using the miScript SYBR green PCR kit (Qiagen) according to the manufacturer's instructions. RT-qPCR was performed in triplicates using the following conditions: 95 °C for 15 min, followed by 40 cycles of 94 °C for 15 s, 55 °C for 30 s, and 70 °C for 30 s. Relative miRNA levels were determined by the $^{\Delta\Delta}$Ct method using the *C.el*-miR-39 as endogenous normalizer.

Data analysis

On pooled samples, RT-qPCR quantifications were performed by using SDS 2.3 (Life Technologies, USA) to generate Ct values.

Gene Arrays data were organized in Excel (Microsoft), and the integrated web-based software package for miScript Arrays analysis was exploited. This software performs quantification using the $^{\Delta\Delta}$Ct method and interpretation of the control assays. Tools are available at the SABiosciences data analysis web portal.

Data on the individual samples are presented as the average of at least three independent experiments ± s.e.. Data Assist 3.1 software packages (Life Technologies, USA) were used to generate relative "fold-change" values. Student's *t* test, performed with the GraphPad Prism 6 software, was used to determine the significance of any difference in the levels of miRNA expression between NW and OW/Ob subjects with alpha <0.05.

Obesity-associated miRNAs were tested using the well-established target prediction tool miRPath v2.0 [33]. miRPath achieves advanced analysis pipelines, such as hierarchical clustering of miRNAs and pathways based on the levels of their interactions. miRNA targets (in CDS or 3′-UTR regions) were predicted by the DIANA-microT-CDS algorithm or even experimentally validated miRNA interactions derived from DIANA-TarBase v6.0. Predicted and/or validated interactions were subsequently combined with merging and meta-analysis algorithms.

All the predicted targets were further analyzed through the use of Kyoto Encyclopedia of Genes and Genomes (KEGG) [34] and QIAGEN's Ingenuity® Pathway Analysis (IPA®, QIAGEN Redwood City, www.qiagen.com/ingenuity). IPA identified lists of genes that satisfy specific biological criteria scoring these genes towards pathways in the Ingenuity Knowledge Base which embraces a large database of biological and chemical relationships extracted from scientific literature.

Competing interests

The authors declare that they have no competing interests.

Authors' contributions

GI participated in the design of the study, performed the molecular and bioinformatic studies, executed the statistical analyses, and drafted the manuscript; PR participated in the design of the study and helped to draft the manuscript; IS performed the miRNA isolation and the molecular studies; FL helped to perform the statistical analysis and to draft the manuscript; PM carried out the sample collection and helped with the miRNA isolation; WA helped to draft the manuscript with critical revision; PDL helped to perform the molecular analyses and to draft the manuscript; AS conceived the study, participated in its design and coordination, and helped to draft the manuscript. All authors read and approved the final manuscript.

Acknowledgements

The work was done as part of the IDEFICS study (http://www.idefics.eu) and the I.Family Study (http://www.ifamilystudy.eu/). We gratefully acknowledge the financial support of the European Community within the Sixth RTD Framework Programme Contract No. 016181 (FOOD) for the IDEFICS study and within the Seventh RTD Framework Programme Contract No. 266044 for the I.Family study.

Author details

[1]Institute of Food Sciences, CNR, Via Roma, 64, 83100 Avellino, Italy. [2]Leibniz Institute for Prevention Research and Epidemiology - BIPS, Bremen, Germany. [3]Institute of Statistics, Faculty of Mathematics and Computer Science, University Bremen, Bremen, Germany. [4]BioGeM, Ariano Irpino, Italy.

References

1. Zimmet P, Alberti KG, Shaw J. Global and societal implications of the diabetes epidemic. Nature. 2001;414:782–7.
2. Kahn SE, Hull RL, Utzschneider KM. Mechanisms linking obesity to insulin resistance and type 2 diabetes. Nature. 2006;444:840–6.
3. Despres J-P, Lemieux I. Abdominal obesity and metabolic syndrome. Nature. 2006;444:881–7.
4. Berndt SI, Gustafsson S, Mägi R, Ganna A, Wheeler E, Feitosa MF, et al. Genome-wide meta-analysis identifies 11 new loci for anthropometric traits and provides insights into genetic architecture. Nat Genet. 2013;45:501–12.
5. Kunej T, Jevsinek Skok D, Zorc M, Ogrinc A, Michal JJ, Kovac M, et al. Obesity gene atlas in mammals. J Genomics. 2013;1:45–55.
6. Loos RJF, Yeo GSH. The bigger picture of FTO: the first GWAS-identified obesity gene. Nat Rev Endocrinol. 2014;10:51–61.
7. Rosen ED, Spiegelman BM. Adipocytes as regulators of energy balance and glucose homeostasis. Nature. 2006;444:847–53.

8. Schaffler A, Muller-Ladner U, Scholmerich J, Buchler C. Role of adipose tissue as an inflammatory organ in human diseases. Endocr Rev. 2006;27:449–67.
9. Kopelman PG. Obesity as a medical problem. Nature. 2000;404:635–43.
10. Kammoun HL, Kraakman MJ, Febbraio MA. Adipose tissue inflammation in glucose metabolism. Rev Endocr Metab Disord. 2014;15:31–44.
11. Kraakman MJ, Murphy AJ, Jandeleit-Dahm K, Kammoun HL. Macrophage polarization in obesity and type 2 diabetes: weighing down our understanding of macrophage function? Front Immunol. 2014;5:470.
12. Tang QQ, Lane MD. Adipogenesis: from stem cell to adipocyte. Annu Rev Biochem. 2012;81:715–36.
13. Xie H, Lim B, Lodish HF. MicroRNAs induced during adipogenesis that accelerate fat cell development are downregulated in obesity. Diabetes. 2009;58:1050–7.
14. Rottiers V, Naar AM. MicroRNAs in metabolism and metabolic disorders. Nat Rev Mol Cell Biol. 2012;13:239–50.
15. Kim HJ, Cho H, Alexander R, Patterson HC, Gu M, Lo KA, et al. MicroRNAs are required for the feature maintenance and differentiation of brown adipocytes. Diabetes. 2014;63:4045–56.
16. Arner P, Kulyte A. MicroRNA regulatory networks in human adipose tissue and obesity. Nat Rev Endocrinol. 2015;11:276–88.
17. Li J, Zhou C, Li J, Su Z, Sang H, Jia E, et al. Global correlation analysis for microRNA and gene expression profiles in human obesity. Pathol Res Pract. 2015;211:361–8.
18. Bartel DP. MicroRNAs: target recognition and regulatory functions. Cell. 2009;136:215–33.
19. Ghildiyal M, Zamore PD. Small silencing RNAs: an expanding universe. Nat Rev Genet. 2009;10:94–108.
20. Ha M, Kim VN. Regulation of microRNA biogenesis. Nat Rev Mol Cell Biol. 2014;15:509–24.
21. Ebert MS, Sharp PA. Roles for microRNAs in conferring robustness to biological processes. Cell. 2012;149:515–24.
22. Krek A, Grün D, Poy MN, Wolf R, Rosenberg L, Epstein EJ, et al. Combinatorial microRNA target predictions. Nat Genet. 2005;37:495–500.
23. Lewis BP, Burge CB, Bartel DP. Conserved seed pairing, often flanked by adenosines, indicates that thousands of human genes are microRNA targets. Cell. 2005;120:15–20.
24. Bartel DP. MicroRNAs: genomics, biogenesis, mechanism, and function. Cell. 2004;116:281–97.
25. van Rooij E. The art of microRNA research. Circ Res. 2011;108:219–34.
26. Mendell JT, Olson EN. MicroRNAs in stress signaling and human disease. Cell. 2012;148:1172–87.
27. Park NJ, Zhou H, Elashoff D, Henson BS, Kastratovic DA, Abemayor E, et al. Salivary microRNA: discovery, characterization, and clinical utility for oral cancer detection. Clin Cancer Res. 2009;15:5473–7.
28. Kosaka N, Iguchi H, Ochiya T. Circulating microRNA in body fluid: a new potential biomarker for cancer diagnosis and prognosis. Cancer Sci. 2010;101:2087–92.
29. Valadi H, Ekstrom K, Bossios A, Sjostrand M, Lee JJ, Lotvall JO. Exosome-mediated transfer of mRNAs and microRNAs is a novel mechanism of genetic exchange between cells. Nat Cell Biol. 2007;9:654–9.
30. Turchinovich A, Samatov TR, Tonevitsky AG, Burwinkel B. Circulating miRNAs: cell-cell communication function? Front Genet. 2013;4:119.
31. McGregor RA, Choi MS. microRNAs in the regulation of adipogenesis and obesity. Curr Mol Med. 2011;11:304–16.
32. Deiuliis JA. MicroRNAs as regulators of metabolic disease: pathophysiologic significance and emerging role as biomarkers and therapeutics. Int J Obes (Lond). 2016;40:88–101.
33. Vlachos IS, Kostoulas N, Vergoulis T, Georgakilas G, Reczko M, Maragkakis M, et al. DIANA miRPath v.2.0: investigating the combinatorial effect of microRNAs in pathways. Nucleic Acids Res. 2012;40(Web Server issue): W498–504.
34. Kanehisa M, Goto S, Sato Y, Kawashima M, Furumichi M, Tanabe M. Data, information, knowledge and principle: back to metabolism in KEGG. Nucleic Acids Res. 2014;42:D199–205.
35. Chen L, Song J, Cui J, Hou J, Zheng X, Li C, et al. microRNAs regulate adipocyte differentiation. Cell Biol Intern. 2013;37:533–46.
36. Zhang R, Wang D, Xia Z, Chen C, Cheng P, Xie H, et al. The role of microRNAs in adipocyte differentiation. Front Med. 2013;7:223–30.
37. Son YH, Ka S, Kim AY, Kim JB. Regulation of adipocyte differentiation via microRNAs. Endocrinol Metab (Seoul). 2014;29:122–35.
38. Linhart HG, Ishimura-Oka K, DeMayo F, Kibe T, Repka D, Poindexter B, et al. C/EBPalpha is required for differentiation of white, but not brown, adipose tissue. Proc Natl Acad Sci U S A. 2001;98:12532–7.
39. Tang YF, Zhang Y, Li XY, Li C, Tian W, Liu L. Expression of miR-31, miR-125b-5p, and miR-326 in the adipogenic differentiation process of adipose-derived stem cells. OMICS. 2009;13:331–6.
40. Li S, Chen X, Zhang H, Liang X, Xiang Y, Yu C, et al. Differential expression of microRNAs in mouse liver under aberrant energy metabolic status. J Lipid Res. 2009;50:1756–65.
41. Novak J, Kruzliak P, Bienertova-Vasku J, Slaby O, Novak M. MicroRNA-206: a promising theranostic marker. Theranostics. 2014;4:119–33.
42. Walden TB, Timmons JA, Keller P, Nedergaard J, Cannon B. Distinct expression of muscle-specific microRNAs (myomirs) in brown adipocytes. J Cell Physiol. 2009;218:444–9.
43. Zhong D, Huang G, Zhang Y, Zeng Y, Xu Z, Zhao Y, et al. MicroRNA-1 and microRNA-206 suppress LXRα-induced lipogenesis in hepatocytes. Cell Signal. 2013;25:1429–37.
44. Bi P, Shan T, Liu W, Yue F, Yang X, Liang XR, et al. Inhibition of Notch signaling promotes browning of white adipose tissue and ameliorates obesity. Nat Med. 2014;20:911–8.
45. Prats-Puig A, Ortega FJ, Mercader JM, Moreno-Navarrete JM, Moreno M, Bonet N, et al. Changes in circulating microRNAs are associated with childhood obesity. J Clin Endocrinol Metab. 2013;98:E1655–60.
46. Can U, Buyukinan M, Yerlikaya FH. The investigation of circulating microRNAs associated with lipid metabolism in childhood obesity. Pediatr Obes. 2015. doi:10.1111/ijpo.12050.
47. Mestdagh P, Hartmann N, Baeriswyl L, Andreasen D, Bernard N, Chen C, et al. Evaluation of quantitative miRNA expression platforms in the microRNA quality control (miRQC) study. Nat Methods. 2014;11:809–15.
48. Cole TJ, Lobstein T. Extended international (IOTF) body mass index cut-offs for thinness, overweight and obesity. Pediatr Obes. 2012;7:284–94.

14

Vitamin A deficiency modulates iron metabolism independent of hemojuvelin (*Hfe2*) and bone morphogenetic protein 6 (*Bmp6*) transcript levels

Juliana Frossard Ribeiro Mendes[1,4*], Egle Machado de Almeida Siqueira[2], João Gabriel Marques de Brito e Silva[3] and Sandra Fernandes Arruda[1,4]

Abstract

Background: Considering that vitamin A deficiency modulates hepcidin expression and consequently affects iron metabolism, we evaluated the effect of vitamin A deficiency in the expression of genes involved in the hemojuvelin (HJV)-bone morphogenetic protein 6 (BMP6)-small mothers against decapentaplegic protein (SMAD) signaling pathway.

Methods: Male Wistar rats were treated: control AIN-93G diet (CT), vitamin A-deficient diet (VAD), iron-deficient diet (FeD), vitamin A- and iron-deficient diet (VAFeD), or 12 mg all-*trans* retinoic acid (atRA)/kg diet.

Results: Vitamin A deficiency (VAD) increased hepatic *Bmp6* and *Hfe2* mRNA levels and down-regulated hepatic *Hamp*, *Smad7*, *Rara*, and intestinal *Fpn1* mRNA levels compared with the control. The FeD rats showed lower hepatic *Hamp*, *Bmp6*, and *Smad7* mRNA levels compared with those of the control, while in the VAFeD rats only *Hamp* and *Smad7* mRNA levels were lower than those of the control. The VAFeD diet up-regulated intestinal *Dmt1* mRNA levels in relation to those of the control. The replacement of retinyl ester by atRA did not restore hepatic *Hamp* mRNA levels; however, the hepatic *Hfe2*, *Bmp6*, and *Smad7* mRNA levels were similar to the control. The atRA rats showed an increase of hepatic *Rara* mRNA levels and a reduction of intestinal *Dmt1* mRNA and *Fpn1* levels compared with those of the control.

Conclusions: The HJV-BMP6-SMAD signaling pathway that normally activates the expression of hepcidin in iron deficiency is impaired by vitamin A deficiency despite increased expression of liver *Bmp6* and *Hfe2* mRNA levels and decreased expression of *Smad7* mRNA. This response may be associated to the systemic iron deficiency and spleen iron retention promoted by vitamin A deficiency.

Keywords: Vitamin A deficiency, Iron status, Hemojuvelin, Bone morphogenetic protein 6, Hepcidin

Background

Iron deficiency affects approximately 20 % of the world population and is the most prevalent nutritional deficiency worldwide (Martínez-Navarrete et al. 2002; Brasil 2007; Assunção et al. 2007). The condition is often considered together with vitamin A deficiency, which affects approximately 250 million people (Strube et al 2002; Zimmermann et al. 2006).

Hepcidin, a peptide hormone secreted by the liver, is an essential molecule for systemic iron homeostasis regulation. The primary role of hepcidin is to control the amount of iron that is released into the circulation from enterocytes and spleen macrophages. Hepcidin binds to ferroportin, which is an iron exporter protein found in most body cell membranes, and triggers the internalization of ferroportin, ubiquitination, and subsequent lysosomal degradation. The result is the prevention of the iron release from enterocytes and splenic macrophages. Hepcidin gene expression is

* Correspondence: jufrossard@gmail.com
[1]Postgraduate Program in Human Nutrition, Faculty of Health Sciences, University of Brasília, Campus Universitário Darcy Ribeiro, POBox 70910-900, Brasília, DF, Brazil
[4]Instituto de Ciências Biológicas, Departamento de Biologia Celular, Laboratório de Bioquímica da Nutrição, Universidade de Brasília, Campus Universitário Darcy Ribeiro, Bloco J, 1 Andar. Asa Norte, Brasília, Distrito Federal CEP: 70910-900, Brasil
Full list of author information is available at the end of the article

regulated by several factors, including body iron status, inflammation, erythropoiesis, and hypoxia (Evstatiev and Gasche 2012).

When body iron stores are high, hepcidin expression is increased, which consequently inhibits iron mobilization from tissues and iron absorption from the diet (Anderson et al. 2009; Hentze et al. 2010). The pathway that modulates hepcidin expression in response to intracellular iron status appears to be dependent on the hemojuvelin (HJV) protein and bone morphogenetic protein 6 (BMP6). The binding of the BMP6 to the BMP receptor (BMPR) and its essential co-receptor HJV leads to the phosphorylation of small mothers against decapentaplegic protein (SMAD) 1, 5, and 8. Phosphorylated SMAD 1/5/8 forms a complex with SMAD 4 that is translocated to the nucleus before activating the hepcidin promoter; this process induces iron retention in tissues (Hentze et al. 2010; Lee et al. 2010; Zhang et al. 2010; Zhang 2010). The BMP6 pathway also induces negative regulators of hepcidin, such as SMAD 7, so that a negative feedback loop that controls hepcidin expression is established. This mechanism prevents excessive hepcidin production, which in turn could lead to iron deficiency (Evstatiev and Gasche 2012).

Recent studies suggest that the metabolism of vitamin A and iron is interrelated (Citelli et al. 2012; Jiang et al. 2012; Tsuchiya et al. 2009). In vitamin A-deficient organisms, systemic iron availability appears to be significantly reduced and iron is accumulated in tissues, especially in the spleen (Tsuchiya et al. 2009; Arruda et al. 2009). Although preliminary data clearly show that vitamin A affects iron homeostasis (Arruda et al. 2009), the mechanism by which retinoids modulate systemic iron homeostasis is unclear. Several physiological processes, such as cell proliferation and differentiation, are modulated by retinoids. The all-trans retinoic acid (atRA), which is the most active form of retinoids, modulates the expression of several genes at the transcriptional level by binding to nuclear receptors, the retinoic acid receptor (RAR), and the retinoid X receptor (RXR), which are transcription factors (Ziouzenkova and Plutzky 2008; Theodosiou et al. 2010).

To explore how vitamin A deficiency alters iron metabolism, the present study evaluated the expression of genes involved in the HJV-BMP6-SMAD signaling pathway. The study also considered the possible involvement of retinoic acid and retinoid X nuclear receptors in the maintenance of iron homeostasis that is mediated by vitamin A.

Methods

Animals

Thirty 21-day-old male Wistar rats (65.7 ± 5.5 g) were housed individually in stainless steel cages and were maintained under a 12 h light cycle at 22 ± 2 °C with free access to water, and food access was allowed only during the dark cycle. The present study was approved by the Animal Care and Use Committee of the University of Brasília (UnBDoc 52606/2011). All applicable national and institutional guidelines for the care and use of animals were followed.

After 7 days of acclimatization, rats were randomly assigned to five groups (six rats per group). The control group (CT) was fed with an AIN-93G diet (Reeves et al. 1993), containing 4000 UI vitamin A/kg; the vitamin A-deficient group (VAD) was fed with an AIN-93G diet without a source of vitamin A; the vitamin A- and iron-deficient group (VAFeD) was fed with an AIN-93G diet without sources of vitamin A and iron; the iron-deficient group (FeD) was fed with an AIN-93G diet without a source of iron; and the retinoic acid group (atRA) was fed with an AIN-93G diet containing 12 mg of atRA/kg as the only source of vitamin A. The animals were weighed weekly, and food intake was recorded daily. After 59 days of feeding the experimental diets, the animals were denied food for 14 h and sacrificed after being anesthetized with 3 % isoflurane. Blood was collected by cardiac puncture into tubes containing 7.0 % ethylenediaminetetraacetic acid (21 μL/mL of blood). The liver, spleen, and small intestine (a 1-cm length of small intestine distal to the pylorus and a 1-cm length proximal to the ileocecal valve were excised, and the lumen was rinsed with saline) were excised and washed in cold 0.9 % NaCl. The samples were frozen in liquid nitrogen (N_2) and stored at −80 °C.

RNA extraction and reverse transcription-polymerase chain reaction analysis (qRT-PCR)

The extraction of total RNA, purity and integrity of the RNA samples, and the cDNA synthesis were performed as described previously (Cunha et al. 2014).

Quantitative real-time PCR was performed using the Fast SYBR Green Master Mix 2x reagent (Applied Biosystems, Foster City, CA, USA) with 2.0 μL of cDNA diluted 50 times (corresponding to 2 ng of total RNA). The final volumes were 10 and 5 μL Fast SYBR Green Master Mix and 10 μmol/L (final concentration) of each primer. The following primers were used for each target genomic region: for hepcidin, *Hamp* TGATGCTGAAGCGAAGGA (forward) and TGTGTTGAGAGGTCAGGAC (reverse); for hemochromatosis type 2 (juvenile) homolog, *Hfe2* GTAGCATCGGGAGCCAAC (forward) and TCAAAGG CTGCAGGAAGATT (reverse); for bone morphogenetic protein 6, *Bmp6* GACAGCAGAGTCGCAATCG (forward) and AGCTCACGTAAAGCTCATGC (reverse); for SMAD family member 7, *Smad7* AGAGGCTGTGTTGCTGTG (forward) and CATCGGGTATCTGGAGTAAGG (reverse); for retinoic acid receptor alpha, *Rara* ACCATTGCCGAC CAGATTACCC (forward) and AAGGTCATTGTGTCTT

GCTCAGGT (reverse); for retinoid X receptor beta, *Rxrβ* CTTCCCAGTCATCAGTTCTTCC (forward) and GGTG GCTTCACATCTTCAGG (reverse); for divalent metal transporter 1, *Dmt1* or solute carrier family 11 member 2, *Scl11a2* CTGATTTACAGTCTGGAGCAG (forward) and CACTTCAGCAAGGTGCAA (reverse); for ferroportin 1, *Fpn1* or solute carrier family 40 member 1, *Slc40a1* TTCCGCACTTTTCGAGATGG (forward) and TACAGT CGAAGCCCAGGACTGT (reverse); and for β-actin, *Actb* GTCGTACCACTGGCATTGTG (forward) and CTCTCA GCTGTGGTGGTGAA (reverse). Quantitative PCR was performed using a 7500 Fast Real-Time PCR System (Applied Biosystems, Cingapura) with 40 cycles at 95 °C for 20 s, 60 °C for 3 s, and 60 °C for 20 s. "The expression of all genes was normalized to the expression of the housekeeping gene β-actin, and the reactions were run in triplicate. The amplification efficiency was determined from the slope obtained from the standard curve relating log [transcribed mRNA] and variation threshold cycle (C_T) with the equation $E = (10 - 1/\text{slope} - 1) \times 100$, and a slope value of the regression line plot of C_T values versus log of input nucleic acid of approximately −3.32 was considered an efficient reaction. PCR efficiency was between 102 and 109 % for all primers. A standard curve was plotted for each gene, which correlated the ΔC_T (C_T target − C_T reference) versus the log of the cDNA amount, and a slope value of the regression line plot of ΔC_T values versus log of input nucleic acid of less than 0.1 was used as a general criterion to accept the validation of the experiment. Based on the data obtained previously, a 1:50 dilution of cDNA was used to analyze qRT-PCR, where the efficiency was higher than 99 %. Melting curve analysis was used to examine the specificity of the products generated for each primer set. The comparative C_T method was used to quantitate the abundance of the target gene mRNA and is given by $2^{-\Delta\Delta C_T}$." This method was performed as described in the tutorial, "Guide to Performing Relative Quantitation of Gene Expression Using Real-Time Quantitative PCR" (Part #: 4371095 Rev B, Applied Biosystems).

Statistical analysis

Statistical analyses were performed using SPSS software (version 19.0, SPSS Inc., Chicago, IL, USA). The normality of data distribution was tested by the Kolmogorov-Smirnov test. Differences between treatment groups were tested by independent sample *t* test. In all tests, a value of $p < 0.05$ was considered statistically significant.

Results

The effect of vitamin A deficiency and atRA on the expression of mRNAs encoding proteins involved in iron homeostasis: *Hamp*, *Hfe2*, *Bmp6*, and *Smad7*

Figure 1 shows the relative transcript levels of hepcidin (*Hamp*), hemochromatosis type 2 (juvenile) homolog (*Hfe2*), bone morphogenetic protein 6 (*Bmp6*), and SMAD family member 7 (*Smad7*) in rat livers, normalized to β-actin (*Actb*) values. Compared to the control group, vitamin A deficiency down-regulated *Hamp* (2.3-fold, $p < 0.001$) and *Smad7* (1.6-fold, $p = 0.027$) mRNA levels in the liver and up-regulated hepatic *Hfe2* (1.2-fold, $p = 0.026$) and *Bmp6* mRNA levels (2.0-fold, $p = 0.0013$). The consumption of atRA, as the only source of dietary vitamin A, resulted in mRNA levels of *Hfe2*, *Bmp6*, and *Smad7* be similar to those values obtained in the control group; however, the atRA diet failed to reverse the inhibitory effect of vitamin A deficiency on *Hamp* mRNA levels (2.8-fold, $p = 0.002$) in the liver. The iron-deficient diet (FeD) down-regulated hepatic levels of *Hamp* (58.7-fold), *Bmp6* (1.6-fold), and *Smad7* mRNA (2.8-fold, $p = 0.000$, 0.002, and 0.005, respectively) compared to those of the control group, and no difference was observed in relation to hepatic *Hfe2* mRNA levels. The VAFeD group showed lower hepatic levels of *Hamp* and *Smad7* mRNA (12.6-fold and 2.4-fold, $p = 0.000$ and 0.006, respectively) relative to the control group, but no difference was observed in the *Hfe2* and *Bmp6* mRNA levels, between these two groups. The VAFeD diet also significantly reduced the hepatic *Hamp*, *Hfe2*, *Bmp6*, and *Smad7* mRNA levels compared to those of the VAD group ($p < 0.001$, 0.035, 0.0003, and 0.002, respectively; Fig. 1), whereas only *Bmp6* mRNA levels were significantly increased in the VAFeD group compared to those in the FeD group ($p = 0.024$).

The effect of vitamin A deficiency and atRA administration on the *Fpn1* and *Dmt1* intestinal mRNA levels

Vitamin A deficiency promoted a decrease in *Fpn1* mRNA levels compared to the control group (1.6-fold, $p = 0.043$; Fig. 2). This response was not reversed when retinyl ester was replaced by all-trans retinoic acid in the diet; instead, the atRA group also showed down-regulation of *Fpn1* mRNA levels in the intestine relative to the control group ($p = 0.020$). The VAFeD group showed higher *Dmt1* mRNA levels than the control group ($p = 0.001$) and the FeD group ($p = 0.002$). No difference was observed on the *Dmt1* mRNA levels in vitamin A- or iron-deficient rats (VAD and FeD groups); however, the association of both deficiencies (VAFeD group) up-regulated *Dmt1* mRNA levels relative to the control (1.8-fold, $p = 0.001$), VAD (1.8-fold, $p = 0.002$), and FeD groups (1.5-fold, $p = 0.002$). The administration of all-trans retinoic acid (atRA) promoted the down-regulation of intestinal *Dmt1* mRNA levels compared to the control group (1.9-fold, $p = 0.014$; Fig. 2).

The effect of vitamin A deficiency and atRA on the *Rarα* and *Rxrβ* mRNA levels in the liver

Vitamin A deficiency reduced the levels of hepatic *Rarα* mRNA (1.2-fold, $p = 0.001$), while the atRA diet

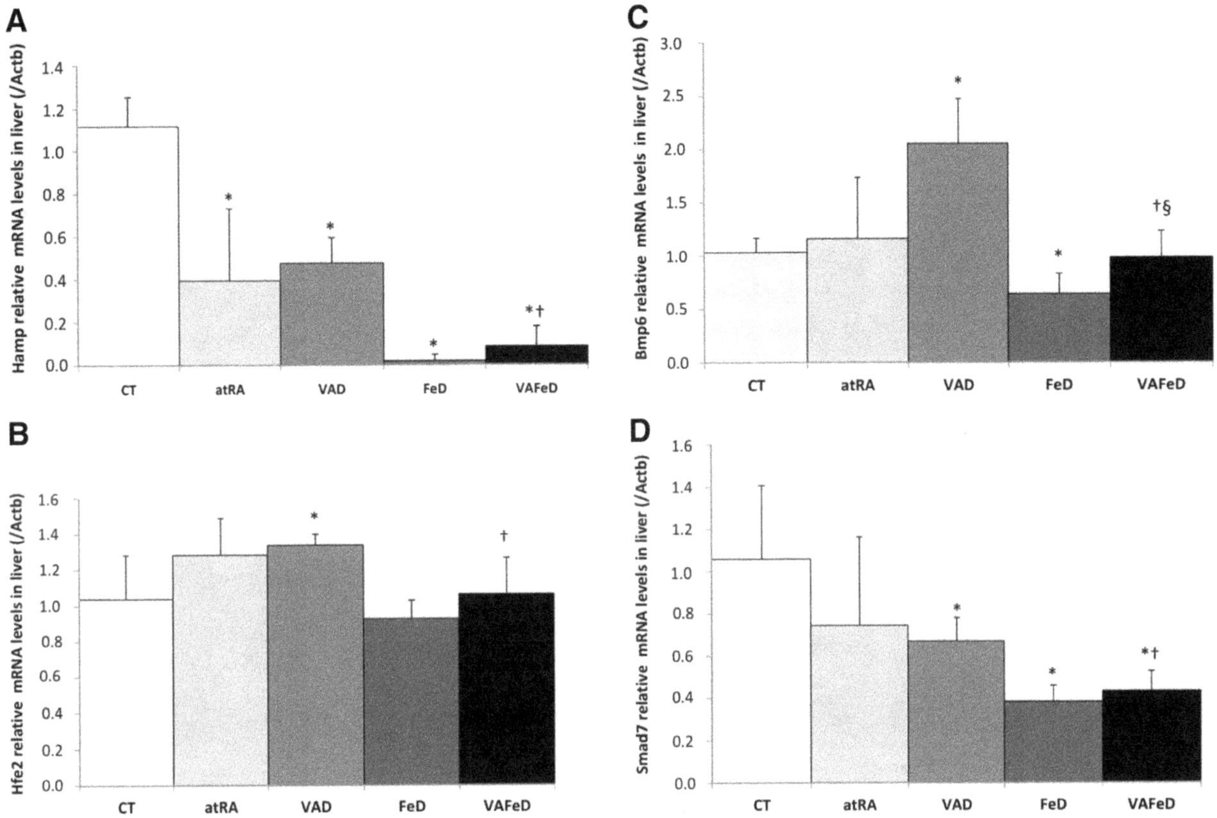

Fig. 1 Relative transcript levels of hepcidin (*Hamp*) (**a**), hemochromatosis type 2 (juvenile) homolog (*Hfe2*) (**b**), bone morphogenetic protein 6 (*Bmp6*) (**c**), and SMAD family member 7 (*Smad7*) (**d**) in the livers normalized to β-actin (Actb) values of rats treated with diets containing different sources and amounts of vitamin A and iron for 59 days. Mean ± standard deviation, *$p < 0.05$ versus the CT group, †$p < 0.05$ versus the VAD group, §$p < 0.05$ versus the FeD group

up-regulated hepatic *Rarα* mRNA, in relation to the control rats. The association between vitamin A and iron deficiency (VAFeD) leads to higher hepatic *Rarα* mRNA levels compared with vitamin A deficiency (VAD), whereas no difference was observed in *Rarα* mRNA levels between the VAFeD and Fe groups. No differences were observed in hepatic *Rxrβ* mRNA levels among the groups (Fig. 3).

Discussion

To explore how vitamin A deficiency alters hepcidin expression and consequently affects iron metabolism, the present study evaluated the expression of genes involved in the HJV-BMP6-SMAD signaling pathway in male Wistar rats treated with diets deficient in vitamin A (VAD) or in iron (FeD) or with diet deficient in both vitamin A and iron (VAFeD). Understanding the mechanisms that control hepcidin gene expression (*Hamp*) is an important goal in the treatment of anemia from chronic diseases.

The iron-deficient group (FeD) showed lower iron concentrations in the liver, spleen, and intestine and lower serum iron status compared to those of the control group (Additional file 1: Figure S1 and Additional file 2: Table S1). The tissue and systemic iron deficiency of FeD rats may have led to the lower levels of hepatic *Bmp6* mRNA and consequent strong down-regulation of *Hamp* mRNA levels compared to those of the control group. These results are consistent with a previous study (Pagani et al. 2011) that found that iron deficiency inhibits hepcidin due to the inhibition of the BMP-SMAD pathway as a consequence of reductions in *Bmp6* mRNA. Corradini et al. (2011) suggested that liver iron concentration was the only factor associated with hepatic *Bmp6* mRNA levels and that it is independent of transferrin saturation and serum iron and hemoglobin concentration, which suggests that hepatic *Bmp6* induction is mediated by liver iron concentration but not by transferrin saturation. Despite hemojuvelin (HJV) acting as a BMP co-receptor in the BMP-signaling pathway that modulates hepatic hepcidin expression (Evstatiev and Gasche 2012), the iron deficiency (FeD) did not alter hepatic *Hfe2* mRNA levels compared with those of the control. Krijt et al (2012) observed no changes in membrane HJV protein levels in rat livers subjected to iron overload and deficiency. The authors suggested that substantial changes

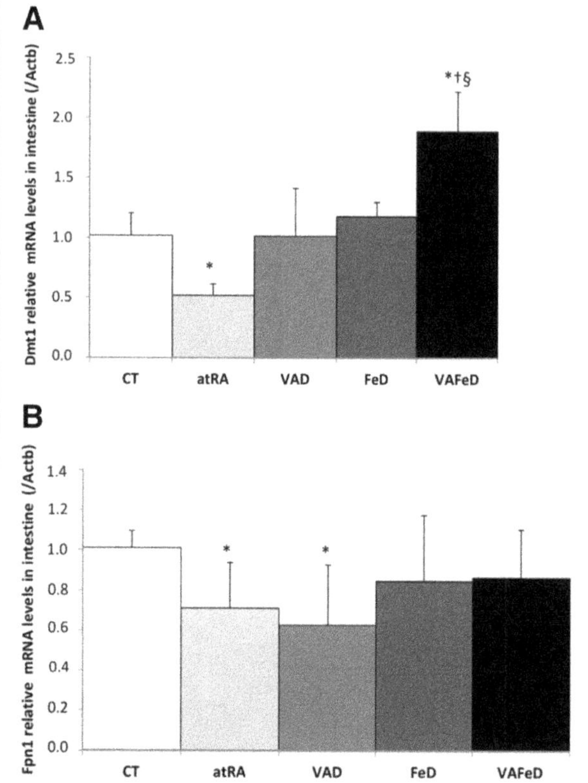

Fig. 2 Relative transcript levels of divalent metal transporter 1 (*Dmt1*) (**a**) and ferroportin 1 (*Fpn1*) (**b**) in the small intestines normalized to β-actin (Actb) values of rats treated with diets containing different sources and amounts of vitamin A and iron for 59 days. Mean ± standard deviation, $*p < 0.05$ versus the CT group, $\dagger p < 0.05$ versus the VAD group, $\S p < 0.05$ versus the FeD group

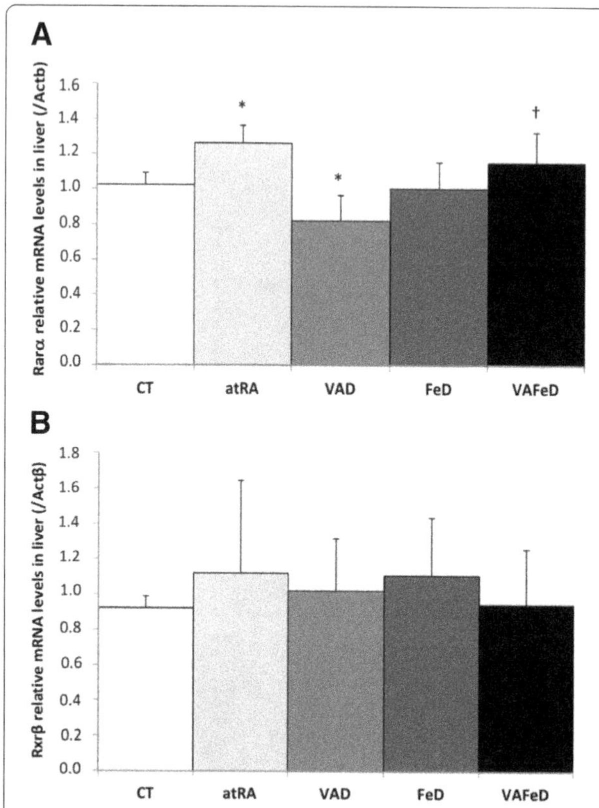

Fig. 3 Relative transcript levels of retinoic acid receptor alpha (*Rara*) (**a**) and retinoid X receptor beta (*Rxrβ*) (**b**) in the livers normalized to β-actin (Actb) values of rats treated with diets containing different sources and amounts of vitamin A and iron for 59 days. Mean ± standard deviation, $*p < 0.05$ versus the CT group, $\dagger p < 0.05$ versus the VAD group, $\S p < 0.05$ versus the FeD group

in *Hamp* mRNA can occur without changes in membrane hemojuvelin content and that this protein is not a limiting step in the control of *Hamp* gene expression.

Although the vitamin A-deficient rats (VAD) have presented systemic iron deficiency (lower serum iron concentration and transferrin saturation) like the iron-deficient groups (FeD and VAFeD), they showed iron retention in the spleen instead of a decrease as would be expected (Additional file 1: Figure S1 and Additional file 2: Table S1). Further, the vitamin A deficiency up-regulated hepatic *Bmp6* and *Hfe* mRNA levels in relation to those of the control group and down-regulated hepatic *Hamp* mRNA levels, despite similar iron levels in the liver, compared to those of the control group (Fig. 1). This contradictory response observed in the VAD group may be associated to an inadequate erythropoiesis promoted by vitamin A deficiency, due to the low availability of iron to expand the erythroid tissue (Evans 2005; Frazer et al. 2012). The inadequate erythropoiesis was characterized in a set of other experiments conducted in these rats (Cunha et al. 2014), where the authors demonstrated that vitamin A deficiency down-regulated renal *Epo* mRNA and up-regulated *Hmox1* in the spleen, suggesting an increased phagocytosis of malformed or undifferentiated erythrocytes and consequent iron accumulation in the spleen, in the heme form. Frazer et al. (2012) observed that a chronic stimulated erythropoiesis led to an increase in liver iron and *Bmp6* mRNA levels and an unexpected decrease in hepatic *Hamp* mRNA levels. A similar profile was also observed in a model of hemolytic anemia, low serum iron status, and high tissue iron concentration, where a reduction in hepcidin expression occurs despite an increase in *Bmp6* expression (Frazer et al. 2012).

Despite all-trans retinoic acid (atRA) being considered the most active form of retinoids, rats treated with 12 mg/kg of atRA to replace retinyl ester presented decreased spleen, gut, and serum iron levels and low transferrin concentrations, in spite of their high liver iron store in relation to that of the control group (Additional file 1: Figure S1 and Additional file 2: Table S1). The low intestinal iron level may lead to the down-regulation of *Fpn1* mRNA levels in the atRA, since during cellular iron deprivation the iron regulatory protein (IRP1 or IRP2)/iron responsive element (IRE) system (IRP/IRE) represses ferroportin translation to reduce iron exportation and preserve cellular iron (Jiang et al. 2012; Galy et al. 2013; Sangokoya et al. 2013). Moreover, the atRA diet did not restore the levels of hepatic *Hamp* mRNA in the atRA group (Fig. 1) compared to those in the control group, and the expression of hepatic *Bmp6* and *Hfe2* genes that are involved in the activation of hepatic hepcidin expression through the BMP-SMAD-HJV pathway was similar to that obtained for the control group. The low systemic iron status of the atRA group in the present study may be responsible for the lower *Hamp* mRNA levels in the liver. Altogether, these contradictory results suggest that the single atRA dose used (12 mg/kg diet) must be suboptimal, either being too high or too low for the physiological needs of rats. Deviations in both directions are likely to induce an abnormal response (Martini et al. 1995).

Different proteins have been identified as negative regulators of hepcidin transcription, including the small mothers against decapentaplegic protein 7 (SMAD 7), which mediate a negative feedback response through the BMP pathway (Mleczko-Sanecka et al. 2010). SMAD 7 and *Hamp* are coregulated in the liver of iron-loaded mice, which suggests that a negative feedback loop is initiated by activating signals (Kautz et al. 2008). Consistent with the coregulation that has been proposed in the literature, the lower levels of hepcidin mRNA that were found in the FeD group were accompanied by down-regulation of hepatic *Smad7* mRNA levels, which corroborates the idea that systemic and tissue iron deficiency lead to low hepcidin concentrations and consequently decrease *Smad7* expression, the inhibitor of the BMP pathway. The down-regulation of hepatic *Smad7* mRNA levels in the VAD group may reflect the inhibition of hepcidin by the systemic iron deficiency, as the levels of *Smad7* and *Hamp* are coregulated in the liver. The association of both deficiencies (VAFeD group) reduced the iron concentrations in the liver, intestine, and spleen (Additional file 1: Figure S1), which may explain the down-regulation of *Hamp*, *Hfe2*, *Bmp6*, and *Smad7* hepatic mRNA levels compared to that of the VAD group (Fig. 1). These results suggest that iron plays a central role in the modulation of the expression of these genes.

Contrary to the present study, in our previous study (Arruda et al. 2009), an up-regulation of *Hamp* expression in VAD rats was observed. However, these apparent contradictory results may be explained by differences in rats' treatment. In the previous study, during the acclimatization period (8 days), the rats were maintained in a commercial rodent diet (Labina Purina/Brazil) with a concentration of vitamin A and iron six- and fivefold higher than the AIN-93G standardized diet, respectively. Considering that vitamin A is fat-soluble, these rats might have higher vitamin A content in the liver at the beginning of the experiment, which may have led to a late establishment of vitamin A deficiency and consequent difference in *Hamp* response, between the studies.

Besides the post-transcriptional regulation of intestinal ferroportin by the iron regulatory protein/iron responsive element (IRE) system in response to cellular iron content, duodenal iron absorption and exportation is also dramatically altered in response to changes in erythropoietic signal and hematological parameters. In the present study, the decrease in intestinal ferroportin mRNA levels in the vitamin A-deficient group may be associated with the decrease in kidney erythropoietin mRNA levels (Cunha et al. 2014) and decreased serum iron status once iron absorption and exportation is altered in response to changes in erythropoietic signal and hematological parameters. Srai et al (2010) showed that a nephrectomy rat model of chronic renal failure had decreased iron transport across the duodenal epithelium compared with sham-operated controls, and the treatment of these rats with Epo significantly increased iron absorption. Their findings suggest that Epo acts directly on intestinal enterocytes to regulate dietary absorption. Similar results were observed in Caco-2 cells treated with Epo, where higher protein and mRNA levels of intestinal DMT-1 and FPN led to increased iron uptake and efflux compared to those of the control cells.

Considering that a transgenic mouse, in which retinoid signaling is impaired specifically in hepatocytes, showed increased expression of hemojuvelin and hepcidin (Tsuchiya et al. 2009), we investigated if modulation of *Hamp* mRNA levels by vitamin A involves retinoic acid receptor (*Rarα*) or retinoid X receptor beta (*Rxrβ*). Although the atRA diet promoted up-regulation and the VAD diet promoted down-regulation of retinoic acid receptor (*Rarα*) mRNA levels in the liver, in both treatments, *Hamp* mRNA levels were reduced (Fig. 3). These results suggest that vitamin A deficiency influences hepcidin expression in an indirect way that does not involve the hepatic *Rarα* receptor.

Conclusions

In conclusion, this study demonstrates that the HJV-BMP6-SMAD signaling pathway that normally activates the expression of hepcidin in iron deficiency is impaired by vitamin A deficiency despite increased expression of liver *Bmp6* and *Hfe2* mRNA levels and decreased expression of Smad7 mRNA. The impairment of HJV-BMP6-SMAD signaling pathway may be associated to the systemic iron deficiency and spleen iron retention promoted by vitamin A deficiency.

Competing interests
Juliana F. R. Mendes, Egle M. de A. Siqueira, João Gabriel M. de B. e Silva, and Sandra F. Arruda declare that they have no conflict of interest.

Authors' contributions
The authors' contributions are as follows: JFRM and JGMBS conducted the animal experiment; JFRM and JGMBS conducted the laboratory work; JFRM, EMAS, and SFA prepared the manuscript; JFRM, EMAS, and SFA were responsible for the experimental design, interpretation of the results, and final version of the manuscript. All authors read and approved the findings of the study.

Acknowledgements
This study was financially supported by the Conselho Nacional de Desenvolvimento Científico e Tecnológico–CNPq, Coordenação de Aperfeiçoamento de Pessoal de Nível Superior (CAPES) and Decanato de Pesquisa e Pós-Graduação (DPP), University of Brasília, Brazil.

Author details
[1]Postgraduate Program in Human Nutrition, Faculty of Health Sciences, University of Brasília, Campus Universitário Darcy Ribeiro, POBox 70910-900, Brasília, DF, Brazil. [2]Cell Biology Department of Biological Sciences Institute, University of Brasília, Campus Universitário Darcy Ribeiro, POBox 70910-900, Brasília, DF, Brazil. [3]Nutrition Department of Health Sciences Faculty, University of Brasília, Campus Universitário Darcy Ribeiro, POBox 70910-900, Brasília, DF, Brazil. [4]Instituto de Ciências Biológicas, Departamento de Biologia Celular, Laboratório de Bioquímica da Nutrição, Universidade de Brasília, Campus Universitário Darcy Ribeiro, Bloco J, 1 Andar. Asa Norte, Brasília, Distrito Federal CEP: 70910-900, Brasil.

References
Anderson GJ, Frazera DM, McLaren GD (2009) Iron absorption and metabolism. Curr Opin Gastroenterol 25:129–135

Arruda SF, Siqueira EMA, Valencia FF (2009) Vitamin A deficiency increases hepcidin expression and oxidative stress in rat. Nutrition 25:472–478

Assunção MCF, Santos IS, Barros AJD et al (2007) Efeito da fortificação de farinhas com ferro sobre anemia em pré-escolares, Pelotas, RS. Rev Saúde Pública 41: 539–548

Brasil (2007) Ministério da Saúde e Unicef Cadernos de atenção básica: Carências de micronutrientes, Bethsáida de Abreu Soares Schmitz. Ministério da Saúde, Brasília

Citelli M, Bittencourt LL, Silva SV, Pierucci APT, Pedrosa C (2012) Vitamin A modulates the expression of genes involved in iron bioavailability. Biol Trace Elem Res 149:64–70

Corradini E, Meynard D, Wu Q, Chen S et al. (2011) Serum and liver iron differently regulate the bone morphogenetic protein 6 (BMP6)-SMAD signaling pathway in mice. Hepatology 54:273–284

Cunha MSB, Siqueira EMA, Trindade LS, Arruda SF (2014) Vitamin A deficiency modulates iron metabolism via ineffective erythropoiesis. J Nutr Biochem 25:1035–1044. doi:10.1016/j.jnutbio.2014.05.005

Evans T (2005) Regulation of hematopoiesis by retinoid signaling. Exp Hematol 33:1055–1061

Evstatiev R, Gasche C (2012) Iron sensing and signaling. Gut 61:933–952

Frazer DM, Wilkins SJ, Darshan D, Badrick AC et al (2012) Stimulated erythropoiesis with secondary iron loading leads to a decrease in hepcidin despite an increase in bone morpho-genetic protein 6 expression. Br J Haematol 157:615–626

Galy B, Ferring-Appel D, Becker C, Gretz N (2013) Iron regulatory proteins control a mucosal block to intestinal iron absorption. Cell Rep 28:844–857

Hentze MW, Muckenthaler MU, Galy B, Camaschella C (2010) Two to tango: regulation of mammalian iron metabolism. Cell 142:24–38

Jiang S, Wang C, Lan L, Zhao D (2012) Vitamin A deficiency aggravates iron deficiency by upregulating the expression of iron regulatory protein-2. Nutrition 28:281–287

Kautz L, Meynard D, Monnier A, Darnaud V et al (2008) Iron regulates phosphorylation of Smad1/5/8 and gene expression of Bmp6, Smad7, Id1, and Atoh8 in the mouse liver. Blood 112:1503–1509

Krijt J, Frýdlová J, Kukačková L, Fujikura Y et al (2012) Effect of iron overload and iron deficiency on liver hemojuvelin protein. PLoS One 7:e37391

Lee DH, Zhou LJ, Zhou Z, Xie JX et al (2010) Neogenin inhibits HJV secretion and regulates BMP-induced hepcidin expression and iron homeostasis. Blood 115:3136–3145

Martínez-Navarrete N, Camacho MM, Martínez-Lahuerta J, Martínez-Monzó J, Fito P (2002) Iron deficiency and iron fortified food—a review. Food Res Int 35:225–231

Martini R, Butler AM, Jiang XM, Murray M (1995) Pretranslational down regulation of cytochrome P450 2C11 in vitamin a-deficient male rat liver: prevention by dietary inclusion of retinoic acid. J Pharmacol Exp Ther 273(1):427–34

Mleczko-Sanecka K, Casanovas G, Ragab A, Breitkopf K et al (2010) SMAD7 controls iron metabolism as a potent inhibitor of hepcidin expression. Blood 115:2657–2665

Pagani A, Nai A, Corna G, Bosurgi L et al (2011) Low hepcidin accounts for the proinflammatory status associated with iron deficiency. Blood 118:736–746

Reeves PG, Nielsen FH, Fahey GC (1993) AIN-93 purified diets for laboratory rodents: final report of the American Institute of Nutrition ad hoc writing committee on the reformulation of the AIN-76a rodent diet. J Nutr 123: 1939–1951

Sangokoya C, Doss JF, Chi JT (2013) Iron-responsive miR-485-3p regulates cellular iron homeostasis by targeting ferroportin. Plos Genet 9:e1003408

Srai SK, Chung B, Marks J (2010) Erythropoietin regulates intestinal iron absorption in a rat model of chronic renal failure. Kidney Int 78:660–667

Strube YNJ, Beard JL, Ross AC (2002) Iron deficiency and marginal vitamin a deficiency affect growth, hematological indices and the regulation of iron metabolism genes in rats. J Nutr 132:3607–15

Theodosiou M, Laudet V, Schubert M (2010) From carrot to clinic: an overview of the retinoic acid signaling pathway. Cell Mol Life Sci 67:1423–1445

Tsuchiya H, Akechi Y, Ikeda R, Nishio R et al (2009) Suppressive effects of retinoids on iron-induced oxidative stress in the liver. Gastroenterology 136:341–350

Zhang AS (2010) Control of systemic iron homeostasis by the hemojuvelin-hepcidin axis. Adv Nutr 1:38–45. b

Zhang AS, Gao J, Koeberl DD, Enns CA (2010) The role of hepatocyte hemojuvelin in the regulation of bone morphogenic protein-6 and hepcidin expression in vivo. J Biol Chem 285:16416–16423. a

Zimmermann MB, Biebinger R, Rohner F, Dib A et al (2006) Vitamin A supplementation in children with poor vitamin A and iron status increases erythropoietin and hemoglobin concentrations without changing total body iron. Am J Clin Nutr 84:580–6

Ziouzenkova O, Plutzky J (2008) Retinoid metabolism and nuclear receptor responses: new insights into coordinated regulation of the PPAR–RXR complex. FEBS Lett 582:32–38

15

Protein-restricted diet during pregnancy after insemination alters behavioral phenotypes of the progeny

Tamio Furuse[1*], Kunio Miyake[2], Takashi Kohda[3], Hideki Kaneda[1], Takae Hirasawa[2], Ikuko Yamada[1], Tomoko Kushida[1], Misho Kashimura[1], Kimio Kobayashi[1], Fumitoshi Ishino[3], Takeo Kubota[2] and Shigeharu Wakana[1]

Abstract

Background: Epidemiological studies suggest that hyponutrition during the fetal period increases the risk of mental disorders such as attention deficit hyperactivity disorder and autism-spectrum disorder, which has been experimentally supported using animal models. However, previous experimental hyponutrition or protein-restricted (PR) diets affected stages other than the fetal stage, such as formation of the egg before insemination, milk composition during lactation, and maternal nursing behavior.

Results: We conducted in vitro fertilization and embryo transfer in mice and allowed PR diet and folic acid-supplemented PR diet to affect only fetal environments. Comprehensive phenotyping of PR and control-diet progenies showed moderate differences in fear/anxiety-like, novelty-seeking, and prosocial behaviors, irrespective of folic-acid supplementation. Changes were also detected in gene expression and genomic methylation in the brain.

Conclusions: These results suggest that epigenetic factors in the embryo/fetus influence behavioral and epigenetic phenotypes of progenies. Significant epigenetic alterations in the brains of the progenies induced by the maternal-protein restriction were observed in the present study. To our knowledge, this is first study to evaluate the effect of maternal hyponutrition on behavioral phenotypes using reproductive technology.

Keywords: Maternal nutrition, In vitro fertilization, Behavioral phenotypes, Gene expression and DNA methylation

Background

Genetic factors are known to influence susceptibility to psychiatric disorders, including schizophrenia, bipolar disorder, major depressive disorder, autism-spectrum disorder (ASD), and attention deficit hyperactivity disorder (AD/HD) [1]. However, recent studies have revealed that environmental and nutritional factors also affect neuronal functions, probably via epigenetic mechanisms [2–5]. In the field of metabolic diseases, "Developmental Origins of Health and Disease" (DOHaD) is the concept that in utero experiences reprogram susceptibility to adult metabolic diseases [6]. It is of interest to test if this concept is applicable to behavioral symptoms in developmental disorders such as AD/HD and ASD. Several studies using rodent models have been conducted to evaluate the effects of maternal hyponutrition on phenotypes of progenies. Restricted feeding in mothers of mice or rats caused body weight restriction, developmental anomalies, changes in metabolic phenotypes, patterns of gene expression, and DNA methylation in progenies [7]. Isocaloric diets, such as the protein restriction (PR) model, are fed in an alternative restriction of the diet [8, 9] by compensating shortage of energy source with carbohydrates [8]. Hence, protein-carbohydrate balance is altered in the PR, making it suitable for evaluating the effects of maternal nutritional imbalance, and not that of calorie shortage [10]. Several reports have examined the interactions between maternal-protein restriction and adult phenotypic/epigenetic alterations [8, 11–13].

* Correspondence: tfuruse@brc.riken.jp
[1]Japan mouse clinic, RIKEN BRC, 3-1-1 Koyadai, Tsukuba, Ibaraki 305-0074, Japan
Full list of author information is available at the end of the article

Maternal PR diet, however, affects not only fetal environments but also formation of the egg before insemination, nutritional condition of maternal milk, and maternal nursing behavior, and therefore, it has potential confounding variables at different stages. In the present study, we performed in vitro fertilization (IVF) to produce neonates and then obtained progenies that were adopted by foster mothers before weaning. This allowed the PR diet to affect only the fetal stage of development.

Methods

Ethics statement of animal experiments

All procedures described here were reviewed and approved by the Institutional Animal Care and Use Committee of RIKEN Tsukuba Branch and were performed in accordance with the RIKEN Guiding Principles for the Care and Use of Laboratory Animals (No. 10-013).

Experimental design

The experimental design is described briefly in Fig. 1. IVF and embryo transfer (ET) techniques were used for mouse production. Female ICR mice, an outbred stock from the Swiss mouse developed in the Institute of Cancer Research [14], were used as recipient and foster mothers. Embryos were generated by fertilizing the eggs and sperm of C57BL/6J (B6) mice that had consumed a normal diet (CE-2, CLEA Japan, Inc., Tokyo, Japan). CE-2 is a rodent diet used for rearing and breeding. The diet consists of crude sources of protein (soybean waste, white-fish meal, and yeast), fat (cereal germ and soybean oil), and carbohydrate (wheat flour and corn). Detailed ingredients of the CE-2 diet are described on the webpage of the supplier (http://www.clea-japan.com/en/diets/diet_a/a_03.html). AIN93G control diet (CD), protein-restricted diet (PR), and protein-restricted diet supplemented with folic acid (FA) were used as experimental diets in recipient mothers beginning 1 month before ET until delivery. The nutrient sources of these experimental diets are described in Table 1. Neonates were adopted by ICR foster mothers immediately after cesarean section. After weaning, we provided the CD to the progenies. The body weight of the mothers and progenies, clinical biochemistry of the recipient mothers, gene expression in the brain of the progenies, and behavioral phenotypes of the progenies were examined.

Experimental diets

The CD was very similar to the standard formation of AIN93G [15]. Test diets were modified from AIN93G formulation as follows: PR, ratio of vitamin-free casein was decreased from 20 to 5%; FA, 0.8 g/kg of folic acid was added to the PR (Table 1). The CD and PR contained 0.02% folic acid (weight composition) and the FA contained 0.1% folic acid (weight composition). Experimental diets were purchased from a commercial supplier (Oriental yeast Co. Ltd, Tokyo, Japan). These diets were isocaloric (4 kcal/g in each feed) and fed to the recipient mothers ad libitum. In addition, only the CD diet was fed to the foster mothers ad libitum.

Mice

All mice used as recipient and foster mothers, as well as for egg and sperm collection, were purchased from a commercial supplier (CLEA Japan, Inc.).

In vitro fertilization and embryo transfer

We conducted IVF and ET as previously described [16] to produce mice for behavioral tests, expression array, and DNA-methylation analysis of brains. In brief, sperm was collected from the caudae epididymides of 25-week-old B6 males and allowed to diffuse in fertilization medium. After preincubation for approximately 1 h to allow for capacitation, the sperm was used for insemination. Meanwhile, 3-week-old female mice ($N = 7$) were superovulated using intraperitoneal injections of PMSG and HCG (serotropin and gonatropin; ASKA Pharmaceutical Co., Tokyo, Japan) with an interval of 48 h between injections. Approximately 15–17 h after the HCG injection, the oocytes-cumulus complexes were collected from the oviducts of superovulated female B6 mice. Then, the complexes from several female mice were placed in fertilization medium. Insemination was performed by adding the preincubated sperm suspension to the fertilization medium containing complexes and cultured at 37 °C with 5% CO_2. 24 h after insemination, 24 2-cell embryos were transferred into the oviducts of pseudopregnant ICR females (CLEA Japan, Inc.) mated to vasectomized ICR males. ICR females that consumed experimental diets were used as pseudopregnant recipients for the ET. Female ICR mice were purchased at 4 to 5 weeks of age, and introduced to the facility for experiments. These mice were split randomly into three groups; CD, PR, and FA. The foster mothers consumed the experimental diets beginning 4 weeks before ET and continuing until delivery. Body weight of recipient mice was measured once per week until delivery via cesarean section [17]. We used only male progeny for behavioral, genomic methylation, and gene expression analyses. Maternal separation in early life alters behavioral phenotypes, gene expression, and brain functions of mice [18, 19]. Hence, newborn male mice had to be adopted by foster mothers immediately after cesarean section (6–7 neonates/foster mother), and body weights were not measured. However, we measured body weights of female neonates to determine the effects of maternal hyponutrition on birth weight of offspring immediately after cesarean section. In order to reduce the number of foster mothers, only males were adopted by foster mothers.

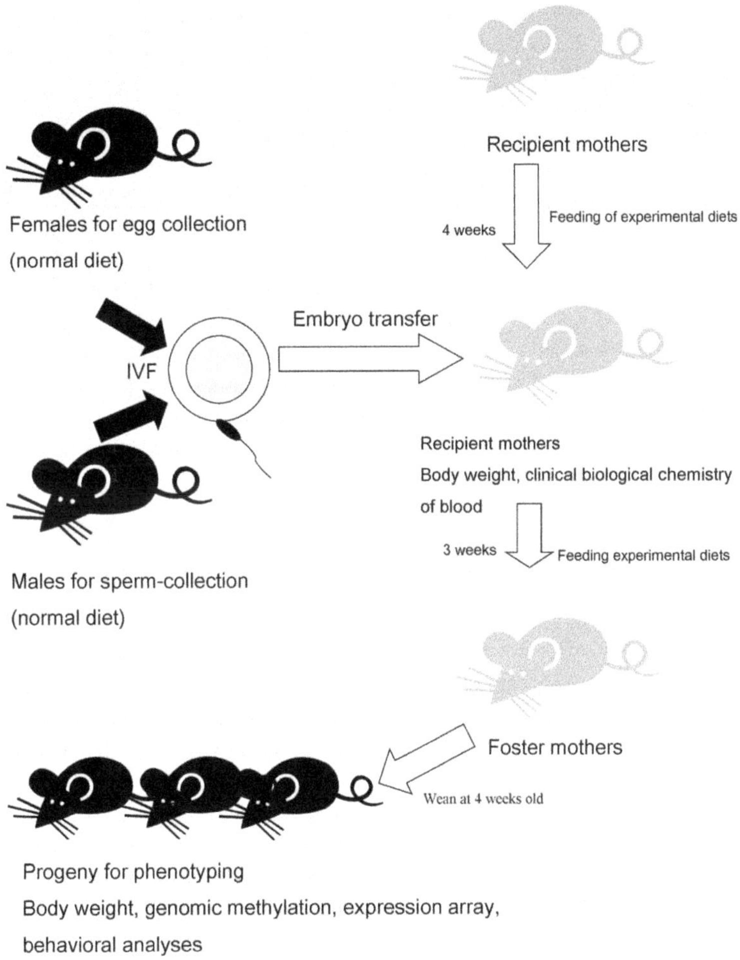

Fig. 1 Experimental strategy. The experimental design of this study is briefly described. Normal diet (CE-2) was fed to females used for oocyte collection and males used for sperm collection. Recipient mothers consumed the control diet (CD) or experimental diet (PR and FA) for 1 month before embryo transfer. Embryos were generated by fertilizing the eggs with sperm of C57BL/6J (B6) mice. After cesarean-section delivery, neonates were fostered by ICR females that had consumed CD, PR, or FA diets. After weaning, offspring consumed the control diet (CD). Serum was separated from blood taken from the ICR females. Brain tissue was collected from offspring after behavioral tests

Clinical-biochemical test

We carried out a clinical-biochemical test using serum collected from ICR females at 13 weeks of age. The mice consumed experimental diets for 7 weeks. Blood collection, separation of serum, and analysis was performed as previously described [20]. In brief, we collected 200 μl of blood from the retro-orbital sinus using a Pasteur pipette (Thermo Fisher Scientific Inc., Waltham, MA). The collected blood was transferred to a microtube containing Coagulant Wako solution (Wako Pure Chemical Industries Co, Osaka, Japan) and serum was separated by centrifuging twice (600–2500×*g* for 5–15 min). We measured total protein (TP), urea nitrogen (UN), albumin (ALB), total cholesterol (T-CHO), HDL-cholesterol (HDL-C), triglyceride (TG), and LDL-cholesterol (LD-C) in the serum with an automatic clinical-biochemistry analyzer (JCA-BM2250, JEOL, Ltd., Tokyo, Japan). Number of subjects: CD, 7; PR, 7; FA, 6.

DNA/RNA extraction

We harvested whole brains from adult male progenies (19 weeks of age) that were used in behavioral analyses, methylation analyses, and expression arrays. Adult males were euthanized via cervical dislocation. Brain samples were rinsed with PBS and frozen immediately using liquid nitrogen. The frozen tissues were stored at −80 °C. RNA and DNA were extracted simultaneously using an AllPrep DNA/RNA Mini Kit (Qiagen, Valencia, CA, USA) from the whole brains, including cerebrum and cerebellum. We then performed gene methylation and expression arrays as described below.

Table 1 Components of experimental diets

Component	Composition (% weight)		
	CD	PR	FA
Vitamin-free casein	20	5.0	5.0
L-cystine	0.3	0.077	0.077
Corn starch	39.7486	51.1716	51.1716
Alpha-corn starch	13.2	17.0	17.0
Sucrose	10.0	10.0	10.0
Soy bean oil	7.0	7.0	7.0
Cellulose powder	5.0	5.0	5.0
AIN-93G mineral mixture	3.5	3.5	3.5
AIN-93 vitamin mixture	1.0	1.0	1.0
Folic acid	0.02	0.02	0.1
Choline bitartrate	0.25	0.25	0.25
Tertiary butylhydroquinone	0.0014	0.0014	0.0014
Total	100.0	100.0	100.0

CD control diet, *PR* protein-restricted diet, *FA* PR diet with supplemental-folic acid

Genomic methylation

Genome-wide DNA methylation analysis was performed as previously reported with slight modification [21]. Genomic DNA was fragmented with methylation-insensitive restriction enzymes (*Mse*I, *Bfa*I, and *CSP*6I) to yield fragments ranging in size from 200 to 1000 base pairs. The enrichment of methylated DNA was performed using the MethylMiner Methylated DNA Enrichment kit (Thermo Fisher Scientific Inc.). Briefly, CpG-dense methylated DNA was isolated from fragmented genomic DNA via binding to the methyl-CpG domain of the MBD2 protein, which is coupled to paramagnetic Dynabeads M-280 streptavidin via a biotin linker. A portion of the fragmented DNA (input) was left untreated and used as a control. DNA was amplified and cleaned using the GenomePlex Complete Whole Genome Amplification (WGA) Kit and GenElute PCR Clean-Up Kit (Sigma-Aldrich St. Louis, MO, USA). For analysis of genomic methylation, we used the Mouse Promoter 1.0R Array (Affymetrix) against methylated (IP) and input DNA (IN). Number of subjects: CD, 3; PR, 4; FA, 4.

Expression array

Expression analysis by DNA microarray was performed with the Agilent system (G4846A; Whole Mouse Genome Microarray Kit (4x44K) Agilent Technologies, Santa Clara, CA, USA). The probes for the microarray were prepared and labeled by Cy3 according to the manufacturer's protocol (Agilent Technologies). Arrays were scanned with a G2505C Microarray Scanner System (Agilent Technologies). Data were normalized using the *R* stats package with the qspline function of the "affy" package in the Bioconductor [22].

Validity of the methylation and expression array data

Results of methylation array analyses have been validated in previous studies [21, 23]. In these studies, the array-based methylation quantification data showed strong concordance with results obtained from bisulfite sequencing ($r = 0.81$ to 0.88) [21, 24]. In addition, expression array data was also validated in previous studies. Expression data obtained by the one color microarray platform showed strong concordance with a TaqMan assay ($r = 0.876$) in a large scale microarray quality control project [25].

Data availability

Expression and methylation array data were deposited in the NCBI gene expression omnibus (http://www.ncbi.nlm.nih.gov/geo/) and accession numbers of the datasets are as follows: GSE79847.

Behavioral tests

We performed the following behavioral tests: open-field test (6-weeks-old), object-exploration test (7-weeks-old), social-interaction test (8-weeks-old), home-cage activity test (9 to 10-weeks-old), light/dark-transition test (11-weeks-old), fear-conditioning test (12-weeks-old), and tail-suspension test (13-weeks-old). Results of the behavioral tests are sensitive to prior experiences [26]. To suppress effects of prior experiences, the behavioral tests were performed in order of less stimulation as described above. We used male mice for the behavioral tests in order to eliminate the effects of the estrous cycle in females. Number of subjects: CD, 10; PR, 10; FA, 7.

Open-field test

Open-field test was performed as previously described [27]. Each mouse was placed in the corner of an open-field apparatus (400 mm wide × 400 mm long × 300 mm high; O'Hara & Co., Ltd., Tokyo, Japan) made of white polyvinyl chloride. The distance traveled by each animal in the open-field was recorded for 20 min with a video-imaging system (Image OF9; O'Hara & Co., Ltd.).

Object-exploration test

We performed an object-exploration test as previously described [27]. Briefly, each mouse was placed in the open-field apparatus without the novel object for 20 min of acclimation before testing. A transparent acrylic tube (bottom diameter, 66 mm; top diameter, 44 mm; height, 154 mm) containing marbles was placed in the center of the open-field. The total time spent exploring the object and frequency of exploration during a 10 min period was determined with a commercial video-imaging system (O'Hara & Co., Ltd.). Exploration was defined as a distance of < 1 cm between the object and the mouse.

Social-interaction test

A social-interaction test was performed as previously described [27]. We used a procedure similar to the object-exploration test to examine social-interaction behavior in mice. A mouse was positioned in the center of the open-field apparatus with an empty transparent acrylic tube and habituated for 20 min. Then, the empty tube was exchanged for another tube containing a novel male mouse, which was placed in the center of the open field. The total time spent exploring the novel mouse and the frequency of exploration during a 10-min period was determined by video-imaging.

Home-cage activity

A home-cage activity test was performed as previously described [27]. Each mouse was placed alone in a testing cage (227 × 329 × 133 mm) under a 12 h light–dark cycle (light on at 08:00 am) and had free access to both food and water. After 1 day of acclimation, spontaneous activity in the cage was measured for 5 days (starting at 08:00 am) using an infrared sensor (activity sensor, O'Hara & Co., Ltd.).

Light/dark transition test

A light/dark transition test was performed as described previously [27]. A commercially available light/dark chamber (O'Hara & Co., Ltd.) consisting of a light chamber (200 mm long × 200 mm wide × 250 mm high) made of white vinyl chloride plates and a dark chamber with the same dimensions made of black vinyl chloride plates was used. The apparatus had an opening (50 mm wide × 30 mm high) in the middle of the wall joining the two chambers. The opening was controlled by a guillotine door. The number of transitions between chambers, time spent in the light chamber, and the total distance traveled by the mouse were measured.

Fear-conditioning test

We performed a fear-conditioning test as previously described [28] with slight modification. On the training day (day 1), each mouse was placed in a shock chamber with white walls (O'Hara & Co. Ltd.) (box A) and 120 s later, 4 tone-shock pairs were given at 90 s intervals. Each tone-shock pair consisted of a tone (70 dB, 10 kHz) for 30 s and a foot shock for 2 s at 0.5 mA. The foot shock was presented to the mice during the last 2 s of the tone. On day 2, each mouse was placed back in box A for 6 min to measure contextual freezing. On day 3, each mouse was placed in a white transparent chamber (box B), and 180 s later, 180 s tones were delivered. Freezing was measured during the first 180 s in box B, representing the response to an unconditioned context, and then during the next 180 s in the presence of the conditioned tone.

Tail-suspension test

In order to examine depression-like behavior in the progenies, a tail-suspension test was performed as described previously [29] with slight modifications. The tail of the mouse was fixed to a metal plate using adhesive tape. Then, the mouse was suspended from the metal plate in an experimental box (400 mm × 400 mm × 300 mm; O'Hara and Co., Ltd.). The duration of immobility of the mouse was measured using a video-analysis system (O'Hara & Co., Ltd.) for 6 min.

Statistical analyses

Body weights, blood biochemistry, and behavioral tests

For the behavioral tests, we analyzed the data obtained from each group using one-way or two-way ANOVA. In case of a significant difference detected by ANOVAs, post-hoc analysis (Fisher's PLSD) was performed.

Methylation analysis

For the methylation analysis, microarray data were analyzed using Partek Genomics Suite software (PGS) 6.6 (Partek, Inc.). Data normalization was performed by the default method, including adjusting the probe sequence, RMA Background Correction, Quantile Normalization, and Log (base 2) transformation [23]. Data quality was assessed using PCA and the application of Partek's quality control workflow. The baseline normalization was performed using the matched-pair normalization tool in PGS, by subtracting the average of IN signals from each IP signal. To detect the MBD binding (methylated) regions in PR or FA relative to CD, we performed a one-way ANOVA and calculated the fold change using geometric mean. Significant region detection (hypermethylation and hypomethylation) was performed using hidden Markov model (HMM) tool in PGS as previously reported [23]. Briefly, in order to capture significant differences in enrichment in PR or FA vs CD across shorter genomic regions (min. ~350 nucleotides) with robust enrichment differences as well as intermediate (min. ~500 nucleotides) and large regions (min. ~1400 nucleotides), three HMM algorithms were applied (s-HMM, m-HMM, and l-HMM). The following cutoffs were used: s-HMM (min. probes: 5, detection states: −5,5, ignore state: 0, max. probability: 0.99, genomic decay: 10000, sigma: 2), m-HMM (min. probes: 10, detection states: −3,3, ignore state: 0, max. probability: 0.99, genomic decay: 10000, sigma: 1), and l-HMM (min. probes: 40, detection states: −1.5,1.5, ignore state: 0, max. probability: 0.99, genomic decay: 10000, sigma: 1).

Gene expression

To determine the genes that showed differential expression among the three experimental groups, Tukey's multiple comparison was performed, and the resultant *P* value was adjusted by Benjamini and Hochberg false discovery rate (BHFDR) to correct multiple tests using the *R* package. Statistical significance was assumed at $P < 0.0001$. The genes that were expressed differently among the groups at the twofold or 0.5-fold change and $P < 0.0001$ level after the BHFDR were regarded as differentially expressed genes. Venn diagrams list of differentially methylated and expressed genes were drawn using the *R* package with the "VennDiagram" function.

Results

Body weight and protein-related parameters of recipient mothers

The experimental design is briefly described in Fig. 1. The three different diets used in this study were protein-restricted (PR), folic acid-supplemented PR (FA), and the control diet (CD) (Table 1). Folic acid is a critical co-enzyme for DNA methylation and may affect epigenetic modification [30]. Oocytes and sperm were obtained from females and males, respectively, which were fed a normal diet (CE-2). In vitro fertilized eggs were transferred to three different kinds of ICR recipient mothers that consumed the PR, FA, or control diet (CD) 1 month before the embryo transfer. Fetuses/neonates were obtained by caesarian section from mothers at 20 days of gestation, and immediately transferred into the care of an ICR foster mother that had consumed the PR, FA, or CD diet. After weaning, offspring consumed the CD. Figure 2a shows average body weights of the recipient mothers of the three different dietary conditions. Similar increases in body weight were observed between the CD and the PR groups at 6–11 weeks of age before ET from B6 mice (two-way ANOVA (Additional file 1)). However, 1 and 2 weeks after the ET (12–13 weeks age), recipient mothers of the PR and FA groups exhibited significantly lower body weights than that of the CD group (two-way ANOVA (Additional file 1)) (Fig. 2a). We performed clinical-biochemical tests in ICR females at 13 weeks of age that consumed experimental diets for 7 weeks. Serum levels of protein-related components such as TP, UN, and ALB (Fig. 2b–d) were significantly lower in the PR and FA groups than in the CD group (one-way ANOVA (Additional file 1)). This may be consistent with differences in body weight. However, as for parameters related to lipid metabolism, levels of total T-CHO and HDL-C were higher in the PR and FA groups than in the CD group (one-way ANOVA (Additional file 1)) (Fig. 2e, f), whereas the TG level was lower (one-way ANOVA (Additional file 1)) (Fig. 2g). We also measured body weights of their progenies from postnatal day 0 and 4 to 12 weeks of age (Additional file 2: Figure S1 A and B). No difference was observed among the three groups with ANOVA, indicating little effect of food components on body weight gain of the progeny (one-way ANOVA (Additional file 1)). In addition, no difference was detected in the performance of embryo transfer among the three groups (Additional file 3: Table S1).

Effects of maternal-protein restriction on behavioral phenotypes of progeny

Several tests were performed to examine the behaviors of progenies, and some showed significant changes due to the maternal metabolic changes described above. The open-field test examining locomotor activity in novel place, an indicator for fear/anxiety-like behavior, showed differences between the study groups. We failed to detect changes in the distance that mice traveled in the open-field arena among the three different progenies (two-way ANOVA (Additional file 1)) (Fig. 3a) but found shorter times or durations spent in the center area (30% of the whole arena) in the PR and FA groups than that in the CD group of mice at 7 weeks of age (two-way ANOVA (Additional file 1)) (Fig. 3b). This indicates increased fear/anxiety like behavior in the PR and FA groups [31]. The object-exploration test examining novelty seeking behavior also showed differences between the study groups. In this test, the duration of active contacts to a novel object was decreased in the PR group relative to that of the CD group (two-way ANOVA (Additional file 1)) (Fig. 3c). In addition, the number of contacts with the object was significantly decreased in the PR and FA groups (two-way ANOVA (Additional file 1)) (Fig. 3d). The social interaction test examining prosocial behavior of mice found that the PR and FA groups exhibited shorter durations of active contacts with a novel mouse than that of the CD group (two-way ANOVA (Additional file 1)) (Fig. 3e), as well as decreased number of contacts (two-way ANOVA (Additional file 1)) (Fig. 3f).

We failed to detect differences in the other tests, such as fear-related behavior in a light/dark-transition test (one-way ANOVA (Additional file 1)) (Additional file 4: Figure S2A–C), contextual and cued learning and memory (one-way ANOVA (Additional file 1)) (Additional file 5: Figure S3A, B), and depressive behavior in a tail-suspension test (one-way ANOVA (Additional file 1)) (Additional file 6: Figure S4) between the three groups. Figure 3g–i shows the effect of supplemented folic acid on locomotor activity, which was measured by the home-cage activity test in a familiar setting and daily activity patterns under a light and dark cycle. The mean activity over 5 days in the home cage is expressed as the activity during the light phase (Fig. 3g), activity during the dark phase (Fig. 3h), and activity patterns during the light/dark cycle (Fig. 3i). During the light phase, no difference was observed in the locomotor activity among all groups (one-way ANOVA (Additional file 1)) (Fig. 3i).

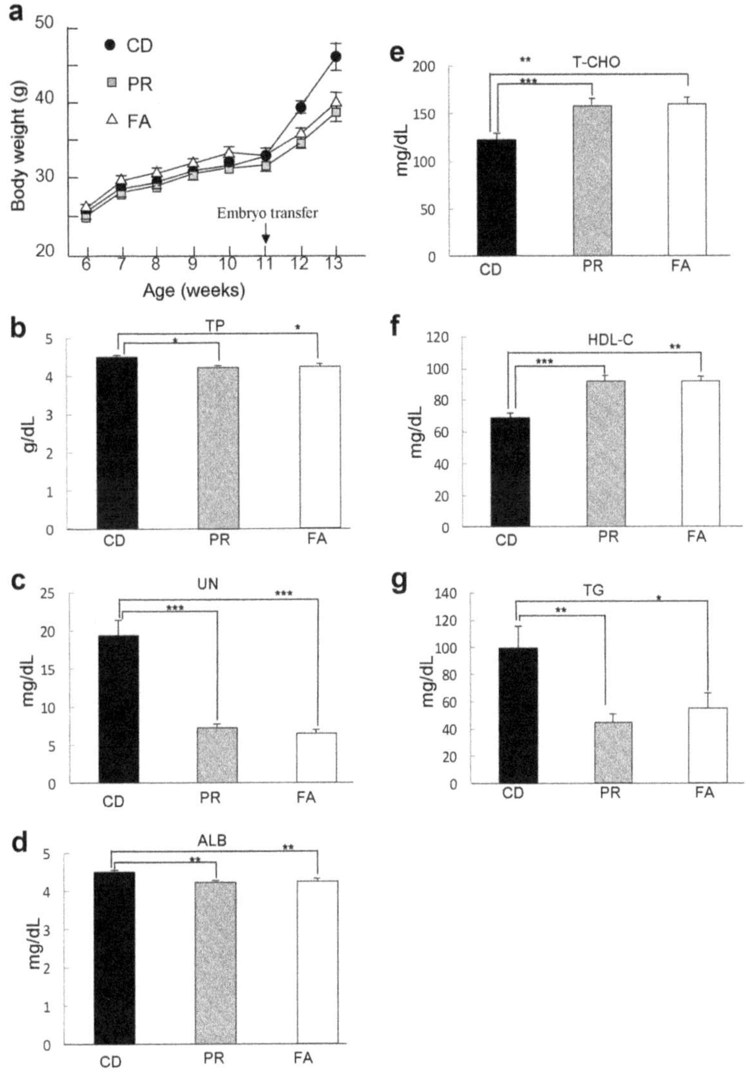

Fig. 2 Body weight changes in recipient mothers and serum levels of clinical-biochemical parameters in ICR females. **a** Body weights of recipient mothers is shown. *Arrowhead* indicates the day of embryo transfer. Number of subjects: CD, 11; PR, 14; FA, 14. **b–h** Serum levels of clinical biochemical parameters in ICR females. (**b**), total protein (TP); (**c**), urea nitrogen (UN); (**d**), albumin (ALB); (**e**), total cholesterol (T-CHO); (**f**), HDL cholesterol (HDL-C); (**g**), triglyceride (TG) in ICR females that consumed CD, PR, and FA for 1 month are shown. Number of subjects, CD, 7; PR, 7; FA, 6. **a–g** *Data* represent the mean ± SEM. *Asterisks* indicate significant differences between groups in post hoc analyses (Fisher's PLSD test, ***: $P < 0.0001$, **: $P < 0.01$, *: $P < 0.05$)

In dark phase, the PR group showed higher locomotor activity than that of the CD groups (one-way ANOVA (Additional file 1)) (Fig. 3h), and interestingly, this increase was abrogated by folic acid supplementation (one-way ANOVA (Additional file 1)) (Fig. 3h). No difference, however, was observed in the locomotor activity patterns between PR and FA groups (Fig. 3i).

Collectively, these results suggest that PR diet in recipient mothers, irrespective of FA supplementation, enhances susceptibility to fear/anxiety-like, novelty seeking, and prosocial behaviors of progenies.

Effect of protein restriction on epigenetic alterations

One may expect to find differences in genomic methylation and gene expression among the three different groups. Thus, we performed genome-wide DNA methylation analysis of the three study groups by MBD-chip. The raw data was analyzed using Partek Genome Suite (PGS) software to detect the significantly differentially enrichment regions, as previously reported (see methods). A total of 292 HMM regions exhibited lower promoter methylation levels in the PR group than in the CD group (Additional file 7), whereas 264 HMM regions were higher in the PR group (Additional file 8). A total

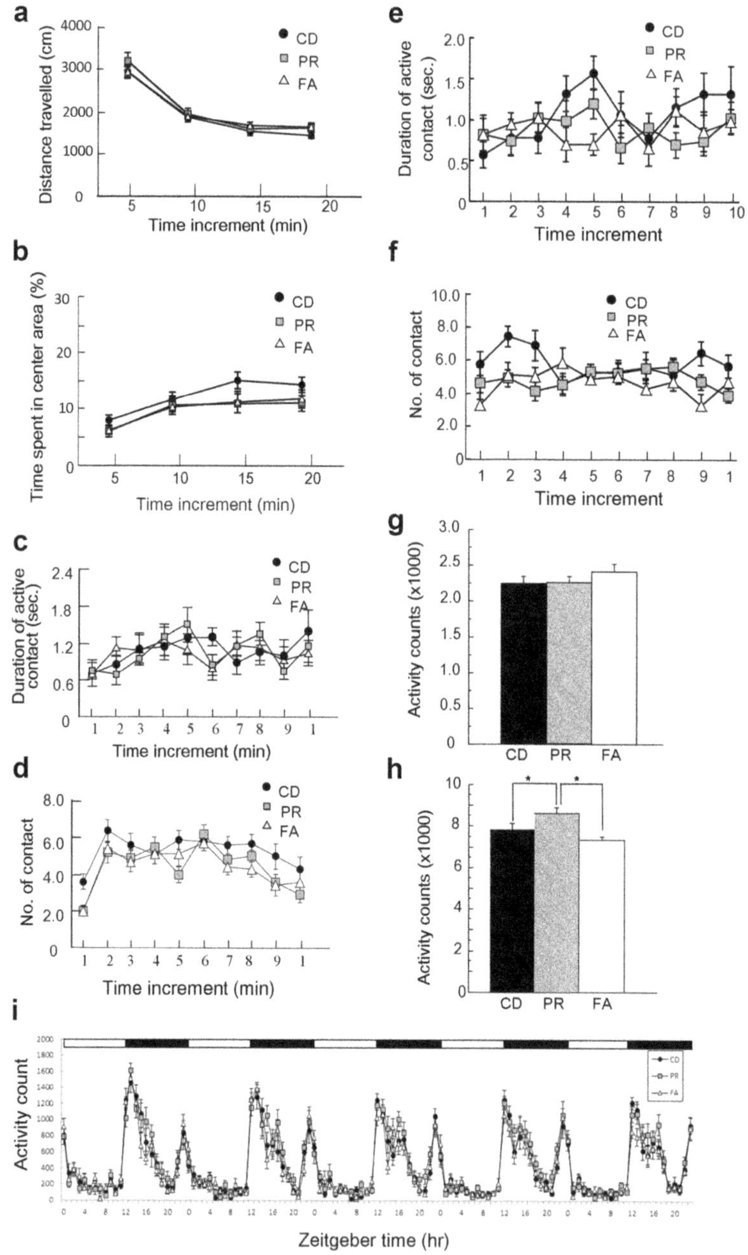

Fig. 3 Results of behavioral tests of progenies. **a**, **b** Results of open-field test at 7 weeks of age. **a** Locomotor activity patterns during the open-field test at 7 weeks of age. **b** Time spent in the center (30% of the open-field arena) at 7 weeks of age. **c**, d Results of object-exploration test. **c** Time spent exploring a novel object. **d** Number of times mice that made contact with a novel object. **e**, **f** Results of social-interaction test. **e** Time spent exploring a novel mouse. Number of subjects: CD, 9; PR, 10; FA, 7. **f** Number of times mice made contact with a novel mouse. **g**–**i** Locomotor activity of mice in their home cages. **g** Mean locomotor activity during the light period. **h** Mean locomotor activity in the home cage during the dark period. **i** Locomotor activity in the home cage during the light/dark cycle. **a**–**i** Number of subjects: CD, 10; PR, 10; FA, 7. *Data* represent the mean ± SEM. *Asterisks* indicate significant differences between groups in post hoc analyses (Fisher's PLSD test, *: $P < 0.05$)

of 392 genes significantly differed between the PR and the CD group in methylation level. A total of 272 HMM regions exhibited lower promoter methylation levels in the FA group than in the CD group (Additional file 9), whereas 222 HMM regions were higher in the PR group (Additional file 10). A total of 383 genes significantly differed between the FA and the CD group in methylation level. A total of 169 HMM regions exhibited lower promoter methylation levels in the FA group than in the PR group (Additional file 11), whereas 127 HMM regions were higher in the PR group (Additional file 12). A total of 211 genes significantly differed between the FA and the CD group in methylation level. In the expression array, there were 25 genes with lower expression levels (less than 0.5 fold change and $P < 0.0001$ level after the BHFDR) and 55 with higher expression levels (greater than 2.0 fold change and $P < 0.0001$ level after the BHFDR) (Additional files 13 and 14) in the PR group relative to the CD group. There were 48 genes with lower expression levels (less than 0.5-fold change and $P < 0.0001$ level after the BHFDR) and 81 with higher expression levels (greater than 2.0-fold change and $P < 0.0001$ level after the BHFDR) (Additional files 15 and 16) in the PR group relative to the CD group. There were 2 genes with lower expression levels (less than 0.5-fold change and $P < 0.0001$ level after the BHFDR) and 3 with higher expression levels (greater than 2.0-fold change and $P < 0.0001$ level after the BHFDR) (Additional files 17 and 18) in the FA group relative to the PR group. In addition, differentially expressed genes in the PR and FA groups relative to the CD group did not intersect with differentially methylated genes in the PR and FA groups relative to the CD group.

Discussion

In the present study, we examined the effect of maternal hyponutrition because of a PR diet on developmental and mental disorders of the progenies by comprehensive phenotyping of behaviors. The examination included seven different assays for fear/anxiety-like, novelty seeking, and prosocial behaviors, as well as others that may be related to AD/HD- and ASD-like behaviors. We found significant differences in the assays for fear/anxiety-like, novelty seeking, and prosocial behaviors, which suggests that environmental factors in the embryo/fetus play an important role in the susceptibility of the progenies to these behaviors. This may be parallel to epidemiological studies showing that environmental or nutritional factors affect behavioral symptoms of AD/HD [32] and ASD [33].

A previous study on diet-induced effects reported an increase in the locomotor activity and a lower birth weight of progeny without weight loss in mothers [9]. However, it was conducted under conditions of natural fecundation that did not exclude confounding variables such as the formation of the egg before insemination, milk composition during lactation, and maternal nursing behavior. To exclude those confounding or additional factors pre and postgestation, we used IVF, which allowed us to examine only the effect of diet-induced environmental changes in utero during implantation and gestation. A similar attempt was performed in a recent study examining a transgenerational effect of diet on metabolic diseases [34]. In addition, we used a PR diet supplemented with folic acid to exclude the effect of folic acid on DNA methylation-mediated epigenetic modification. In fact, Lillycrop et al. reported that FA supplementation prevents epigenetic modification of hepatic gene expression in offspring [8]. As expected, the PR and FA diets caused differences in gene expression and genomic methylation in the brains of adult progenies. However, only a moderate proportion of the differences between PR and CD diets were abrogated by FA supplementation. In addition, the FA group showed a different methylation pattern relative to that of the PR group, whereas adult progenies of FA group exhibited behavioral alterations similar to those in the PR group. These results suggest a moderate contribution of FA to the effects of PR on behaviors. Analysis of recipient mothers showed decreases in protein-related components in serum such as TP, UN, and ALB, as well as the triglyceride levels, which were consistent with a decrease in body weight of the mothers, and increases in levels of total cholesterol, HDL-C, and LDL-C. These changes may underlie environmental changes in utero during implantation and gestation, which could cause susceptibility of the offspring.

Several reports have examined AD/HD and ASD mouse models lacking certain gene functions [35–38]. AD/HD models lacking genes related to the dopaminergic system clearly exhibited a deficiency in sustained attention and elevated locomotor activity [35, 38], whereas ASD models lacking genes related with functions of GABAergic and oxytocin related neurons showed decreased social approach [39] and increased fear/anxiety-like behaviors [40]. These behavioral alterations were observed in this study, but the level of differences was moderate. In a previous report, the progenies of B6 mothers that consumed a protein-restricted diet were found to have a lower birth weight relative to the control group; however, the body weight of the mothers were not altered [9]. In the study, the B6 strain was used for mothers and DBA/2 strain was used for fathers of progenies [9], whereas in the present study we used ICR females as recipient mothers and B6 as the source of the embryo. We provided experimental diets to pre-pregnant and pregnant ICR females, and the females that consumed the PR and FA diets exhibited abnormal metabolism of protein relative to the CD group in a clinical-biochemical test. This did not result in lower body weight of these pre-pregnant females; however, pregnant females of the PR group exhibited significantly lower body weight relative to the CD group. Additionally, the progenies of the PR group did not exhibit lower birth weights. Although the amount of protein in the PR group was sufficient for development in newborn mice, it might have been insufficient for body weight gain in the pregnant females. According to the observed phenotype of mice in our previous study [41], the body mass of the ICR strain is much larger than that of the B6 strain. Thus, accumulated protein source in the ICR females may have compensated for the insufficient protein diet in the fetuses of the PR group. In addition, neonates from the ICR females that were fed experimental diets were nursed by the foster mothers that were fed the CD. IVF and ET, which are assisted reproductive technologies, are thought to induce epigenetic changes in the embryo and to alter the adult phenotype in humans [42]. Hence, these differences in experimental conditions resulted in different behavioral phenotypes exhibited by the progenies in the present and previous studies. Therefore, pre-insemination and postnatal/lactation effects of maternal hyponutrition may play a similarly important part in determining offspring behavioral phenotypes.

As in a previous study [9], the present study used only male mice for the behavioral tests in order to eliminate phenotypic variation in female mice caused by the desynchronization of the estrous cycle. The B6 mouse exhibits sex dimorphisms in several behavioral phenotypes, including motor function in the rotarod test, learning and memory in the Morris water-maze test and the fear conditioning test, and locomotor activity in the open-field test [43]. The moderate effects of maternal protein restriction on behavioral phenotypes of the progenies observed in the present study may be gender-specific phenomena.

The methylation levels of promoters in these genes were not correlated with expression levels of the genes. The epigenetic alterations in the brain of the progenies induced by the maternal-protein restriction were clearly observed in the present study. A causal link between epigenetic and behavioral alterations remains to be investigated.

The results of the present study suggest that although maternal protein restriction during pregnancy is a moderate risk factor for developmental or mental disorders of the progeny, it may be substantiated by interaction with genetic factors, including specific mutations or genetic variations. In addition, pre-insemination and postnatal/lactation effects of maternal hyponutrition may significantly contribute to the phenotype.

To verify this hypothesis, it may be necessary to examine the effect of hyponutritional exposure in utero on known developmental disorder models, such as AD/HD and ASD models, or other mouse strains, and to clarify the additive consequences or interaction for behavioral phenotypes.

Conclusions

The PR group exhibited fear/anxiety related behaviors and inattention to a novel object or a novel mouse more than those of the control diet group. As might be expected, adult brains of the PR group exhibited differences in patterns of the expression array analysis and of genomic-methylation.

Environmental factors in the embryo/fetus play an important role in susceptibility to alteration of progenies' behaviors. The present study is, to our knowledge, the first to evaluate the effect of maternal hyponutrition on behavioral phenotypes using reproductive technology.

Additional files

Additional file 1: Values of the statistical analysis.

Additional file 2: Figure S1. Body-weight changes in progeny. (A) Body weight of progeny immediately after delivery with caesarean section is shown. Number of subjects: CD, 9; PR, 6; FA, 5. Female neonates were used. (B) Body weight of progeny at 4 to 12 weeks of age is shown. Number of subjects: CD, 10; PR, 10; FA, 7. Male mice were used. Data represent the mean ± SEM.

Additional file 3: Table S1. Performance of embryo transfer in recipient mothers. Mean litter sizes of offspring from each recipient mother are shown. Twenty-four embryos (2-cell) were transferred to each recipient mother. Results of ANOVA analysis, main effect of diet, $F(2, 36) = 0.874$, $P > 0.42$.

Additional file 4: Figure S2. Light/dark transition test. (A) The number of transition between the light and dark chambers. (B) Time spent in light chamber. (C) Total distance traveled. (A-C) Number of subjects: CD, 10; PR, 10; FA, 7. Data represent the mean ± SEM.

Additional file 5: Figure S3. Results of fear conditioning test. (A) Freezing responses pre- and post-training with three tone-shock pairs in box A. Pre-train indicates the freezing levels in box A (the shocking chamber) before the onset of training. Context indicates the freezing level after training. (B) Freezing responses with no tone and during tone in box B. (A, B) Number of subjects: CD, 6; PR, 10; FA, 7; Data represent the mean ± SEM.

Additional file 6: Figure S4. Tail-suspension test. Percent of immobility time in five minutes is shown. Data represent the mean ± SEM. Number of subjects: CD, 6; PR, 10; FA, 7.

Additional file 7: Supplemental information 1. HMM regions in which methylation levels were lower in PR group relative to CD group. Table also includes identifiers such as gene symbol, Transcript ID, Distance to TSS, percent overlap with region, precise chromosome location of the region, region length, PGS region ID, markers (number of probes), mean enrichment level across the region (fold enrichment), and HMM state (s-HMM: -5, m-HMM: -3, l-HMM: -1.5).

Additional file 8: HMM regions in which methylation levels were higher in PR group relative to CD group. Table also includes identifiers such as gene symbol, Transcript ID, Distance to TSS, percent overlap with region, precise chromosome location of the region, region length, PGS region ID, markers (number of probes), mean enrichment level across the region (fold enrichment), and HMM state (s-HMM: +5, m-HMM: +3, l-HMM: +1.5).

Additional file 9: HMM regions in which methylation levels were lower in FA group relative to CD group. Table also includes identifiers such as gene symbol, Transcript ID, Distance to TSS, percent overlap with region, precise chromosome location of the region, region length, PGS region ID, markers (number of probes), mean enrichment level across the region (fold enrichment), and HMM state (s-HMM: -5, m-HMM: -3, l-HMM: -1.5).

Additional file 10: HMM regions in which methylation levels were higher in FA group relative to CD group. Table also includes identifiers such as gene symbol, Transcript ID, Distance to TSS, percent overlap with region, precise chromosome location of the region, region length, PGS region ID, markers (number of probes), mean enrichment level across the region (fold enrichment), and HMM state (s-HMM: +5, m-HMM: +3, l-HMM: +1.5).

Additional file 11: HMM regions in which methylation levels were lower in FA group relative to PR group. Table also includes identifiers such as gene symbol, Transcript ID, Distance to TSS, percent overlap with region, precise chromosome location of the region, region length, PGS region ID, markers (number of probes), mean enrichment level across the region (fold enrichment), and HMM state (s-HMM: -5, m-HMM: -3, l-HMM: -1.5).

Additional file 12: HMM regions in which methylation levels were higher in FA group relative to PR group. Table also includes identifiers such as gene symbol, Transcript ID, Distance to TSS, percent overlap with region, precise chromosome location of the region, region length, PGS region ID, markers (number of probes), mean enrichment level across the region (fold enrichment), and HMM state (s-HMM: +5, m-HMM: +3, l-HMM: +1.5).

Additional file 13: List of genes that exhibited lower expression level in PR group relative to CD group in adult brain. Table also includes identifiers such as probe name, PrimaryAccession ID, GeneSymbol, Gene ontology (GO), Gene description, chromosome number, P value in Tukey's multiple comparison test adjusted by FDR, and mean fold change of expression level.

Additional file 14: List of genes that exhibited higher expression level in PR group relative to CD group in adult brain. Table also includes identifiers such as probe name, PrimaryAccession ID, GeneSymbol, Gene ontology (GO), Gene description, chromosome number, P value in Tukey's multiple comparison test adjusted by FDR, and mean fold change of expression level.

Additional file 15: List of the genes which exhibited lower expression levels in FA group relative to CD group. Table also includes identifiers such as probe name, PrimaryAccession ID, GeneSymbol, Gene ontology (GO), Gene description, chromosome number, P value in Tukey's multiple comparison test adjusted by FDR, and mean fold change of expression level.

Additional file 16: List of the genes which exhibited higher expression levels in FA group relative to CD group. Table also includes identifiers such as probe name, PrimaryAccession ID, GeneSymbol, Gene ontology (GO), Gene description, chromosome number, P value in Tukey's multiple comparison test adjusted by FDR, and mean fold change of expression level.

Additional file 17: List of genes that exhibited lower expression level in FA group relative to PR group in adult brain. Table also includes identifiers such as Probe name, PrimaryAccession ID, GeneSymbol, Gene ontology (GO), Gene description, chromosome number, P value in Tukey's multiple comparison test adjusted by FDR, and mean fold change of expression level.

Additional file 18: List of genes that exhibited higher expression level in FA group relative to PR group in adult brain. Table also includes identifiers such as Probe name, PrimaryAccession ID, GeneSymbol, Gene ontology (GO), Gene description, chromosome number, P value in Tukey's multiple comparison test adjusted by FDR, and mean fold change of expression level.

Abbreviations
DOHaD: Developmental origins of health and diseases; ET: Embryo transfer; IVF: In vitro fertilization; PMSG: Pregnant mare serum gonadotropin

Acknowledgements
The authors thank Dr. Ryo Kominani for his helpful advice, members of the animal facility at RIKEN for providing the animals used in this study, and technical staff for their assistance with the experiments.

Funding
This work was supported by JSPS KAKENHI Grant Numbers 24700440 and 26430098 for TF.

Authors' contributions
TF, TK*, and SW conceived and supervised the study; TF, KM, and TK** designed the experiments; TF, KM, TK**, HK, TH, IY, TK***, KK, and MK performed the experiments; TF, TK**, KM, and HK wrote the manuscript. *TKub; **, TKoh; ***, TKush. All authors read and approved the final manuscript.

Competing interests
The authors declare that they have no competing interests.

Author details
[1]Japan mouse clinic, RIKEN BRC, 3-1-1 Koyadai, Tsukuba, Ibaraki 305-0074, Japan. [2]Department of Epigenetic Medicine, University of Yamanashi, 1110 Shimokato, Chuo, Yamanashi 409-3898, Japan. [3]Department of Epigenetics, Medical Research Institute, Tokyo Medical and Dental University, 1-5-45 Yushima, Bunkyoku, Tokyo 113-8510, Japan.

References
1. Lee SH, Ripke S, Neale BM, Faraone SV, Purcell SM, Perlis RH, et al. Genetic relationship between five psychiatric disorders estimated from genome-wide SNPs. Nat Genet. 2013;45:984–94.
2. Clair D, Xu M, Wang P, Yu Y, Fang Y, Zhang F, et al. Rates of adult Schizophrenia following prenatal exposure to the Chinese famine of 1959–1961. JAMA. 2005;294:557–62.
3. Lahti J, Räikkönen K, Kajantie E, Heinonen K, Pesonen A, Järvenpää A, et al. Small body size at birth and behavioural symptoms of ADHD in children aged five to six years. J Child Psychol Psychiatry. 2006;47:1167–74.
4. Schendel D, Bhasin T. Birth weight and gestational age characteristics of children with autism, including a comparison with other developmental disabilities. Pediatrics. 2008;121:1155–64.
5. Susser E, Clair D, He L. Latent effects of prenatal malnutrition on adult health. Ann Ny Acad Sci. 2008;1136:185–92.
6. McNamara B, Gubhaju L, Chamberlain C, Stanley F, Eades S. Early life influences on cardio-metabolic disease risk in aboriginal populations—what is the evidence? A systematic review of longitudinal and case-control studies. Int J Epidemiol. 2012;41:1661–82.
7. Zheng J, Xiao X, Zhang Q, Yu M. DNA methylation: the pivotal interaction between early-life nutrition and glucose metabolism in later life. Brit J Nutr. 2014;112:1850–57.
8. Lillycrop K, Phillips E, Jackson A, Hanson M, Burdge G. Dietary protein restriction of pregnant rats induces and folic acid supplementation prevents epigenetic modification of hepatic gene expression in the offspring. J Nutr. 2005;135:1382–6.
9. Vucetic Z, Totoki K, Schoch H, Whitaker K, Hill-Smith T, Lucki I, et al. Early life protein restriction alters dopamine circuitry. Neuroscience. 2010;168:359–70.
10. Armitage J, Khan I, Taylor P, Nathanielsz P, Poston L. Developmental programming of the metabolic syndrome by maternal nutritional imbalance: how strong is the evidence from experimental models in mammals? J Physiol. 2004;561:355–77.
11. Bautista CJ, Boeck L, Larrea F, Nathanielsz PW. Effects of a maternal low protein isocaloric diet on milk leptin and progeny serum leptin concentration and appetitive behavior in the first 21 days of neonatal life in the First 21 Days of Neonatal Life in the Rat. Pediatri Res. 2008;63:358–63.
12. Burdge GC, Slater-Jefferies J, Torrens C, Phillips ES, Hanson MA, Lillycrop KA. Dietary protein restriction of pregnant rats in the F0 generation induces altered methylation of hepatic gene promoters in the adult male offspring in the F1 and F2 generations. Br J Nutr. 2007;97:435–9.
13. Geraghty AA, Lindsay KL, Alberdi G, McAuliffe FM, Gibney ER. Nutrition during pregnancy impacts offspring's epigenetic status-evidence from human and animal studies. Nutr Metab Insights. 2015;8:41–7.
14. Eaton GJ, Johnson FN, Custer RP, Crane AR. The Icr:Ha(ICR) mouse: a current account of breeding, mutations, diseases and mortality. Lab Anim. 1980;14:17–24.
15. Reeves P, Nielsen F, Fahey GC. AIN-93 purified diets for laboratory rodents: final report of the American Institute of Nutrition ad hoc writing committee on the reformulation of the AIN-76A rodent diet. J Nutr. 1993;123:1939–51.
16. Kaneda H, Taguma K, Suzuki C, Ozaki A, Nakamura C, Hachisu A, et al. An Optimal embryo transfer condition for the effective production of DBA/2J Mice. Exp Anim. 2007;56:385–88.
17. Yoshii A, Kitahara S, Ueta H, Matsuno K, Ezaki T. Role of uterine contraction in regeneration of the murine postpartum endometrium. Biol Reprod. 2014;91:32.
18. Nishi M, Horii-Hayashi N, Sasagawa T. Effects of early life adverse experiences on the brain: implications from maternal separation models in rodents. Front Neurosci. 2014;8:166.

19. Holmes A, le Guisquet AM, Vogel E, Millstein RA, Leman S, Belzung C. Early life genetic, epigenetic and environmental factors shaping emotionality in rodents. Neurosci Biobehav Rev. 2005;29:1335–46.
20. Inoue M, Sakuraba Y, Motegi H, Kubota N, Toki H, Matsui J, et al. A series of maturity onset diabetes of the young, type 2 (MODY2) mouse models generated by a large-scale ENU mutagenesis program. Hum Mol Genet. 2004;13:1147–57.
21. Robinson MD, Stirzaker C, Statham AL, Coolen MW, Song JZ, Nair SS, et al. Evaluation of affinity-based genome-wide DNA methylation data: effects of CpG density, amplification bias, and copy number variation. Genome Res. 2010;20:1719–29.
22. Gautier L, Cope L, Bolstad BM, Irizarry RA. affy–analysis of Affymetrix GeneChip data at the probe level. Bioinformatics. 2004;20:307–15.
23. Sadikovic B, Yoshimoto M, Al-Romaih K, Maire G, Zielenska M, Squire J. In vitro analysis of integrated global high-resolution DNA methylation profiling with genomic imbalance and gene expression in osteosarcoma. PLoS One. 2008;3:e2834.
24. Roessler J, Ammerpohl O, Gutwein J, Hasemeier B, Anwar SL, Kreipe H, et al. Quantitative cross-validation and content analysis of the 450k DNA methylation array from Illumina, Inc. BMC Res Notes. 2012;5:210.
25. Patterson TA, Lobenhofer EK, Fulmer-Smentek SB, Collins PJ, Chu T-MM, Bao W, et al. Performance comparison of one-color and two-color platforms within the MicroArray Quality Control (MAQC) project. Nat Biotechnol. 2006; 24:1140–50.
26. Crawley JN. Behavioral phenotyping strategies for mutant mice. Neuron. 2008;57:809–18.
27. Furuse T, Wada Y, Hattori K, Yamada I, Kushida T, Shibukawa Y, et al. Phenotypic characterization of a new Grin1 mutant mouse generated by ENU mutagenesis. Eur J Neurosci. 2010;31:1281–91.
28. Zeng H, Chattarji S, Barbarosie M, Rondi-Reig L, Philpot B, Miyakawa T, et al. Forebrain-specific calcineurin knockout selectively impairs bidirectional synaptic plasticity and working/episodic-like memory. Cell. 2001;107:617–29.
29. Tomida S, Mamiya T, Sakamaki H, Miura M, Aosaki T, Masuda M, et al. Usp46 is a quantitative trait gene regulating mouse immobile behavior in the tail suspension and forced swimming tests. Nat Genet. 2009;41:688–95.
30. Waterland RA, Jirtle RL. Transposable elements: targets for early nutritional effects on epigenetic gene regulation. Mol Cell Biol. 2003;23:5293–300.
31. Buccafusco KR, Crawley JN. Methods of behavior analysis in neuroscience. 2nd ed. Boca Raton: CRC Press; 2009. p. 97–102.
32. Jo H, Schieve LA, Sharma AJ, Hinkle SN, Li R, Lind JN. Maternal prepregnancy body mass index and child psychosocial development at 6 years of age. Pediatrics. 2015;135:e1198–209.
33. Lyall K, Schmidt RJ, Hertz-Picciotto I. Maternal lifestyle and environmental risk factors for autism spectrum disorders. Int J Epidemiol. 2014;43:443–64.
34. Huypens P, Sass S, Wu M, Dyckhoff D, Tschöp M, Theis F, et al. Epigenetic germline inheritance of diet-induced obesity and insulin resistance. Nat Genet. 2016;48:497–9.
35. Braz BY, Galiñanes GL, Taravini IR, Belforte JE, Murer GM. Altered corticostriatal connectivity and exploration/exploitation imbalance emerge as intermediate phenotypes for a neonatal dopamine dysfunction. Neuropsychopharmacology. 2015;40:2576–87.
36. Engel, Creson, Hao, Shen, Maeng, Nekrasova, et al. The extracellular signal-regulated kinase pathway contributes to the control of behavioral excitement. Mol Psychiatry. 2009;14:448–61.
37. Russell V, Sagvolden T, Johansen E. Animal models of attention-deficit hyperactivity disorder. Behav Brain Funct. 2005;1:9.
38. Sagvolden, Russell, Aase, Johansen. Rodent models of attention-deficit/hyperactivity disorder. Biol Psychiatry. 2005;57:1239–47.
39. Silverman J, Yang M, Lord C, Crawley J. Behavioural phenotyping assays for mouse models of autism. Nat Rev Neurosci. 2010;11:490–502.
40. Spencer CM, Alekseyenko O, Hamilton SM, Thomas AM, Serysheva E, Yuva-Paylor LA, et al. Modifying behavioral phenotypes in Fmr1KO mice: genetic background differences reveal autistic-like responses. Autism Res. 2011;4:40–56.
41. Suzuki T, Furuse T, Yamada I, Motegi H, Kozawa Y, Masuya H, et al. Pheno-Pub: a total support system for the publication of mouse phenotypic data on the web. Mamm Genome. 2013;24:473–83.
42. Feuer S, Rinaudo P. From Embryos to Adults: A DOHaD Perspective on In Vitro Fertilization and Other Assisted Reproductive Technologies. Healthcare (Basel). 2016;4:E51.
43. Ashworth A, Bardgett ME, Fowler J, Garber H, Griffith M, Curran CP. Comparison of neurological function in males and females from two substrains of C57BL/6 mice. Toxics. 2015;3:1–17.

16

Methyl group donors abrogate adaptive responses to dietary restriction in *C. elegans*

Maja Klapper[1], Daniel Findeis[2], Harald Koefeler[3,4] and Frank Döring[1*]

Abstract

Background: Almost all animals adapt to dietary restriction through alternative life history traits that affect their growth, reproduction, and survival. Economized management of fat stores is a prevalent type of such adaptations. Because one-carbon metabolism is a critical gauge of food availability, in this study, we used *Caenorhabditis elegans* to test whether the methyl group donor choline regulates adaptive responses to dietary restriction. We used a modest dietary restriction regimen that prolonged the fecund period without reducing the lifetime production of progeny, which is the best measure of fitness.

Results: We found that dietary supplementation with choline abrogate the dietary restriction-induced prolongation of the reproductive period as well as the accumulation and delayed depletion of large lipid droplets and whole-fat stores and increased the survival rate in the cold. By contrast, the life span-prolonging effect of dietary restriction is not affected by choline. Moreover, we found that dietary restriction led to the enlargement of lipid droplets within embryos and enhancement of the cold tolerance of the progeny of dietarily restricted mothers. Both of these transgenerational responses to maternal dietary restriction were abrogated by exposing the parental generation to choline.

Conclusions: In conclusion, supplementation with the methyl group donor choline abrogates distinct responses to dietary restriction related to reproduction, utilization of fat stored in large lipid droplets, cold tolerance, and thrifty phenotypes in *C. elegans*.

Keywords: Dietary restriction, Lipid droplet, Choline, Methyl group donor, Thrifty phenotype, Life history traits, *C. elegans*

Background

Dietary restriction (DR) induces several adaptations, including the extension of the reproductive period, prolongation of the adult life span, and the reduction of energy turnover (Fontana and Partridge 2015). Although the life span-prolonging effect of DR and the mechanisms involved have been extensively studied in a variety of organisms, the impact of DR on the regulation of lipid droplet (LD) homeostasis is limited (Baumeier et al. 2015; Bouwman et al. 2009; Miersch and Doring 2013; Palgunow et al. 2012). LDs are evolutionarily conserved fat storage organelles containing a triacylglyceride core surrounded by a phospholipid monolayer composed mainly of phosphatidylcholine and phosphatidylethanolamine (Zhang et al. 2010b). In addition to this classical function, LDs were recently recognized to function as storage organelles for histones during embryogenesis (Cermelli et al. 2006; Li et al. 2012), assembly platforms for specific viruses (Welte 2015), and intracellular antibacterial defense systems (Anand et al. 2012). During periods of reduced food availability and/or growth, fatty acids are effectively delivered from LDs to maintain key energy-consuming processes (Barbosa et al. 2015; Lee et al. 2014; Narbonne and Roy 2009).

Functional genomic screens of the model organisms *Caenorhabditis elegans* and *Drosophila melanogaster* have been performed to identify genes that regulate LD formation and utilization (Ashrafi et al. 2003; Guo et al. 2008). These screens established that Arf1-COPI-mediated vesicular transport and the phosphatidylcholine synthesis pathway play important roles in the morphology and

* Correspondence: sek@molprev.uni-kiel.de
[1]Institute of Human Nutrition and Food Science, Molecular Prevention, Christian-Albrechts University of Kiel, Heinrich-Hecht-Platz 10, 24118 Kiel, Germany
Full list of author information is available at the end of the article

functionality of LDs. Many LD regulatory genes are conserved from worms to humans. Moreover, it has been shown that dietary factors, such as vaccenic acid, also regulate LD functionality (Zhang et al. 2010a). We have previously reported that in *C. elegans*, DR leads to the enlargement of LDs in the intestine and hypodermis (Miersch and Doring 2013; Palgunow et al. 2012), which are the main fat storage tissues of nematodes. However, little is known about the underlying cellular mechanism and the physiological role of this DR-induced LD phenotype. Because one-carbon metabolism regulates the homeostasis of phosphatidylcholine synthesis, lipogenesis, lipid droplet size, and lipolytic efficacy (Ehmke et al. 2014; Li et al. 2011), in this study, we used *C. elegans* to determine whether the methyl group donor choline plays a regulatory role in the enlargement of LDs and other adaptive phenotypes that are induced by DR.

Results

Intake of the methyl group donor choline abrogates both the enlargement of intestinal lipid droplets and the increase in the fat content of dietarily restricted worms

Consistent with the results of our previous studies (Miersch and Doring 2013; Palgunow et al. 2012), DR was observed to cause enlargement of LDs in the intestine, which is one of the main fat storage tissues of *C. elegans* (Fig. 1a, a vs b). Because one-carbon metabolism plays a critical role in the regulation of both LD size and the extent of fat storage (Ehmke et al. 2014; Li et al. 2011), we supplemented the diet of the DR worms with the methyl group donor choline. We found that choline supplementation abrogates the enlargement of the intestinal LDs in DR worms (Fig. 1a, b vs d). Supplementation with the essential amino acid methionine, another methyl group donor, also reduced the size of the LDs in the intestine of DR worms (Fig. 1a, b vs f). Quantitative analysis revealed that the increased mean (Fig. 1b) and maximal (Fig. 1c) LD volume and the higher proportion of LDs >5 μm^3 (Fig. 1d/e) were completely abrogated, or even overcompensated, in DR worms provided with supplemental choline. Choline supplementation also prevented the increase in the total LD volume (Fig. 1f) of DR worms. Because this LD parameter may serve as a proxy indicator of the extent of fat storage, we determined the triacylglyceride (TAG) contents of the worms. Consistent with the results of the LD analysis, the increase in the TAG content of DR worms was also abrogated by choline supplementation (Fig. 1g). The analysis of lipid classes revealed that choline supplementation increased the phosphatidylcholine content, which was reduced in worms subjected to DR (Fig. 1h). Taken together, our results showed that both the enlargement of intestinal lipid droplets and the increase in the fat content of dietarily restricted worms are abolished by dietary supplementation with the methyl group donor choline.

Choline does not abrogate the enlargement of hypodermal lipid droplets induced by dietary restriction

In addition to the intestine, the hypodermis functions as a major fat storage tissue in *C. elegans*. Confocal microscopy of the mid-segments (Fig. 1a, g–i) and heads (Fig. 2a, a–f) of the worms revealed that neither choline nor methionine supplementation prevented the enlargement of the hypodermal LDs in these regions of DR worms. Quantitative analyses of the hypodermal LDs localized in the head region of the worms showed that DR increased the mean LD volume (Fig. 2b), the number of LDs (Fig. 2c), the total LD volume (Fig. 2d)—a proxy indicator of the extent of fat storage—and the proportion of LDs >5 μm^3 (Fig. 2e/f). None of these effects of DR was prevented by choline supplementation. Therefore, choline does not affect the DR-mediated enlargement of hypodermal LDs.

Choline abrogates the delayed depletion of the fat stores of dietarily restricted worms

Economized management of fat stores is a common adaptation to DR conditions. We therefore evaluated whether DR worms retain their fat stores more effectively than AL-fed worms (AL, ad libitum). In response to starvation (24 or 72 h), the contents of the LDs in the mid-segment of the worms were exhausted in the AL condition (Fig. 3a, a vs c), but not in the DR condition (Fig. 3a, b vs d). Quantitative analysis revealed that the large LDs (5–10 μm^3, >10 μm^3) of DR worms were more resistant to starvation-induced fat depletion than those of the AL-fed worms (Fig. 3b–d). Next, we evaluated the fat stores of the worms by analyzing both LD volume (Fig. 3e) and lipid content (Fig. 3f). It was consistently found using both methods of evaluation that the DR worms retained approximately 60–70 % of their initial fat stores in response to starvation, whereas the AL-fed worms retained approximately 40 % (Fig. 3e/f) of these stores. Finally, we examined whether choline supplementation would prevent the occurrence of the fat-retaining phenotype of DR worms. We found that the decrease in LD exhaustion (Fig. 3a, b vs d) and the delay in the depletion of both the large LDs >5 μm^3 (Fig. 3b–d) and fat stores (Fig. 3e/f) in the DR worms were abolished by choline supplementation. Taken together, our results indicate that DR worms preserve fat stores more efficiently than AL-fed animals, with the larger LDs being particularly resistant to lipolysis. These adaptive responses are abolished when the diet of DR worms is supplemented with the methyl group donor choline.

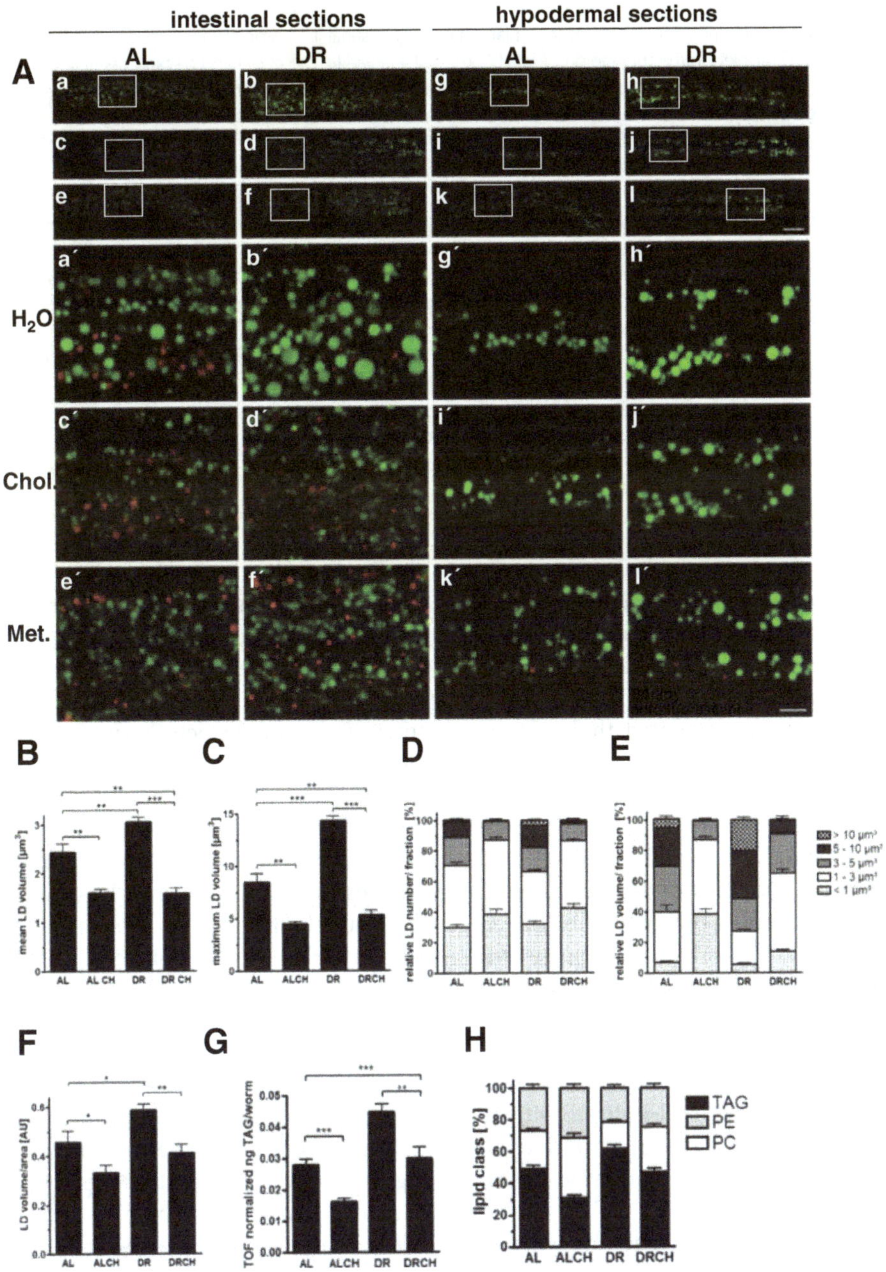

Fig. 1 (See legend on next page.)

(See figure on previous page.)

Fig. 1 Choline and methionine supplementation abrogates the enlargement of intestinal lipid droplets and increase in fat content observed in dietarily restricted worms. **a** Lipid droplets in the mid-region of ad libitum-fed L4 larvae (*a, c, e, g, i, k*) and dietarily restricted L4 larvae (*b, d, f, h, j, l*), without (H_2O vehicle control; *a, b, g, h*) or with choline (*c, d, i, j*) or methionine (*e, f, k, l*) supplementation, were visualized after short-term (20 min) vital BODIPY™ $^{493/503}$ staining using a ×63 objective and Zeiss Apotome equipment. Image stacks with a depth of 10 µm, consisting of 21 planes at 0.5-µm intervals, were captured and rendered as maximal projections (*a–f*). Images *a–f* show intestinal lipid droplets. In *g–l*, only the first six to eight images of the respective stacks are projected to demonstrate the lipid droplets in the upper hypodermal segment. The BODIPY™ $^{493/503}$ fluorescence signals (*green*) and the auto-fluorescence signals of lysosome-related organelles (*red*) are shown to study possible co-localizations of the signals. Scale bars, 20 and 10 µm (magnifications). **b–f** Images of intestinal lipid droplets were analyzed using the 3D spot segmentation plug-in of ImageJ software. The mean LD volume (**b**), maximum LD volume (**c**), and total LD volume are shown. The distributions of the relative number of LDs (**d**) and relative LD volume (**e**) per LD size category (<1, 1–3, 3–5, 5–10, and >10 µm^3) are shown. **f** The summarized LD volume per area (AU, arbitrary units), a proxy indicator of the extent of fat storage, is shown (**f**). The data were derived from six to nine individual worms per feeding condition in three independent experiments. **g, h** The triacylglyceride (TAG), phosphatidylethanolamine (PE), and phosphatidylcholine (PC) contents of L4 larvae were assessed using thin-layer chromatography (TLC). **g** TAG content was normalized to the TOF value (time of flight), a proxy indicator of the worm's body length. Five-microliter samples containing lipids from equal numbers of worms (166 or 333) were dotted onto each lane to ensure that the amounts of triacylglycerides and phospholipids were in the linear range of the triolein and phospholipid standard curve, respectively. The assays were conducted in duplicate, and the results of six to eight independent experiments are summarized. *AL* ad libitum, *AL CH* ad libitum condition with choline supplementation, *DR* dietary restriction, *DR CH* dietary restriction condition with choline supplementation, *TOF* time of flight, a proxy measurement of the length of the worms

Choline abrogates the enlargement of the lipid droplets of progeny (F_1) produced by dietarily restricted mothers (P_o)

Because the increased LD size, higher fat content, and less depleted fat stores observed in DR worms are thrifty phenotypic traits, we speculated that maternal DR would affect LD size and fat-related phenotypes in the descendent F_1 progeny. Differential lipid analysis revealed similar changes in both the triacylglyceride-to-phospholipid ratio and the composition of the phosphatidylcholine fatty acid species of the restricted P_0 generation and the F_1 embryos (F_1 generation) of DR mothers (Additional file 1: Figure S1). These results indicate that quantitative as well as qualitative aspects of lipid metabolism are transmitted to the embryos of DR mothers. Remarkably, the F_1 embryos showed enlarged vesicles localized throughout their bodies in utero (Fig. 4a, a vs b). These vesicles co-localized with the LD marker protein ATGL (Fig. 4b, a), but not with VIT-2, a yolk marker (Fig. 4b, b). The large vesicles of isolated embryos were BODIPY™ $^{493/503}$-positive (Fig. c). These results confirmed that the enlarged vesicles observed in DR-derived embryos are true LDs. A higher proportion of large LDs >5 µm^3 were still present in DR-derived AL-fed L1/2 larvae (AL-DR, 24/30) compared with AL-derived AL-fed L1/2 larvae (AL-AL, 24/30) (Fig. 4d). This persistent effect was not observed in DR-derived L4 larvae (Fig. 4d). Importantly, enlarged LDs did not occur in the embryos (F_1 generation) of DR mothers (P_0 generation) that were provided a diet supplemented with either choline or methionine (Fig. 4a, b vs c, d). Taken together, the results show that maternal DR causes enlargement of the LDs of offspring and that this transgenerational effect is abolished by providing methyl group donors to the mothers.

Choline abrogates the increased survival rates observed in the cold in dietarily restricted worms and in the larvae produced by dietarily restricted mothers

In nature, DR is often coincident with lower temperatures. Thus, for the ectotherm *C. elegans* in particular, it would be favorable for DR worms to provoke adaptations that are beneficial under cold conditions. Consistent with this theory, DR worms survived the cold for longer periods than do AL-fed worms (Fig. 5a). This DR response was also abolished by choline supplementation (Fig. 5a). Similar to the persistence of the LD phenotype, DR-derived AL-fed L2 larvae (DR-AL) (Fig. 5b), but not the respective L4 larvae (Fig. 5c), were more resistant to cold than the AL-derived AL-fed L2 larvae (AL-AL). As observed for LD size, the transgenerational effect of DR on cold survival was abrogated by choline supplementation of the mothers' diet (Fig. 5b, DRCH-AL). Thus, both DR worms and the progeny of DR mothers show higher survival rates in the cold compared with their AL-fed counterparts. These cold-adaptive responses of DR animals are abrogated by choline supplementation.

Choline abrogates the extension of the reproductive period, but not the increase in the life span of dietarily restricted worms

The altered lipid composition, increased LD size, and higher survival rates in the cold observed in embryos derived from DR mothers might indicate that the reproduction of mothers subjected to DR is altered. As expected, DR prolonged the fecund period of the worms compared with those exposed to the AL conditions (Fig. 5d). The resulting lifetime progeny production rate, which is the best indicator of fitness, was not reduced and was even slightly increased by DR (Fig. 5e). The DR-induced extension of the reproductive period was

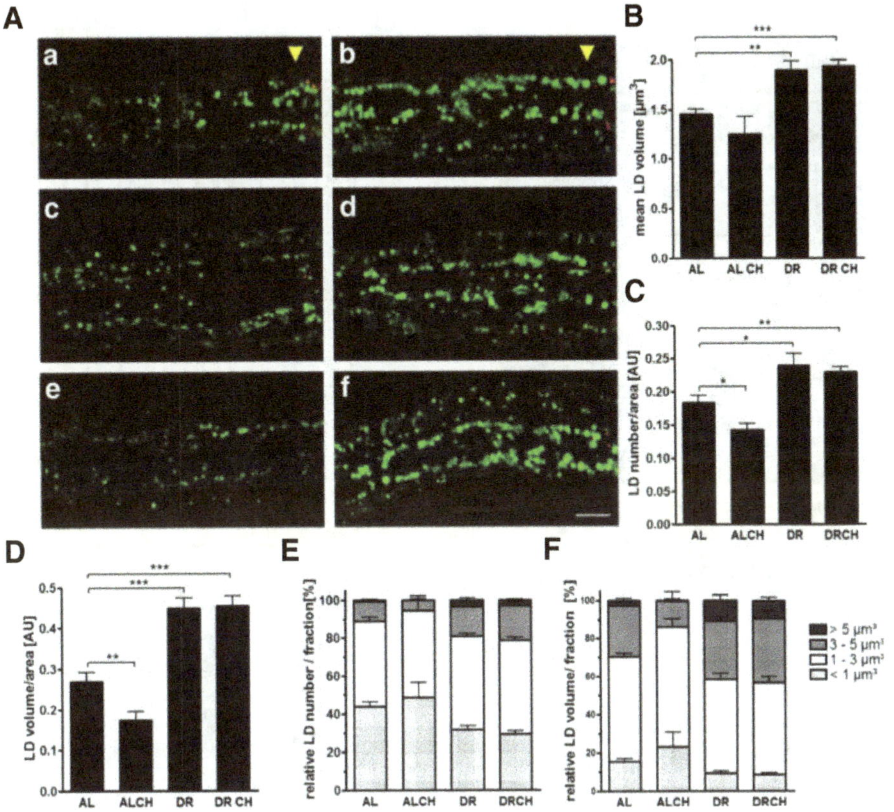

Fig. 2 Choline and methionine supplementation do not abrogate the enlargement of the hypodermal lipid droplets of dietarily restricted worms. **a** Hypodermal lipid droplets in the heads of ad libitum-fed L4 larvae (*a, c, e*) and dietarily restricted L4 larvae (*b, d, f*) without (H_2O vehicle control; *a, b*) or with choline (*c, d*) and methionine (*e, f*) supplementation were visualized using short-term vital BODIPY™ 493/503 staining. Image stacks with a depth of 10 µm, consisting of 21 focal planes at 0.5-µm intervals, were captured and rendered as maximum projections. *Yellow arrowheads* indicate the beginning of the intestine. The BODIPY™ 493/503 fluorescence signals (*green*) and the auto-fluorescence signals of lysosome-related organelles (*red*) are shown to study possible co-localizations of the signals. Scale bars, 20 and 10 µm (magnifications). **b–f** Quantification of hypodermal lipid droplets in the head using the 3D spot segmentation plug-in of ImageJ software. The mean LD volume (**b**), the summarized LD number/area (AU, arbitrary unit) (**c**), and the summarized LD volume/area (AU, arbitrary unit), a proxy indicator of the extent of fat storage (**D**), are shown. The distributions of the relative LD number **e** and LD volume **f** per LD size category (<1, 1–3, 3–5, >5 µm^3) are shown. The data were derived from six to nine individual worms per feeding condition in three independent experiments. *AL* ad libitum, *AL CH* ad libitum condition with choline supplementation, *DR* dietary restriction, *DR CH* dietary restriction condition with choline supplementation

completely abrogated by either choline or methionine supplementation (Fig. 5d). Surprisingly, the DR-mediated life span extension was only slightly reduced by choline or methionine supplementation (Fig. 5f), indicating that these methyl group donors exert specific effects on LD size, fat storage, survival in the cold, and reproduction.

Discussion

Almost all organisms respond to reduced food intake, or DR, via alternative life history traits that ensure survival, growth, and reproduction. In the present study, we applied a standardized DR regime (Miersch and Doring 2013; Palgunow et al. 2012) during postembryonic development. As this DR regime prevents developmental delay and growth retardation, it mimics a moderate, but sufficient food intake. The phenotypes resulting from implementing this DR regime include the accumulation of fat in large LDs, delayed depletion of fat stores, and prolongation of the fecund period without a reduction of the lifetime progeny production rate. Thus, the observed DR-induced phenotypes are highly consistent with the life history theory. Another basic theory argues that a food-restricted mother modifies the phenotype of her progeny such that they are prepared for survival in a poor nutritional environment (Barker 2001). The enlargement of the LDs and the accumulation of triacylglycerides in embryos derived from DR mothers might represent such a thrifty phenotype, assuming that the accumulated, larger embryonic LDs are more resistant to starvation-induced depletion, as observed in the mothers.

As mentioned above, our findings regarding the DR-induced phenotypes are in good agreement with the life history theory and the thrifty phenotype theory. These types of ultimate explanations are insufficient to explain

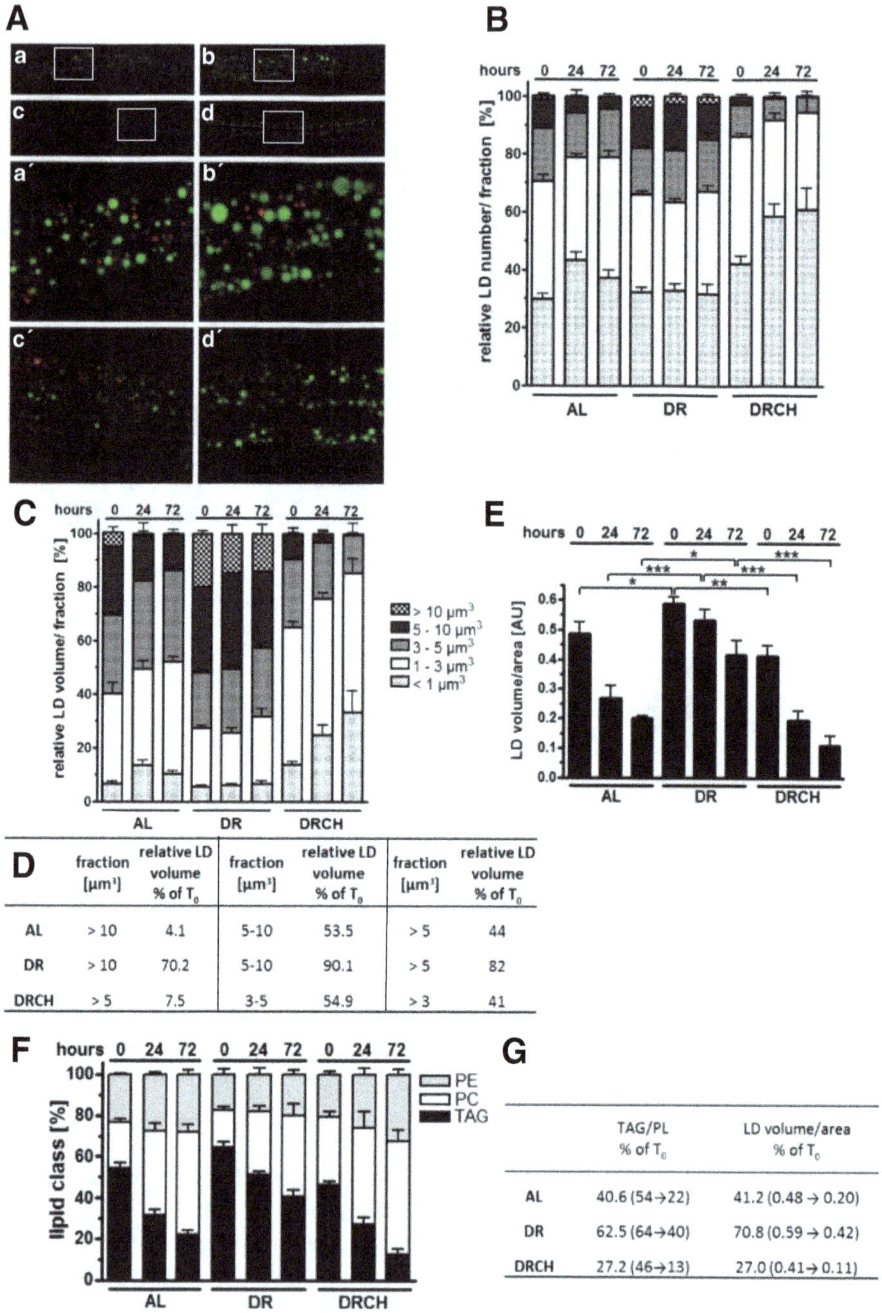

D

	fraction [μm³]	relative LD volume % of T_0	fraction [μm³]	relative LD volume % of T_0	fraction [μm³]	relative LD volume % of T_0
AL	> 10	4.1	5-10	53.5	> 5	44
DR	> 10	70.2	5-10	90.1	> 5	82
DRCH	> 5	7.5	3-5	54.9	> 3	41

G

	TAG/PL % of T_0	LD volume/area % of T_0
AL	40.6 (54→22)	41.2 (0.48 → 0.20)
DR	62.5 (64→40)	70.8 (0.59 → 0.42)
DRCH	27.2 (46→13)	27.0 (0.41→ 0.11)

Fig. 3 (See legend on next page.)

(See figure on previous page.)
Fig. 3 Choline abrogates the delayed depletion of the fat stores of dietarily restricted worms. **a** Depletion of lipid droplets in response to starvation (24 h) in ad libitum-fed L4 larvae (*a, c*) and dietarily restricted L4 larvae (*b, d*), without (H_2O vehicle control; *a, b*), or with choline (*c, d*) supplementation. Lipid droplets were visualized after short-term (20 min) vital BODIPY™ 493/503 staining using a ×63 objective and Zeiss Apotome equipment. Image stacks with a depth of 10 µm, consisting of 21 focal planes at 0.5-µm intervals, were captured and rendered as maximum projections. The images show intestinal lipid droplets in the mid-regions of the worms. The BODIPY™ 493/503 fluorescence signals (*green*) and the auto-fluorescence signals of lysosome-related organelles (*red*) are shown to study possible co-localizations of the signals. Scale bars, 20 and 10 µm (magnifications). **b–e** Quantification of intestinal lipid droplets using the 3D spot segmentation plug-in of ImageJ software. The lipid droplets of ad libitum-fed (AL) and dietarily restricted (DR) L4 larvae were analyzed at time point T_0 (0 h, no starvation) and in response to starvation for 24 or 72 h. The distributions of the relative lipid droplet number/fraction (**b**) and the relative lipid droplet volume/fraction (**c**) per lipid droplet size category (<1, 1–3, 3–5, 5–10, >10 µm^3) are shown. Table **d** shows the relative lipid droplet volume in response to 72 h of starvation (% of T_0) among different lipid droplet size categories (>10, 5–10, >5 µm^3). **e** shows the summarized LD volume/area (AU, arbitrary unit), a proxy indicator of the extent of fat storage. The data were derived from six to nine individual worms per feeding condition in three independent experiments. **f, g** Triacylglyceride (TAG), phosphatidylethanolamine (PE), and phosphatidylcholine (PC) contents were assessed using thin-layer chromatography (TLC). The lipid contents of ad libitum-fed (AL) and dietarily restricted (DR) L4 larvae were analyzed at time point T_0 (0 h, no starvation) and in response to starvation for 24 or 72 h. Table **g** shows the relative ratio of the TAG and phospholipid (PL; PE+PC) contents in response to 72 h of starvation (% of T_0). These ratios correspond to the lipid droplet volume/area. Five-microliter samples containing lipids from equal numbers of worms (166 or 333) were dotted onto each lane to ensure that the amounts of triacylglycerides and phospholipids were in the linear range of the triolein and phospholipid standard curve, respectively. The assays were conducted in duplicate, and six to eight independent experiments are summarized. *AL* ad libitum, *DR* dietary restriction, *DR CH* dietary restriction condition supplemented with choline

the biological functions of the phenotypes in terms of immediate physiological or environmental factors. In searching for such factors, we consider that animals with a genetic deficiency in methyl group donors phenocopies the observed DR-induced effects. For example, *C. elegans* mutants deficient in the synthesis of SAM, the main methyl group donor found in most organisms, show enlarged LDs during both the adult and embryonic stages, increased fat stores, reduced levels of phosphatidylcholine, and delayed depletion of fat stores (Ehmke et al. 2014; Hansen et al. 2005; Walker et al. 2011). Several animal- and patient-based studies have suggested that a diet deficient in methyl group donors is an important factor in the etiology of non-alcoholic fat liver (Leermakers et al. 2015). For example, a choline-deficient diet causes hepatic fat accumulation (Rinella and Green 2004; Zeisel et al. 1991). We suggest that endogenous and exogenous methyl group donors are critical under DR conditions and that the resulting activity of one-carbon metabolism in turn regulates LD size and fat storage. This phenomenon is particularly true for *C. elegans* and other nematodes because their food source, *Escerichia coli*, does not contain phosphatidylcholine. Accordingly, we found that dietary supplementation with choline as well as methionine abrogates the DR-induced fat-related phenotypes. Interestingly, folic acid and vitamin B_{12} are also involved in determining the activity of one-carbon metabolism. Restriction of these vitamins may be related to the fat-related phenotypes observed under DR. A study in rats has shown that vitamin B_{12} deficiency causes increased fatty acid synthesis (Matlib et al. 1979). All of these findings support the view that one-carbon metabolism is a critical gauge of food availability and a key pathway involved in regulating the adaptive storage and utilization of fat.

The most abundant phospholipid in the LD monolayer is PC, which can be synthesized from choline (via the Kennedy pathway), or via the SAM-dependent methylation of phosphoethanolamine (in nematodes and plants) or phosphatidylethanolamine (in mammals) (Brendza et al. 2007; Palavalli et al. 2006). It has been shown that depletion of PC or loss-of-function mutations of the genes that mediate methylation-dependent PC synthesis (*sams-1* and *pmt-1*) leads to enlargement of LDs (Bartz et al. 2007; Guo et al. 2008; Szymanski et al. 2007; Walker et al. 2011). Further studies revealed that LD enlargement occurs when there is a reduced level of PC due to fusion of the existing LDs (Guo et al. 2008; Krahmer et al. 2011; Li et al. 2011; Walker et al. 2011). Based on these findings, we propose that the expansion of LDs induced by DR is caused by the decreased availability of methyl group donors and subsequent reduction of PC levels, which in turn promotes LD fusion. This hypothesis is supported by the observation that dietary supplementation with the methyl group donors choline and methionine increases the PC content and decreases LD size in DR worms.

Remarkably, embryos derived from DR mothers also exhibit a decreased PC content and very large LDs. Both of these phenotypes can be abolished by choline or methionine supplementation of the restricted diet of the mothers, indicating that these methyl group donors are provided to the embryos maternally. Consistent with this conclusion, the embryos of a methyl group donor-deficient mutant (*sams-1*) also exhibit large LDs. As enlarged embryonic LDs as well as cold tolerance are also

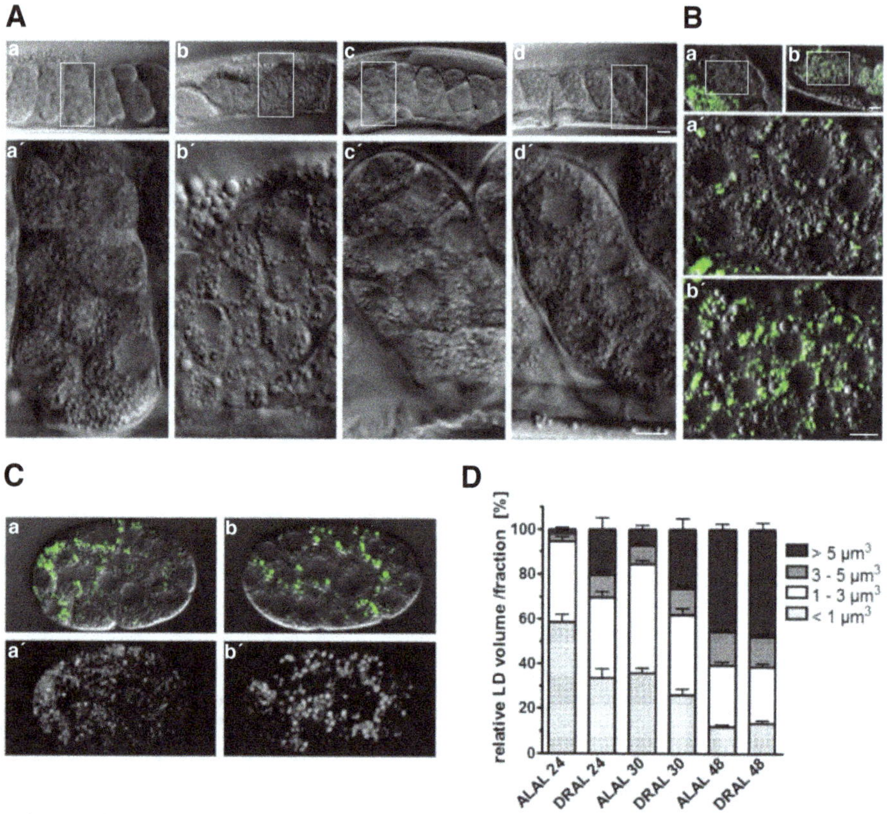

Fig. 4 Choline and methionine abrogate the enlargement of the lipid droplets of in utero embryos (F_1) produced by dietarily restricted mothers (P_0). **a** DIC images of in utero embryos (F_1 generation) derived from ad libitum-fed (AL, *a*) and dietarily restricted (DR, *b*) adult worms (P_0 generation) supplemented with choline (*c*) or methionine (*d*). Images were captured using a ×63 objective. Scale bar, 20 µm. Enlargements of the framed areas are shown in *a´–d´* (×5, scale bar, 10 µm). **b** The lipid droplet marker ATGL::GFP (*a, a´*) and the vitellogenin marker Vit-2::GFP (*b, b´*) are shown. Images were captured using a ×100 objective. Scale bar, 20 µm; ×5 magnification *a´, b´*, scale bar, 10 µm. **c** Lipid droplets from isolated embryos obtained from ad libitum-fed (AL, *a*) and dietarily restricted (DR, *b*) adult worms were visualized using short-term vital BODIPY™ 493/503 staining. Merged DIC and BODIPY™ 493/503 fluorescence images (*a, b*) and fluorescence images (*a´, b´*) are shown. Image stacks (*a´, b´*) with a depth of 10 µm, consisting of 21 focal planes at 0.5 µm intervals, were captured and rendered as maximum projections of the BODIPY™ 493/503 signals. **d** Quantification of intestinal lipid droplets in ad libitum-fed (AL) L1 larvae (F_1 generation; 24 h after hatching), L1/L2 larvae (F_1 generation; 30 h after hatching), and L4 (F_1 generation; 48 h after hatching) obtained from ad libitum-fed (AL) and dietarily restricted (DR) adult worms (P_0 generation). Analyses were performed using the 3D spot segmentation plug-in of ImageJ software. The distribution of the relative lipid-droplet volume/fraction ratio per lipid droplet size category (<1, 1–3, 3–5, >5 µm³) is shown. The data were derived from six to nine individual worms per feeding condition in three independent experiments. ALAL24/30/48, ad libitum feeding of the P_0 generation and ad libitum feeding of F_1 larvae 24, 30, or 48 h after hatching; DRAL24/30/48, dietary restriction of the P_0 generation and ad libitum feeding of F_1 larvae 24, 30, or 48 h after hatching

observed in DR mother-derived L1/2 larvae, we suggest that the maternally provided methyl group donors persist in the progeny. Thus, the existence of a relationship between the availability of methyl group donors, PC contents, and LD size provides an explanation for the observed DR-induced fat-related phenotypes and their abolishment through choline or methionine supplementation. As the reduced PC content, increased LD size, and adaptation to cold are inherited by the next generation and can be abolished by supplementation with methyl group donors, the one-carbon metabolism of the mothers may play an important role in the occurrence of these thrifty phenotypes. Nevertheless, we cannot exclude that the inherited effect has something to do with histone methylation and subsequent gene expression. This should be studied in future experiments focusing on epigenetic effects.

We found that the starvation-induced depletion of fat stores, particularly that of the large LDs, is reduced in DR worms. This fat-sparing effect can also be abolished by supplementation with methyl group donors. In *Drosophila*, it has been shown that DR increases starvation resistance (Burger et al. 2007). Because the surface-to-volume ratio is lower in larger LDs than in smaller LDs, the rate of degradation of the former by lipases might be decreased. Consistent with this hypothesis, a *C. elegans* mutant (*dhs-28*) deficient in peroxisomal β-oxidation is characterized by extremely large LDs that

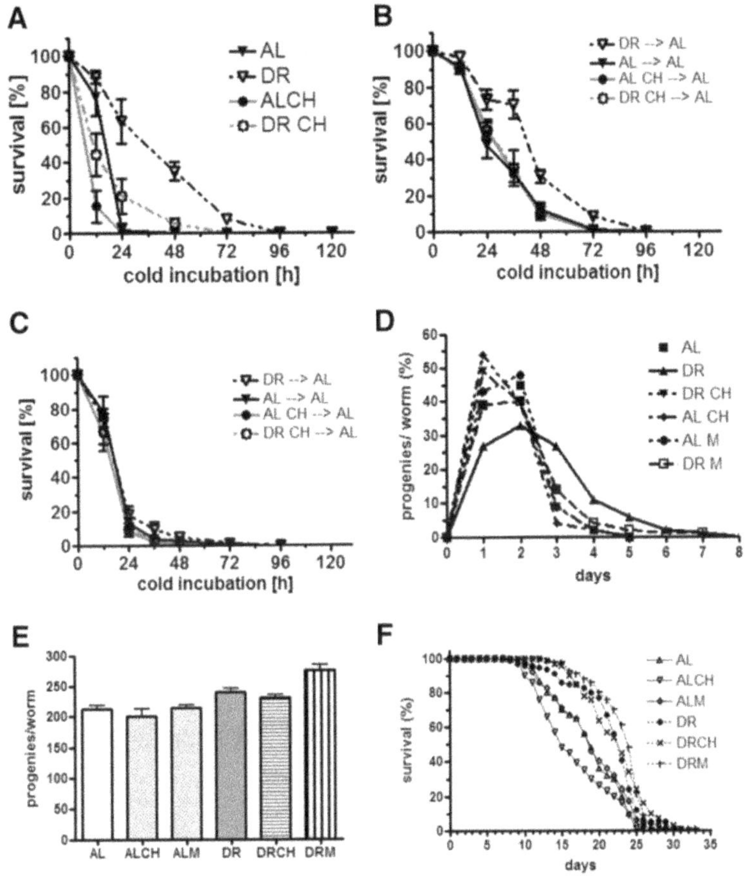

Fig. 5 Choline abrogates the extension of the reproductive period and increased survival rate in the cold in the P_0 and F_1 generations, but not the increase in the life span of dietarily restricted worms. **a** Survival curves of ad libitum-fed (AL) and dietarily restricted (DR) young adult worms without (H_2O vehicle control; AL, DR) or with choline (AL CH, DR CH) supplementation, following their transfer from 20 to 0 °C. The data were obtained in three independent experiments. **b, c** Survival curves of AL-fed L1 larvae (**b**) or AL-fed L4 larvae (**c**) obtained from either AL-fed or DR adult worms, without (H_2O vehicle control; AL, DR) or with choline (AL CH, DR CH) supplementation, following their direct transfer from 20 to 0 °C. The data were obtained in three independent experiments. DR/AL→AL, DR/AL) of the P_0 generation and AL of F_1 larvae; DR CH →AL, DR with choline supplementation of the P_0 generation and AL feeding of F_1 larvae. **d–f** Time-course of the progeny production (**d**), length of the reproductive period (**e**), and lifetime progeny production rate (**f**) of ad libitum-fed (AL) and dietarily restricted (DR) worms, without (H_2O vehicle control; AL, DR) or with choline (AL CH, DR CH) or methionine (AL M, DR M) supplementation. **g** Life span curves representing the typical results of two to four independent experiments using ad libitum-fed (AL) and dietarily restricted (DR) worms, without (H_2O vehicle control; AL, DR) or with choline (AL CH, DR CH) or methionine (AL M, DR M) supplementation

are more resistant to lipase-mediated lipolysis compared with smaller LDs (Zhang et al. 2010a). Moreover, studies in flies have shown that the large LDs that form due to reduced PC levels are more resistant to lipolysis (Guo et al. 2008; Krahmer et al. 2011). In mutant mice, the generation of small LDs leads to enhanced lipolysis (Nishino et al. 2008). The size of LDs is functionally important in the supply of fatty acids. From this point of view, a decreased rate of supply of fatty acids derived from large LDs may contribute to the prolonged reproductive period of DR worms. This hypothesis should be tested in future studies using mutants that are not responsive to starvation-induced fat depletion.

Conclusions

We have demonstrated that subjecting *C. elegans* to a moderate DR regime during the postembryonic period induces the prolongation of the reproductive period, the accumulation and delayed depletion of large LDs and whole-fat stores, an increased survival rate in the cold, the enlargement of LDs, and a higher level of cold resistance in the filial generation. Because all of these effects are prevented by dietary supplementation with methyl group donors, we conclude that one-carbon metabolism is a critical gauge of food availability, a key pathway in regulating the adaptive storage and utilization of fat, and an important determinant for the induction of thrifty phenotypes.

Methods

Worm strains, culture, dietary restriction

The wild-type strain used in this study was Bristol N2. A VS20 strain expressing an ATGL-1::GFP fusion protein [atgl-1p::atgl-1::GFP] was used as a lipid droplet reporter strain. The strain pwls[vit-2p::vit-2::GFP] was used for the visualization of vitellogenin-containing yolk granules. The worms were cultured at 20 °C on nematode growth medium (NGM) plates using *E. coli* OP50 as the food source, following standard methods (Brenner 1974). For the supplementation experiments, solutions of choline (10 mM), ethanolamine (10 mM), betaine (10 mM), or methionine (1 mM) were spread on the bacterial lawn. Age synchronization of the nematodes was achieved through hypochlorite treatment of gravid adults. Dietary restriction of the worms was achieved as previously described (Palgunow et al. 2012). In short, adjusted optical densities (250 µl, OD_{600} 0.7 or 1.5) of the *E. coli* strain OP50 were spread onto antibiotic-free agar plates (without peptone) and incubated for 16 h at 37 °C. This leads to different amounts of bacteria per agar plate depending on the OD of seeded OP50. To further standardize food availability per worm, 500 synchronized embryos were sorted onto AL and dDR agar plates by flow cytometry and were cultivated at 20 °C until reaching the L4 or adult stage. To exclude starvation, L4 larvae and adult worms were transferred daily to fresh agar plates.

Number of progeny and reproductive period

To determine the number of progeny, 48 h after synchronization and cultivation under a particular condition, L4 larvae were placed on plates containing a ring of palmitic acid to prevent their escape. Five worms per plate were cultivated for an additional 48 h. This time point was considered day 1 of adulthood and progeny production. The animals were subsequently transferred to new plates at 24-h intervals until the end of their reproductive period. The progeny on the residual plates were counted the day after the adults were transferred. Three plates were analyzed for each condition in three independent experiments. The reproductive period was calculated as the period during which 95 % of the progeny were produced.

Survival rate under cold conditions

Immediately before the worms were shifted to 0 °C, the NGM plates were divided into four segments that were placed in different positions in the incubator. The nematodes were transferred to 0 °C as larvae or young adults, and survival was monitored at specific time points. The samples were analyzed in triplicate for each condition and time point. The survival rate was calculated as the percentage of dead individuals after 24 h of recovery at 20 °C among the total number of worms that had been counted immediately after incubation at 0 °C. Worms were scored as dead if they did not respond when gently touched with a platinum wire.

Starvation experiments

Synchronized worms were grown for 48 h on NGM agar plates until reaching the L4 stage. Approximately 4000 worms were harvested from 10 to 12 NGM plates/condition and were washed three times with M9 buffer. Control worms (0 h of starvation) with or without choline supplementation were immediately sorted using a COPAS Biosort flow cytometric system into Precellys vials (1000 worms/sample) and were stored at −80 °C until further processing. To induce starvation, worms were cultivated in 15-ml Falcon tubes in a Nutator mixer in 3 ml of M9 buffer supplemented with an antibiotic (dilution: 1:100, Cell Culture Guard, AppliChem) and choline or the vehicle (H_2O). After 24 and 72 h of starvation, the worms were collected as described above for the control worms (0 h of starvation). The samples were used for TLC and protein quantification. An aliquot of live worms grown under each condition (0, 24, or 72 h of starvation) was subjected to vital BODIPY™ 493/503 staining for analysis of the number and size of the lipid droplets.

BODIPY™ 493/503 vital staining and fluorescence imaging

To visualize fat storage in worms and embryos, vital BODIPY™ 493/503 (Invitrogen, Darmstadt, Germany) staining was performed as previously described (Klapper et al. 2011). Briefly, freshly harvested worms were washed three times with M9 buffer and were incubated in 500 µL of BODIPY™ 493/503 solution (6.7 µg/µl in M9 buffer) for 20 min. After washing twice with M9, the worms were anesthetized using sodium azide (1 %) and immediately examined via microscopy. BODIPY™ 493/503 fluorescence was visualized using an Axio Imager system and a Z1 microscope equipped with a 38 HE filter (excitation: BP 470/40, beam splitter: FT 495, emission: BP 525/50), coupled to an apotome-sectioning system (ApoTome.2, Zeiss). To distinguish between BODIPY™ 493/503-positive structures and auto-fluorescent lysosome-related organelles, auto-fluorescence was imaged using the DAPI channel. GFP fluorescence was visualized with a 38 HE filter (excitation BP 470/40; beam splitter FT 495; emission BP 525/50).

Analysis of the number and size of lipid droplets

BODIPY™ 493/503-stained lipid droplets localized in selected regions were imaged via 3D fluorescence microscopy using an Axio Imager Z1 microscope and a Plan-Apochromat ×63/1.3 oil immersion objective. The apotome-sectioning system was used to collect z-stacks with a step size of 0.5 µm. The z-stacks comprised 21 planar images (format, 138.4 × 104 μm; 692 × 520 pixels). Images were captured using an AxioCam MRm (Zeiss) system. ImageJ software (version 1.47 h) and the 3D spot segmentation plug-in were used to analyze the z-stacks. BODIPY™ 493/503-positive structures were automatically identified, and the volume of each droplet was evaluated by totaling the number of voxels per droplet. If necessary, the brightness and contrast levels were manually adjusted before performing the calculations.

Thin-layer chromatography

After thawing worms stored at −80 °C, worms collected using the COPAS Biosort system were analyzed by thin-layer chromatography (Matyash et al. 2008). Lipids were extracted from 1000 or 2000 homogenized worms (*Precellys24* homogenizer; full speed; 3 × 10 s) using a solution containing 375 μl of methanol, 1250 μl of methyl-tert-butyl-ether [63], and 312 μl of H2O (3:10:2.5 [v]) and were dissolved in 30 μl of chloroform. Probes were applied to *Polygram SIL G* pre-coated TLC sheets (20 × 20 cm; 0.2-mm silica gel; Macherey-Nagel) using hexane/diethyl-ether/formic acid (20:20:1 [v]) as the mobile phase for TAG and phospholipids. A 5-μl aliquot of worm extract was applied to each lane to ensure that the amounts of TAGs and phospholipids were within the linear range of the standard curves. The assays were conducted in duplicate. The lipid spots were stained for 20 s in a dip solution containing 10 % copper (II) sulfate, 8 % phosphor acid, and 5 % methanol. Quantification was achieved by calculating the spot intensity per area (pixel/μm^2) using *AlphaEaseFC* (BioRad) software. Triolein (Sigma Aldrich, Germany) and a phospholipid mixture (Sigma Aldrich, P3817) were used as standards. All of the results are presented as the mean values for the standard and diluted probes.

Lipid composition analysis

Embryos were washed three times with M9 buffer supplemented with Tween 20 (1:100,000) to prevent the embryos from attaching to the tubes. Defined numbers of embryos that were sorted using the COPAS Biosort system were then transferred to chloroform-rinsed Pyrex tubes and were immediately frozen at −80 °C until being utilized for mass spectroscopy. The contents of the fatty acids triacylglyceride, phosphatidylcholine, and plasmalogen were analyzed using a high-resolution LC-MS/MS platform (Fauland et al. 2011) equipped with a Lipid Data Analyzer (Hartler et al. 2011). The results were normalized according to the contents of different fatty acid classes, the sample weight, and the protein content.

Statistical analysis

Statistical analysis was performed using Microsoft Excel (2003) and GraphPad Prism (Version 4.0) software. Unless otherwise noted, the data represent the mean ± SEM of at least three independent experiments. The significance of the differences was calculated using an unpaired two-tailed *t* test. Welch's correction was applied if the variances were different. Differences were considered significant at $p < 0.05$ (*), $p < 0.01$ (**), and $p < 0.001$ (***).

Competing interests

The authors declare that they have no competing interests.

Authors' contributions

MK carried out the DR assays, choline supplementation studies, lipid droplet analyses, and all other experiments regarding fat metabolism. MK helped to draft the manuscript. DF carried out F1 experiments regarding cold resistance and lipid droplet size. HK carried out lipodomic analyses. FD conceived of the study and participated in its design and coordination. FD drafted and finalized the manuscript. All authors read and approved the final manuscript.

Acknowledgements

We thank Astrid Reinke and Fabian Neumann for high throughput processing of plates and reagents. The study was funded by the University of Kiel and the leisure time of the authors.

Author details

[1]Institute of Human Nutrition and Food Science, Molecular Prevention, Christian-Albrechts University of Kiel, Heinrich-Hecht-Platz 10, 24118 Kiel, Germany. [2]Institute of Genetics, TU Braunschweig, 38106 Braunschweig, Germany. [3]ZMF—Center for Medical Research, University of Graz, Core Facility for Mass Spectrometry, Lipidomics and Metabolomics, A-8010 Graz, Austria. [4]Omics Center Graz, A-8010 Graz, Austria.

References

Anand P, Cermelli S, Li Z, Kassan A, Bosch M, Sigua R, Huang L, Ouellette AJ, Pol A, Welte MA, Gross SP (2012) A novel role for lipid droplets in the organismal antibacterial response. eLife 1:e00003. doi:10.7554/eLife.00003

Ashrafi K, Chang FY, Watts JL, Fraser AG, Kamath RS, Ahringer J, Ruvkun G (2003) Genome-wide RNAi analysis of Caenorhabditis elegans fat regulatory genes. Nature 421(6920):268–272

Barbosa AD, Savage DB, Siniossoglou S (2015) Lipid droplet-organelle interactions: emerging roles in lipid metabolism. Curr Opin Cell Biol 35:91–97. doi:10.1016/j.ceb.2015.04.017

Barker DJP (2001) Type 2 diabetes: the thrifty phenotype—preface. Br Med Bull 60:1–3. doi:10.1093/Bmb/60.1.1

Bartz R, Li WH, Venables B, Zehmer JK, Roth MR, Welti R, Anderson RG, Liu P, Chapman KD (2007) Lipidomics reveals that adiposomes store ether lipids and mediate phospholipid traffic. J Lipid Res 48(4):837–847

Baumeier C, Kaiser D, Heeren J, Scheja L, John C, Weise C, Eravci M, Lagerpusch M, Schulze G, Joost HG, Schwenk RW, Schurmann A (2015) Caloric restriction and intermittent fasting alter hepatic lipid droplet proteome and diacylglycerol species and prevent diabetes in NZO mice. Biochim Biophys Acta 1851(5):566–576. doi:10.1016/j.bbalip.2015.01.013

Bouwman FG, Claessens M, van Baak MA, Noben JP, Wang P, Saris WH, Mariman EC (2009) The physiologic effects of caloric restriction are reflected in the in vivo adipocyte-enriched proteome of overweight/obese subjects. J Proteome Res 8(12):5532–5540. doi:10.1021/pr900606m

Brendza KM, Haakenson W, Cahoon RE, Hicks LM, Palavalli LH, Chiapelli BJ, McLaird M, McCarter JP, Williams DJ, Hresko MC, Jez JM (2007) Phosphoethanolamine N-methyltransferase (PMT-1) catalyses the first reaction of a new pathway for phosphocholine biosynthesis in Caenorhabditis elegans. Biochem J 404(3):439–448. doi:10.1042/BJ20061815

Brenner S (1974) The genetics of Caenorhabditis elegans. Genetics 77(1):71–94
Burger JM, Hwangbo DS, Corby-Harris V, Promislow DE (2007) The functional costs and benefits of dietary restriction in Drosophila. Aging Cell 6(1):63–71. doi:10.1111/j.1474-9726.2006.00261.x
Cermelli S, Guo Y, Gross SP, Welte MA (2006) The lipid-droplet proteome reveals that droplets are a protein-storage depot. Curr Biol 16(18):1783–1795. doi:10.1016/j.cub.2006.07.062
Ehmke M, Luthe K, Schnabel R, Doring F (2014) S-Adenosyl methionine synthetase 1 limits fat storage in Caenorhabditis elegans. Genes Nutr 9(2): 386. doi:10.1007/s12263-014-0386-6
Fauland A, Kofeler H, Trotzmuller M, Knopf A, Hartler J, Eberl A, Chitraju C, Lankmayr E, Spener F (2011) A comprehensive method for lipid profiling by liquid chromatography-ion cyclotron resonance mass spectrometry. J Lipid Res 52(12):2314–2322. doi:10.1194/jlr.D016550
Fontana L, Partridge L (2015) Promoting health and longevity through diet: from model organisms to humans. Cell 161(1):106–118. doi:10.1016/j.cell.2015.02.020
Guo Y, Walther TC, Rao M, Stuurman N, Goshima G, Terayama K, Wong JS, Vale RD, Walter P, Farese RV (2008) Functional genomic screen reveals genes involved in lipid-droplet formation and utilization. Nature 453(7195):657–661. doi:10.1038/nature06928
Hansen M, Hsu AL, Dillin A, Kenyon C (2005) New genes tied to endocrine, metabolic, and dietary regulation of lifespan from a Caenorhabditis elegans genomic RNAi screen. PLoS Genet 1(1):119–128. doi:10.1371/journal.pgen.0010017
Hartler J, Trotzmuller M, Chitraju C, Spener F, Kofeler HC, Thallinger GG (2011) Lipid data analyzer: unattended identification and quantitation of lipids in LC-MS data. Bioinformatics 27(4):572–577. doi:10.1093/bioinformatics/btq699
Klapper M, Ehmke M, Palgunow D, Bohme M, Matthaus C, Bergner G, Dietzek B, Popp J, Doring F (2011) Fluorescence-based fixative and vital staining of lipid droplets in Caenorhabditis elegans reveal fat stores using microscopy and flow cytometry approaches. J Lipid Res 52(6):1281–1293. doi:10.1194/jlr.D011940
Krahmer N, Guo Y, Wilfling F, Hilger M, Lingrell S, Heger K, Newman HW, Schmidt-Supprian M, Vance DE, Mann M, Farese RV Jr, Walther TC (2011) Phosphatidylcholine synthesis for lipid droplet expansion is mediated by localized activation of CTP:phosphocholine cytidylyltransferase. Cell Metab 14(4):504–515. doi:10.1016/j.cmet.2011.07.013
Lee JH, Kong J, Jang JY, Han JS, Ji Y, Lee J, Kim JB (2014) Lipid droplet protein LID-1 mediates ATGL-1-dependent lipolysis during fasting in Caenorhabditis elegans. Mol Cell Biol 34(22):4165–4176. doi:10.1128/MCB.00722-14
Leermakers ET, Moreira EM, Kiefte-de Jong JC, Darweesh SK, Visser T, Voortman T, Bautista PK, Chowdhury R, Gorman D, Bramer WM, Felix JF, Franco OH (2015) Effects of choline on health across the life course: a systematic review. Nutr Rev 73(8):500–522. doi:10.1093/nutrit/nuv010
Li Y, Na K, Lee HJ, Lee EY, Paik YK (2011) Contribution of sams-1 and pmt-1 to lipid homoeostasis in adult Caenorhabditis elegans. J Biochem 149(5):529–538. doi:10.1093/jb/mvr025
Li Z, Thiel K, Thul PJ, Beller M, Kuhnlein RP, Welte MA (2012) Lipid droplets control the maternal histone supply of Drosophila embryos. Curr Biol 22(22): 2104–2113. doi:10.1016/j.cub.2012.09.018
Matlib MA, Frenkel EP, Mukherjee A, Henslee J, Srere PA (1979) Enzymatic properties of mitochondria isolated from normal and vitamin B12-deficient rats. Arch Biochem Biophys 197(2):388–395
Matyash V, Liebisch G, Kurzchalia TV, Shevchenko A, Schwudke D (2008) Lipid extraction by methyl-tert-butyl ether for high-throughput lipidomics. J Lipid Res 49(5):1137–1146. doi:10.1194/jlr.D700041-JLR200
Miersch C, Doring F (2013) Sex differences in body composition, fat storage, and gene expression profile in Caenorhabditis elegans in response to dietary restriction. Physiol Genomics 45(13):539–551. doi:10.1152/physiolgenomics.00007.2013
Narbonne P, Roy R (2009) Caenorhabditis elegans dauers need LKB1/AMPK to ration lipid reserves and ensure long-term survival. Nature 457(7226):210–214. doi:10.1038/nature07536
Nishino N, Tamori Y, Tateya S, Kawaguchi T, Shibakusa T, Mizunoya W, Inoue K, Kitazawa R, Kitazawa S, Matsuki Y, Hiramatsu R, Masubuchi S, Omachi A, Kimura K, Saito M, Amo T, Ohta S, Yamaguchi T, Osumi T, Cheng J, Fujimoto T, Nakao H, Nakao K, Aiba A, Okamura H, Fushiki T, Kasuga M (2008) FSP27 contributes to efficient energy storage in murine white adipocytes by promoting the formation of unilocular lipid droplets. J Clin Invest 118(8): 2808–2821. doi:10.1172/JCI34090
Palavalli LH, Brendza KM, Haakenson W, Cahoon RE, McLaird M, Hicks LM, McCarter JP, Williams DJ, Hresko MC, Jez JM (2006) Defining the role of phosphomethylethanolamine N-methyltransferase from Caenorhabditis elegans in phosphocholine biosynthesis by biochemical and kinetic analysis. Biochemistry 45(19):6056–6065. doi:10.1021/bi060199d
Palgunow D, Klapper M, Doring F (2012) Dietary restriction during development enlarges intestinal and hypodermal lipid droplets in Caenorhabditis elegans. PLoS One 7(11):e46198. doi:10.1371/journal.pone.0046198
Rinella ME, Green RM (2004) The methionine-choline deficient dietary model of steatohepatitis does not exhibit insulin resistance. J Hepatol 40(1):47–51
Szymanski KM, Binns D, Bartz R, Grishin NV, Li WP, Agarwal AK, Garg A, Anderson RG, Goodman JM (2007) The lipodystrophy protein seipin is found at endoplasmic reticulum lipid droplet junctions and is important for droplet morphology. Proc Natl Acad Sci USA 104(52):20890–20895
Walker AK, Jacobs RL, Watts JL, Rottiers V, Jiang K, Finnegan DM, Shioda T, Hansen M, Yang F, Niebergall LJ, Vance DE, Tzoneva M, Hart AC, Naar AM (2011) A conserved SREBP-1/phosphatidylcholine feedback circuit regulates lipogenesis in metazoans. Cell 147(4):840–852. doi:10.1016/j.cell.2011.09.045
Welte MA (2015) Expanding roles for lipid droplets. Curr Biol 25(11):R470–R481. doi:10.1016/j.cub.2015.04.004
Zeisel SH, Da Costa KA, Franklin PD, Alexander EA, Lamont JT, Sheard NF, Beiser A (1991) Choline, an essential nutrient for humans. FASEB J 5(7):2093–2098
Zhang SO, Box AC, Xu N, Le Men J, Yu J, Guo F, Trimble R, Mak HY (2010a) Genetic and dietary regulation of lipid droplet expansion in Caenorhabditis elegans. Proc Natl Acad Sci U S A 107(10):4640–4645. doi:10.1073/pnas.0912308107
Zhang SO, Trimble R, Guo F, Mak HY (2010b) Lipid droplets as ubiquitous fat storage organelles in C. elegans. BMC Cell Biol 11:96. doi:10.1186/1471-2121-11-96

17

FTO genotype, dietary protein intake, and body weight in a multiethnic population of young adults

David C. Merritt[†], Joseph Jamnik[†] and Ahmed El-Sohemy[*]

Abstract

Background: Variation in the fat mass and obesity-associated gene (*FTO*) has been associated with susceptibility to obesity, but the association appears to be modified by diet. We investigated whether dietary protein intake modifies the association between *FTO* variant rs1558902 and body mass index (BMI) and waist circumference in young adults ($n = 1491$) from the cross-sectional Toronto Nutrigenomics and Health Study.

Results: Lifestyle, genetic, anthropometric, and biochemical data were collected and diet was assessed using a Toronto-modified Willett Food Frequency Questionnaire. General linear models stratified by ethnicity and adjusted for age, sex, and total energy intake were used to examine the association between FTO genotypes and measures of body weight, and whether protein intake modified any of the associations. East Asians who were homozygous for the rs1558902 risk allele (A) had a greater BMI ($p = 0.004$) and waist circumference ($p = 0.03$) than T allele carriers. This association was not observed in individuals of Caucasian or South Asian ancestry. Among East Asians, a significant FTO-protein interaction was observed for BMI ($p = 0.01$) and waist circumference ($p = 0.007$). Those with low protein intake (≤ 18% total energy intake) who were homozygous for the rs1558902 risk allele (A) had significantly higher BMI ($p < 0.0001$) and waist circumference ($p = 0.0006$) compared to carriers of the T allele. These associations were absent in the high protein intake group (> 18% total energy intake). Compared to Caucasians and South Asians, East Asians consumed a significantly higher ratio of animal-to-plant protein ($p < 0.05$).

Conclusions: These findings suggest that high dietary protein intake may protect against the effects of risk variants in the *FTO* gene on BMI and waist circumference.

Keywords: Nutrigenomics, *FTO*, Obesity, Protein, Diet, Weight loss, BMI

Background

Despite increasing emphasis on the importance of health promotion, worldwide obesity rates and their associated health and economic burdens continue to rise. A recent systemic review of data collected from over 9 million individuals representing 199 countries reported that mean body mass index (BMI) has increased significantly worldwide since 1980 [1]. Associated with premature death, linked to cardiovascular disease, type 2 diabetes, and cancer, the widespread obesity epidemic has evolved into one of the most serious public health concerns of the century [2].

* Correspondence: a.el.sohemy@utoronto.ca
[†]Equal contributors
Department of Nutritional Sciences, University of Toronto, 150 College Street, Room 350, Toronto, Ontario M5S 3E2, Canada

Obesity is known to have a significant genetic component alongside various lifestyle and environmental factors [3–6]. Socioeconomic status, education, physical activity, ethnicity, and dietary patterns have all been reported as significant environmental influences [5, 7, 8]. Strongly linked with the development of obesity, the fat mass and obesity-associated (*FTO*) gene was one of the first genetic loci identified as being associated with body weight [9–17]. Studies have reported a range of 0.25–0.41 kg/m^2 increase in BMI per *FTO* risk allele, and a corresponding 20–40% increased risk of obesity [18]. Individuals homozygous for *FTO* risk variants are, on average, 3 kg heavier than those without such alleles [9]. Risk alleles are most prevalent in European populations (~ 42%) and least prevalent in African populations (~ 12%), accounting for 0.3 and 0.1% of total BMI variance, respectively [18, 19]. In Asian populations, the *FTO* risk allele frequency and explained variation in BMI is estimated to be 30 and 0.2%, respectively [20]. While there have been a large number of loci identified in addition to *FTO* which collectively explain a larger portion of total variation in BMI [21], the potential for effect modification by diet has been most extensively studied with *FTO*.

The association between *FTO* and dietary intake has been investigated in a number of studies. Variation in *FTO* has been associated with increased energy, fat, and protein intake [22–25]. Furthermore, it has been shown that the effects of several *FTO* polymorphisms on body weight can be modified by various dietary parameters [26–30]. Recently, a large randomized intervention trial investigated anthropometric measures and fat distribution in response to weight loss diets over a 2-year period [27]. Those who carried at least one copy of the *FTO* rs1558902 risk allele (A) experienced significantly greater reductions in body mass and fat distribution in response to a high-protein diet compared to T allele homozygotes, while this effect of *FTO* genotype was not observed in the low-protein treatment group. This interaction between dietary protein and *FTO* genotype on weight loss has been replicated in a population of obese adults in Spain [31]. However, the majority of participants in these studies were Caucasian, and it is unclear whether the *FTO* variants interact with dietary protein intake to influence measures of body weight in individuals of diverse ethnocultural backgrounds. The objective of the present study was to examine the association between genetic variation in *FTO* and measures of body weight and to determine whether protein intake modifies any observed associations in a cross-sectional population of ethnically diverse young adults.

Methods

Study population

Subjects ($n = 1639$) were individuals from the cross-sectional Toronto Nutrigenomics and Health (TNH) Study. Recruitment for the TNH study began in 2004 and ended in fall of 2010. The study was approved by the University of Toronto Ethics Review Board and informed consent was obtained from all individuals included in the study. Participants were males and females between 20 and 29 years of age. Individuals provided a self-reported account of their ancestry and were classified into one of four major ethnocultural groups—Caucasian, East Asian, South Asian, and "others"—as described previously [32]. All participants completed a 1-month 196-item semi-quantitative food frequency questionnaire (FFQ), a 63-item food preference checklist, and a general health and lifestyle questionnaire (GHLQ). The GHLQ included questions about physical activity, lifestyle habits, medication, dietary supplements, demographic status, dietary restrictions, education, and place of birth. Details of the Toronto-modified Willett FFQ used in the present study have been described previously [32]. Subjects provided a fasting blood sample from which DNA was isolated. Pregnant or nursing women and individuals who could not provide a blood sample were excluded from the study. We also excluded individuals with diabetes ($n = 3$), highly muscular subjects ($n = 10$), individuals missing *FTO* genotype, anthropometric, or dietary data ($n = 20$), and those belonging to the "other" ethnocultural group ($n = 115$). After exclusions, 1491 individuals (468 men and 1023 women) remained.

Dietary assessment

A 1-month 196-item semi-quantitative FFQ (Toronto-modified Willet) was used to estimate each subject's daily dietary protein intake. Subjects were given instructions and visual aids of common portion sizes to assist them in completing the FFQ. The base Willett FFQ has previously been validated for energy-adjusted protein intake against multiple 24-h recalls [33]. Protein intake was adjusted for total energy intake and expressed as percentage of total energy intake in all analyses in the present study.

Anthropometric/biochemical measurements and genotyping

Anthropometric measurements including height, weight, blood pressure, and waist circumference were determined as previously described [32]. BMI (kg/m^2) was calculated, and physical activity was measured by questionnaire and expressed as metabolic equivalent hours per week (MET), as described previously [32]. Blood samples were collected after a 12-h minimum fast by LifeLabs Medical Laboratory Services (Toronto, Canada) for DNA isolation and biochemical analysis using previously described methods [34]. Subjects were genotyped for rs1558902, a common single nucleotide polymorphism (SNP) in *FTO* at Princess Margret Hospital (Toronto, Canada) using Sequenom MassARRAY® technology.

Statistical analysis

All analyses were conducted using SAS Statistical Analysis Software v.9.2 (SAS Institute Inc., Cary, NC, USA). Variables that were not normally distributed were appropriately $\log_{e-}$ or square root transformed prior to analysis in order to satisfy the requirements of the statistical methods utilized, but the mean values and standard errors are reported in tables and figures without transformation to facilitate interpretation. Outcome variables BMI and waist circumference were log-transformed in all analyses. The α error was set at 0.05 and reported p values are two-sided.

Subject characteristics by rs1558902 genotype were compared using χ^2 tests for categorical variables and ANCOVAs adjusted for age, sex, ethnicity, BMI, and total energy intake for continuous variables. The associations between rs1558902 genotype and BMI as well as waist circumference were explored using general linear models (GLMs) in each ethnocultural group. Analyses were adjusted for age, sex, and total energy intake. The Tukey-Kramer procedure was used to account for multiple comparisons when assessing differences in means between genotypes. Median energy-adjusted protein intakes were established for each ethnocultural subgroup and individuals were classified as either having "low" (≤ median) or "high" (> median) energy-adjusted protein intake. GLMs were then used to determine whether stratification by median values of energy-adjusted protein intake modified the association between rs1558902 genotype and BMI or waist circumference in each ethnocultural group. A test for the interaction between rs1558902 genotype and energy-adjusted dietary protein intake was performed on BMI and waist circumference. Macronutrient intakes were compared between those consuming "low" and "high" protein within each ethnocultural group. GLMs adjusted for age and sex were used to assess differences in energy-adjusted macronutrient intakes. GLMs adjusted for age and sex were also used to compare differences in the ratio of animal-to-plant protein consumption within each ethnocultural group.

Results

Subject characteristics by FTO genotype are summarized in Table 1. The minor allele (A) frequency of rs1558902 was 30% for the total population, 42% in Caucasians, 13% in East Asians, and 29% in South Asians. Genotype frequencies were significantly different between ethnocultural groups, with the prevalence of risk allele (A) carriers being highest in Caucasians and lowest in East Asians ($p < 0.0001$). Significant associations were observed between rs1558902 and BMI ($p = 0.02$), physical activity ($p = 0.005$), homeostatic model assessment of insulin resistance (HOMA-IR) ($p = 0.02$), homeostatic model assessment of β cell function (HOMA-β) ($p = 0.02$), and triglycerides ($p = 0.01$) after adjusting for age, sex, ethnicity, BMI, and energy intake. No associations between rs1558902 and waist circumference ($p = 0.07$) or total energy intake ($p = 0.17$) were observed.

Subgroup analysis by ethnicity revealed a significant association between rs1558902 genotype and BMI ($p = 0.004$) and waist circumference ($p = 0.03$) in East Asians (Table 2), where risk allele homozygotes (AA, $n = 11$) had a higher BMI and waist circumference than T allele carriers (TT, $n = 422$; TA, $n = 125$). In Caucasians, TA heterozygotes ($n = 367$) at rs1558902 had a significantly greater waist circumference than TT homozygotes ($n = 256$), while AA homozygotes ($n = 136$) had a similar waist circumference to both TT ($n = 256$) and TA individuals. There was no association between rs1558902 genotype and BMI or waist circumference in South Asians. There was no significant interaction between *FTO* genotype and sex on BMI or waist circumference in any ethnocultural group. Further subgroup analyses were performed for Caucasians, East Asians, and South Asians to determine the relationship between protein intake, FTO genotype, and measures of obesity (Table 3). Median energy-adjusted protein intake in Caucasians, East Asians, and South Asians were determined to be 17, 18, and 17% of total energy intake, respectively. East Asians in the low-protein group (≤ 18% total energy intake) who were homozygous risk allele carriers (AA) had significantly higher BMI ($p < 0.0001$) and waist circumference ($p = 0.0006$) than carriers of the T allele. This association between rs1558902 genotype and BMI or waist circumference was not observed in the high protein intake group ($p > 0.05$). There were significant interactions between rs1558902 genotype and energy-adjusted protein intake on both BMI ($p = 0.01$) and waist circumference ($p = 0.007$) in East Asians. There was no significant interaction between rs1558902 genotype and dietary protein intake on BMI or waist circumference in Caucasian or South Asian individuals ($p > 0.05$).

Energy-adjusted macronutrient intakes in "low"- and "high"-protein consumers are shown in Table 4. High protein consumption was associated with significantly ($p < 0.05$) lower intake of total carbohydrates, sugars, and starches in all three major ethnocultural groups. High protein consumption was also associated ($p < 0.05$) with greater consumption of saturated fat in all ethnocultural groups. High protein intake was also associated ($p < 0.05$) with lower polyunsaturated fat intake in Caucasians, and greater total fat and monounsaturated fat in East Asians and South Asians. High total protein consumption was associated ($p < 0.05$) with greater intake of protein from animal sources across all ethnocultural groups, and lower intakes of protein from plant sources in Caucasians and East Asians. The ratio of animal-to-plant protein intakes across ethnocultural groups is shown in Fig. 1. East Asians had a higher ratio of animal-to-plant protein intake than Caucasians or South Asians ($p < 0.05$).

Discussion

Although *FTO* is an established genetic susceptibility locus for obesity, the extent to which dietary factors modify this association has been unclear. Several studies have examined the effects of different dietary

Table 1 Subject characteristics by *FTO* genotype

	rs1558902 genotype			
	TT	TA	AA	*p*
Subjects [*n*(%)]	762 (51)	569 (38)	160 (11)	
Age (year)	22.5 ± 0.1	22.8 ± 0.1	22.7 ± 0.2[a]	0.11
Sex [*n*(%)]				0.78
Male	233 (50)	184 (39)	51 (11)	
Female	529 (52)	385 (38)	109 (10)	
Ethnicity [*n*(%)]				< 0.0001
Caucasian	256 (34)	367 (48)	136 (18)	
East Asian	422 (76)	125 (22)	11 (2)	
South Asian	84 (48)	77 (44)	13 (8)	
BMI (kg/m^2)	22.3 ± 0.1b	23.2 ± 0.2a	23.6 ± 0.3a	0.02
Systolic blood pressure (mmHg)	112.6 ± 0.4	114.7 ± 0.5	115.2 ± 0.8	0.77
Diastolic blood pressure (mmHg)	69.0 ± 0.3	69.7 ± 0.3	69.3 ± 0.6	0.73
Waist circumference (cm)	72.8 ± 0.3	75.1 ± 0.4	75.9 ± 0.7	0.07
Physical activity (METs)	7.7 ± 0.1b	7.6 ± 0.1b	8.4 ± 0.2a	0.005
Glucose (mmol/L)	4.79 ± 0.01	4.78 ± 0.02	4.77 ± 0.03	0.92
Insulin (pmol/L)	46.2 ± 1.0	47.6 ± 1.9	45 ± 2.6	0.39
HOMA-IR	1.39 ± 0.03	1.43 ± 0.06	1.34 ± 0.09	0.02
HOMA-β	107.2 ± 4.2	106.9 ± 3.8	101.7 ± 5.6	0.02
Cholesterol				
Total (mmol/L)	4.25 ± 0.03	4.26 ± 0.03	4.25 ± 0.06	0.93
HDL (mmol/L)	1.54 ± 0.01	1.54 ± 0.02	1.53 ± 0.03	0.28
LDL (mmol/L)	2.27 ± 0.02	2.28 ± 0.03	2.31 ± 0.05	0.71
Total/HDL (mmol/L)	2.89 ± 0.03	2.92 ± 0.04	2.88 ± 0.05	0.64
Triglycerides (mmol/L)	0.99 ± 0.02	0.97 ± 0.02	0.91 ± 0.03	0.01
hs-CRP (mg/L)	1.0 ± 0.1	1.5 ± 0.1	1.4 ± 0.2	0.59
Free fatty acids (μmol/L)	487.2 ± 9.1	483.8 ± 10.8	475.5 ± 20.8	0.82
Dietary intake				
Energy (kcal/day)	2033 ± 33	2116 ± 98	2017 ± 68	0.17
Protein (g/day)	89.9 ± 1.6	89.6 ± 1.7	84.0 ± 3.0	0.39
Total fat (g/day)	67.5 ± 1.2	71.0 ± 1.5	69.8 ± 3.0	0.96
Carbohydrates (g/day)	267.7 ± 4.5	279.6 ± 5.3	262.6 ± 8.7	0.52

Differences between groups assessed using χ^2 test for categorical variables and ANCOVA adjusted for age, sex, ethnicity, BMI, and energy intake for continuous variables. Groups without a common letter differ after a Tukey-Kramer post hoc test ($p < 0.05$)
METs metabolic equivalent hours per week, *HOMA-IR* homeostasis model of insulin resistance, *HOMA-β* homeostasis model of β-cell function, *HDL* high-density lipoprotein, *LDL* low-density lipoprotein, *hs-CRP* high-sensitivity C-reactive protein
[a]Mean ± SE (all such values)

interventions on measures of body weight and composition, but the results remain inconsistent. We examined the interaction between *FTO* variant rs1558902 and dietary protein intake on BMI and waist circumference in a cross-sectional population of young adults of diverse ethnocultural backgrounds. Our findings indicate that protein intake modifies the effect of *FTO* risk variants in East Asian individuals, but not Caucasians or South Asians. East Asian individuals homozygous for the risk allele (A) of rs1558902 who had a low dietary protein intake had significantly higher BMI and waist circumference than T allele carriers. No association was observed between *FTO* genotype and BMI or waist circumference among those consuming higher amounts of protein. These findings suggest that dietary protein intake protects against the effect of the *FTO* risk variants on BMI and waist circumference. Our findings are based on East Asians living in North America, whereas almost all other studies evaluating *FTO* variants in Asian populations are based in Asia [35]. We did not observe a clear

Table 2 *FTO* genotype and measures of body weight stratified by ethnicity

	rs1558902 genotype			
	TT	TA	AA	*p*
Caucasians				
Subjects (*n*)	256	367	136	
BMI (kg/m^2)	22.9 ± 0.2[a]	23.6 ± 0.2	23.4 ± 0.3	0.07
Waist circumference (cm)	74.7 ± 0.5a	76.4 ± 0.5b	75.6 ± 0.8ab	0.03
East Asians				
Subjects (*n*)	422	125	11	
BMI (kg/m^2)	21.7 ± 0.1b	22.0 ± 0.2b	24.5 ± 1.2a	0.004
Waist circumference (cm)	71.0 ± 0.4b	71.4 ± 0.6b	77.0 ± 3.0a	0.03
South Asians				
Subjects (*n*)	84	77	13	
BMI (kg/m^2)	23.7 ± 0.4	23.6 ± 0.5	24.8 ± 1.8	0.93
Waist circumference (cm)	76.4 ± 1.1	75.2 ± 1.5	77.2 ± 3.8	0.96

Differences between groups assessed using GLMs adjusted for age, sex, and energy intake
Groups without a common letter differ after a Tukey-Kramer post hoc test (p<0.05)
[a]Mean ± SE (all such values)

association between *FTO* and BMI or waist circumference, or any significant *FTO*-protein interaction on measures of body weight in Caucasians or South Asians.

The prevalence of the rs1558902 risk allele in the present study population is in agreement with previous reported values for Caucasian, East Asian, and South Asian populations [18–20]. The rs1558902 genotype has been robustly associated with body weight across multiple ethnicities and is in strong linkage disequilibrium with other *FTO* variants such as rs9939609 and rs9930506 [13, 18, 36, 37]. Using rs1558902 as a proxy for widespread variation in the *FTO* gene, we replicated the association between *FTO* risk variants and BMI [18]. Carriers of the risk allele had a significantly higher BMI

Table 3 *FTO* genotype and measures of body weight stratified by ethnicity and protein intake

	Low protein (≤ median intake)[a]				High protein (> median intake)[a]				
	rs1558902 genotype				rs1558902 genotype				Interaction
	TT	TA	AA	*p*[b]	TT	TA	AA	*p*[b]	*p*[c]
Caucasian									
Subjects (*n*)	115	197	68		141	170	68		
Body mass index (kg/m^2)	22.4 ± 0.3[d]	23.1 ± 0.2	23.1 ± 0.4	0.2	23.3 ± 0.3	24.1 ± 0.3	23.7 ± 0.4	0.17	0.95
Waist circumference (cm)	73.6 ± 0.7	76.2 ± 0.6	75.4 ± 1.1	0.07	75.5 ± 0.7	76.6 ± 0.8	75.9 ± 1.0	0.17	0.99
East Asian									
Subjects (*n*)	215	55	9		207	70	2		
Body mass index (kg/m^2)	21.5 ± 0.2c	22.5 ± 0.3b	25.0 ± 1.3a	< 0.0001	21.8 ± 0.2	21.5 ± 0.3	22.4 ± 1.9	0.58	0.01
Waist circumference (cm)	70.6 ± 0.5b	72.0 ± 0.9b	78.9 ± 3.4a	0.0006	71.4 ± 0.5	71.0 ± 0.8	68.1 ± 1.3	0.34	0.007
South Asian									
Subjects (*n*)	42	40	5		42	37	8		
Body mass index (kg/m^2)	23.8 ± 0.7	23.4 ± 0.7	24.4 ± 2.3	0.83	23.5 ± 0.5	23.9 ± 0.8	25.0 ± 2.7	0.86	0.86
Waist circumference (cm)	76.8 ± 1.7	74.4 ± 1.8	76.3 ± 5.2	0.75	76.0 ± 1.3	75.9 ± 2.5	77.8 ± 5.4	0.98	0.76

Groups without a common letter differ after a Tukey-Kramer post hoc test (p<0.05)
[a]Low and high protein intakes determined using ethnicity-specific medians: Caucasians (17% energy intake), East Asians (18% energy intake), South Asians (17% energy intake)
[b]Determined using GLMs adjusted for age and sex
[c]Interactions between rs1558902 genotype and energy-adjusted protein intake on markers of body mass determined using GLMs adjusted for age and sex
[d]Mean ± SE (all such values)

Table 4 Macronutrient intake in high- and low-protein consumers stratified by ethnicity

	Low protein (≤ median intake)[a]	High protein (> median intake)[a]	p^b
Caucasian (*n*)	380	379	
Carbohydrates			
Total carbohydrates (% energy intake)	54.3 ± 0.4[d]	50.0 ± 0.4	< .0001
Sugars[c] (% energy intake)	25.0 ± 0.4	23.1 ± 0.3	0.0001
Fiber (g/day)	27.1 ± 0.7	26.2 ± 0.7	0.57
Starches (% energy intake)	24.2 ± 0.3	21.8 ± 0.3	< .0001
Carbohydrates from whole grains (% energy intake)	8.4 ± 0.3	9.2 ± 0.3	0.05
Fat			
Total fats (% energy intake)	30.5 ± 0.4	30.9 ± 0.3	0.70
Saturated fat (% energy intake)	9.4 ± 0.1	10.2 ± 0.1	< .0001
Monounsaturated fat (% energy intake)	12.5 ± 0.2	12.2 ± 0.2	0.38
Polyunsaturated fat (% energy intake)	5.9 ± 0.1	5.6 ± 0.1	0.01
Protein			
Total protein (% energy intake)	14.4 ± 0.1	19.1 ± 0.1	< .0001
Animal protein intake (% energy intake)	7.6 ± 0.1	12.7 ± 0.2	< .0001
Plant protein intake (% energy intake)	6.7 ± 0.1	6.4 ± 0.1	0.01
East Asian (*n*)	279	279	
Carbohydrates			
Total carbohydrates (% energy intake)	56.8 ± 0.4	49.6 ± 0.4	< .0001
Sugars[c] (% energy intake)	24.7 ± 0.5	21.1 ± 0.4	< .0001
Fiber (g/day)	24.0 ± 0.9	20.8 ± 0.7	0.08
Starches (% energy intake)	27.5 ± 0.4	24.1 ± 0.4	< .0001
Carbohydrates from whole grains (% energy intake)	5.8 ± 0.3	6.1 ± 0.3	0.68
Fat			
Total fats (% energy intake)	28.4 ± 0.4	30.1 ± 0.3	0.0002
Saturated fat (% energy intake)	9.0 ± 0.1	9.8 ± 0.1	< .0001
Monounsaturated fat (% energy intake)	11.1 ± 0.2	11.6 ± 0.1	0.01
Polyunsaturated fat (% energy intake)	5.6 ± 0.1	5.6 ± 0.1	0.64
Protein			
Total protein (% energy intake)	15.5 ± 0.1	20.9 ± 0.1	< .0001
Animal protein intake (% energy intake)	9.1 ± 0.1	14.9 ± 0.2	< .0001
Plant protein intake (% energy intake)	6.4 ± 0.1	6.1 ± 0.1	0.01
South Asian (*n*)	87	87	
Carbohydrates			
Total carbohydrates (% energy intake)	60.5 ± 0.9	50.4 ± 0.9	< .0001
Sugars[c] (% energy intake)	27.7 ± 0.8	21.3 ± 0.6	< .0001
Fiber (g/day)	23.2 ± 1.5	23.2 ± 1.5	0.77
Starches (% energy intake)	27.7 ± 1.0	24.4 ± 0.7	0.01
Carbohydrates from whole grains (% energy intake)	7.9 ± 1.1	8.2 ± 0.7	0.07
Fat			
Total fats (% energy intake)	27.2 ± 0.9	30.0 ± 0.7	0.01
Saturated fat (% energy intake)	8.6 ± 0.3	9.9 ± 0.3	0.004
Monounsaturated fat (% energy intake)	10.9 ± 0.6	11.6 ± 0.3	0.04
Polyunsaturated fat (% energy intake)	5.4 ± 0.2	5.7 ± 0.2	0.32

Table 4 Macronutrient intake in high- and low-protein consumers stratified by ethnicity *(Continued)*

	Low protein (≤ median intake)[a]	High protein (> median intake)[a]	p^b
Protein			
Total protein (% energy intake)	14.0 ± 0.2	20.6 ± 0.3	< .0001
Animal protein intake (% energy intake)	7.4 ± 0.3	14.3 ± 0.4	< .0001
Plant protein intake (% energy intake)	6.6 ± 0.2	6.3 ± 0.2	0.39

[a]Low and high protein intakes determined using ethnicity-specific medians: Caucasians (17% energy intake), East Asians (18% energy intake), South Asians (17% energy intake)
[b]Determined using GLMs adjusted for age and sex
[c]Mean ± SE (all such values)
[d]Includes glucose, fructose, sucrose, lactose, and maltose

($p = 0.02$) than non-carriers and, although not significant, a similar trend was observed for waist circumference ($p = 0.07$).

Recently, there has been increased interest in determining whether dietary macronutrient composition interacts with variation in *FTO* to influence measures of body weight. The POUNDS LOST trial, a 2-year randomized weight loss intervention program, investigated the effects of different dietary treatments in a large population of obese individuals [27]. The authors observed that subjects with the risk allele (A) at rs1558902 who were placed on high-protein diets experienced greater positive changes in body composition and fat distribution than those on low-protein diets. No such effect of protein was observed among carriers of the T allele. These results suggest that dietary protein can mitigate the genetic risk associated with *FTO*. These findings were replicated in a recent weight loss trial which found that those with the *FTO* risk allele had greater weight loss and greater improvement in various metabolic parameters when placed on a high-protein diet [31]. However, a study of over 16,000 children from 14 study populations found that the adverse effects of variation in *FTO* on BMI were attenuated by low, rather than high, protein intake [38]. It is notable that the majority of subjects in the aforementioned studies were Caucasian, with only limited representation of other ethnocultural groups. Despite high prevalence of the risk allele and strong genetic effects reported in European populations, we were unable to detect an interaction between variation in *FTO* and protein intake on measures of body weight in young Caucasian individuals in the present study population. This is in agreement with analyses from the DiOGenes project, a European program focused on dietary components, genetics, and behavioral factors involved in the prevention of weight gain, which found no interaction between *FTO* and dietary protein intake on change in body weight or waist circumference at baseline or during the 6.8-year follow-up period [39]. They did, however, confirm an association between *FTO* variation and BMI and waist circumference at baseline. Furthermore, a recent meta-analysis evaluated 40 cross-sectional studies and found no interaction between *FTO* variants and protein intake on BMI [35]. That study did, however, identify an association between rs9939609 (or proxy SNPs) and higher dietary protein intakes, a relationship that was absent in the present investigation. However, the authors acknowledged that 87% of studies analyzed were based on Caucasian populations, and examinations of more diverse ethnic groups are clearly warranted.

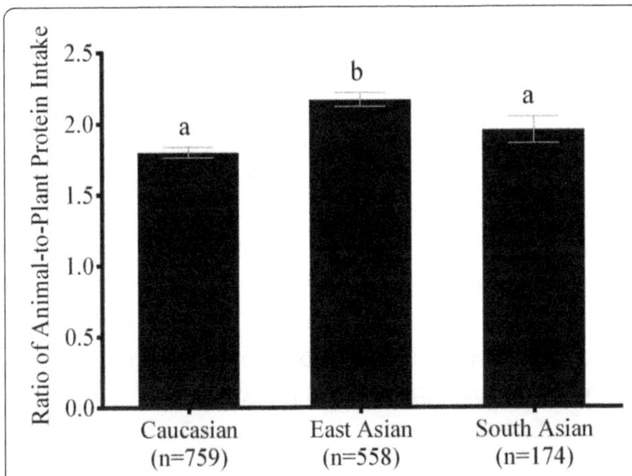

Fig. 1 Ratio of animal-to-plant protein intake across ethnocultural groups. Differences in the ratio of animal-to-plant protein intake between groups were compared using GLMs adjusted for age and sex. Groups without a common superscript letter differ after a Tukey-Kramer post hoc test ($p < 0.05$)

We observed elevated BMI and waist circumference in East Asian risk allele (A) homozygotes at rs1558902 in the low protein intake group, but not in those consuming higher amounts of protein. The mean BMI of risk allele homozygotes in those consuming low amounts of protein was 25.0 ± 1.3 kg/m^2, which makes them overweight, according to the United States Department of Health [40]. Furthermore, the average waist circumference for this group of participants was 78.9 ± 3.4 cm. Elevated BMI and waist circumference are established risk factors for cardiovascular disease [41, 42]. In the high protein intake group, all means were within normal ranges, and no significant differences in BMI or waist circumference were observed between genotypes. This would suggest that higher protein intakes may attenuate the association between *FTO* risk variants and adiposity and thus improve cardiovascular health outcomes in certain ethnocultural groups. We identified significant interactions between *FTO* genotypes and protein intake on both anthropometric outcomes in East Asians. Among East Asians, high total protein consumption was associated with lower intake of total carbohydrates, sugars, and starches. High total protein consumption was additionally associated with increased intake of total fats, saturated fat, and monounsaturated fat. High total protein consumption among East Asians was associated with greater animal protein intake, but less intake of protein from plant sources. Furthermore, compared to Caucasians and South Asians, East Asians consumed a significantly greater ratio of animal-to-plant protein. This suggests a potential effect of protein source on the observed interaction between *FTO* genotype and protein intake on body weight. Further investigation is needed to determine the clinical significance of these findings and potential applications as part of weight management interventions.

It has been established that *FTO* influences food intake rather than energy expenditure, yet many aspects of the association between variations in *FTO* and diet remain unclear. Many studies have identified an association between *FTO* risk variants and greater energy intake, especially in children and adolescents [23, 24, 38, 43, 44]. However, a large-scale multiethnic meta-analysis found an overall association between *FTO* risk variants and lower energy intake [35]. Interestingly, we observed no significant association between *FTO* variant rs1558902 and energy intake ($p = 0.17$). Additionally, contradictory to other studies that identified no association between variation in *FTO* and energy expenditure [22, 45], we identified a significant association between self-reported activity and rs1558902 genotype, where AA homozygotes were more physically active than T allele carriers in the overall population. However, this association was not observed in any ethnocultural group upon stratification by ethnicity (data not shown), and the self-reported measure of physical activity in the present study cannot be equated to direct measures of total energy expenditure.

Several limitations need to be considered when interpreting results from the present study. Although the total number of subjects included was relatively large, there were only 160 risk allele homozygotes (AA) for *FTO* variant rs1558902. Of these 160 individuals, 85% were Caucasian, so there was a limited subset of South and East Asian risk allele homozygotes. We were able to detect an association between rs1558902 and measures of body weight in East Asians in the low protein intake group; however, there were only two East Asian individuals with the AA genotype at rs1558902 genotype in the high protein intake group, and it is unclear if the lack of association in the high intake group was solely due to the modifying effects of protein intake, or whether a lack of statistical power could have played a role. Results of the present study should, therefore, be interpreted with caution. It is also possible that the lack of *FTO*-protein interaction on measures of body weight in Caucasians and South Asians was a result of FFQ-associated measurement error in assessing dietary protein intake, in addition to FFQ measurement error for individual food items as well as total energy intake. However, any measurement errors would likely occur equally across the different *FTO* genotypes and would not likely explain the observed associations. Moreover, despite its widespread use as a measure of body composition and adiposity, BMI does not take bone structure into account and cannot differentiate between lean and fat mass. For this reason, BMI is considered to be a poor surrogate measure of adiposity in some populations, which can lead to misclassification of obesity status [46]. While ethnicity-specific criteria for the classification of BMI have been suggested, BMI was treated as a continuous variable in the present study and all analyses were stratified by ethnocultural status, minimizing the potential effects of such differences. Waist circumference may be a better estimate of visceral body fat and can be a strong indicator of cardiovascular disease risk [47, 48]. In the present study, the analysis of BMI in conjunction with waist circumference minimized the risk of misclassification associated with the use of BMI as a measure of adiposity. Although analyses in the present study were adjusted for age, sex, and energy intake and stratified by ethnicity, it is possible that unaccounted for residual confounders influenced the results observed. Finally, the cross-sectional nature of our study precludes the establishment of causality in any of the associations we observed.

Conclusions

Our findings suggest that dietary protein intake modifies the association between genetic variation in *FTO* and measures of body weight in certain ethnocultural groups. Higher dietary protein intakes might protect against the obesogenic effects of certain *FTO* genotypes and lead to improved individual metabolic profiles. The benefits of high-protein diets for weight management have been previously demonstrated [49, 50], and our results have further suggested a link between *FTO*, protein intake, and body weight. Elucidating the mechanism governing this gene-diet interaction is a clear direction for future research. Further studies should also focus on evaluating the viability of this nutritional strategy in personalized weight loss interventions.

Abbreviations

BMI: Body mass index; FFQ: Food frequency questionnaire; *FTO*: Fat mass and obesity-associated gene; GHLQ: General health and lifestyle questionnaire; GLM: General linear model; HOMA: Homeostatic model assessment; MET: Metabolic equivalent hours per week; SNP: Single nucleotide polymorphism; TNH: Toronto Nutrigenomics and Health

Funding

Funding for this study was provided by the Canadian Institute for Health Research (CIHR).

Authors' contributions

AE-S and JJ designed the research. DCM and JJ conducted the statistical analysis. DCM wrote the paper. AE-S had the primary responsibility for the final content. All authors read and approved the final manuscript.

Competing interests

AE-S holds shares in Nutrigenomix Inc., a genetic testing company for personalized nutrition. DCM and JJ declare that they have no competing interests.

References

1. Finucane MM, Stevens GA, Cowan MJ, Danaei G, Lin JK, Paciorek CJ, Singh GM, Gutierrez HR, Lu Y, Bahalim AN, et al. National, regional, and global trends in body-mass index since 1980: systematic analysis of health examination surveys and epidemiological studies with 960 country-years and 9.1 million participants. Lancet. 2011;377:557–67.
2. Kopelman P. Health risks associated with overweight and obesity. Obes Rev. 2007;8(Suppl 1):13–7.
3. Loos RJ. Genetic determinants of common obesity and their value in prediction. Best Pract Res Clin Endocrinol Metab. 2012;26:211–26.
4. Wardle J, Carnell S, Haworth CM, Plomin R. Evidence for a strong genetic influence on childhood adiposity despite the force of the obesogenic environment. Am J Clin Nutr. 2008;87:398–404.
5. Kopelman PG. Obesity as a medical problem. Nature. 2000;404:635–43.
6. Bouchard C. Genetic factors in obesity. Med Clin North Am. 1989;73:67–81.
7. Malik VS, Willett WC, Hu FB. Global obesity: trends, risk factors and policy implications. Nat Rev Endocrinol. 2013;9:13–27.
8. Wang Y, Beydoun MA. The obesity epidemic in the United States—gender, age, socioeconomic, racial/ethnic, and geographic characteristics: a systematic review and meta-regression analysis. Epidemiol Rev. 2007;29:6–28.
9. Frayling TM, Timpson NJ, Weedon MN, Zeggini E, Freathy RM, Lindgren CM, Perry JR, Elliott KS, Lango H, Rayner NW, et al. A common variant in the FTO gene is associated with body mass index and predisposes to childhood and adult obesity. Science. 2007;316:889–94.
10. Vasan SK, Karpe F, Gu HF, Brismar K, Fall CH, Ingelsson E, Fall T. FTO genetic variants and risk of obesity and type 2 diabetes: a meta-analysis of 28,394 Indians. Obesity (Silver Spring). 2014;22:964–70.
11. Dina C, Meyre D, Gallina S, Durand E, Korner A, Jacobson P, Carlsson LM, Kiess W, Vatin V, Lecoeur C, et al. Variation in FTO contributes to childhood obesity and severe adult obesity. Nat Genet. 2007;39:724–6.
12. Hinney A, Nguyen TT, Scherag A, Friedel S, Bronner G, Muller TD, Grallert H, Illig T, Wichmann HE, Rief W, et al. Genome wide association (GWA) study for early onset extreme obesity supports the role of fat mass and obesity associated gene (FTO) variants. PLoS One. 2007;2:e1361.
13. Hotta K, Nakata Y, Matsuo T, Kamohara S, Kotani K, Komatsu R, Itoh N, Mineo I, Wada J, Masuzaki H, et al. Variations in the FTO gene are associated with severe obesity in the Japanese. J Hum Genet. 2008;53:546–53.
14. Hunt SC, Stone S, Xin Y, Scherer CA, Magness CL, Iadonato SP, Hopkins PN, Adams TD. Association of the FTO gene with BMI. Obesity (Silver Spring). 2008;16:902–4.
15. Tonjes A, Zeggini E, Kovacs P, Bottcher Y, Schleinitz D, Dietrich K, Morris AP, Enigk B, Rayner NW, Koriath M, et al. Association of FTO variants with BMI and fat mass in the self-contained population of Sorbs in Germany. Eur J Hum Genet. 2010;18:104–10.
16. Villalobos-Comparán M, Teresa Flores-Dorantes M, Teresa Villarreal-Molina M, et al. The FTO gene is associated with adulthood obesity in the Mexican population. Obesity (Silver Spring). 2008;16:2296–301.
17. Peeters A, Beckers S, Verrijken A, Roevens P, Peeters P, Van Gaal L, Van Hul W. Variants in the FTO gene are associated with common obesity in the Belgian population. Mol Genet Metab. 2008;93:481 4.
18. Loos RJ, Yeo GS. The bigger picture of FTO: the first GWAS-identified obesity gene. Nat Rev Endocrinol. 2014;10:51–61.
19. Speliotes EK, Willer CJ, Berndt SI, Monda KL, Thorleifsson G, Jackson AU, Lango Allen H, Lindgren CM, Luan J, Magi R, et al. Association analyses of 249,796 individuals reveal 18 new loci associated with body mass index. Nat Genet. 2010;42:937–48.
20. Li H, Kilpelainen TO, Liu C, Zhu J, Liu Y, Hu C, Yang Z, Zhang W, Bao W, Cha S, et al. Association of genetic variation in FTO with risk of obesity and type 2 diabetes with data from 96,551 East and South Asians. Diabetologia. 2012;55:981–95.
21. Locke AE, Kahali B, Berndt SI, Justice AE, Pers TH, Day FR, Powell C, Vedantam S, Buchkovich ML, Yang J, et al. Genetic studies of body mass index yield new insights for obesity biology. Nature. 2015;518:197–206.
22. Speakman JR, Rance KA, Johnstone AM. Polymorphisms of the FTO gene are associated with variation in energy intake, but not energy expenditure. Obesity (Silver Spring). 2008;16:1961–5.
23. Lee HJ, Kim IK, Kang JH, Ahn Y, Han BG, Lee JY, Song J. Effects of common FTO gene variants associated with BMI on dietary intake and physical activity in Koreans. Clin Chim Acta. 2010;411:1716–22.
24. Timpson NJ, Emmett PM, Frayling TM, Rogers I, Hattersley AT, McCarthy MI, Davey Smith G. The fat mass- and obesity-associated locus and dietary intake in children. Am J Clin Nutr. 2008;88:971–8.
25. Ahmad T, Lee IM, Pare G, Chasman DI, Rose L, Ridker PM, Mora S. Lifestyle interaction with fat mass and obesity-associated (FTO) genotype and risk of obesity in apparently healthy U.S. women. Diabetes Care. 2011;34:675–80.
26. Sonestedt E, Roos C, Gullberg B, Ericson U, Wirfalt E, Orho-Melander M. Fat and carbohydrate intake modify the association between genetic variation in the FTO genotype and obesity. Am J Clin Nutr. 2009;90:1418–25.
27. Zhang X, Qi Q, Zhang C, Smith SR, Hu FB, Sacks FM, Bray GA, Qi L. FTO genotype and 2-year change in body composition and fat distribution in response to weight-loss diets: the POUNDS LOST Trial. Diabetes. 2012;61:3005–11.
28. Huang T, Qi Q, Li Y, Hu FB, Bray GA, Sacks FM, Williamson DA, Qi L. FTO genotype, dietary protein, and change in appetite: the Preventing Overweight Using Novel Dietary Strategies trial. Am J Clin Nutr. 2014;99:1126–30.
29. Grau K, Hansen T, Holst C, Astrup A, Saris WH, Arner P, Rossner S, Macdonald I, Polak J, Oppert JM, et al. Macronutrient-specific effect of FTO rs9939609 in response to a 10-week randomized hypo-energetic diet among obese Europeans. Int J Obes. 2009;33:1227–34.
30. Moleres A, Ochoa MC, Rendo-Urteaga T, Martinez-Gonzalez MA, Azcona San Julian MC, Martinez JA, Marti A, Genoi. Dietary fatty acid distribution modifies obesity risk linked to the rs9939609 polymorphism of the fat mass and obesity-associated gene in a Spanish case-control study of children. Br J Nutr. 2012;107:533–8.
31. de Luis DA, Aller R, Izaola O, Primo D, Urdiales S, Romero E. Effects of a high-protein/low-carbohydrate diet versus a standard hypocaloric diet on weight and cardiovascular risk factors: role of a genetic variation in the rs9939609 FTO gene variant. J Nutrigenet Nutrigenomics. 2015;8:128–36.
32. Garcia-Bailo B, Brenner DR, Nielsen D, Lee HJ, Domanski D, Kuzyk M, Borchers CH, Badawi A, Karmali MA, El-Sohemy A. Dietary patterns and ethnicity are associated with distinct plasma proteomic groups. Am J Clin Nutr. 2012;95:352–61.
33. Subar AF, Thompson FE, Kipnis V, Midthune D, Hurwitz P, McNutt S, McIntosh A, Rosenfeld S. Comparative validation of the Block, Willett, and National Cancer Institute food frequency questionnaires: the Eating at America's Table Study. Am J Epidemiol. 2001;154:1089–99.
34. Cahill L, Corey PN, El-Sohemy A. Vitamin C deficiency in a population of young Canadian adults. Am J Epidemiol. 2009;170:464–71.
35. Qi Q, Kilpelainen TO, Downer MK, Tanaka T, Smith CE, Sluijs I, Sonestedt E, Chu AY, Renstrom F, Lin X, et al. FTO genetic variants, dietary intake and body mass index: insights from 177,330 individuals. Hum Mol Genet. 2014;23:6961–72.
36. Monda KL, Chen GK, Taylor KC, Palmer C, Edwards TL, Lange LA, Ng MC, Adeyemo AA, Allison MA, Bielak LF, et al. A meta-analysis identifies new loci associated with body mass index in individuals of African ancestry. Nat Genet. 2013;45:690–6.
37. Liu C, Mou S, Cai Y. FTO gene variant and risk of overweight and obesity among children and adolescents: a systematic review and meta-analysis. PLoS One. 2013;8:e82133.
38. Qi Q, Downer MK, Kilpelainen TO, Taal HR, Barton SJ, Ntalla I, Standl M, Boraska V, Huikari V, Kiefte-de Jong JC, et al. Dietary intake, FTO genetic variants, and adiposity: a combined analysis of over 16,000 children and adolescents. Diabetes. 2015;64:2467–76.
39. Vimaleswaran KS, Angquist L, Hansen RD, van der AD B-NN, Holst C, Tjonneland A, Overvad K, Jakobsen MU, Boeing H, et al. Association between FTO variant and change in body weight and its interaction with dietary factors: the DiOGenes study. Obesity (Silver Spring). 2012;20:1669–74.
40. Clinical guidelines on the identification, evaluation, and treatment of overweight and obesity in adults—the evidence report. National Institutes of Health. Obes Res. 1998;6 Suppl 2:51S–209S.

41. Dobbelsteyn CJ, Joffres MR, MacLean DR, Flowerdew G. A comparative evaluation of waist circumference, waist-to-hip ratio and body mass index as indicators of cardiovascular risk factors. The Canadian Heart Health Surveys. Int J Obes Relat Metab Disord. 2001;25:652–61.
42. Janssen I, Katzmarzyk PT, Ross R. Body mass index, waist circumference, and health risk: evidence in support of current National Institutes of Health guidelines. Arch Intern Med. 2002;162:2074–9.
43. Cecil JE, Tavendale R, Watt P, Hetherington MM, Palmer CN. An obesity-associated FTO gene variant and increased energy intake in children. N Engl J Med. 2008;359:2558–66.
44. Haupt A, Thamer C, Staiger H, Tschritter O, Kirchhoff K, Machicao F, Haring HU, Stefan N, Fritsche A. Variation in the FTO gene influences food intake but not energy expenditure. Exp Clin Endocrinol Diabetes. 2009;117:194–7.
45. Berentzen T, Kring SI, Holst C, Zimmermann E, Jess T, Hansen T, Pedersen O, Toubro S, Astrup A, Sorensen TI. Lack of association of fatness-related FTO gene variants with energy expenditure or physical activity. J Clin Endocrinol Metab. 2008;93:2904–8.
46. Kennedy AP, Shea JL, Sun G. Comparison of the classification of obesity by BMI vs. dual-energy X-ray absorptiometry in the Newfoundland population. Obesity (Silver Spring). 2009;17:2094–9.
47. Savva SC, Tornaritis M, Savva ME, Kourides Y, Panagi A, Silikiotou N, Georgiou C, Kafatos A. Waist circumference and waist-to-height ratio are better predictors of cardiovascular disease risk factors in children than body mass index. Int J Obes Relat Metab Disord. 2000;24:1453–8.
48. Han TS, van Leer EM, Seidell JC, Lean ME. Waist circumference action levels in the identification of cardiovascular risk factors: prevalence study in a random sample. BMJ. 1995;311:1401–5.
49. Leidy HJ, Clifton PM, Astrup A, Wycherley TP, Westerterp-Plantenga MS, Luscombe-Marsh ND, Woods SC, Mattes RD. The role of protein in weight loss and maintenance. Am J Clin Nutr. 2015;101(Suppl):1320S-9S.
50. Johnstone AM. Safety and efficacy of high-protein diets for weight loss. Proc Nutr Soc. 2012;71:339–49.

18

ONS: an ontology for a standardized description of interventions and observational studies in nutrition

Francesco Vitali[1,4†], Rosario Lombardo[2*†], Damariz Rivero[4], Fulvio Mattivi[5,12], Pietro Franceschi[5], Alessandra Bordoni[6], Alessia Trimigno[6], Francesco Capozzi[6], Giovanni Felici[7], Francesco Taglino[7], Franco Miglietta[1], Nathalie De Cock[3], Carl Lachat[3], Bernard De Baets[8], Guy De Tré[9], Mariona Pinart[10], Katharina Nimptsch[10], Tobias Pischon[10], Jildau Bouwman[11], Duccio Cavalieri[1,4*] and the ENPADASI consortium

Abstract

Background: The multidisciplinary nature of nutrition research is one of its main strengths. At the same time, however, it presents a major obstacle to integrate data analysis, especially for the terminological and semantic interpretations that specific research fields or communities are used to. To date, a proper ontology to structure and formalize the concepts used for the description of nutritional studies is still lacking.

Results: We have developed the Ontology for Nutritional Studies (ONS) by harmonizing selected pre-existing de facto ontologies with novel health and nutritional terminology classifications. The ONS is the result of a scholarly consensus of 51 research centers in nine European countries. The ontology classes and relations are commonly encountered while conducting, storing, harmonizing, integrating, describing, and searching nutritional studies. The ONS facilitates the description and specification of complex nutritional studies as demonstrated with two application scenarios.

Conclusions: The ONS is the first systematic effort to provide a solid and extensible formal ontology framework for nutritional studies. Integration of new information can be easily achieved by the addition of extra modules (i.e., nutrigenomics, metabolomics, nutrikinetics, and quality appraisal). The ONS provides a unified and standardized terminology for nutritional studies as a resource for nutrition researchers who might not necessarily be familiar with ontologies and standardization concepts.

Keywords: Ontology, Nutrition, Health, Intervention study, Observational study, Metabolomics, Food intake, Biomarker, Databases

Background

Human Nutritional Science studies the effects of food components on metabolism, health, performance, and disease resistance of humans, also encompassing the study of human behavior related to food choices. Nutritional epidemiology, on the other hand, assesses the relations between diet, nutrients and health, and disease outcomes [1]. Yet, there is a major disconnection between the description of nutrition-based prevention of disease and the understanding of the complex network of interactions by which nutrition modulates health. To fill this gap, a set of nutrition-related sub-disciplines (e.g., nutritional biochemistry, clinical nutrition, nutritional epidemiology, nutrigenetics, and nutrimetabolomics) provide fundamental evidence at different levels and from different perspectives, contributing to the expansion of nutritional science as a more systematic and complex discipline [2, 3]. As nutrition data are heterogeneous in terms of quality and nature, a comprehensive consideration of all aspects is challenging [4], even if substantial advance has been made to improve

* Correspondence: lombardo@cosbi.edu; duccio.cavalieri@unifi.it
†Equal contributors
[2]The Microsoft Research - University of Trento Centre for Computational and Systems Biology (COSBI), Piazza Manifattura, 1, I-38068 Rovereto, TN, Italy
[1]Institute of Biometeorology (IBIMET), National Research Council (CNR), Via Giovanni Caproni, 8, 50145 Florence, FI, Italy

the reporting of findings and the data quality [5] of nutrition research [6], which is one of the prerequisites for integrated analysis.

To integrate evidence, a systematic re-organization of concept definitions is needed. Currently, concept definitions are often derived from multiple sources, with the drawback that slight variations can lead to misleading interpretations [7]. Since in bioscience in general, and in nutritional science in particular, the same concept can be referred to by multiple synonymous terms, abbreviations, or acronyms [8], as well as using different languages, term classifications such as the Medical Subject Headings (MeSH) [9] or the NCI Thesaurus [10] provide fundamental resources. However, thesauri or controlled vocabularies for biomedical information do not specify relations between concepts. Although those efforts can be used to standardize general study descriptions, considerable advances would arise from the use of resources that, in addition to standardizing the vocabulary, also include connections/relations between classes, such as ontologies, specifically tailored to the nutritional sciences.

Often biomedical researchers refer to ontologies using the terminologies more appropriately pertaining to "controlled vocabularies," "thesauri" (i.e., a list, often organized in a hierarchy or taxonomy, of concepts and their textual descriptions), or "taxonomies" (i.e., a hierarchy consisting of terms denoting classes linked by sub- and super-class relations). A proper ontology, however, is defined as a formal representation of knowledge in a certain reality (i.e., a certain domain of knowledge), in a way that different people—and, notably, computers—can understand the concepts it contains and learn about the reality that is being represented [8, 11]. Ontologies consist of defined classes of entities, typically structured within a knowledge hierarchy where concepts are connected by standardized [12] semantic relationships (i.e., "is-a," "part-of") formally specifying knowledge relations such as generalizations of specifications of the reality of interest [13].

Open Biomedical Ontologies (OBO), established in 2001, is a platform for developing interoperable ontologies for biomedical research [14]. Efforts have been made in the agricultural field to develop nutrition-oriented ontologies focused on the description of food components such as "the food classification and description system" [15] developed by European Food Safety Authority (EFSA). Other notable efforts in developing food-focused ontologies were reviewed elsewhere [16]. Based on literature search and public ontological repository queries (OBO Foundry searched using ONTOBEE, and Bioportal), a single example of a nutritional ontology was found (the Bionutrition Ontology—BNO, http://purl.bioontology.org/ontology/BNO). The latter represents a controlled vocabulary of nutritional terms, without a proper annotation of terms or definition of properties, and lacks orthogonality (i.e., no terms are imported or refer to external ontologies). To the authors' knowledge, a proper ontology integrating the terms related to food description, medical science, genetics, genomics data, and nutritional science methods for diet and health research is not available to date. To fill this gap, we present the Ontology for Nutritional Studies (ONS) to facilitate the harmonization and integration of biological samples collected using different methodologies, referred to by differing terminologies in various fast-growing sub-disciplines in the dietary and health research.

The ONS was developed within the European Nutritional Phenotype Assessment and Data Sharing Initiative (ENPADASI) consortium [17], which joins scientists from 51 research centers in nine countries of Europe with the common effort to handle and make available big nutritional data through the open access nutritional database Data Sharing In Nutrition (DASH-IN) [17, 18]. DASH-IN is a distributed pan-European infrastructure and supports the storage of both interventional and observational studies and provides the tools for distributed management and search and analysis of the data [19]. The development of this infrastructure requires an ontology to harmonize biochemical, genetic, clinical, and nutritional concepts typically found in intervention and observational studies. The ontology would provide a coherent means of data annotation and data querying over the distributed infrastructure. Further developments of the project led to a stronger need for a proper conceptual framework such as the ONS that could be used by a broader nutrition community to build upon for annotating general nutritional studies. The ENPADASI framework gathered researchers from different nutrition-related fields (health sciences, biology, genetics, microbiology, agricultural sciences, food technology, science of materials, chemistry, metabolomics, genomics, bioinformatics, and metagenomics) and offered the ideal milieu for creating the first ontology in nutrition.

Methods

Terms to be included in the ONS were collected among partners of the ENPADASI consortium, as well as from templates for data and metadata upload into the DASH-IN databases. In compliance with the OBO Foundry principles [14], the ONS has been developed to be as follows: (i) Interoperable with other ontologies, as it has been formalized using the latest OWL 2 Web Ontology Language [20] and RDF specifications [21] and edited using Protégé [22]; the hermit reasoner (http://hermit-reasoner.com/) was used for consistency checking. (ii) Accessible, under the Creative Commons license (CC BY 4.0), published on GitHub (https://github.com/enpadasi/Ontology-for-Nutritional-Studies) and at NCBO BioPortal (http://bioportal.bioontology.org/ontologies/

ONS). (iii) Orthogonal to other ontologies by reusing existing terms. Besides assuring compliance with the OBO Foundry principles, we also ensured that the ONS followed the increasingly established FAIR principles [23]. As such, the ONS is also published in the FAIR-sharing database (https://fairsharing.org/bsg-s001068).

To enhance interoperability with other ontologies, the ONS builds on a subset of the Ontology for Biomedical Investigations (OBI) [24]. The subset was created using the ONTODOG tool [25] and is composed of all terms relevant to nutritional investigations and extended also in accordance with the bioinformatics infrastructure of ENPADASI. Moreover, this assured the adoption of a well-defined and widely adopted structure for the top and mid-level classes and principally the adherence to the Basic Formal Ontology (BFO) [26] as upper ontology.

Additional relevant ontologies were used orthogonally in the ONS as discussed in the results. To ensure and enhance orthogonality, all terms were first searched using the ONTOBEE [27] web service and catalogued with their URIs. ONTOFOX [28] was then used to import all terms with related annotations and axioms (option includeAllAnnotations). Newly defined terms, specific to the ONS, have been labeled with "ONS_" followed by a 7-digit number. Terms related to food description were also included by importing a subset of terms from the FOODON ontology [29]. All intermediate files of this development process (i.e., template files used for web services or imported ontologies) were stored on GitHub repository. Additional file 1 contains instruction on how to browse, download, and contribute to ONS. The same instruction is also present online at the wiki page of the GitHub repository (https://github.com/enpadasi/Ontology-for-Nutritional-Studies/wiki). In this development process, terms from a number of different ontologies were imported. Table 1 reports a summary of the classes that were imported in the ONS (excluding individuals) and their ontology of origin.

Results

The initial ontological curation identified a large number of relevant terms to consider. The terms were then

Table 1 Prefix and URL of the ontology of origin of the classes imported in ONS

	Prefix	No. of terms in ONS	URL
Basic Formal Ontology	BFO	45	http://ifomis.uni-saarland.de/bfo/
Chemical Entities of Biological Interest	CHEBI	14	https://www.ebi.ac.uk/chebi/
Clinical Measurement Ontology	CMO	5	https://bioportal.bioontology.org/ontologies/CMO
EMBRACE Data And Methods Ontology	EDAM	12	http://edamontology.org/page
Experimental Factor Ontology	EFO	30	https://www.ebi.ac.uk/efo/
eagle-i Research Resource Ontology	ERO	2	https://open.med.harvard.edu/wiki/display/eaglei/Ontology
Food Ontology	FOODON	2809	https://foodontology.github.io/foodon/
Human Phenotype Ontology	HP	2	http://human-phenotype-ontology.github.io/
The Information Artifact Ontology	IAO	63	https://github.com/information-artifact-ontology/IAO
Informed Consent Ontology	ICO	5	https://github.com/ICO-ontology/ICO
NCBITaxon ontology	NCBITaxon	17	http://www.obofoundry.org/ontology/ncbitaxon.html
The NCI Thesaurus	NCIT	26	http://www.obofoundry.org/ontology/ncit.html
Ontology of Biological and Clinical Statistics	OBCS	5	https://github.com/obcs/obcs
Ontology for Biomedical Investigations	OBI	265	http://obi-ontology.org/
Ontology for Biobanking	OBIB	4	http://www.obofoundry.org/ontology/obib.html
Ontology for General Medical Science	OGMS	11	http://www.obofoundry.org/ontology/ogms.html
The Ontology of Host-Microbiome Interactions	OHMI	4	https://github.com/OHMI-ontology/OHMI
Ontological Minimum Information About Biobank data Sharing	OMIABIS	3	http://www.obofoundry.org/ontology/omiabis.html
The Ontology of Medically Related Social Entities	OMRSE	1	https://github.com/ufbmi/OMRSE
The Semanticscience Integrated Ontology	SIO	33	https://github.com/micheldumontier/semanticscience
STATistics Ontology	STATO	4	http://stato-ontology.org/
An ontology of units of measurements	UO	18	https://github.com/bio-ontology-research-group/unit-ontology

either imported from existing ontologies, redefined from existing concepts, or annotated de novo. By merging 3334 terms imported from already existing ontologies and 100 newly defined terms, the ONS describes both intervention and observational studies in nutrition.

Central nutritional concepts

In the ONS, relevant nutritional concepts have been related to each other to offer a well-organized synopsis of the knowledge in health and nutrition sciences. The ONS harmonizes all pertinent concepts from different domains, defining appropriate relationships and improving and simplifying the process of conceptual organization of the many facets of real studies. Here, we present (Fig. 1) how diet, food, and food component concepts, which can be considered central for an ontology aimed at effectively assisting researchers in the standardized description of the nutritional study they are conducting, were included, defined, and connected in the ONS.

Diet is defined as the regular course of eating and drinking adopted by a person or animal (ONS_0000080). For the purpose of the nutritional community, we further detailed the diet concept into three sub-classes: (i) Usual diet is defined as the regular course of eating and drinking adopted by a population in a certain geographical area, or in a certain cultural setting, or following certain common eating behavior. It is also intended as the diet a person would follow without further prescription or indications, i.e., vegetarian diet (ONS_0000083). (ii) Prescribed diet is defined as a diet prescribed by a physician/nutritionist to meet specific nutritional needs of a person (ONS_0000082). (iii) Intervention diet is defined as the diet administered during an intervention study. It usually comprises the adoption of a certain nutritional intervention (ERO_0000347), intended as the prescription of consuming or not consuming certain food, and follows a precise study design. Intervention studies usually compare at least two subgroups of a population, one control group receiving a null nutritional intervention and one or more test groups receiving the intervention (ONS_0000081).

Food component is defined as any substance that is distributed in foodstuffs. It includes materials derived from plants or animals, such as vitamins or minerals, as well as environmental contaminants (CHEBI_78295, ONS_0000073). Starting from this definition, we further detailed the food component concept into different subclasses: (i) Nutrient (ONS_0000077): A nutrient is a food component used by the body for normal physiological functions that guarantee survival and growth. It must be supplied in adequate and defined amounts from foods consumed within a diet. Malnutrition occurs when the right amount of nutrient is not provided. (ii) Food bioactive (ONS_0000076): A food bioactive is a food

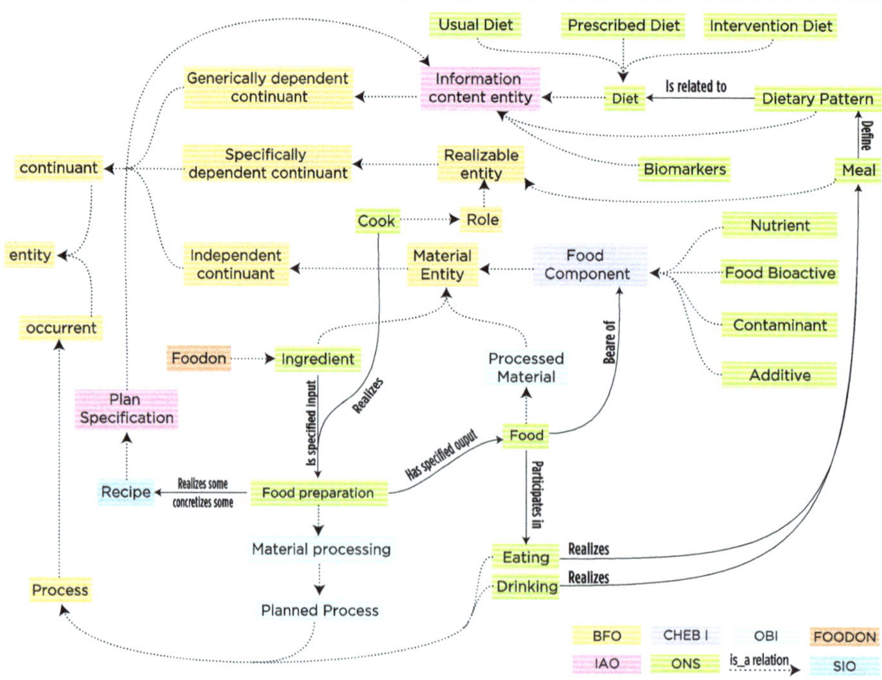

Fig. 1 Upper and mid-level hierarchical structure of the ONS showing how relevant nutritional concepts have been related to each other. Considering the large number of concepts and relations defined in the ONS, further detailed relations are not shown here. The terms in green boxes are ONS-specific terms, while terms in other color boxes are imported from existing ontologies (i.e., BFO, OBI, IAO, CHEBI, SIO, FOODON). Dotted arrows represent "is_a" semantic relations, while solid arrows represent other types of semantic relations

component other than those needed to meet basic human nutritional needs (nutrients). Food bioactives modulate one or more metabolic processes, possibly resulting in the promotion of better health. The daily required intake for food bioactives is not established yet, and there is no demonstration that malnutrition occurs when the right amount is not provided. (iii) Contaminant: Contaminant is unwanted food component that makes the food no longer suitable for use (ONS_0000075). (iv) Additive: Additive is a component added to food to improve or preserve it (ONS_0000074).

Multiple definitions can be found for the food concept. As an example, CHEBI (CHEBI:33290) defines "Any material that can be ingested by an organism" and MESH (MeSH D005502) defines "Any substances taken in by the body that provides nourishment." For the purposes of the nutritional community, the concept of food was expanded as food is defined as a complex matrix that is consumed by a person through the process of eating or drinking (ONS_0000079). Foods are bearer of the nutrients, bioactives, and, sometimes, other food components. Food consumption, through the meal consumption, follows a certain dietary pattern, which define the diet. Nutrients and bioactives contained in food can be exploited by the human organism thanks to the process of digestion (ONS_0000101), absorption (ONS_0000102), metabolization (ONS_0000103), or through the intervention of the gut microflora (OHMI_0000020). The concept of food can be split into the following: (i) Raw food: A raw food is an uncooked, unprocessed food that is consumed in its natural state (ONS_0000099); (ii) Processed food: A processed food is the result of the process of home or industrial food preparation (ONS_0000100).

In nutritional science, biomarkers are increasingly being used to provide objective results and to avoid biases (e.g., reporting bias and recall bias). Three groups of biomarkers were identified for use in nutrition science [30], along with the dietary biomarker development framework: "exposure biomarker" for dietary intake and nutrient status, "effect biomarker" for measuring biological effects of food components, and "susceptibility biomarker" for assessing the effects of diet on human health. In the ONS, we are presenting the first formal ontology application for the biomarker class (ONS_0000095) and its sub-classes, using the definition from the commentary [30]. ONTOBEE query for the "biomarker" returned multiple results mainly from the Experimental Factor Ontology (EFO), all having the class "Measurement" (EFO_0001444) as super-class (a measurement is an information entity that is a recording of the output of a measurement such as produced by an instrument). However, it has to be noted that a similar class can also be found in the Information Artifact Ontology (IAO) named "Measurement datum" (IAO_0000109, a measurement datum is an information content entity that is a recording of the output of a measurement such as produced by a device). In the ONS, the biomarker class was defined as a sub-class of the "Measurement datum" class (IAO_0000109) in line with the OBI ontology, which uses the IAO class.

Integrated analysis of data and joint pooled analysis are strongly promoted in nutrition by research funders, though raise scientists' concern, as the scientific interest in the open access to nutritional data often conflicts with the General Data Protection Regulation. When fully achieved, integrated analysis will lead to new discoveries and maximize use of public funds. In ENPADASI, this problem was broadly dealt with from both legal and technical aspects, and a recommendation on minimal information to be added as metadata to studies to boost integration capacity has been developed [19]. The identification of minimal requirements, essential to connect existing and future study (meta) databases, facilitates data exchange and data interpretation, helping to increase the robustness of results from future joint data analysis in nutritional epidemiology [31]. In fact, joint data analysis has already started helping to achieve new discoveries [32]. In the ONS, we have included the minimal required study information in the growing conceptual/ontological framework. Each minimal required study term was placed at the appropriate hierarchical level in the ontology. To easily identify terms pertaining to the minimal study information, an annotation property ("in_minimal_requirements_subset") was created.

Application scenarios

The ONS is designed to enable the description of both intervention and observational studies in human nutrition. Here, we present two application scenarios based on published nutritional studies, one for the observational study design and one for the interventional study design. Figures 2 and 3 illustrate how the ONS was built to support the standardized annotation of most descriptors of a nutritional study, starting from initial phases of a study (i.e., formalizing the definition of population stratum) to finally connect to the specific results and how they were obtained. Figures and descriptions have to be intended at the single instance level (i.e., specific for the study object of description). For this reason, we introduced the use of individuals (and their connections) for very study-specific element alongside concepts in classes. In the text below, the italic notation indicates the properties, while the notation PREFIX:CLASS is used to indicate classes in the ontology, for example the notation "ONS:Diet" indicates the class with label "Diet" in the ONS ontology. For abbreviation of the ontologies, we refer the reader to the list of imported ontologies in the "Methods" section.

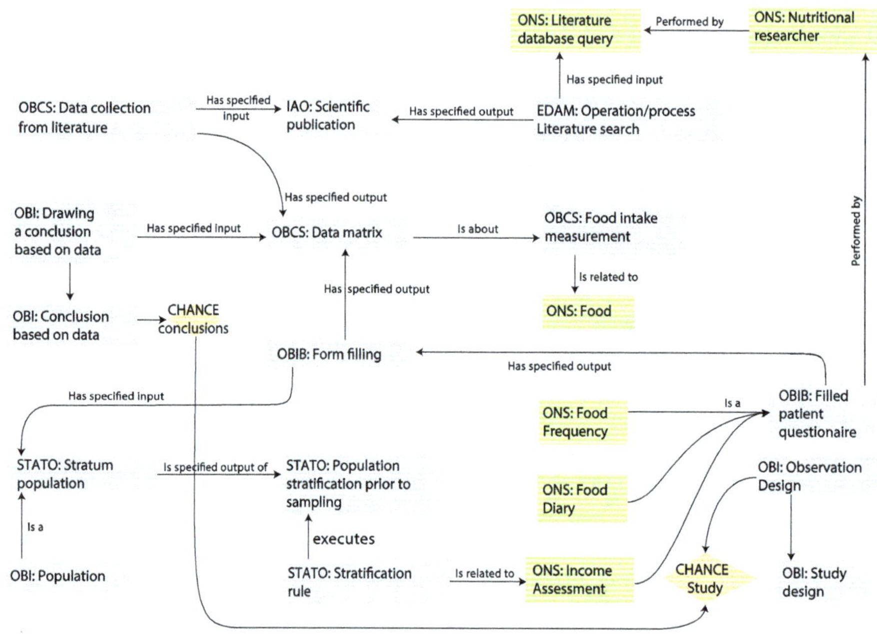

Fig. 2 Application scenario to the description of an observational study: modeling of the CHANCE study with the ONS. Terms in rhombus indicate instance-level terms specific to the CHANCE study (i.e., the specific conclusion of the CHANCE study), while terms in rectangular boxes represent general concept in the ONS. The presented semantic representation should be intended at the single instance level for the purpose of specifically describe CHANCE study

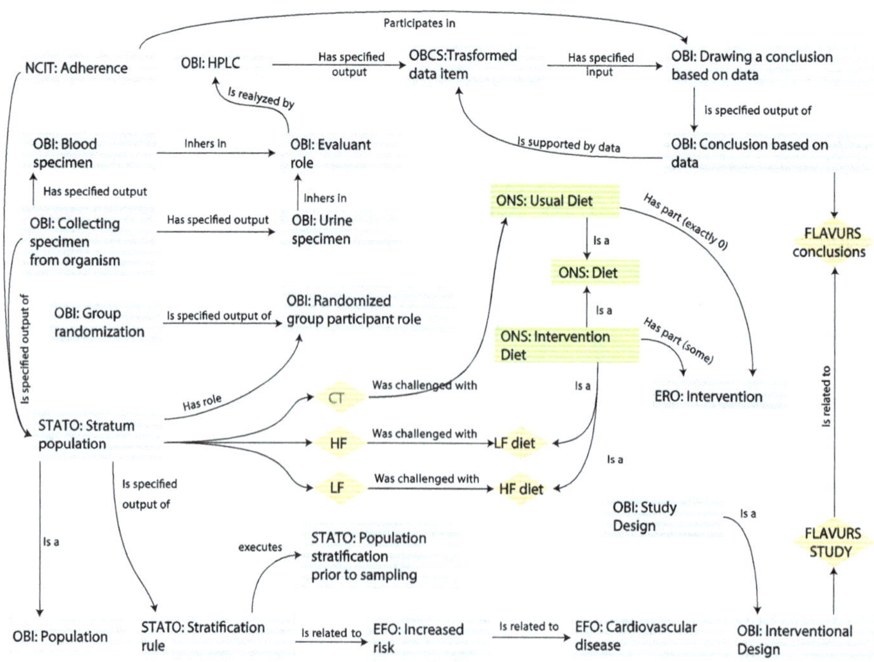

Fig. 3 Application scenario to the description of an intervention study: modeling of the FLAVURS study with the ONS. Terms in rhombus indicate instance-level terms specific to the FLAVURS study (i.e., the specific conclusion of the FLAVURS study), while terms in rectangular boxes represent general concept in the ONS. The presented semantic representation should be intended at the single instance level for the purpose of specifically describe FLAVURS study

Observational studies

The first application scenario is represented by the CHANCE study [33]. Figure 2 illustrates how the ONS can be used to formalize information on how the study was conducted. This observational study aims at developing novel and affordable nutritious foods to optimize the diet and reduce the risk of diet-related diseases among groups at risk of poverty (ROP). The CHANCE study uses two different approaches to draw its final conclusion. The first is a literature search process (EDAM:Literature search), performed with a specific textual literature database query (i.e., an instance of the class ONS:Literature database query). Output of the literature search process is a number of scientific publications (IAO:Scientific publication) which are subject to analysis and review to extract data (OBCS:data collection from literature), a process that ultimately results in an organized data matrix (OBCS:Data matrix). CHANCE also included an observational study approach. In this case, a population was firstly divided into sub-populations based on their economic income. This stratification (STATO:Population stratification prior to sampling) was carried out following a specific stratification rule (STATO:Stratification rule), based on the risk of poverty (ROP) of the subjects assessed with a questionnaire (ONS:Income assessment). The stratified population was then challenged with (i.e., *is specified input of*) two nutritional questionnaires (ONS:Food frequency and ONS: Food diary) aimed at assessing the foods consumed by the subjects and producing results finally organized in a data matrix. In both cases, the data matrices (OBCS:Data matrix) specific for this study contain information about the nutrients and food consumed by the population and represent the specified data object on which conclusions are drawn (OBI:drawing a conclusion based on data).

Intervention studies

The second application scenario is represented by the FLAVURS (impact of increasing doses of flavonoid-rich and flavonoid-poor fruit and vegetables on cardiovascular risk factors in an 'at risk' group) study [34]. Figure 3 illustrates how the ONS can be used to formalize the information on how the study was conducted. This interventional study aimed to investigate the effects of high and low flavonoid diets on the vascular function and other cardiovascular disease risk factors. In this study, a population, selected on the basis of the stratification rule (STATO:Stratification rule) of having a relative risk of developing cardiovascular disease higher than 1.5, has been randomly divided (OBI:Group randomization and OBI:Randomized group participant role) into three groups: control group (CT), high flavonoid group (HF), and low flavonoid group (LF). Each of the groups was challenged with a different diet (ONS:Diet): CT followed the usual diet (ONS:Usual Diet), which is defined to *have exactly 0* interventions (ERO:Intervention); in the HF and the LF groups, individuals were challenged with two different types of intervention diet (ONS:Intervention diet) encompassing two different intervention (ERO:Intervention) protocols. In HF diet, the intervention was performed by the prescription of consuming fruit and vegetables with high flavonoid content, while in the LF diet the intervention was concretized by the prescription of consuming fruit and vegetables with low flavonoid content.

Urine and blood (OBI:Urine specimen and OBI:Blood specimen) were collected from individuals (OBI:Collecting specimen from organism) and analyzed (i.e., they *inherited* the evaluant role OBI:Evaluant role) by an HPLC assay (HPLC class) including untargeted metabolomics [35]. Output of the analysis was a data item in the form of a matrix (OBCS:Transformed data item) that is used to draw specific FLAVURS conclusions (OBI: Drawing a conclusion based on data and OBI:conclusion based on data).

Discussion and conclusions

The ONS is the first systematic effort to provide a formal ontology framework for the description of nutritional studies. In this context, the main aim of the ONS is the establishment of an ontological framework that can assist nutrition researchers by selecting the appropriate terms from the wide range of existing ontologies and creating the relevant missing key concepts for the field. Nutrition researchers, who might not necessarily be familiar with ontologies and concept standardization, can find in the ONS a single knowledge entry point for a unified and standardized terminology without having to resort to numerous ontology sources. In addition to standardizing concept descriptions and assisting in annotation, the ONS will structure querying of nutritional studies stored in public databases (such as the resources developed in the ENPADASI project). Finding the suitable studies (i.e., those more directly comparable regarding design, employed stratification criteria, or type of intervention diet employed) represents the basis for integrated analysis. Such a query, in fact, cannot be efficiently based on string matching, but rather on more complex textual analysis and machine learning methodologies for which ontology is crucial. A well-established nutritional ontology would also enable more accurate search for required data as well as the automated integration and analysis of data from multiple sources [36].

Diet, nutrient, and food are indeed central concepts for nutritional sciences, and they were included and connected with higher level concepts in ONS. Moreover, the ONS supports the research needs identified by other initiatives such as the Food Biomarkers Alliance (FoodBAll) by including for the first time in a formal ontology the concept of biomarker in nutrition, and its sub-classes, as defined in [30].

Besides acquiring widespread utilization, an ontology can be considered successful only if (i) continuous development and (ii) constant contribution/updates from researchers with specific knowledge is ensured. We invite and encourage researchers in the nutritional field to contribute to the further development, adoption, and promotion of the ONS. Contributions are already possible using the GitHub tracking/issues system (Additional file 1) and an online community platform to facilitate the process of curation and extension of the ONS will be developed for this purpose. As a next challenge, the ONS aims to integrate nutritional studies with non-life sciences such as economy, psychology, and sociology, which also influence the nutritional status of individuals [37–39].

Abbreviations

DASH-IN: Data Sharing In Nutrition; EFSA: European Food Safety Authority; ENPADASI: European Nutritional Phenotype Assessment and Data Sharing Initiative; FLAVURS: Impact of increasing doses of flavonoid-rich and flavonoid-poor fruit and vegetables on cardiovascular risk factors in an "at risk" group; FoodEx2: Version 2 of the EFSA Food classification and description system for exposure assessment; HPLC: High-performance liquid chromatography; MeSH: Medical Subject Headings; OBO: Open Biomedical Ontologies; ONS: Ontology for Nutritional Studies; OWL: Web Ontology Language; RDF: Resource Description Framework; ROP: Risk of poverty

Funding

This work was supported by the Italian Ministry of University and Research (MIUR) [decreto n. 2224, 05/10/2015 and n.2027, 11/09/2015] and by the European Nutritional Phenotype Assessment and Data Sharing Initiative (ENPADASI) and its infrastructure as part of the Joint Programming Initiative "A Healthy Diet for a Healthy Life" (JPI-HDHL).

Authors' contributions

FV, RL, and DC led the content creation, ontology development, and manuscript drafting. MP curated the link between the ONS and the minimal study requirements. DR, FM, PF, AB, AT, FC, GF, FT, FM, NDC, CL, BDB, GDT, MP, KN, TP, JB, and DC contributed to the curation of the ONS-specific terms and critically commented the manuscript. DC coordinated the ontology development and manuscript drafting. All other authors critically commented the manuscript. All authors read and approved the final manuscript.

Competing interests

The authors declare that they have no competing interests.

Author details

[1]Institute of Biometeorology (IBIMET), National Research Council (CNR), Via Giovanni Caproni, 8, 50145 Florence, FI, Italy. [2]The Microsoft Research - University of Trento Centre for Computational and Systems Biology (COSBI), Piazza Manifattura, 1, I-38068 Rovereto, TN, Italy. [3]Department of Food Technology, Safety and Health, Ghent University, Coupure links 653, 9000 Ghent, Belgium. [4]Department of Biology, University of Florence, Via Madonna del Piano, 6, 50019 Sesto F, FI, Italy. [5]Food Quality and Nutrition Department, Research and Innovation Centre, Edmund Mach Foundation, Via Edmund Mach, 1, 38010 San Michele all'Adige, TN, Italy. [6]Department of Agri-Food Sciences and Technologies, University of Bologna, Piazza Goidanich 60, Cesena, FC, Italy. [7]Institute for Systems Analysis and Computer Science (IASI), National Research Council (CNR), Via dei Taurini, 19, 00185 Rome, RM, Italy. [8]KERMIT, Department of Data Analysis and Mathematical Modelling, Ghent University, Coupure links 653, 9000 Ghent, Belgium. [9]Department of Telecommunications and Information Processing, Ghent University, Coupure links 653, 9000 Ghent, Belgium. [10]Molecular Epidemiology Research Group, Max Delbrück Center for Molecular Medicine, Berlin, Germany. [11]Microbiology and Systems Biology, TNO, Utrechtseweg 48, 3704HE Zeist, The Netherlands. [12]Center Agriculture Food Environment, University of Trento, San Michele all'Adige, Italy.

References

1. Leaf A, Weber PC. A new era for science in nutrition. Am J Clin Nutr. 1987; 45(5 Suppl):1048–53.
2. Wahlqvist ML. The new nutrition science: sustainability and development. Public Health Nutr. 2005;8:766–72. https://doi.org/10.1079/PHN2005780
3. Bordoni A, Capozzi F. Foodomics for healthy nutrition. Curr Opin Clin Nutr Metab Care. 2014;17:418–24. https://doi.org/10.1097/MCO.0000000000000089.
4. Serra-Majem L, MacLean D, Ribas L, Brulé D, Sekula W, Prattala R, et al. Comparative analysis of nutrition data from national, household, and individual levels: results from a WHO-CINDI collaborative project in Canada, Finland, Poland, and Spain. J Epidemiol Community Health. 2003;57:74–80. https://doi.org/10.1136/JECH.57.1.74.
5. Yang C, Pinart M, Kolsteren P, Van Camp J, De Cock N. Perspective: essential study quality descriptors for data from nutritional epidemiologic research. Adv Nutr. 2017;8(5):639–51.
6. Lachat C, Hawwash D, Ocké MC, Berg C, Forsum E, Hörnell A, et al. Strengthening the Reporting of Observational Studies in Epidemiology-nutritional epidemiology (STROBE-nut): an extension of the STROBE statement. PlosMed. 2016;13:6. https://doi.org/10.1371/journal.pmed.1002036
7. Lange MC, Lemay DG, German JB. A multi-ontology framework to guide agriculture and food towards diet and health. J Sci Food Agric. 2007;87: 1427–34. https://doi.org/10.1002/jsfa.2832.
8. Rubin DL, Shah NH, Noy NF. Biomedical ontologies: a functional perspective. Brief Bioinform. 2007;9:75–90. https://doi.org/10.1093/bib/bbm059.
9. Lipscomb CE. Medical subject headings (MeSH). Bull Med Libr Assoc. 2000;88: 265–6. http://www.ncbi.nlm.nih.gov/pubmed/10928714. Accessed 13 Dec 2017
10. Hartel FW, de Coronado S, Dionne R, Fragoso G, Golbeck J. Modeling a description logic vocabulary for cancer research. J Biomed Inform. 2005;38: 114–29. https://doi.org/10.1016/J.JBI.2004.09.001.
11. Arp R, Smith B, Spear AD. Building ontologies with basic formal ontology: MIT Press; 2015.
12. Relations Ontology. http://www.obofoundry.org/ontology/ro.html. Accessed 14 Dec 2017.
13. Groß A, Pruski C, Rahm E. Evolution of biomedical ontologies and mappings: overview of recent approaches. Comput Struct Biotechnol J. 2016;14:333–40. https://doi.org/10.1016/J.CSBJ.2016.08.002.
14. Smith B, Ashburner M, Rosse C, Bard J, Bug W, Ceusters W, et al. The OBO Foundry: coordinated evolution of ontologies to support biomedical data integration. Nat Biotechnol. 2007;25:1251–5. https://doi.org/10.1038/nbt1346.
15. The food classification and description system FoodEx 2 (revision 2). EFSA Support Publ. 2015;12. doi:https://doi.org/10.2903/sp.efsa.2015.EN-804.
16. Boulos M, Yassine A, Shirmohammadi S, Namahoot C, Brückner M. Towards an "Internet of Food": food ontologies for the internet of things. Futur Internet. 2015;7:372–92. https://doi.org/10.3390/fi7040372.
17. ENPADASI. http://www.enpadasi.eu/. Accessed 14 Dec 2017.
18. Dragsted L, Hm Dijk-stroeve J, Dobre I, Priami C, Cavalieri D, Laville M, Brennan L, Bouwman J. The data sharing initiative for nutrition (DASH-IN) under ENPADASI. Ann Nutr Metab. 2015;67:35–6.
19. Pinart M, Nimptsch K, Bouwman J, Dragsted LO, Lachat C, Perozzi G, Canali R Lombardo R, D'Archivio M, Guillaume M, Donneau A.F, Jeran S, Linseisen J, Kleiser C, Nöthlings U, Barbaresko J, Boeing H, Stelmach-Mardas M, Heuer T, Laird E, . Walton J, Gasparini P, Robino A, Castaño L, Rojo-Martínez G, Merino J, Masana L, Standl M, Schulz H, Biagi E, Nurk E, Matthys C, Gobbetti M, de Angelis M, Windler E, Zyriax BC, Tafforeau J, Pischon T. Joint data analysis in nutritional epidemiology: identification of observational studies and minimal requirements. J Nutr, 2018 148(2):285-297. https://doi.org/10.1093/jn/nxx037
20. Hitzler P, Patel-Schneider PF. OWL 2 web ontology language primer W3C proposed recommendation. 2009. https://www.w3.org/TR/2009/PR-owl2-primer-20090922/all.pdf. Accessed 14 Dec 2017.

21. Lassila O, Swick RR. Resource Description Framework (RDF) model and syntax specification. World Wide Web Internet and Web Information Systems. 1999. https://www.w3.org/TR/1999/REC-rdf-syntax-19990222/. Accessed 14 Dec 2017.
22. Musen MA, Protégé Team the P. The Protégé project: a look back and a look forward. AI matters. 2015;1:4–12. https://doi.org/10.1145/2757001.2757003.
23. Wilkinson MD, Dumontier M, Aalbersberg IJ, Appleton G, Axton M, Baak A, Blomberg N, Boiten JW, da Silva Santos LB, Bourne PE, Bouwman J. The FAIR Guiding Principles for scientific data management and stewardship. Scientific data. 2016;3 https://doi.org/10.1038/sdata.2016.18.
24. Bandrowski A, Brinkman R, Brochhausen M, Brush MH, Bug B, Chibucos MC, et al. The ontology for biomedical investigations. PLoS One. 2016;11: e0154556. https://doi.org/10.1371/journal.pone.0154556.
25. Zheng J, Xiang Z, Stoeckert CJ, He Y. Ontodog: a web-based ontology community view generation tool. Bioinformatics. 2014;30:1340–2. https://doi.org/10.1093/bioinformatics/btu008.
26. Basic Formal Ontology (BFO) | Home. http://ifomis.uni-saarland.de/bfo/. Accessed 14 Dec 2017.
27. Ong E, Xiang Z, Zhao B, Liu Y, Lin Y, Zheng J, et al. Ontobee: a linked ontology data server to support ontology term dereferencing, linkage, query and integration. Nucleic Acids Res. 2017;45:D347–52. https://doi.org/10.1093/nar/gkw918.
28. Xiang Z, Courtot M, Brinkman RR, Ruttenberg A, He Y. OntoFox: web-based support for ontology reuse. BMC Res Notes. 2010;3:175. https://doi.org/10.1186/1756-0500-3-175.
29. Griffiths E, Brinkman F, Dooley D, Hsiao W, Buttigieg P, Hoehndorf R. FoodON: a global farm-to-fork food ontology. The Development of a Universal Food Vocabulary. http://ceur-ws.org/Vol-1747/IP21_ICBO2016.pdf. Accessed 14 Dec 2017.
30. Dragsted LO, Gao Q, Praticò G, Manach C, Wishart DS, Scalbert A, et al. Dietary and health biomarkers—time for an update. Genes Nutr. 2017;12:24. https://doi.org/10.1186/s12263-017-0578-y.
31. NCD Risk Factor Collaboration (NCD-RisC), Zhou B, Bentham J, Di CM, Bixby H, Danaei G, Cowan MJ, et al. Worldwide trends in blood pressure from 1975 to 2015: a pooled analysis of 1479 population-based measurement studies with 19·1 million participants. Lancet. 2017;389:37–55. https://doi.org/10.1016/S0140-6736(16)31919-5.
32. Wu JHY, Marklund M, Imamura F, Tintle N, Ardisson Korat AV, de Goede J, et al. Omega-6 fatty acid biomarkers and incident type 2 diabetes: pooled analysis of individual-level data for 39 740 adults from 20 prospective cohort studies. Lancet Diabetes Endocrinol. 2017;5:965–74. https://doi.org/10.1016/S2213-8587(17)30307-8.
33. Nikolić M, Glibetić M, Gurinović M, Milešević J, Khokhar S, Chillo S, et al. Identifying critical nutrient intake in groups at risk of poverty in Europe: the CHANCE project approach. Nutrients. 2014;6:1374–93. https://doi.org/10.3390/nu6041374.
34. Chong MF, George TW, Alimbetov D, Jin Y, Weech M, Macready AL, et al. Impact of the quantity and flavonoid content of fruits and vegetables on markers of intake in adults with an increased risk of cardiovascular disease: the FLAVURS trial. Eur J Nutr. 2013;52:361–78. https://doi.org/10.1007/s00394-012-0343-3.
35. Ulaszewska MM, Trost K, Stanstrup J, Tuohy KM, Franceschi P, Chong MF-F, George T, Minihane AM, Lovegrove JA, Mattivi F. Urinary metabolomic profiling to identify biomarkers of a flavonoid-rich and flavonoid-poor fruits and vegetables diet in adults: the FLAVURS trial. Metabolomics. 2016;12:1–22.
36. Lemay DG, Zivkovic AM, German JB. Building the bridges to bioinformatics in nutrition research. Am J Clin Nutr. 2007;86:1261–9.
37. Ramos-Elorduy BJ. The importance of edible insects in the nutrition and economy of people of the rural areas of Mexico. Ecol Food Nutr. 1997;36: 347–66. https://doi.org/10.1080/03670244.1997.9991524.
38. Germanov J, Williams L. The epidemic of dieting women: the need for a sociological approach to food and nutrition. Appetite. 1996;27:97–108. https://doi.org/10.1006/appe.1996.0038.
39. Hollis JF, Carmody TP, Connor SL, Fey SG, Matarazzo JD. The Nutrition Attitude Survey: associations with dietary habits, psychological and physical well-being, and coronary risk factors. Health Psychol. 1986;5:359–74.

19

High-fat diet modifies expression of hepatic cellular senescence gene p16(INK4a) through chromatin modifications in adult male rats

Xiyuan Zhang[1], Guanying Bianca Xu[2], Dan Zhou[4] and Yuan-Xiang Pan[2,3,5*]

Abstract

Background: Liver is the crucial organ as a hub for metabolic reactions. p16(INK4a) is a well-established cyclin-dependent kinase (CDK) inhibitor that plays important role in the molecular pathways of senescence, which lead to irreversible cell cycle arrest with secretion of proinflammatory cytokines and mitochondrial dysfunction. This study tested the hypothesis that cellular senescence regulated by p16(INK4a) is associated with high-fat diet in adult male rats.

Methods: Sprague Dawley rats were fed a high-fat (HF) diet or a control (C) diet for 9 weeks after weaning. At 12 weeks of age, liver samples of male rats were collected to investigate the key genes and liver physiological status.

Results: Both mRNA and protein expression level of cellular senescence marker, p16(INK4a), was increased significantly in HF group when compared to C group. A decrease of tri-methylated histone H3 lysine 27 (H3K27Me3) in the coding region of p16(INK4a) was observed. On the other hand, mRNA and protein expression of another inhibitor of cyclin-dependent kinase, p21(Cip1), was decreased significantly in HF group; however, no significant chromatin modification was found in this gene. Histological analysis demonstrated hepatic steatosis in HF group as well as severe fat accumulation.

Conclusions: Our study demonstrated that HF diet regulated cellular senescence marker p16(INK4a) through chromatin modifications, which may promote hepatic fat accumulation and steatosis.

Keywords: High-fat diet, p21(Cip1), Fatty liver, Hepatic cellular senescence, Chromatin modification

Background

Dietary factors play pivotal role in modulating liver function and physiology as well as in the development of hepatic cells: a high-fat (HF) diet can increase hepatic lipid content and plasma insulin concentration, causing insulin resistance in obese animals [1–3], while maternal high-fat diet leads to altered regulation of liver development in offspring through DNA methylation, which may cause early hepatic dysfunction [4]. Several animal models have been reported to establish the association between high-fat diet and the physiological changes in the liver [5–10].

* Correspondence: yxpan@illinois.edu
[2]Department of Food Science and Human Nutrition, University of Illinois Urbana-Champaign, 461 Bevier Hall, MC-182, 905 South Goodwin Avenue, Urbana, IL 61801, USA
[3]Division of Nutritional Sciences (DNS), University of Illinois Urbana-Champaign, 461 Bevier Hall, MC-182, 905 South Goodwin Avenue, Urbana, IL 61801, USA
Full list of author information is available at the end of the article

Among the annotated genes using the Gene Oncology database, cell cycle control genes were the second largest group of altered genes associated with HF diet-induced changing [11], and this link between HF diet and cell cycle regulation has also been reported in other studies using either cell or animal models [4, 12, 13]. p16(INK4a) is a biomarker of cellular senescence and aging [14, 15], and its expression has been linked to replicative hypofunction in many types of cells, including hematopoietic progenitors [16], lymphocytes [17, 18], neural stem cells [19], and pancreatic beta cells [20]. Pervious study has shown that high-fat diet induced increasing level of p16(INK4a) transcription rate in an obese rat model, which was associated with a higher acetylation levels of histone H4 and lower methylation level of histone H3 lysine 27 in p16(INK4a) promoter and coding region [21]. p21(Cip1), on the other hand, belongs to the family of CDK inhibitor proteins and is a universal inhibitor of CDKs which include cyclin D-, E-, and A-dependent kinases [22, 23]. Upregulation of p21(Cip1) protein was proved to be involved in impaired regeneration of fatty livers in obese mice [4]. Although literature indicates that p16(INK4a) and p21(Cip1) alteration may not be necessary for either exogenous or endogenous liver carcinogenesis [24], it remains unclear how high-fat diet affects expressions of these CDK inhibitors and how the expression changes affect liver function as well as hepatic physiology.

As briefly mentioned before, the expressions of p16(INK4a) gene is regulated through epigenetic modifications. Hypermethylation of DNA in promoter CpG islands is associated with the transcriptional silencing of p16(INK4a) gene, and the di-methylation of histone H3 lysine 9 (H3K9) correlates with the DNA methylation status in colon cancer development [25]. High-fat diet was proved to alter DNA methylation in genes related to liver lipid metabolism and hepatic steatosis: for example, *Ndufb9*, or NADH dehydrogenase 1 beta subcomplex 9, was found hyper-methylated in CpG sites in the HFD group, which downregulates its expression [26]. However, few studies have been done to investigate the role of dietary high fat in regulation of p16(INK4a) expression through epigenetic modifications.

This study was designed to investigate the expression and chromatin modifications of CKIs p16(INK4a) and p21(Cip1) in adult male rat model induced by high-fat diet and its effects on hepatic cellular senescence as well as liver physiology. We hypothesized that high-fat diet regulates hepatic cellular senescence in male adult rats by regulating p16(INK4a) and p21(Cip1) expression through chromatin modifications, which may promote hepatic fat accumulation and steatosis.

Methods

Animal study

Sprague Dawley rats were fed a high-fat diet (HF) or a control (C) diet for 9 weeks after weaning. All information regarding the diets (Research Diets, Inc., New Brunswick, NJ) is listed in Table 1. Animals were individually housed in standard polycarbonate cages in a humidity- and temperature-controlled room on a 12-h light-dark cycle and had free access to food and water. At 12 weeks of age, the animals were sacrificed and the left lobe of the liver was collected, rapidly frozen in liquid nitrogen, and stored in − 70 °C for future use. We confirm that all applicable institutional and governmental regulations regarding the ethical use of animals were followed during this research (University of Illinois Institutional Animal Care and Use Committee approval #09112).

Table 1 Diet formula

Diet formula	C	HF
Total energy, kJ/g	16.75	19.68
Protein, g/kg	20	24
Carbohydrate, g/kg	64	41
Fat, g/kg	7	24
Ingredient, g/kg		
Casein	200	200
L-Cystine	3	3
Corn starch	437.2	72.8
Maltodextrin	100	100
Sucrose	102	172.8
Cellulose	50	50
Soybean oil	25	25
Lard	47	177.5
Mineral mix[a]	10	10
DiCalcium phosphate	13	13
Calcium carbonate	5.5	5.5
Potassium citrate	16.5	16.5
Vitamin mix[b]	10	10
Choline bitartrate	2	2
Yellow dye #5	0.025	N/A
Red dye #40	0.0025	0.05

The diet formula is provided by http://www.researchdiets.com/
[a]Mineral mix (AIN-93): (research diets) product no. S10026 for rodents
[b]Vitamin mix (AIN-93): (research diets) product no. V10001 for rodents

RNA isolation and cDNA synthesis

Frozen liver samples (50–100 mg) were ground using mortar and pestle with liquid nitrogen, and total RNA was extracted with TRI reagent (Sigma, St. Louis, MO). RNA samples were incubated with DNase I (Roche, Mannheim, Germany) at room temperature for 20 min, followed by 10 min in 90 °C heat block to prevent contamination of genomic DNA. High-capacity cDNA Reverse Transcription Kit (Applied Biosystems, Foster City, CA) was used for reverse transcription of 2 μg of total RNA. Reverse transcription was performed in a 2720 Thermal Cycler (Applied Biosystems) with 20 μL reaction volume with the following program: heated at 25 °C for 10 min, incubated at 37 °C for 2 h, and then heated at 85 °C for 5 s. The 20 μL of final product was diluted to 400 μL for 5 ng/μL using RNase free water (Fisher, Fair Lawn, NJ) and stored at − 20 °C.

Real-time quantitative PCR

To measure the relative transcriptional level of target genes, qPCR was performed in a 96-well plate using a

7300 real-time PCR System (Applied Biosystems). Five microliters of cDNA, with the final concentration of 5 ng/μL, was mixed with 10 μL SYBR Green master mix (Quanta Biosciences Inc., Gaithersburg, MD) and 1 μL of each 5 nmol/L primer (forward and reverse). The reaction was incubated using the following program: 95 °C for 10 min, followed by 35 cycles of 95 °C for 15 s and 60 °C for 1 min. High efficiency of the machine and the presence of a unique product were ensured by checking that the slope of the standard was in the range of −3.3 ± 0.3 and the *R* square to be larger than 0.98. Kinetic analysis was conducted to detect the exponential phase of amplification in each well with 25 ng template cDNA. mRNA level of ribosomal protein L7a was utilized as the internal control. In order to determine the gene transcription rate, primers were designed to amplify a region including both exon and intron of that gene. The relative expression level of this region can indicate the pre-mRNA rate of the gene and further present the transcription rate. Primers used for qPCR were designed using Vector NTI software (InforMax Inc., Frederick, MD), and all the primers used for real-time PCR are listed in Table 3.

Triacylglycerol and non-esterified fatty acid assay in plasma and liver tissues

One hundred milligrams of frozen liver samples were ground using a mortar and pestle with liquid nitrogen and mixed with 0.3 mL saline (0.9% *w*/*v* NaCl). Homogenized samples were quickly frozen in liquid nitrogen and kept in − 70 °C until analysis. The samples were quickly thawed in 37 °C and diluted five times to 1.5 mL. Twenty microliters of the diluted samples was incubated with 20 μL 1% deoxycholate in 37 °C for 5 min, and 10 μL of the samples was analyzed via the Thermo Infinity Triglycerides Liquid Stable Reagent (Thermo Fisher Scientific, Rockford, IL) following company protocol and using a commercially available standard reference kit (Verichem Laboratories, Providence, RI). Lowry assay was performed to determine the protein concentration, which was used to normalize the triacylglycerol (TAG) concentration in the liver. To determine plasma TAG levels, plasma samples were thawed on ice and analyzed accordingly following company protocol as for liver samples. Non-esterified fatty acid concentration in the liver was determined using a commercially available kit (HR-2 Series, Wako Diagnostics, Richmond, VA).

Liver histology

Frozen liver samples from offspring were embedded in O.C.T. compound (Gentaur, Kampenhout, Belgium) prior to sectioning. All sections were then stained with hematoxylin and eosin (H&E) or oil red O (ORO, Newcomer Supply, Middleton, WI) and evaluated for steatosis, fat accumulation, and inflammation, by a pathologist blind to the identity of the experimental groups.

Chromatin immunoprecipitation (ChIP)

To determine the specific chromatin modification and transcription factor binding, ChIP analysis was employed according to a modified protocol [27]. Two hundred milligrams of frozen liver samples were ground using a mortar and pestle with liquid nitrogen and washed with PBS. The samples were resuspended in PBS and cross-linked in 1% formaldehyde for 10 min at room temperature. After centrifugation, the pellet was resuspended in nuclei swelling buffer (5 mmol/L Pipes [NaOH] pH 8.0, 85 mmol/L KCl, 0.5% NP40) containing protease inhibitor and phosphorylation inhibitor. The nuclei were lysed in SDS lysis buffer (50 mol/L Tris-HCl pH 8.1, 10 mmol/L EDTA, 1% SDS) containing protease inhibitor and phosphorylation inhibitor. The chromatin was sonicated (Fisher Scientific model 100 Sonic Dismembrator, Pittsburgh, PA) on ice with six bursts for 40 s at power setting 5 with 2 min cooling between each burst. After removing the cell debris by centrifuging the sonicated product at 13,000 rpm in 4 °C for 10 min, sheared chromatin was diluted in ChIP Dilution Buffer to 10 mL to perform 10 immunoprecipitations (IPs). One milliliter of the diluted lysate was incubated overnight on a hematology mixer (Model 346, Fisher Scientific) with 2 μg of primary antibodies at 4 °C (all the antibody information is listed in Table 2). Sixty microliters of pre-blocked salmon sperm DNA/protein G agarose beads (60 μl, 50% slurry; Upstate Biotechnology, Lake Placid, NY) was then added to each chromatin sample, followed by 2 h of incubation at 4 °C. The mixture was then centrifuged at 2000 rpm for 1 min at 4 °C. Supernatant of normal rabbit IgG was saved as input control. The pellets containing immunoprecipitated complexes were washed sequentially with 1 mL of low-salt solution (0.1% SDS, 1% triton X-100, 2 mM EDTA, 20 mmol/L Tris-HCl pH 8.0, 150 mmol/L NaCl), high-salt solution (0.1% SDS, 1% triton X-100, 2 mM EDTA, 20 mmol/L Tris-HCl pH 8.0, 500 mmol/L NaCl), and LiCl solution (0.25 mol/L LiCl, 1% NP40, 1% sodium deoxycholate, 1 mM EDTA, 10 mmol/L Tris-HCl pH 8.0) and twice with

Table 2 Antibodies used in ChIP

Antibody	Species	Company	Catalog no.
IgG	Rabbit	Santa Cruz	sc-2027
H3Ac	Rabbit	Millipore	06-599
H4Ac	Rabbit	Upstate	06-866
H3K9Me2	Rabbit	Millipore	07-030
H3K9Me3	Rabbit	Upstate	07-442
H3K27Me3	Rabbit	Upstate	07-449
Pol II		Millipore	05-623

TE (pH 8.0). Antibody/protein/DNA complexes were eluted from Protein G beads by adding twice 250 μL of the elution buffer (1% SDS and 50 mmol/L $NaHCO_3$) followed by shaking at 37 °C for 15 min at 300 rpm and flash spinning down at room temperature. The combined supernatants were incubated at 65 °C for 5 h with 20 μL 5 mol/L NaCl and 1 μg of RNase A (Qiagen, Hilden, Germany) to reverse the formaldehyde cross-linking and release the DNA fragments. Samples were then treated with proteinase K (Sigma) at 37 °C for 1 h to remove protein. DNA was purified with a DNA miniprep system (Qiagen). Five percent of immunoprecipitated DNA was used for real-time PCR reaction to detect promoter and coding regions of the p16(INK4a) and p21(Cip1) genes. Primers were designed using Vector NTI software (InforMax Inc., Frederick, MD) and are listed in Table 3.

Immunofluorescent staining

Unfixed, frozen colon sections were embedded in Tissue-Tek OCT compound (VWR, Radnor, PA) and cut to 8-μm-thick sections using Leica CM3050 S cryostat (Leica Microsystems, Inc., IL) at − 24 °C; sections were stored in − 80 °C before immunofluorescence staining. When conducting an immunofluorescent staining, slides were first washed in 1× PBS and fixed in 4% formaldehyde. Then, slides were blocked with blocking buffer (1× PBS/5% normal goat serum/0.05% Triton X-100) and incubated with p21 antibody (F-5) Alexa Fluor 488 (1:50, sc6246 AF488, Santa Cruz Biotechnologies, Dallas, TX) and anti-CDKN2A/p16INK4a antibody (1:100, ab211542, Abcam, Cambridge, UK) at 4 °C overnight. After primary incubation, slides were washed again with 1× PBS and then incubated with Goat anti-Rabbit IgG (H+L) Highly Cross-Adsorbed Secondary Antibody, Alexa Fluor 647 (1:100, Thermo Fisher Scientific, Eugene, OR) at room temperature for 1 h. All slides were then rinsed in 1× PBS again and incubated with DyLight 554 Phallioidin (1:50, Cell Signaling Technology, Danvers, MA) and Hoechst 33342 (Thermo Fisher Scientific, Eugene, OR), respectively, for 15 min in dark at room temperature. After

Table 3 Primers, locations, and functions

Gene	Sequence	Function	Ensembl ID
p16(INK4a)	Forward (p16(INK4a) + 12F) 5′-TGCAGATAGACTAGCCAGGGGA-3′ Reverse (p16(INK4a) + 76R) 5′-CTTCCAGCAGTGCCCGCA-3′	mRNA	ENSRNOT00000066011
p16(INK4a)	Forward (p16(INK4a) − 61F) 5′-ACTGGGCGGGCACTGAATCTC-3′ Reverse (p16(INK4a) + 101R) 5′-TCCGGGGCGTTTGGTGAAG-3′	ChIP promoter	
p16(INK4a)	Forward (p16(INK4a) + 5829F) 5′-CGGGTCACCGACAGGCATAA-3′ Reverse (p16(INK4a) + 5889R) 5′-TTGGACCACCCATGCTCACC-3′	ChIP coding and transcription rate	
p16(INK4a)	Forward (p16(INK4a) + 7947F) 5′-TCCGAGTCCCCATCTGTGACTGT-3′ Reverse (p16(INK4a) + 8016R) 5′-TGGAGGATGGATTGGAGCACC-3′	ChIP downstream	
p21(Cip1)	Forward (p21(Cip1) + 5100F) 5′-CCGAGAACGGTGGAACTTTGAC-3′ Reverse (p21(Cip1) + 5171R) 5′-GAACACGCTCCCAGACGTAGTTG-3′	mRNA and ChIP	ENSRNOT00000000628
p21(Cip1)	Forward (p21(Cip1) − 320F) 5′-GACAGACCTGTAAACGCTCAAC-3′ Reverse (p21(Cip1) − 233R) 5′-ACACCTGCTTGTCACGCA-3′	ChIP promoter	
p21(Cip1)	Forward (p21(Cip1) − 5200F) 5′-GGCTCACTTACACTTCCCAG-3′ Reverse (p21(Cip1) − 5125R) 5′-GGTTTCATTGGCTGGAGC-3′	ChIP upstream	
p21(Cip1)	Forward (p21(Cip1) + 6388F) 5′-AAAACGGAGGCAGACCAG-3′ Reverse (p21(Cip1) + 6450R) 5′-TCCCGCAGTATCTTGCCT-3′	Transcription rate	
L7a	Forward (L7a + 67F) 5′-GAGGCCAAAAAGGTGGTCAAT-3′ Reverse (L7a + 127R) 5′-CCTGCCCAATGCCGAAGTTCT-3′	mRNA	ENSRNOT00000006754

incubation, slides were washed with 1× PBS, mounted with Prolong-Gold Antifade Reagent (Molecular Probes by Life Technologies, Carlsbad, CA), and dried in dark overnight at 4 °C. Pictures were taken using the Confocal LSM 700 microscope (Carl Zeiss Microscopy, LLC, United States) with Zen software (Carl Zeiss AG, Ontario, CA) at magnification of × 10. To quantify protein expression, five 350 μm × 350 μm captured pictures in each group were analyzed. ImageJ Software (NIH, Bethesda, MD) was applied to separate the nucleus spheres and p16 or p21 protein spheres by channel (blue, red and green) and to measure sphere areas. Protein expression is calculated by the protein spheres (μm^2) ratio to nucleus sphere area (μm^2).

Statistical analysis

Results are presented as mean ± SEM (animal numbers of specific experiments are descripted in the figure legends). Comparison of food intake and body weight during treatment period and chromatin modifications at p16 and p21 genes between HF and C groups were performed by one-way analysis of variance (ANOVA) using proc GLM program in SAS v. 9.1 (SAS Institute, Cary, NC). Comparison of other physiological outcomes, mRNA expression, and protein expression were performed by two-trailed t test using proc GLM program in SAS v. 9.1 (SAS Institute, Cary, NC). Significance (*) was set at $p < 0.05$ level.

Results

Physiological outcomes

Food intake and body weight

The body weight (g) of rats fed HF diet was significantly higher than those fed C diet after 7 weeks of feeding (Fig. 1a). Energy intake (kCal) in HF group was significantly different from that in the C group (Fig. 1b).

Plasma and liver triacylglyceride (TAG) and non-esterified fatty acid (NEFA)

Plasma TAG levels were not different between the HF and C groups, while liver TAG significantly increased in the rats of HF group when compared to the C group. No significant difference was observed in liver NEFA level between C and HF groups (Fig. 2a).

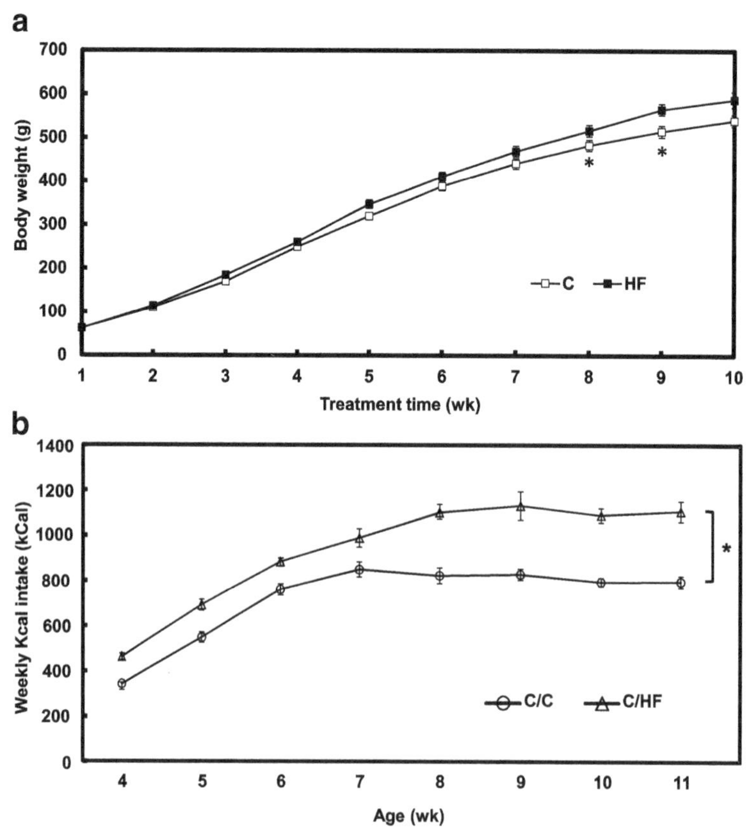

Fig. 1 Physiological outcome of rats fed high-fat diet and control diet. **a** Effect of different diets on body weight of C and HF rats through 9 weeks of feeding. Values are mean ± SEM, $p < 0.05$*. **b** Energy intake graph of rats fed with different diets: control (C, $n = 10$) diet, and high-fat (HF, $n = 10$) diet. Values are mean ± SEM. $p < 0.05$*

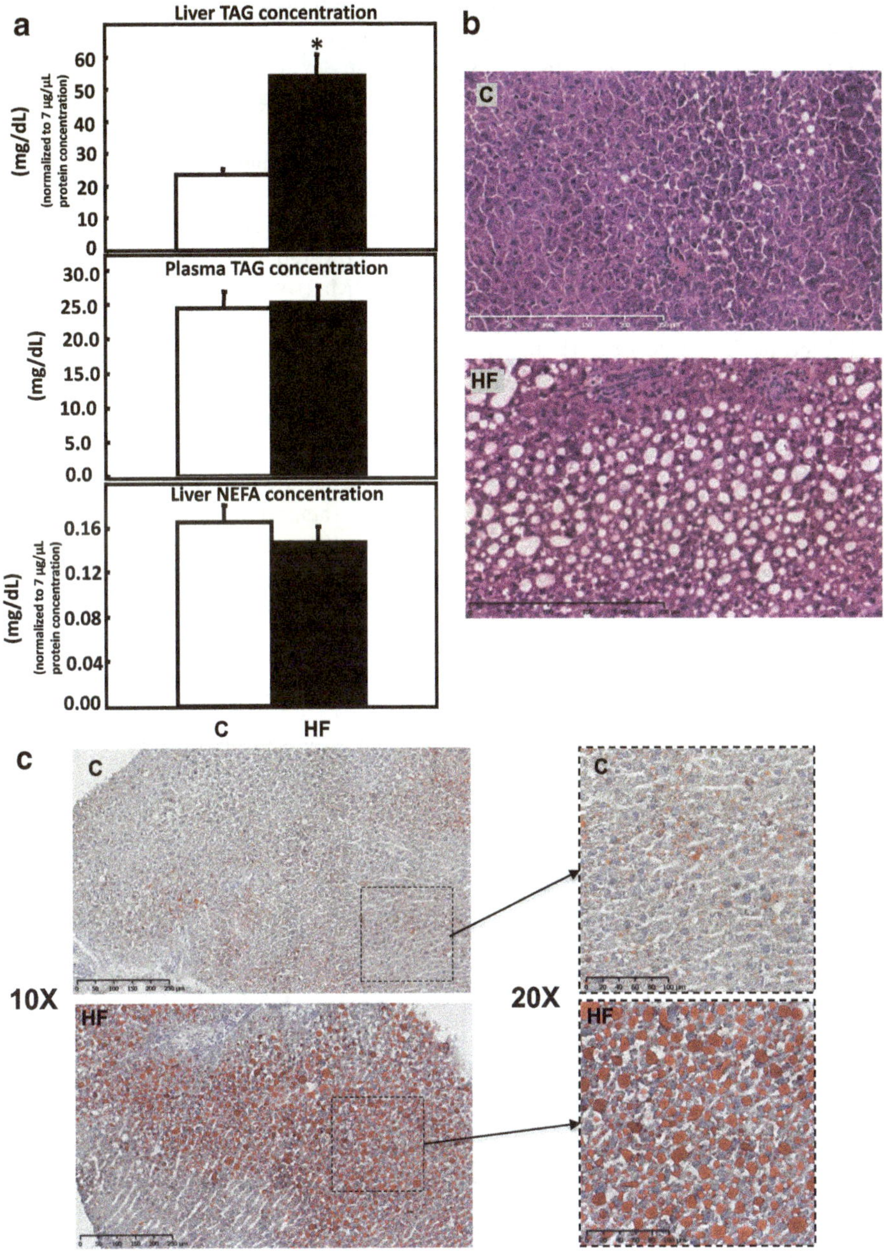

Fig. 2 Liver histological outcome rats fed HF and C diets. **a** Triglyceride (TAG) concentration in plasma and liver, non-esterified fatty acid (NEFA) concentration in the liver. Data are presented in arbitrary units as relative liver TAG or NEFA abundance normalized to protein abundance. Values are mean ± SEM, $P < 0.05$*. **b** H&E stain of representative liver sections (× 20). **c** ORO stain of representative liver sections (× 10 left and × 20 right)

Hematoxylin and eosin (H&E) stain and oil-red-O (ORO) stain

Photomicrographs of liver sections stained with hematoxylin and eosin are shown in Fig. 2b. As expected, based on observations made by previous studies [6, 28–31], comparing to liver tissue collected from C group, liver tissue from HF group showed development of hepatic steatosis and extensive degenerative ballooning, which was predominantly microvascular and involved zone 3 (perivenular) hepatocytes [21]. ORO staining suggests that liver tissue collected from HF group has increased fat accumulation with larger lipid droplets (Fig. 2c). Together, these observations indicated that high-fat diet triggered significant histological changes in the liver, increased hepatic lipid accumulation, and hence induced fatty liver.

Cellular senescence parameters

Gene expression

mRNA level of p16(INK4a) gene, as a marker of cellular senescence, increased significantly in livers of rats in HF group when compared to the C group, while the mRNA level of p21(Cip1), another inhibitor of cyclin-dependent kinase, was significantly lower in HF group than in C group (Fig. 3a). Transcription rate of p16(INK4a) gene was accordingly significantly increased in HF group, while the transcription rate of p21(Cip1) gene did not change between the two groups (Fig. 3b).

Protein level of p16 (INK4a) and p21 (Cip1) by immunofluorescent staining

Immunofluorescent pictures suggest that there is a difference in protein expression of p16 (INK4a) and p21 (Cip1) between C and HF groups (Fig. 4a). Consistent with mRNA expression, protein level of p16 (INK4a) increased significantly in livers of rats in HF group when compared to the C group, while protein level of p21 (Cip1) was significantly lower in HF group than in C group (Fig. 4b, c).

Chromatin modifications in p16(INK4a) and p21(Cip1) genes

ChIP assay was performed to investigate the possible chromatin modifications occurring in the livers of C and HF adult male rats that affected gene transcription. Results showed that methylation level of histone H3 lysine 27 (H3K27Me3) was significantly lowered in the p16(INK4a) coding region in HF rats compared with C rats. Lowered methylation level of histone H3 lysine 4 (H3K4Me2) was also observed at promoter region and in the coding region of p16(INK4a) in HF rats compared with C rats; however, no significance was detected (Fig. 5).

On the other hand, as for gene p21(Cip1), the methylation level of histone H3 lysine 4 (H3K4Me2) was increased at the promoter region in HF rats compared with C rats, while decreased in the coding region, with no significance detected. Meanwhile, the methylation level of histone H3 lysine 27 (H3K27Me3) was almost

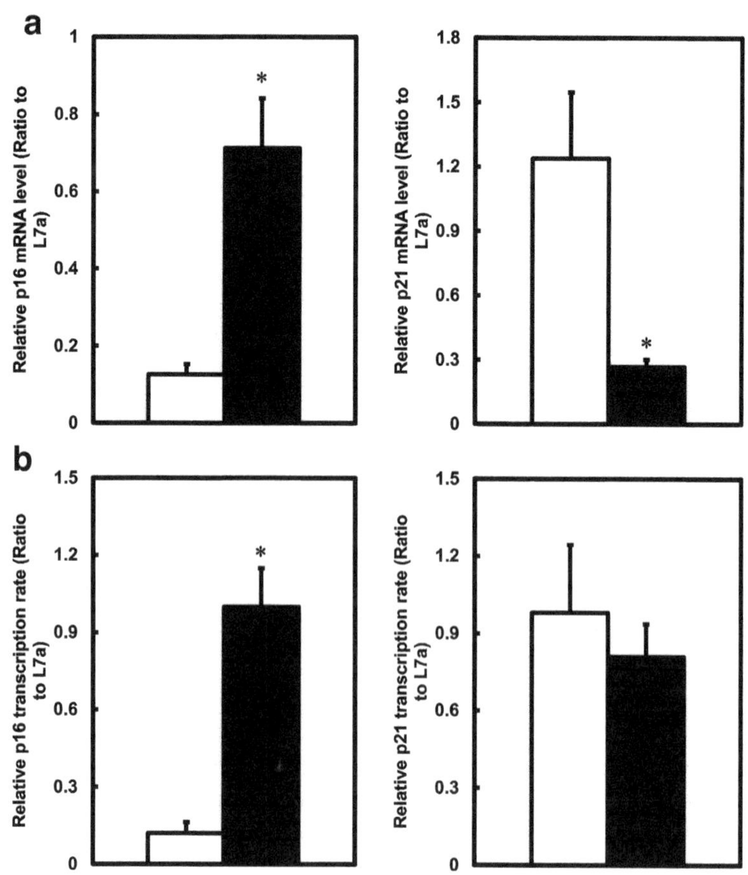

Fig. 3 Effects of different diets on hepatic cellular senescence genes in male rats. **a** p16(INK4a) and p21(Cip1) mRNA level in C and HF rats as determined by quantitative real-time PCR. Data are presented in arbitrary units as relative mRNA abundance normalized to rL7a transcript abundance ($n = 10$). Values are mean ± SEM, $P < 0.05$*. **b** p16(INK4a) and p21(Cip1) transcription rate under different maternal diets in male offspring rats as determined by quantitative real-time PCR ($n = 10$). Values are mean ± SEM, $P < 0.05$*

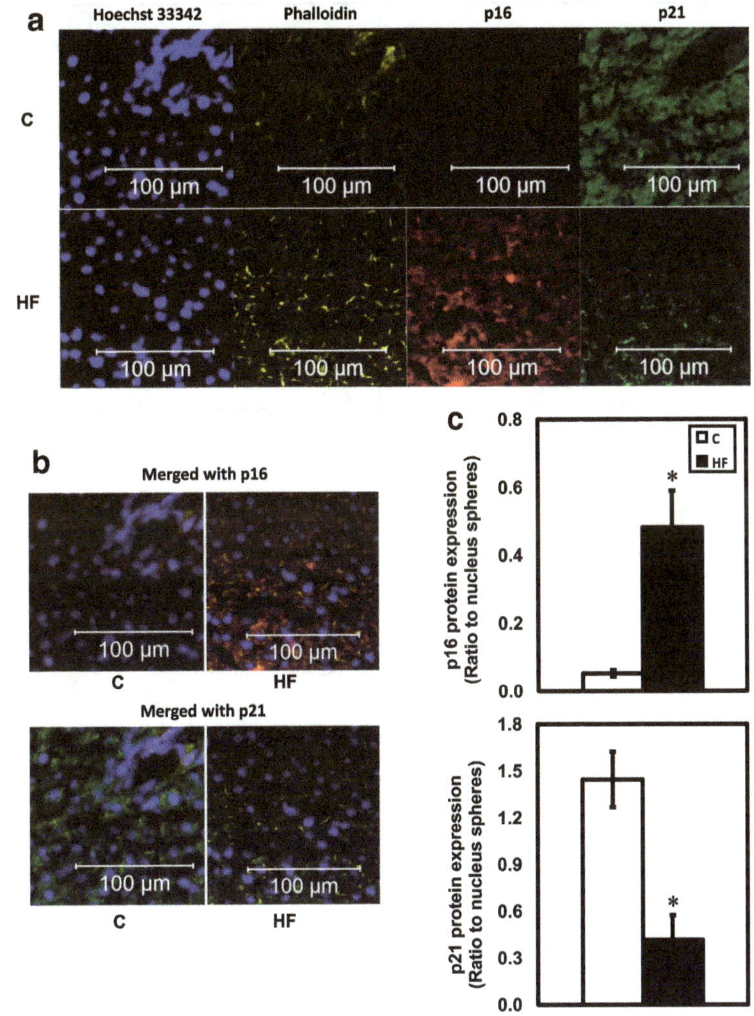

Fig. 4 Confocal immunofluorescent pictures (× 10) of rat livers and protein expression analysis. **a** Single channel pictures of stained nucleus (blue), actin filament (yellow), p16 INK4a antibody Alexa Flour 647 conjugated (red), and p21 Cip1 antibody Alexa Flour 488 conjugated (green). **b** Merged pictures (p16 INK4a/actin/nucleus and p21 Cip1/actin/nucleus, respectively) are selected and presented respectively to visualize protein quantification and localization. **c** p16 (INK4a) and p21 (Cip1) quantified protein level in C and HF rats as determined by immunofluorescence signal intensity ratio to nucleus signal intensity ($n = 5$). Data are presented as protein immunofluorescent sphere area to nucleus sphere area. Values are mean ± SEM, $P < 0.05$*

same at the promoter region and in the coding region of p21(Cip1) in HF rats compared with C rats (Fig. 6).

Discussion

The purpose of the present study was to determine the mRNA expressions of CKIs p16(INK4a) and p21(Cip1) genes and to investigate the chromatin modification in these two genes induced by HF diet in livers of adult male rats and their effects on inducing hepatic physiological changes. Here, we reported that significantly increased mRNA expression of p16(INK4a) and significantly decreased p21(Cip1) mRNA expression were observed in livers of adult rats fed HF diet, comparing to rats fed C diet. The protein levels of p16 (INK4a) and p21 (Cip1) were confirmed by immunofluorescence, and the results were consistent with mRNA expression. We further investigated and discovered that expression of p16(INK4a) was regulated by chromatin modifications in the coding region. Also, we reported that HF diet induced physiological outcomes in adult rats including significantly increased energy intake and body weight, as well as significantly increased liver TAG concentration, which induced fatty liver in adult rats.

Lipid accumulation has been confirmed to be associated with fatty liver development and prevention [32]. In previous studies, an increased liver TAG concentration in animal models fed HF diet or in their offspring [33–35] was observed, as well as increased lipid accumulation (indicated by larger lipid droplets from ORO staining in animals fed HF diet) and extensive ballooning degeneration

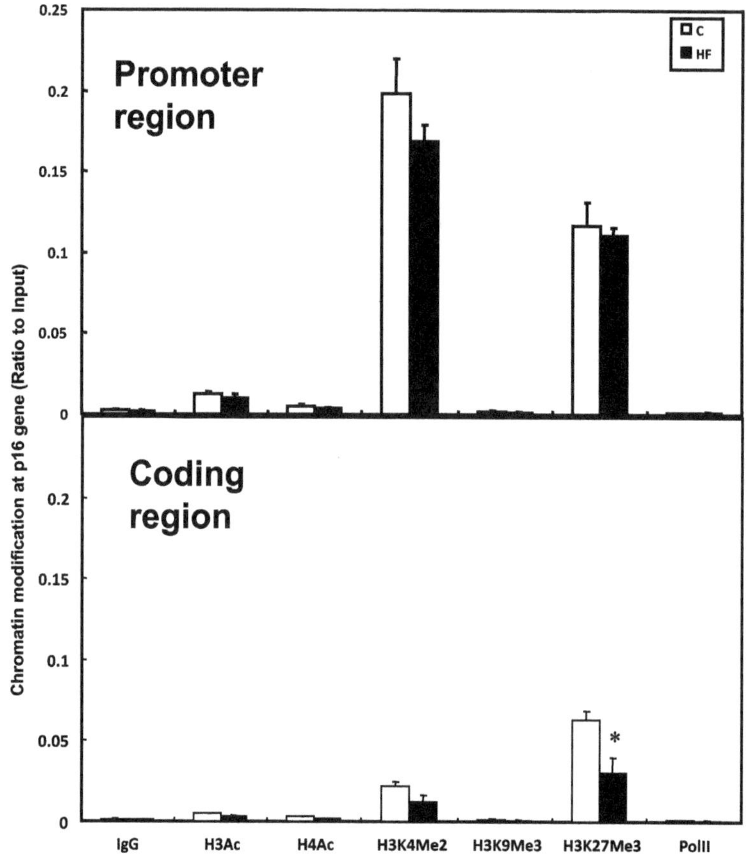

Fig. 5 Chromatin modification at coding region and promoter region in p16(INK4a) gene in livers of rats fed C and HF diets respectively. Chromatin modification on p16(INK4a) gene at different regions in HF ($n = 10$) and C ($n = 10$) rats as determined by chromatin immunoprecipitation (ChIP) assay. Data are presented in arbitrary units as relative DNA abundance normalized to DNA of input abundance. Values are means ± SEM, $P < 0.05$*

[36, 37], which is consistent with our results, indicating that HF diet induced fatty liver in rats in this current study.

We also found mRNA and protein expression of both p16(INK4a) and p21(Cip1), two well-established cell cycle inhibitors, biomarkers of aging and cellular senescence [38–40] have been altered significantly by HF diet in livers of adult rats, however, in opposite direction. The increase of p16(INK4a) mRNA can be partially explained by the decrease of tri-methylated histone H3 lysine 27 (H3K27Me3) in the coding region of p16(INK4a) that was observed in this present study, as H3K27Me3 has been considered as a suppressor of gene transcription [41–43]. On the other hand, a significantly decreased mRNA expression of p21(Cip1) was observed in HF rats; however, there was no significant difference on transcription rate of this gene between two diet groups. Further, an increased methylation level of histone H3 lysine 4 (H3K4Me2) in promoter region of p21 (Cip1) in HF rats was observed, as well as a decreased methylation level in the coding region, although no significance was detected. Consistent with our results, a declined amount of p21(Cip1)1 with an elevated expression of p16(INK4a) were observed in human diploid fibroblasts after cell achieve senescence by an early research [44]. The same research also demonstrated that p16(INK4a) and p21(Cip1) have very different age-related accumulation patterns, and the downregulation of p21(Cip1) might be a necessary part for putative differentiation program in late senescent cells. Thus, the decrease of p21(Cip1) mRNA might be explained by the differential role it plays in the mechanisms of senescence in cells. Histone H3 lysine 4 methylation (H3K4me) may also contribute to p21(Cip1) transcription [45]. Another study suggests that the absence of H3K4me2 in coding region induces increased of H3K4ac, while the degree of H3K4ac enrichment is proportional to the rate of transcription [46]. The two studies together may be used to explain the results gained from current study: in the liver of adult rats fed HF diet, a higher level of H3K4me2 in promoter region of p21(Cip1) repressed its expression; meanwhile, a lower level of H3K4me2 in coding region maintained its transcription rate, keeping it at almost the same level as in C group rats.

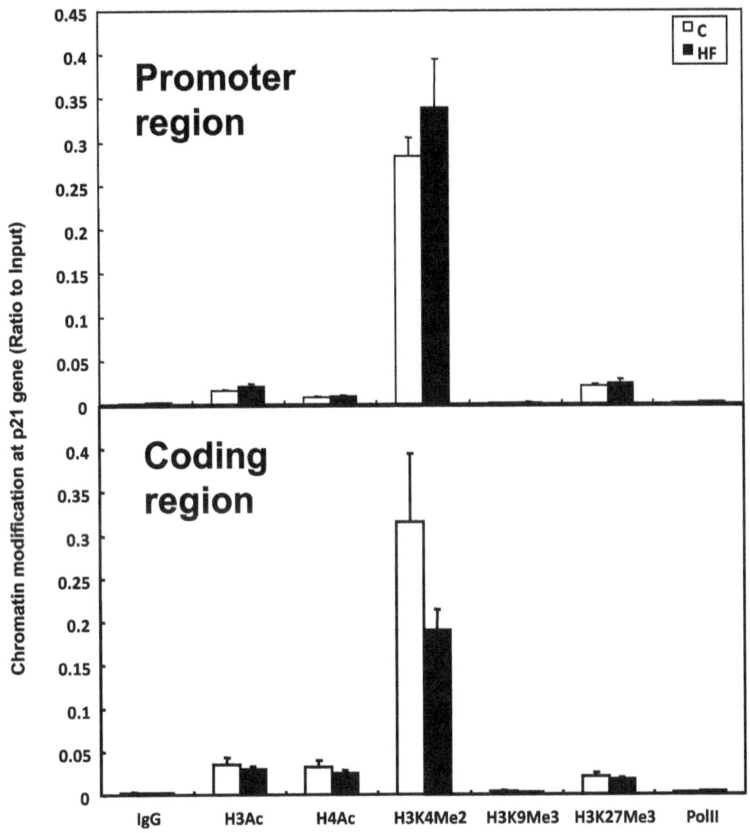

Fig. 6 Chromatin modification at coding region and promoter region in p21(Cip1) gene in livers of rats fed C and HF diets respectively. Chromatin status in p21(Cip1) gene at different regions in HF and C rats as determined by ChIP assay. Data are presented in arbitrary units as relative DNA abundance normalized to DNA of input abundance. Values are means ± SEM

The regulatory mechanisms of p16(INK4a) and p21(Cip1) on cellular senescence remain unclear at this point. Previous study demonstrated that p16(INK4a) regulates cell senescence through both CDK4/6-dependent and CDK4/6-independent mechanisms. Under CDK4/6-dependent mechanism, enhanced p16(INK4a) expression disassociates and releases p21(Cip1) from cyclinD-CDK4/6 complexes, inhibiting CDK4/6 activity, and therefore promotes cell senescence and decreases regenerative capacity. However, the study also suggests that mechanism through which p16(INK4a) induces senescence varies, depending on aging condition, cell type and species [47]. Meanwhile, it is reported that lowered p21(Cip1) expression causes lower serum adiponectin, a protein that inhibits proliferation of liver cancer cells, and therefore impairs apoptosis and/or induces cell cycle progression in the liver [48, 49]. On the other hand, an enhanced p21(Cip1) expression in the liver is usually linked to accelerated hepatocyte senescence [50–52].

Conclusion

Overall, our study demonstrates that, in adult rats fed HF diet, it activates cellular senescence through interplay between p16(INK4a) and p21(Cip1) in the liver. This is accompanied by elevated TAG accumulation. The increased expression of p16(INK4a) was associated with histone modifications, in particular, the trimethylation of histone 3 lysine 27 and the demethylation of histone 3 lysine 4, happened in promoter and coding regions respectively.

Abbreviations

C: Control; CDK: Cyclin-dependent kinase; ChIP: Chromatin immunoprecipitation; CKI: CDK inhibitor; H&E: Hematoxylin and eosin; H3K27Me3: Trimethylation histone H3 lysine 27; H3K4: Histone H3 lysine 4; H3K4Me2: Demethylation histone H3 lysine 4; H3K9: Histone H3 lysine 9; HF: High fat; HFD: High-fat diet; NEFA: Non-esterified fatty acid; ORO: Oil red O; qPCR: Quantitative real-time polymerase chain reaction; Rb: Retinoblastoma; TAG: Triacylglycerol; TSA: Trichostatin A

Funding

This project was supported by the United States Department of Agriculture Cooperative State Research, Education, and Extension Service, Hatch project no. ILLU-698-374.

Authors' contributions

The experiments were performed in the laboratory of Y-XP at the University of Illinois at Urbana-Champaign. Y-XP, XZ, and DZ were responsible for the conception and design of the experiments. XZ and DZ conducted the experiments and collected the data. XZ and GX analyzed the data, performed the statistical analysis, and wrote the manuscript. Y-XP, XZ, and GX had the primary responsibility for the final content. All authors read and approved the final manuscript.

Competing interests

The authors declare that they have no competing interests.

Author details

[1]Pediatric Oncology Branch (POB), National Cancer Institute (NCI), National Institute of Health (NIH), Bethesda, MD 20892, USA. [2]Department of Food Science and Human Nutrition, University of Illinois Urbana-Champaign, 461 Bevier Hall, MC-182, 905 South Goodwin Avenue, Urbana, IL 61801, USA. [3]Division of Nutritional Sciences (DNS), University of Illinois Urbana-Champaign, 461 Bevier Hall, MC-182, 905 South Goodwin Avenue, Urbana, IL 61801, USA. [4]Hongqiao International Institute of Medicine, Shanghai Tongren Hospital/Faculty of Public Health, Shanghai Jiao Tong University School of Medicine, Shanghai 200025, China. [5]Illinois Informatics Institute, University of Illinois at Urbana-Champaign, 461 Bevier Hall, MC-182, 905 South Goodwin Avenue, Urbana, IL 61801, USA.

References

1. Vilar L, Oliveira CP, Faintuch J, Mello ES, Nogueira MA, Santos TE, Alves VA, Carrilho FJ. High-fat diet: a trigger of non-alcoholic steatohepatitis? Preliminary findings in obese subjects. Nutrition. 2008;24:1097–102.
2. Jornayvaz FR, Jurczak MJ, Lee HY, Birkenfeld AL, Frederick DW, Zhang D, Zhang XM, Samuel VT, Shulman GI. A high-fat, ketogenic diet causes hepatic insulin resistance in mice, despite increasing energy expenditure and preventing weight gain. Am J Physiol Endocrinol Metab. 2010;299: E808–15.
3. Liu Z, Patil IY, Jiang T, Sancheti H, Walsh JP, Stiles BL, Yin F, Cadenas E. High-fat diet induces hepatic insulin resistance and impairment of synaptic plasticity. PLoS One. 2015;10:e0128274.
4. Dudley KJ, Sloboda DM, Connor KL, Beltrand J, Vickers MH. Offspring of mothers fed a high fat diet display hepatic cell cycle inhibition and associated changes in gene expression and DNA methylation. PLoS One. 2011;6:e21662.
5. Gao M, Ma Y, Liu D. High-fat diet-induced adiposity, adipose inflammation, hepatic steatosis and hyperinsulinemia in outbred CD-1 mice. PLoS One. 2015;10:e0119784.
6. Nakamura A, Terauchi Y. Lessons from mouse models of high-fat diet-induced NAFLD. Int J Mol Sci. 2013;14:21240–57.
7. Shearn CT, Mercer KE, Orlicky DJ, Hennings L, Smathers-McCullough RL, Stiles BL, Ronis MJ, Petersen DR. Short term feeding of a high fat diet exerts an additive effect on hepatocellular damage and steatosis in liver-specific PTEN knockout mice. PLoS One. 2014;9:e96553.
8. Ishimoto T, Lanaspa MA, Rivard CJ, Roncal-Jimenez CA, Orlicky DJ, Cicerchi C, McMahan RH, Abdelmalek MF, Rosen HR, Jackman MR, et al. High-fat and high-sucrose (western) diet induces steatohepatitis that is dependent on fructokinase. Hepatology. 2013;58:1632–43.
9. Ganz M, Csak T, Szabo G. High fat diet feeding results in gender specific steatohepatitis and inflammasome activation. World J Gastroenterol. 2014; 20:8525–34.
10. Tan X, Xie G, Sun X, Li Q, Zhong W, Qiao P, Sun X, Jia W, Zhou Z. High fat diet feeding exaggerates perfluorooctanoic acid-induced liver injury in mice via modulating multiple metabolic pathways. PLoS One. 2013;8:e61409.
11. Kirpich IA, Gobejishvili LN, Bon HM, Waigel S, Cave M, Arteel G, Barve SS, McClain CJ, Deaciuc IV. Integrated hepatic transcriptome and proteome analysis of mice with high-fat diet-induced nonalcoholic fatty liver disease. J Nutr Biochem. 2011;22:38–45.
12. Wu Y, Zhang Z, Liao X, Wang Z. High fat diet triggers cell cycle arrest and excessive apoptosis of granulosa cells during the follicular development. Biochem Biophys Res Commun. 2015;466:599–605.
13. Zhu QC, Gao RY, Wu W, Guo BM, Peng JY, Qin HL. Effect of a high-fat diet in development of colonic adenoma in an animal model. World J Gastroenterol. 2014;20:8119–29.
14. Krishnamurthy J, Torrice C, Ramsey MR, Kovalev GI, Al-Regaiey K, Su L, Sharpless NE. Ink4a/Arf expression is a biomarker of aging. J Clin Invest. 2004;114:1299–307.
15. Campisi J, d'Adda di Fagagna F. Cellular senescence: when bad things happen to good cells. Nat Rev Mol Cell Biol. 2007;8:729–40.
16. Janzen V, Forkert R, Fleming HE, Saito Y, Waring MT, Dombkowski DM, Cheng T, DePinho RA, Sharpless NE, Scadden DT. Stem-cell ageing modified by the cyclin-dependent kinase inhibitor p16INK4a. Nature. 2006;443:421–6.
17. Signer RA, Montecino-Rodriguez E, Witte ON, Dorshkind K. Aging and cancer resistance in lymphoid progenitors are linked processes conferred by p16Ink4a and Arf. Genes Dev. 2008;22:3115–20.
18. Liu Y, Johnson SM, Fedoriw Y, Rogers AB, Yuan H, Krishnamurthy J, Sharpless NE. Expression of p16(INK4a) prevents cancer and promotes aging in lymphocytes. Blood. 2011;117:3257–67.
19. Molofsky AV, Slutsky SG, Joseph NM, He S, Pardal R, Krishnamurthy J, Sharpless NE, Morrison SJ. Increasing p16INK4a expression decreases forebrain progenitors and neurogenesis during ageing. Nature. 2006;443:448–52.
20. Krishnamurthy J, Ramsey MR, Ligon KL, Torrice C, Koh A, Bonner-Weir S, Sharpless NE. p16INK4a induces an age-dependent decline in islet regenerative potential. Nature. 2006;443:453–7.
21. Zhang X, Zhou D, Strakovsky R, Zhang Y, Pan YX. Hepatic cellular senescence pathway genes are induced through histone modifications in a diet-induced obese rat model. Am J Physiol Gastrointest Liver Physiol. 2012;302:G558–64.
22. Sherr CJ, Roberts JM. CDK inhibitors: positive and negative regulators of G1-phase progression. Genes Dev. 1999;13:1501–12.
23. Xiong Y, Hannon GJ, Zhang H, Casso D, Kobayashi R, Beach D. p21 is a universal inhibitor of cyclin kinases. Nature. 1993;366:701–4.
24. Sasaki Y, Tsujiuchi T, Murata N, Kubozoe T, Tsutsumi M, Konishi Y. Absence of p16, p21 and p53 gene alterations in hepatocellular carcinomas induced by N-nitrosodiethylamine or a choline-deficient L-amino acid-defined diet in rats. Cancer Lett. 2000;152:71–7.
25. Yoruker EE, Mert U, Bugra D, Yamaner S, Dalay N. Promoter and histone methylation and p16(INK4A) gene expression in colon cancer. Exp Ther Med. 2012;4:865–70.
26. Yoon A, Tammen SA, Park S, Han SN, Choi SW. Genome-wide hepatic DNA methylation changes in high-fat diet-induced obese mice. Nutr Res Pract. 2017;11:105–13.
27. Chen H, Pan YX, Dudenhausen EE, Kilberg MS. Amino acid deprivation induces the transcription rate of the human asparagine synthetase gene through a timed program of expression and promoter binding of nutrient-responsive basic region/leucine zipper transcription factors as well as localized histone acetylation. J Biol Chem. 2004;279:50829–39.
28. Chao J, Huo TI, Cheng HY, Tsai JC, Liao JW, Lee MS, Qin XM, Hsieh MT, Pao LH, Peng WH. Gallic acid ameliorated impaired glucose and lipid homeostasis in high fat diet-induced NAFLD mice. PLoS One. 2014;9:e96969.
29. Sasidharan SR, Joseph JA, Anandakumar S, Venkatesan V, Madhavan CN, Agarwal A. Ameliorative potential of Tamarindus indica on high fat diet induced nonalcoholic fatty liver disease in rats. ScientificWorldJournal. 2014;2014:507197.
30. Ragab SM, Abd Elghaffar S, El-Metwally TH, Badr G, Mahmoud MH, Omar HM. Effect of a high fat, high sucrose diet on the promotion of non-alcoholic fatty liver disease in male rats: the ameliorative role of three natural compounds. Lipids Health Dis. 2015;14:83.
31. Wu J, Zhang H, Zheng H, Jiang Y. Hepatic inflammation scores correlate with common carotid intima-media thickness in rats with NAFLD induced by a high-fat diet. BMC Vet Res. 2014;10:162.
32. Deminice R, da Silva RP, Lamarre SG, Kelly KB, Jacobs RL, Brosnan ME, Brosnan JT. Betaine supplementation prevents fatty liver induced by a high-fat diet: effects on one-carbon metabolism. Amino Acids. 2015;47:839–46.
33. Benatti RO, Melo AM, Borges FO, Ignacio-Souza LM, Simino LA, Milanski M, Velloso LA, Torsoni MA, Torsoni AS. Maternal high-fat diet consumption modulates hepatic lipid metabolism and microRNA-122 (miR-122) and microRNA-370 (miR-370) expression in offspring. Br J Nutr. 2014;111:2112–22.
34. Heden TD, Morris EM, Kearney ML, Liu TW, Park YM, Kanaley JA, Thyfault JP. Differential effects of low-fat and high-fat diets on fed-state hepatic triacylglycerol secretion, hepatic fatty acid profiles, and DGAT-1 protein expression in obese-prone Sprague-Dawley rats. Appl Physiol Nutr Metab. 2014;39:472–9.
35. Seet EL, Yee JK, Jellyman JK, Han G, Ross MG, Desai M. Maternal high-fat-diet programs rat offspring liver fatty acid metabolism. Lipids. 2015;50:565–73.
36. Jung CH, Cho I, Ahn J, Jeon TI, Ha TY. Quercetin reduces high-fat diet-induced fat accumulation in the liver by regulating lipid metabolism genes. Phytother Res. 2013;27:139–43.

37. Wang Y, Ziogas DC, Biddinger S, Kokkotou E. You deserve what you eat: lessons learned from the study of the melanin-concentrating hormone (MCH)-deficient mice. Gut. 2010;59:1625–34.
38. Coppe JP, Rodier F, Patil CK, Freund A, Desprez PY, Campisi J. Tumor suppressor and aging biomarker p16(INK4a) induces cellular senescence without the associated inflammatory secretory phenotype. J Biol Chem. 2011;286:36396–403.
39. Capparelli C, Chiavarina B, Whitaker-Menezes D, Pestell TG, Pestell RG, Hulit J, Ando S, Howell A, Martinez-Outschoorn UE, Sotgia F, Lisanti MP. CDK inhibitors (p16/p19/p21) induce senescence and autophagy in cancer-associated fibroblasts, "fueling" tumor growth via paracrine interactions, without an increase in neo-angiogenesis. Cell Cycle. 2012;11:3599–610.
40. Bernardes de Jesus B, Blasco MA. Assessing cell and organ senescence biomarkers. Circ Res. 2012;111:97–109.
41. Di Croce L, Helin K. Transcriptional regulation by Polycomb group proteins. Nat Struct Mol Biol. 2013;20:1147–55.
42. Simon JA, Kingston RE. Occupying chromatin: Polycomb mechanisms for getting to genomic targets, stopping transcriptional traffic, and staying put. Mol Cell. 2013;49:808–24.
43. Hon GC, Hawkins RD, Ren B. Predictive chromatin signatures in the mammalian genome. Hum Mol Genet. 2009;18:R195–201.
44. Stein GH, Drullinger LF, Soulard A, Dulic V. Differential roles for cyclin-dependent kinase inhibitors p21 and p16 in the mechanisms of senescence and differentiation in human fibroblasts. Mol Cell Biol. 1999;19:2109–17.
45. Pinskaya M, Morillon A. Histone H3 lysine 4 di-methylation: a novel mark for transcriptional fidelity? Epigenetics. 2009;4:302–6.
46. Guillemette B, Drogaris P, Lin HH, Armstrong H, Hiragami-Hamada K, Imhof A, Bonneil E, Thibault P, Verreault A, Festenstein RJ. H3 lysine 4 is acetylated at active gene promoters and is regulated by H3 lysine 4 methylation. PLoS Genet. 2011;7:e1001354.
47. LaPak KM, Burd CE. The molecular balancing act of p16(INK4a) in cancer and aging. Mol Cancer Res. 2014;12:167–83.
48. Healy ME, Chow JD, Byrne FL, Breen DS, Leitinger N, Li C, Lackner C, Caldwell SH, Hoehn KL. Dietary effects on liver tumor burden in mice treated with the hepatocellular carcinogen diethylnitrosamine. J Hepatol. 2015;62:599–606.
49. Saxena NK, Fu PP, Nagalingam A, Wang J, Handy J, Cohen C, Tighiouart M, Sharma D, Anania FA. Adiponectin modulates C-Jun N-terminal kinase and mammalian target of rapamycin and inhibits hepatocellular carcinoma. Gastroenterology. 2010;139:1762–73. 1773 e1761-1765
50. Serra MP, Marongiu F, Sini M, Marongiu M, Contini A, Wolff H, Rave-Frank M, Krause P, Laconi E, Koenig S. Hepatocyte senescence induced by radiation and partial hepatectomy in rat liver. Int J Radiat Biol. 2014;90:876–83.
51. Aini W, Miyagawa-Hayashino A, Ozeki M, Adeeb S, Hirata M, Tamaki K, Uemoto S, Haga H. Accelerated telomere reduction and hepatocyte senescence in tolerated human liver allografts. Transpl Immunol. 2014;31:55–9.
52. Toshima T, Shirabe K, Fukuhara T, Ikegami T, Yoshizumi T, Soejima Y, Ikeda T, Okano S, Maehara Y. Suppression of autophagy during liver regeneration impairs energy charge and hepatocyte senescence in mice. Hepatology. 2014;60:290–300.

20

Plasma fatty acid levels and gene expression related to lipid metabolism in peripheral blood mononuclear cells

Sunniva V. Larsen[1], Kirsten B. Holven[1,2], Inger Ottestad[1], Kine N. Dagsland[3], Mari C. W. Myhrstad[3] and Stine M. Ulven[1*]

Abstract

Background: Solid evidence indicates that intake of marine n-3 fatty acids lowers serum triglycerides and that replacing saturated fatty acids (SFA) with polyunsaturated fatty acids (PUFA) reduces plasma total cholesterol and LDL cholesterol. The molecular mechanisms underlying these health beneficial effects are however not completely elucidated. The aim of this study was therefore to investigate the expression of genes related to lipid metabolism in peripheral blood mononuclear cells (PBMC) depending on the plasma levels of n-6 and n-3 fatty acids and the SFA to PUFA ratio.

Methods: Fifty-four healthy subjects were grouped into tertiles ($n = 18$) based on plasma levels of n-6 and n-3 fatty acids and the SFA to PUFA ratio. The PBMC gene expression levels among subjects in the highest versus the lowest tertiles were compared. In total, 285 genes related to cholesterol and triglyceride metabolism were selected for this explorative study.

Results: Among the 285 selected genes, 161 were defined as expressed in the PBMCs. The plasma SFA to PUFA ratio was associated with the highest number of significantly different expressed genes (25 gene transcripts), followed by plasma n-6 fatty acid level (15 gene transcripts) and plasma n-3 fatty acid level (8 gene transcripts). In particular, genes involved in cholesterol homeostasis were significantly different expressed among subjects with high compared to low plasma SFA to PUFA ratio.

Conclusion: Genes involved in lipid metabolism were differentially expressed in PBMCs depending on the plasma fatty acid levels. This finding may increase our understanding of how fatty acids influence lipid metabolism at a molecular level in humans.

Keywords: Cardiovascular risk factors, Nutrition, Fat quality, Plasma fatty acids, Lipid metabolism, Gene expression, Peripheral blood mononuclear cells

Background

Cardiovascular disease (CVD) is the leading cause of morbidity and mortality worldwide [1]. Dyslipidemia, including elevated levels of plasma total cholesterol (total-C), low-density lipoprotein cholesterol (LDL-C), and triglycerides (TG), is a major risk factor for CVD. Dietary fatty acids play a significant role in modulating plasma lipids, thereby influencing the CVD risk [2]. Solid evidence indicates that intake of marine n-3 fatty acids, and replacing saturated fatty acids (SFA) with polyunsaturated fatty acids (PUFA), prevents CVD and CVD mortality [3–7]. One of the CVD reducing effects of marine n-3 fatty acids is the TG lowering effect, while replacing SFAs with PUFAs has been shown in several randomized controlled trials to reduce plasma total- and LDL-C [8–10]. Animal studies and in vitro experiments have demonstrated different molecular mechanisms of how marine n-3 fatty acids reduce hepatic very low-

* Correspondence: smulven@medisin.uio.no
[1]Department of Nutrition, Institute for Basic Medical Sciences, University of Oslo, P.O. Box 1046, Blindern, 0317 Oslo, Norway
Full list of author information is available at the end of the article

density lipoprotein (VLDL) production and increase the VLDL clearance [11, 12]. The molecular mechanisms behind the total- and LDL-C lowering effects of replacing SFAs with PUFAs are however less clear. Therefore, studies investigating the molecular mechanisms underlying the health effects of SFAs and PUFAs in humans are warranted.

In humans, linoleic acid (LA; 18:2n-6) and alpha-linolenic acid (ALA; 18:3n-3) are not biosynthesized de novo. Since the conversion of these fatty acids into long chain PUFAs is limited, plasma PUFA levels have been shown to be objective biomarkers of dietary intake [13, 14]. Hence, using plasma fatty acids is an alternative approach to examine the association between dietary fat quality and CVD risk.

The ability of fatty acids to regulate gene transcription may account for their effects on lipid metabolism. Fatty acids regulate gene transcription directly by binding as ligands to specific transcription factors, thereby controlling the activity of the transcription factor, or indirectly by regulating different signaling pathways controlling the nuclear abundance of transcription factors [15–17]. In particular, there is considerable evidence that PUFAs modulate the transcription of genes involved in lipid metabolism by regulating the activity of the nuclear receptors peroxisome proliferator activated receptors (PPAR) and liver x receptors (LXR) or by suppressing the nuclear abundance of the sterol regulatory binding proteins (SREBP) [17, 18]. Our understanding of how SFAs modulate the expression of genes encoding proteins related to lipid metabolism is however more limited [19].

In order to get a comprehensive understanding of how dietary fat quality affect lipid metabolism, to prevent dyslipidemia in humans, we need a suitable model system. Changes in gene expression occur prior to changes in protein levels, and gene expression analysis is therefore a valuable and sensitive technique measuring early changes related to diet [20, 21]. Peripheral blood mononuclear cells (PBMC) include lymphocytes and monocytes which circulate around in the body and are exposed to both environmental factors and metabolic tissues. Studies have shown that PBMCs may be used as a surrogate model for liver metabolism since these cells reflect hepatic regulation of cholesterol metabolism as well as metabolic and immune responses [22–26].

Some postprandial studies have examined the effect of fat intake on the mRNA level of genes involved in lipid metabolism in PBMCs [26, 27]. To our knowledge, no studies have particularly focused on the impact of plasma fatty acid levels on PBMC gene expression related to lipid metabolism. The aim of the present study was therefore to investigate the relation of plasma levels of n-6 and n-3 fatty acids, and SFA to PUFA ratio, to PBMC gene expression specifically related to lipid metabolism using cross-sectional data from a human intervention study [28].

Methods

Study design and participants

Fifty-four healthy, non-smoking men and women aged 18–50 years were included in this cross-sectional sub-study of a randomized controlled trial designed to investigate the health effects of fish oil with different quality focusing on lipids, oxidative stress, and inflammation [28, 29]. In addition, we have analyzed the plasma lipidomic profile, the PBMC gene expression profile, and the effects on lipoprotein subclasses from this dietary intervention study [30–33]. A detailed description of the protocol, participant recruitment and enrolment, inclusion and exclusion criteria, and compliance is described elsewhere [28]. In the present study, data from the end of intervention was utilized.

The study population was grouped into tertiles three times according to the plasma fatty acid levels and the SFA to PUFA ratio by arranging samples from the highest to the lowest value. First, the subjects were grouped according to the plasma level of total n-3 fatty acids which included ALA, eicosapentaenoic acid (EPA; 20:5n-3), docosapentaenoic acid (DPA; 22:5n-3), and docosahexaenoic acid (DHA; 22:6n-3). Second, the subjects were grouped according to the plasma level of total n-6 fatty acids which included LA and arachidonic acid (AA; 20:4n-6). Finally, the subjects were grouped according to the plasma SFA to PUFA ratio, which included the SFAs myristic acid (14:0), palmitic acid (16:0), and stearic acid (18:0), and the PUFA included the sum of plasma total levels of n-3 and n-6 fatty acids. The subjects in the highest ($n = 18$) and the lowest ($n = 18$) tertile were compared.

The intervention study was conducted according to the guidelines laid down in the Declaration of Helsinki, and all procedures involving human subjects were approved by the Regional Committee of Medical Ethics (approval no. 6.2008.2215) and the Norwegian Social Science Data Services (approval no. 21924). Written informed consent was obtained from all participants. The study was registered at www.clinicaltrials.gov (ID no. NCT01034423).

Clinical and biochemical measurements

Procedures regarding clinical and biochemical measurements have been described earlier [28]. In brief, fasting venous blood samples were collected after an overnight fast (≥ 12 h). Serum was obtained from silica gel tubes (Becton Dickinson Vacutainer Systems, UK) and kept at room temperature for 30 min before centrifugation (1500*g*, 12 min). Plasma was obtained from EDTA tubes (Becton Dickinson Vacutainer Systems, UK), immediately placed on ice and centrifuged within 10 min (1500*g*, 4 °C, 10 min). EDTA tubes with whole blood were kept at room temperature for a maximum of 48 h before counting the total number of lymphocytes and monocytes. Fasting serum concentrations of total-C, LDL-C, HDL-C, and TGs, as well as lymphocyte and monocyte counts, were measured by standard methods in a routine clinical laboratory (Fürst Medical Laboratory, Oslo, Norway).

Fatty acid analysis

Plasma lipids were extracted by use of the Bligh and Dyer method [34], as described by Ottestad et al. [28]. Fatty acids in Bligh and Dyer extract were derivatized and analyzed as methyl esters on a GC (HP 6890) equipped with a BPX-70 column (SGE Analytical Science Private Limited, Melbourne, Australia). The plasma level of the individual fatty acids is expressed as mass percentage (%wt) of total fatty acids in plasma.

PBMC and RNA isolation

PBMCs were isolated by using the BD Vacutainer Cell Preparation tubes according to the manufacturer's instructions (Becton, Dickinson San Jose, CA, USA), as described previously [31]. This is a well-documented and standardized method to collect mononuclear cells with high purity (above 90%), and according to the manufacturer, approximately 80% of the cells are lymphocytes and 12% are monocytes. Pellets were stored at − 80 °C for further RNA analysis. Total RNA was isolated from the PBMC samples using RNeasy Mini Kit (Qiagen). RNA quantity and quality were measured using the ND 1000 Spectrophotometer (Seven Werner AB) and Agilent bioanalyser (Agilent Technologies Inc.), respectively.

Microarray analysis and selection of genes

Gene expression was analyzed by hybridization to an Illumina HumanHT-12 v4 Expression BeadChip and scanned on an Illumina HiSCan microarray scanner (Illumina Inc., CA 92122). Illumina GenomeStudio was used to transform bead-level data to probe-level intensities and statistics, which were exported raw for bioinformatics analysis. Quantile normalization of the Illumina intensities was performed, and probes without a detectable expression (detection $P > 0.01$) in at least 10% of the samples were excluded from further analyses. From the 48,000 probes presented on the Illumina array, 21,236 probes were defined as expressed in the current study. A more detailed description of the protocol is given elsewhere [31]. The raw data are available from the Gene Expression Ominbus (GEO) (accession number GSE111567).

A total of 285 genes encoding proteins related to cholesterol and TG metabolism were selected for this explorative study. The genes were selected based on relevant gene sets related to cholesterol and TG metabolism (26 gene sets) in the Molecular Signature Database v6.0 [35] limited to collection C5 (Gene ontology, GO), as well as literature summarizing loci associated with different lipid traits [36]. Out of the 285 genes, 161 genes were defined as expressed on the HumanHT-12 v4 microarray and included in the statistical analyses (Additional file 1). The list of the differentially expressed genes was based on the lowest P values for genes containing multiple probe set. The expression levels of the differentially expressed genes which were expressed by more than one probe are shown in Additional files 2, 3, and 4.

Statistical analysis

Differences in Log2 gene expression between subjects in the highest and lowest tertiles were compared by independent samples t test. No adjustment for multiple testing was performed because of the explorative design of the study. Significantly different expressed genes were further correlated with clinical and biochemical parameters by Pearson's correlation. Differences in subject characteristics and plasma fatty acid levels between subjects in the highest and lowest tertiles were compared by independent samples t test or Mann-Whitney U test when normally and not normally distributed, respectively. All statistical analyses were performed using R open source software version 3.4.1 [37]. P values < 0.05 were considered significant.

Results

Subject characteristics and plasma fatty acid levels

The subjects included in the study were young and middle-aged adults with a median age of 25 (22-30) years and BMI (22.6 ± 2.6 kg/m^2) and serum lipids within the normal range as shown in Table 1. There was a skewed distribution of men and women (15 men and 39 women) among the subjects. The plasma levels of fatty acids in the study population are shown in Table 1.

The characteristics and plasma fatty acid levels of subjects in the highest ($n = 18$) and lowest ($n = 18$) tertiles based on plasma levels of n-6 and n-3 fatty acids, and SFA to PUFA ratio, are presented in Table 2. The serum level of TG was significantly lower among subjects in the highest compared to subjects in the lowest plasma n-6 fatty acid tertile ($P < 0.01$). In contrast, the serum level of TG was significantly higher among subjects in the highest compared to subjects in the lowest plasma SFA to PUFA ratio tertile ($P < 0.01$). There were no significant differences in any markers between subjects in the highest and the lowest plasma n-3 fatty acid tertile.

As expected, the plasma levels of EPA, DPA, and DHA were significantly higher among subjects in the highest compared to subjects in the lowest plasma n-3 fatty acid tertile ($P < 0.01$, $P < 0.01$, and $P < 0.01$, respectively) (Table 2). The plasma levels of myristic and palmitic acid were significantly higher among subjects in the highest

Table 1 Characteristics and plasma fatty acid profile of the study population

	n 54
Male/female (*n*)	15/39
Age (years)	25 (22-30)
BMI (kg/m^2)	22.7 ± 2.6
Total-C (mmol/l)	4.8 ± 0.9
LDL-C (mmol/l)	2.7 ± 0.8
HDL-C (mmol/l)	1.5 ± 0.4
TG (mmol/l)	0.9 (0.7–1.1)
Plasma level of fatty acids (wt%)	
Total SFA	30.7 (29.5–31.9)
Myristic acid (14:0)	0.9 (0.7–1.1)
Palmitic acid (16:0)	21.5 (20.6–23.3)
Stearic acid (18:0)	7.9 ± 1.0
Total n-6	34.7 ± 3.9
LA (18:2n-6)	28.8 ± 3.6
AA (20:4n-6)	5.9 ± 1.1
Total n-3	6.3 ± 2.4
ALA (18:3n-3)	0.5 (0.5–0.6)
EPA (20:5n-3)	1.94 (0.7–2.7)
DPA (22:5n-3)	0.6 ± 0.2
DHA (22:6n-3)	3.2 ± (2.1–4.1)
Total PUFA	40.1 (38.9–48.1)
SFA to PUFA ratio	0.8 ± (0.7–0.8)

Values are presented as frequency, mean ± SD or median and 25th–75th percentiles

BMI body mass index, *Total-C* total cholesterol, *LDL-C* low-density lipoprotein cholesterol, *HDL-C* high-density lipoprotein cholesterol, *TG* triglyceride, *SFA* saturated fatty acid, *LA* linoleic acid, *AA* arachidonic acid, *ALA* alpha-linolenic acid, *EPA* eicosapentaenoic acid, *DPA* docosapentaenoic acid, *DHA* docosahexaenoic acid, *PUFA* polyunsaturated fatty acid

compared to subjects in the lowest plasma SFA to PUFA ratio tertile ($P < 0.01$ and $P < 0.01$, respectively) and significantly lower among subjects in the highest compared to subjects in the lowest plasma n-6 fatty acid tertile ($P < 0.01$ and $P < 0.01$, respectively). In addition, the plasma levels of LA and AA were significantly higher among subjects in the highest compared to subjects in the lowest plasma n-6 fatty acid tertile ($P < 0.01$ and $P = 0.02$, respectively). The percentage of monocytes and lymphocytes did not significantly differ among subjects in the highest compared to the lowest plasma n-3 fatty acid tertile, n-6 fatty acid tertile, and the SFA to PUFA ratio tertile, respectively (Table 2).

PBMC gene expression

Out of the 161 mRNA transcripts included in the study, 41 were significantly differently expressed depending on plasma fatty acid levels and the SFA to PUFA ratio (Fig. 1). The plasma SFA to PUFA ratio was associated with the highest number of significantly different expressed genes (25 gene transcripts, $P < 0.05$), followed by plasma n-6 fatty acid level (15 gene transcripts, $P < 0.05$), and n-3 fatty acid level (8 gene transcripts, $P < 0.05$), as shown in Fig. 1. Seven gene transcripts were associated with both plasma n-6 fatty acid level and plasma SFA to PUFA ratio, and one gene transcript was associated with both plasma n-3 fatty acid level and plasma SFA to PUFA ratio (Fig. 2). No gene transcripts were shared across plasma n-6 and n-3 fatty acid levels and plasma SFA to PUFA ratio. Differentially expressed genes associated with the plasma levels of n-6 and n-3 fatty acids and the SFA to PUFA ratio are presented in Tables 3, 4, and 5, respectively.

Differentially expressed genes between subjects in the highest and lowest plasma SFA to PUFA ratio tertile included genes encoding proteins involved in cholesterol homeostasis (Table 5). The mRNA levels of *insulin-induced gene 2* (INSIG2), *ER lipid raft associated 2* (ERLIN2), *Caveolin 1* (CAV1), and *COPII subunit SEC24* (SEC24) were significantly higher expressed among subjects in the highest compared to subjects in the lowest plasma SFA to PUFA ratio tertile. The mRNA levels of *scavenger receptor class B member 1* (SCARB1,) *ATP binding-cassette subfamily A member 2* (ABCA2), and *3-hydroxy-3-methylglutaryl-CoA reductase* (HMGCR) were significantly lower expressed among subjects in the highest compared to subjects in the lowest plasma SFA to PUFA ratio tertile. Interestingly, several of the differentially expressed genes associated with plasma SFA to PUFA ratio, including CAV1 and HMGCR, were opposite differentially expressed when comparing subjects in the highest versus the lowest plasma n-6 fatty acid tertile.

In order to examine whether the differentially expressed genes were associated with BMI or serum lipids, correlation analyses were performed (Table 6). BMI was significantly positively correlated to the expression levels of two genes (LACTB and SNX13) and significantly negatively correlated to the expression levels of five genes (ERLIN2, GSK3B, KLHL8, SCARB1, and SELS). The serum level of TG was significantly negatively correlated to the expression levels of five genes (DAGLB, GSK3B, KAT5, KLHL8, and SCARB1). The serum levels of total-C and LDL-C were significantly negatively correlated to the expression levels of two genes (FAM117B and KAT5) and one gene (LRP5), respectively.

Even though the percentage number of lymphocytes and monocytes was constant in the three comparisons, we also checked if cell subset-specific genes were differently expressed between the groups (data not shown). We did not observe any significant alterations in the gene expression levels of the B cell-specific gene *CD20*, the T helper cell-specific gene *CD4*, and the monocyte-specific gene *CD14* between the subjects in any of the groups. These findings suggest that there is no indication that there is a

Table 2 Characteristics and plasma fatty acid profile of subjects in the highest and lowest tertiles

	n-6 level			n-3 level			SFA/PUFA ratio		
	Highest tertile (n 18)	Lowest tertile (n 18)	*P*	Highest tertile (n 18)	Lowest tertile (n 18)	*P*	Highest tertile (n 18)	Lowest tertile (n 18)	*P*
Male/female	5/13	5/13		3/15	5/13		5/13	6/12	
Age (years)	28 (23–33)	26 (21–29)	0.31	27 (21–31)	27 (21–28)	0.80	27 (22–29)	29 (23–33)	0.38
BMI (kg/m^2)	22.5 ± 2.9	22.6 ± 2.6	0.94	22.2 ± 2	22.7 ± 3.3	0.57	23.3 ± 2.7	22.6 ± 2.6	0.41
Total-C (mmol/l)	4.9 ± 0.9	4.7 ± 1.1	0.65	4.9 ± 1	4.9 ± 1	0.96	4.7 ± 0.8	5.0 ± 0.9	0.25
LDL-C (mmol/l)	2.7 ± 0.8	2.6 ± 0.9	0.79	2.6 ± 0.9	2.8 ± 0.6	0.71	2.5 ± 0.6	2.8 ± 0.9	0.16
HDL-C (mmol/l)	1.6 ± 0.4	1.4 ± 0.3	0.15	1.6 ± 0.3	1.4 ± 0.4	0.28	1.5 ± 0.4	1.6 ± 0.3	0.74
TG (mmol/l)	0.8 (0.6–0.9)	1.4 (0.9–1.7)	*0.01*	0.9 (0.6–1.1)	1.2 (0.7–1.2)	0.30	1.3 (0.8–1.6)	0.8 (0.6–0.9)	*0.01*
Lymphocytes (%)	38.4 ± 6.8	43.0 ± 8.5	0.08	42.2 ± 10.0	37.6 ± 4	0.09	42.1 ± 8.7	37.4 ± 8.4	0.11
Monocytes (%)	8.5 ± 1.8	8.1 ± 1.9	0.49	8.1 ± 1.7	8.6 ± 2.3	0.42	8.8 ± 2.2	8.48 ± 2.0	0.71
Plasma level of fatty acids (wt%)									
Total SFA	29.6 (28.8–30.5)	32.7 (31.1–33.2)	*< 0.01*	30.7 (29.3–32.3)	31.3 (29.8–31.8)	0.78	33.0 (31.5–33.2)	29.1 (28.7–29.5)	*< 0.01*
Myristic acid (14:0)	0.8 (0.6–1.0)	1.2 (0.8–1.2)	*< 0.01*	0.9 (0.6–1.1)	1.0 (0.7–1.1)	0.57	1.2 (0.9–1.2)	0.7 (0.6–0.9)	*< 0.01*
Palmitic acid (16:0)	20.8 (20.2–21.6)	23.5 (21.4–24.2)	*< 0.01*	21.9 (20.4–23.7)	22.2 (20.9–22.6)	0.39	23.8 (21.8–24.5)	20.7 (20.2–20.7)	*< 0.01*
Stearic acid (18:0)	8.1 ± 0.7	8.1 ± 1.1	0.86	8.2 ± 1.1	8.0 ± 1.0	0.65	8.0 ± 1.1	7.7 ± 0.8	0.37
Total n-6	38.6 ± 1.3	30.3 ± 2.9	*< 0.01*	31.0 ± 4.0	31.5 ± 4.5	0.74	30.8 ± 3.4	38.0 ± 2.0	*< 0.01*
LA (18:2n-6)	32.3 ± 1.6	24.9 ± 2.5	*< 0.01*	27.8 ± 3.8	29.2 ± 4.1	0.29	24.8 ± 2.5	31.8 ± 2.1	*< 0.01*
AA (20:4n-6)	6.2 ± 1.1	5.4 ± 0.9	*0.02*	5.8 ± 0.7	6.2 ± 1.2	0.32	5.9 ± 1.3	6.2 ± 1. 1	0.58
Total n-3	5.8 ± 2.5	7.0 ± 2.3	0.12	9.0 ± 0.9	3.6 ± 0.49	*< 0.01*	6.1 ± 2.5	6.8 ± 2.4	0.44
ALA (18:3n- 3)	0.6 (0.5–0.6)	0.5 (0.4–0.6)	0.46	0.5 (0.5–0.6)	0.5 (0.5–0.6)	0.79	0.5 (0.5–0.6)	0.5 (0.5–0.5)	0.95
EPA (20:5n-3)	1.7 (0.6–2.3)	2.3 (1.8–2.9)	0.14	3.2 (2.8–3.7)	0.6 (0.5–0.6)	*< 0.01*	1.8 (0.7–2.6)	2.2 (1.3–3.2)	0.46
DPA (22:5n-3)	0.6 ± 0.1	0.7 ± 0.2	0.26	0.8 ± 0.1	0.5 ± 0.1	*< 0.01*	0.6 ± 0.2	0.6 ± 0.1	0.80
DHA (22:6n-3)	3.0 (1.9–4.1)	3.6 (3.1–4.1)	0.14	4.3 (4.1–4.7)	1.9 (1.8–2.1)	*< 0.01*	3.2 (2.0–4.1)	3.4 (2.8–4.3)	0.48
Total PUFA	44.4 (42.1–47.3)	37.3 (35.8–39.7)	*< 0.01*	42.6 (39.5–46.7)	40.4 (37.7–41.5)	*0.05*	36.9 (35.8–39.1)	44.7 (43.1–47.3)	*< 0.01*
SFA to PUFA ratio	0.7 (0.6–0.7)	0.8 (0.8–0.9)	*< 0.01*	0.7 (0.6–0.8)	0.8 (0.7–0.8)	0.13	0.9 (0.8–0.9)	0.7 (0.6–0.7)	*< 0.01*

Lymphocytes and monocytes are given as percentage of total white cell count. Differences between tertiles were analyzed using the independent samples *t* test when normally distributed or the Mann-Whitney *U* test when not normally distributed. *P* values < 0.05 were considered significant and are presented in italic. Values are presented as mean ± SD or medians and 25th–75th percentile

BMI body mass index, *Total-C* total cholesterol, *LDL-C* low-density lipoprotein cholesterol, *HDL-C* high-density lipoprotein cholesterol, *TG* triglycerides, *SFA* saturated fatty acid, *LA* linoleic acid, *AA* arachidonic acid, *ALA* alpha-linolenic acid, *EPA* eicosapentaenoic acid, *DPA* docosapentaenoic acid, *DHA* docosahexaenoic acid, *PUFA* polyunsaturated fatty acid

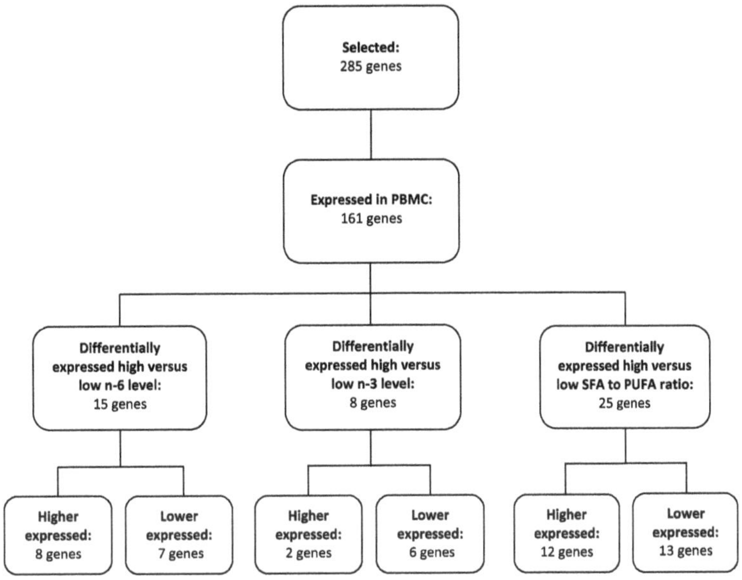

Fig. 1 Flowchart of gene selection and number of differentially expressed genes between subjects in the highest and lowest tertile of plasma n-6 level, plasma n-3 level and plasma SFA to PUFA ratio. Differences in Log2 gene expression between subjects in the highest and lowest tertiles were compared by independent samples *t* test. *P* values < 0.05 were considered significant

difference in B lymphocyte/monocyte ratio in the comparisons. However, we observed a significant lower mRNA level of the cytotoxic T lymphocyte-specific gene *CD8A* in the high versus low plasma n-6 level group, and significant higher mRNA levels of *CD8A* and *CD8B* in the high versus low plasma SFA to PUFA ratio group. This may indicate that plasma fatty acids may influence the T lymphocyte/monocyte ratio.

Discussion

In this explorative study, we investigated the potential relation of plasma n-6 and n-3 fatty acid levels, and plasma SFA to PUFA ratio, to PBMC gene expression related to lipid metabolism in healthy subjects. The plasma SFA to PUFA ratio was associated with the highest number of differentially expressed genes, followed by plasma n-6 and n-3 fatty acid level. In particular, genes involved in cholesterol metabolism were differentially expressed.

PBMCs have previously been shown to reflect hepatic lipid metabolism during fasting [23]. In addition, genes related to lipid metabolism have been shown to be differentially expressed in PBMCs after acute meal studies with different fat qualities [26, 27]. In the present study, we used a targeted approach to investigate whether 285 genes encoding proteins related to cholesterol and TG metabolism were differentially expressed depending on plasma fatty acid levels. Among the 285 genes, a total of 161 genes were expressed in the PBMCs. Interestingly, it seems like the plasma SFA to PUFA ratio is a stronger determinant than the plasma levels of n-6 and n-3 fatty acids alone regarding the potential of influencing gene expression levels in PBMCs. PBMCs may therefore function as a good model system to get a better understanding of how genes involved in lipid metabolism are regulated by the plasma fatty acid levels and in particular the SFA to PUFA ratio.

Genes involved in the regulation of cholesterol homeostasis were differentially expressed among subjects with high compared to low plasma SFA to PUFA ratio. ABCA2 encodes a member of the ATP-binding cassette (ABC) transporters, a subfamily of transporters that have been functionally linked to intracellular lipid transport [38]. The mRNA level of ABCA2 was significantly lower among subjects with high compared to low plasma SFA to PUFA ratio. It has been demonstrated that ABCA2 positively regulates low-density lipoprotein receptor (LDLR) mRNA expression and negatively regulates cholesterol esterification in hamster ovary cells [39]. In addition, it has been shown that overexpression of ABCA2 in neuroblastoma cells results in decreased cellular cholesterol levels [40]. Thus, our findings suggest that a lower ABCA2 expression level may lead to lower uptake and lower synthesis of cholesterol.

Because most cells in the periphery of the body do not express pathways for catabolizing cholesterol, efflux of cholesterol is critical for maintaining cholesterol homeostasis. SCARB1 and CAV1 are genes encoding proteins involved in cholesterol efflux. The mRNA level of CAV1 was significantly higher among subjects with high compared to low plasma SFA to PUFA ratio. It has been shown that CAV1 regulates the ATP-binding cassette subfamily G member 1 (ABCG1)-mediated efflux of

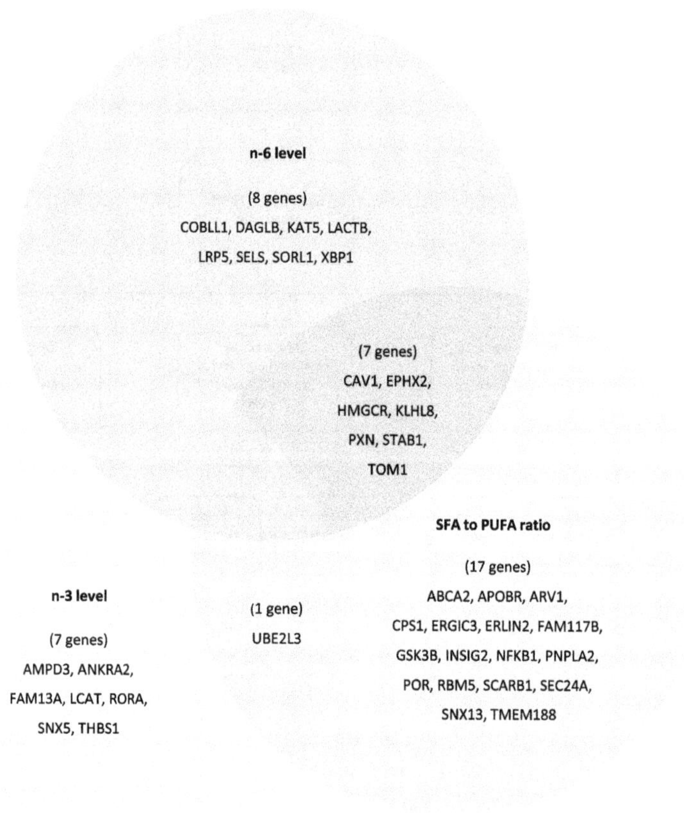

Fig. 2 Differently expressed genes associated with plasma fatty acid levels and SFA to PUA ratio. Number of differentially expressed genes associated with n-3 level (8 gene transcripts), n-6 level (15 gene transcripts), and SFA to PUFA ratio (25 gene transcripts). Seven differentially expressed genes were associated with both n-6 level and SFA to PUFA ratio, and one differently expressed gene was associated with both n-3 level and SFA to PUFA ratio. Differences in Log2 gene expression between subjects in the highest and lowest tertiles were compared by independent samples *t* test. *P* values < 0.05 were considered significant

cholesterol, probably by regulating ABCG1 trafficking to the cell surface [41], and a potential increase in CAV1 will subsequently lead to increased cholesterol efflux through ABCG1. Interestingly, there was also a significantly lower mRNA level of CAV1 among subjects with high compared to low plasma n-6 fatty acid level. As n-6 fatty acids are the majority of total plasma PUFAs, this finding may suggest that SFAs and PUFAs may exert different effects on cholesterol efflux pathways. We did not observe a significant difference in the mRNA level of ABCG1 among subjects with high compared to low plasma SFA to PUFA ratio. However, there was a significantly lower mRNA level of SCARB1, which encodes another plasma membrane receptor mediating cholesterol transfer to and from HDL. In contrast to ABCG1, which mediate cholesterol efflux via active transport, SCARB1 mediates cholesterol transport to and from HDL via passive facilitated diffusion [42]. In cholesterol-loaded mouse macrophages incubated with diluted human serum, it has been shown that cholesterol efflux is mainly mediated by active transport [43]. We therefore speculate that there may be a higher efflux of cholesterol via active transport than by passive transport in response to a high intracellular cholesterol load, which may explain the lower expression level of SCARB1 in subjects with high compared to low plasma SFA to PUFA ratio.

In addition, there was a significantly lower mRNA level of HMGCR among subjects with high compared to low SFA to PUFA ratio, and the mRNA level of HMGCR was significantly higher among subjects with high compared to low plasma n-6 PUFA level. HMGCR encodes the rate limiting step in the cholesterol biosynthesis pathway, and a lower expression of this gene will subsequently lead to reduced synthesis of cholesterol. The finding in the present study is in line with a recent postprandial study investigating the effects of SFA in lean and obese subjects [27]. It is interesting that although the abovementioned study investigated the acute effects of a high fat meal, we were able to observe a similar change in the mRNA level of HMGCR among subjects

Table 3 Differentially expressed genes between subjects in the highest and lowest plasma n-6 tertile

Gene	Highest tertile (n 18)	Lowest tertile (n 18)	Mean difference	P
STAB1*	8.66 ± 0.30	8.30 ± 0.47	0.36	0.011
SORL1	*10.25 ± 0.27*	*10.06 ± 0.27*	*0.19*	*0.039*
*KLHL8**	*9.13 ± 0.25*	*8.94 ± 0.19*	*0.18*	*0.020*
DAGLB	9.21 ± 0.30	9.03 ± 0.19	0.18	0.040
*TOM1**	*9.78 ± 0.24*	*9.62 ± 0.20*	*0.16*	*0.037*
PXN*	8.14 ± 0.19	8.00 ± 0.18	0.14	0.030
HMGCR*	8.85 ± 0.14	8.76 ± 0.11	0.09	0.036
KAT5	*7.45 ± 0.09*	*7.39 ± 0.09*	*0.06*	*0.047*
LRP5	6.79 ± 0.09	6.87 ± 0.09	− 0.08	0.013
LACTB	*7.15 ± 0.12*	*7.24 ± 0.12*	*− 0.09*	*0.027*
SELS	*9.66 ± 0.12*	*9.83 ± 0.27*	*− 0.18*	*0.020*
XBP1	*10.63 ± 0.23*	*10.85 ± 0.37*	*− 0.22*	*0.042*
EPHX2*	8.18 ± 0.32	8.40 ± 0.30	− 0.22	0.043
CAV1*	6.88 ± 0.11	7.13 ± 0.32	− 0.25	0.005
COBLL1	7.98 ± 0.23	8.28 ± 0.49	− 0.30	0.028

Expression of genes is given as mRNA level. Values are presented as mean ± SD and are log2 transformed. Differences between tertiles were analyzed using the independent samples *t* test. *P* values < 0.05 were considered significant
*Genes differentially expressed between subjects in the highest and lowest n-6 tertile and between subjects in the highest and lowest SFA to PUFA ratio tertile. The genes presented in italics are expressed by more than one probe (shown in Additional file 2: Table S2). The probe with lowest *p*-value is shown in Table 3

with higher plasma SFA to PUFA ratio compared to subjects with lower plasma SFA to PUFA ratio. The transcription of HMGCR is regulated by sterol regulatory element-binding proteins (SREBPs) [44]. SREBP2 stimulates the transcription of genes involved in cholesterol biosynthesis and uptake [45]. We did not observe a significant difference in the mRNA level of SREBP2 among subjects with high compared to low SFA to PUFA ratio, nor did we observe a significant difference in the expression level of the *LDL receptor* (LDLR) which is also regulated by SREBP2. However, several genes involved in the proteolytic regulation of SREBP2, including INSIG2 and ERLIN2, were significantly higher expressed among subjects with high compared to low SFA to PUFA ratio. INSIG2 binds to cholesterol-loaded sterol binding proteins (SCAPs) in the endoplasmic reticulum (ER) and prevents the movement of the SCAP-SREBP complex to the Golgi apparatus for further

Table 4 Differentially expressed genes between subjects in the highest and lowest plasma n-3 tertile

Gene	Highest tertile (n 18)	Lowest tertile (n 18)	Mean Difference	P
SNX5	*8.53 ± 0.13*	*8.43 ± 0.14*	*0.10*	*0.029*
AMPD3	6.94 ± 0.06	6.88 ± 0.06	0.06	0.012
LCAT	6.93 ± 0.07	6.99 ± 0.07	− 0.06	0.013
RORA	*7.11 ± 0.13*	*7.21 ± 0.10*	*− 0.10*	*0.018*
FAM13A	*7.33 ± 0.14*	*7.43 ± 0.15*	*− 0.10*	*0.049*
*UBE2L3**	*7.16 ± 0.16*	*7.28 ± 0.17*	*− 0.12*	*0.035*
ANKRA2	9.10 ± 0.20	9.25 ± 0.17	− 0.15	0.017
THBS1	7.29 ± 0.32	7.62 ± 0.43	− 0.32	0.016

Expression of genes is given as mRNA level. Values are presented as mean ± SD and are log2 transformed. Differences between tertiles were analyzed using the independent samples *t* test. *P* values < 0.05 were considered significant
*Genes differentially expressed between subjects in the highest and lowest n-3 tertile and between subjects in the highest and lowest SFA to PUFA ratio tertile. The genes presented in italics are expressed by more than one probe (shown in Additional file 3: Table S3). The probe with lowest *p*-value is shown in Table 4

Table 5 Differentially expressed genes between subjects in the highest and lowest plasma SFA to PUFA ratio tertile

Gene	Highest tertile (n 18)	Lowest tertile (n 18)	Mean difference	P
EPHX2*	8.41 ± 0.33	8.18 ± 0.31	0.23	0.036
FAM117B	*8.58 ± 0.33*	*8.36 ± 0.09*	*0.22*	*0.012*
CAV1*	7.09 ± 0.27	6.87 ± 0.23	0.22	0.014
SEC24A	7.72 ± 0.26	7.56 ± 0.17	0.16	0.038
*UBE2L3***	*7.24 ± 0.18*	*7.09 ± 0.13*	*0.15*	*0.010*
ARV1	8.07 ± 0.16	7.95 ± 0.11	0.12	0.011
NFKB1	11.09 ± 0.10	11.00 ± 0.15	0.09	0.037
SNX13	7.49 ± 0.15	7.40 ± 0.10	0.09	0.045
INSIG2	8.14 ± 0.09	8.07 ± 0.07	0.06	0.025
TMEM188	7.01 ± 0.07	6.95 ± 0.09	0.06	0.034
ERLIN2	*6.99 ± 0.06*	*6.93 ± 0.06*	*0.05*	*0.034*
CPS1	6.84 ± 0.07	6.79 ± 0.07	0.05	0.033
*TOM1**	*7.04 ± 0.08*	*7.13 ± 0.10*	*− 0.09*	*0.006*
POR	7.75 ± 0.14	7.85 ± 0.11	− 0.10	0.037
GSK3B	8.22 ± 0.15	8.32 ± 0.13	− 0.10	0.021
HMGCR*	8.76 ± 0.19	8.88 ± 0.13	− 0.12	0.015
RBM5	10.81 ± 0.12	10.93 ± 0.15	− 0.12	0.033
ERGIC3	*10.54 ± 0.18*	*10.67 ± 0.13*	*− 0.12*	*0.031*
PXN*	8.00 ± 0.14	8.13 ± 0.15	− 0.13	0.014
SCARB1	7.49 ± 0.23	7.62 ± 0.12	− 0.14	0.025
APOBR	8.11 ± 0.18	8.25 ± 0.17	− 0.14	0.038
*KLHL8**	*8.96 ± 0.21*	*9.13 ± 0.25*	*− 0.17*	*0.042*
ABCA2	7.41 ± 0.25	7.61 ± 0.30	− 0.20	0.042
PNPLA2	8.28 ± 0.28	8.48 ± 0.30	− 0.20	0.050
STAB1*	8.31 ± 0.50	8.67 ± 0.38	− 0.35	0.023

Expression of genes is given as mRNA level. Values are presented as mean ± SD and are log2 transformed. Differences between tertiles were analyzed using the independent samples *t* test. *P* values < 0.05 were considered significant
*Genes differentially expressed between subjects in the highest and lowest n-6 tertile and between subjects in the highest and lowest SFA to PUFA ratio tertile
**Genes differentially expressed between subjects in the highest and lowest n-3 tertile and between subjects in the highest and lowest SFA to PUFA ratio tertile. The genes presented in italics are expressed by more than one probe (shown in Additional file 4: Table S4). The probe with lowest *p*-value is shown in Table 5

Table 6 Correlations between subject characteristics and differentially expressed genes associated with plasma n-6 level and/or SFA to PUFA ratio (n 54)

	BMI	TG	Total-C	LDL-C
DAGLB		− 0.31 (*P* 0.020)		
ERLIN2	− 0.31 (*P* 0.021)			
FAM117B			− 0.29 (*P* 0.034)	
GSK3B	− 0.28 (*P* 0.042)	− 0.31 (*P* 0.024)		
KAT5		− 0.33 (*P* 0.016)	− 0.32 (*P* 0.017)	
KLHL8	− 0.29 (*P* 0.034)	− 0.30 (*P* 0.026)		
LACTB	0.31 (*P* 0.023)			
LRP5				− 0.30 (*P* 0.027)
SCARB1	− 0.26 (*P* 0.059)	− 0.27 (*P* 0.045)		
SELS	− 0.32 (*P* 0.033)			
SNX13	0.42 (*P* < 0.01)			

Correlations were analyzed using Pearson's *r*. *P* values < 0.05 were considered significant
BMI body mass index, *TG* triglycerides, *Total-C* total cholesterol, *LDL-C* low-density lipoprotein cholesterol

processing and eventually transcription of HMGCR and other SREBP target genes. In addition, INSIG proteins play an important role in oxysterol-regulated cleavage of SREBPs [46]. ERLIN2 encodes a cholesterol-sensing protein which has been suggested to stabilize the SREBP-SCAP-INSIG complex in the ER [47]. This gene was also significantly negatively correlated with BMI, thereby implicating that BMI impact on intracellular cholesterol levels. Thus, a higher mRNA level of INSIG2 and ERLIN2 is in line with the lower mRNA level of HMGCR observed in the present study. Additionally, we observed a higher mRNA level of SEC24 among subjects with high compared to low plasma SFA to PUFA ratio. SEC24 is a component of the COP11-coated vesicles, which transport the SREBP-SCAP complex to the Golgi. When ER cholesterol rises above a threshold of total lipids, the cholesterol binds to SCAP, which triggers a conformational change in the protein that occludes the binding of the COPII proteins [48]. We speculate that a higher expression level of SEC24 may be a response to a higher intracellular cholesterol level among subjects with high compared to low plasma SFA to PUFA ratio.

Although we did not observe differences in serum cholesterol levels among subjects with high compared to low plasma SFA to PUFA ratio, the differentially expressed genes observed in the present study may reflect an intracellular status of excess cholesterol. Changes in the expression of genes occur prior to changes at protein level, and these findings may therefore reflect early changes related to diet. The question remains how the abovementioned genes are potentially regulated by changes in the plasma SFA to PUFA ratio. It is well known that dietary intake of PUFA, in particular of LA, AA, EPA, and DHA, correlate with their respective percentages in plasma total fatty acids [14]. However, the total plasma fatty acid profile may not reflect the total dietary intake of fat as the fatty acid composition in different lipid fractions differs depending on the fat intake [49]. However, we have shown recently in a dietary intervention study where SFA were replaced with PUFA that the total plasma fatty acid profile reflected dietary fat intake changes [8]. It is clear that fatty acids have the ability to regulate the expression of genes involved in lipid metabolism. PUFAs have been shown to decrease nuclear SREBP-1 protein levels in part by inhibition of the interaction of oxysterols with LXR; however, this mechanism does not seem to affect SREBP2 [50]. The findings in the present study may therefore be explained by the plasma levels of SFAs. Recent findings suggest that SFAs may decrease SREBP activity directly, but the exact mechanisms whereby SFAs may exert their effects on SREBP and its downstream targets remain to be established [19].

The present study has several strengths. Gene expression profiling in PBMCs has been shown to be more sensitive to dietary changes than the traditional biochemical parameters in the circulation, and we specifically choose genes involved in biological processes related to TG and cholesterol metabolism. In the present study, we have compared the mRNA levels with plasma levels of n-3, n-6, and the SFA to PUFA ratio. Since intake of the n-3 and the n-6 fatty acids are reflected in the plasma total fatty acid composition, our data indicate that intake of these fatty acids may cause differences in gene expression. The major limitation of the present study is the limited number of subjects. Due to the small number of subjects, the subjects were separated into groups based on tertiles, which may have had an impact on the number of significantly differentially expressed genes observed between the highest and lowest tertiles. However, since we used end of study samples from a fish oil intervention, we could at least expect a larger variation in plasma n-3 fatty acid level among the subjects. Another limitation is that that there may be a different T lymphocyte/monocyte ratio in the n-6 tertile groups and the SFA to PUFA tertile groups. Whether the mRNA levels of CD8A and CD8B are linked to the plasma level of the fatty acids or by the change in the number of subset cells cannot be determined by this cross-sectional study. Another limitation is the lack of PBMC material to perform protein measurements to validate our mRNA results. Since this was an explorative study, we did not adjust for multiple testing. Although no causal relationship can be made due to the cross-sectional design of the study, the current study shows that the plasma fatty acid levels can influence the PBMC expression of genes involved in lipid metabolism.

Conclusion

In conclusion, the main findings in the present study were that PBMCs express genes involved in hepatic lipid metabolism and that the expression of several of the genes was influenced by plasma fatty acid levels. This finding supports the use of PBMCs as a model system for investigating the role dietary n-3 and n-6 fatty acids on gene expression related to lipid metabolism. The plasma SFA to PUFA ratio seems to be more important than the plasma n-6 and n-3 fatty acid level alone with regard to influencing mRNA levels. In particular, genes involved in cholesterol homeostasis were significantly differently expressed among subjects with high compared to low plasma SFA to PUFA ratio. This may reflect an intracellular status of excess cholesterol among subjects with high plasma SFA to PUFA ratio. The current findings should be further studied in experimental studies and tested in well-controlled human dietary intervention studies.

Acknowledgements
We thank the participants of the study and Einar Ryeng at NTNU for technical help with the microarray analysis.

Funding
This study was funded by the University of Oslo, Oslo and Akershus University College of Applied Science, the research council of Norway, and the Throne-Holst Foundation for Nutrition Research, Oslo, Norway.

Authors' contributions
SVL designed the research, selected the genes, performed the statistical analyses, analyzed the data, and drafted the manuscript. KBH designed the research, analyzed the data, and drafted the manuscript. IO designed the research, coordinated the intervention study, and drafted the manuscript. KND designed the research and selected the genes. MCWM designed the research, performed the microarray analysis, analyzed the data, and drafted the manuscript. SMU designed the research, was responsible for the intervention study, analyzed the data, and drafted the manuscript. All authors read and approved the final manuscript.

Competing interests
Dr. Holven has received research grants and/or personal fees from Tine SA, Mills SA, Olympic Seafood, Kaneka, Amgen, Sanofi, and Pronova, none of which are related to the content of this manuscript. Dr. Ulven has received research grants from Tine DA, Mills DA, and Olympic Seafood, none of which are related to the content of this manuscript. The other authors declare that they have no competing interests.

Author details
[1]Department of Nutrition, Institute for Basic Medical Sciences, University of Oslo, P.O. Box 1046, Blindern, 0317 Oslo, Norway. [2]Norwegian National Advisory Unit on Familial Hypercholesterolemia, Department of Endocrinology, Morbid Obesity and Preventive Medicine, Oslo University Hospital, P.O. Box 4950, Nydalen, 0424 Oslo, Norway. [3]Department of Health, Nutrition and Management, Faculty of Health Sciences, Oslo and Akershus University College of Applied Sciences, P.O. Box 4, St. Olavs plass, 0130 Oslo, Norway.

References
1. Benjamin EJ, Blaha MJ, Chiuve SE, Cushman M, Das SR, Deo R, et al. Heart disease and stroke statistics-2017 update: a report from the American Heart Association. Circulation. 2017;135:e146–603. https://doi.org/10.1161/cir.0000000000000485.
2. Schwab U, Lauritzen L, Tholstrup T, Haldorssoni T, Riserus U, Uusitupa M, et al. Effect of the amount and type of dietary fat on cardiometabolic risk factors and risk of developing type 2 diabetes, cardiovascular diseases, and cancer: a systematic review. Food Nutr Res. 2014;58 https://doi.org/10.3402/fnr.v58.25145.
3. Hu FB, Bronner L, Willett WC, Stampfer MJ, Rexrode KM, Albert CM, et al. Fish and omega-3 fatty acid intake and risk of coronary heart disease in women. JAMA. 2002;287:1815–21.
4. He K, Song Y, Daviglus ML, Liu K, Van Horn L, Dyer AR, et al. Accumulated evidence on fish consumption and coronary heart disease mortality: a meta-analysis of cohort studies. Circulation. 2004;109:2705–11.
5. Jakobsen MU, O'Reilly EJ, Heitmann BL, Pereira MA, Bälter K, Fraser GE, et al. Major types of dietary fat and risk of coronary heart disease: a pooled analysis of 11 cohort studies. Am J Clin Nutrition. 2009;89:1425–32.
6. Mozaffarian D, Micha R, Wallace S. Effects on coronary heart disease of increasing polyunsaturated fat in place of saturated fat: a systematic review and meta-analysis of randomized controlled trials. PLoS Med. 2010;7:e1000252.
7. Casula M, Soranna D, Catapano AL, Corrao G. Long-term effect of high dose omega-3 fatty acid supplementation for secondary prevention of cardiovascular outcomes: a meta-analysis of randomized, placebo controlled trials [corrected]. Atheroscler Suppl. 2013;14:243–51. https://doi.org/10.1016/s1567-5688(13)70005-9.
8. Ulven SM, Leder L, Elind E, Ottestad I, Christensen JJ, Telle-Hansen VH, et al. Exchanging a few commercial, regularly consumed food items with improved fat quality reduces total cholesterol and LDL-cholesterol: a double-blind, randomised controlled trial. Brit J Nutrition. 2016;116:1383–93. https://doi.org/10.1017/s0007114516003445.
9. Schwab U, Lauritzen L, Tholstrup T, Haldorsson TI, Riserus U, Uusitupa M, et al. Effect of the amount and type of dietary fat on cardiometabolic risk factors and risk of developing type 2 diabetes, cardiovascular diseases, and cancer: a systematic review. Food Nutrition Res. 2014;58 https://doi.org/10.3402/fnr.v58.25145, https://doi.org/10.3402/fnr.v58.25145.
10. Mensink RP, Zock PL, Kester AD, Katan MB. Effects of dietary fatty acids and carbohydrates on the ratio of serum total to HDL cholesterol and on serum lipids and apolipoproteins: a meta-analysis of 60 controlled trials. Am J Clin Nutrition. 2003;77:1146–55.
11. Shearer GC, Savinova OV, Harris WS. Fish oil—how does it reduce plasma triglycerides? Biochim Biophys Acta. 1821;2012:843–51. https://doi.org/10.1016/j.bbalip.2011.10.011.
12. Harris WS. N-3 fatty acids and serum lipoproteins: human studies. Am J Clin Nutrition. 1997;65:1645S–54S.
13. Arab L. Biomarkers of fat and fatty acid intake. J Nutr. 2003;133 Suppl 3:925s–32s.
14. Astorg P, Bertrais S, Laporte F, Arnault N, Estaquio C, Galan P, et al. Plasma n-6 and n-3 polyunsaturated fatty acids as biomarkers of their dietary intakes: a cross-sectional study within a cohort of middle-aged French men and women. Eur J Clin Nutrition. 2008;62:1155–61. https://doi.org/10.1038/sj.ejcn.1602836.
15. Jump DB. Fatty acid regulation of gene transcription. Critical Rev Clin Lab Sci. 2004;41:41–78.
16. Desvergne B, Michalik L, Wahli W. Transcriptional regulation of metabolism. Physiol Rev. 2006;86:465–514. https://doi.org/10.1152/physrev.00025.2005.
17. Afman LA, Muller M. Human nutrigenomics of gene regulation by dietary fatty acids. Progress Lipid Res. 2012;51:63–70. https://doi.org/10.1016/j.plipres.2011.11.005.
18. Georgiadi A, Kersten S. Mechanisms of gene regulation by fatty acids. Adv Nutrition (Bethesda, Md). 2012;3:127–34. https://doi.org/10.3945/an.111.001602.
19. Vallim T, Salter AM. Regulation of hepatic gene expression by saturated fatty acids. Prostaglandins Leukot Essent Fat Acids. 2010;82:211–8. https://doi.org/10.1016/j.plefa.2010.02.016
20. Afman L, Milenkovic D, Roche HM. Nutritional aspects of metabolic inflammation in relation to health—insights from transcriptomic biomarkers in PBMC of fatty acids and polyphenols. Mol Nutrition Food Res. 2014;58:1708–20. https://doi.org/10.1002/mnfr.201300559.

21. de Mello VDF, Kolehmanien M, Schwab U, Pulkkinen L, Uusitupa M. Gene expression of peripheral blood mononuclear cells as a tool in dietary intervention studies: what do we know so far? Mol Nutrition Food Res. 2012;56:1160–72.
22. Caimari A, Oliver P, Keijer J, Palou A. Peripheral blood mononuclear cells as a model to study the response of energy homeostasis-related genes to acute changes in feeding conditions. Omics : a journal of integrative biology. 2010;14:129–41. https://doi.org/10.1089/omi.2009.0092.
23. Bouwens M, Afman LA, Müller M. Fasting induces changes in peripheral blood mononuclear cell gene expression profiles related to increases in fatty acid β-oxidation: functional role of peroxisome proliferator-activated receptor α in human peripheral blood mononuclear cells. Am J Clin Nutrition. 2007;86:1515–23.
24. Myhrstad MC, Narverud I, Telle-Hansen VH, Karhu T, Lund DB, Herzig KH, et al. Effect of the fat composition of a single high-fat meal on inflammatory markers in healthy young women. Br J Nutr. 2011;106:1826–35. https://doi.org/10.1017/s0007114511002510.
25. Bouwens M, van de Rest O, Dellschaft N, Bromhaar MG, de Groot LC, Geleijnse JM, et al. Fish-oil supplementation induces antiinflammatory gene expression profiles in human blood mononuclear cells. Am J Clin Nutrition. 2009;90:415–24.
26. Bouwens M, Grootte Bromhaar M, Jansen J, Muller M, Afman LA. Postprandial dietary lipid-specific effects on human peripheral blood mononuclear cell gene expression profiles. Am J Clin Nutrition. 2010;91: 208–17. https://doi.org/10.3945/ajcn.2009.28586.
27. Esser D, van Dijk SJ, Oosterink E, Lopez S, Muller M, Afman LA. High fat challenges with different fatty acids affect distinct atherogenic gene expression pathways in immune cells from lean and obese subjects. Mol Nutrition Food Res. 2015;59:1563–72. https://doi.org/10.1002/mnfr.201400853.
28. Ottestad I, Vogt G, Retterstøl K, Myhrstad MC, Haugen J-E, Nilsson A, et al. Oxidised fish oil does not influence established markers of oxidative stress in healthy human subjects: a randomised controlled trial. Brit J Nutrition. 2012;108:315–26.
29. Ottestad I, Retterstøl K, Myhrstad M, Andersen L, Vogt G, Nilsson A, et al. Intake of oxidised fish oil does not affect circulating levels of oxidised LDL or inflammatory markers in healthy subjects. Nutrition, Metabol Cardiovasc Dis. 2013;23:e3–4.
30. Ottestad I, Hassani S, Borge GI, Kohler A, Vogt G, Hyotylainen T, et al. Fish oil supplementation alters the plasma lipidomic profile and increases long-chain PUFAs of phospholipids and triglycerides in healthy subjects. PLoS One. 2012;7:e42550. https://doi.org/10.1371/journal.pone.0042550.
31. Myhrstad MC, Ulven SM, Gunther CC, Ottestad I, Holden M, Ryeng E, et al. Fish oil supplementation induces expression of genes related to cell cycle, endoplasmic reticulum stress and apoptosis in peripheral blood mononuclear cells: a transcriptomic approach. J Intern Med. 2014;276:498–511. https://doi.org/10.1111/joim.12217.
32. Myhrstad MC, Ottestad I, Gunther CC, Ryeng E, Holden M, Nilsson A, et al. The PBMC transcriptome profile after intake of oxidized versus high-quality fish oil: an explorative study in healthy subjects. Genes Nutrition. 2016;11:16. https://doi.org/10.1186/s12263-016-0530-6.
33. Rundblad A, Holven KB, Ottestad I, Myhrstad MC, Ulven SM. High-quality fish oil has a more favourable effect than oxidised fish oil on intermediate-density lipoprotein and LDL subclasses: a randomised controlled trial. Brit J Nutrition. 2017;117:1291–8. https://doi.org/10.1017/s0007114517001167.
34. Bligh EG, Dyer WJ. A rapid method of total lipid extraction and purification. Canadian J Biochem Physiol. 1959;37:911–7.
35. Subramanian A, Tamayo P, Mootha VK, Mukherjee S, Ebert BL, Gillette MA, et al. Gene set enrichment analysis: a knowledge-based approach for interpreting genome-wide expression profiles. Proceed Nat Acad Sci. 2005; 102:15545–50. https://doi.org/10.1073/pnas.0506580102.
36. Lange LA, Willer CJ, Rich SS. Recent developments in genome and exome-wide analyses of plasma lipids. Current Opinion Lipidol. 2015;26:96–102.
37. Team RC. R: A language and environment for statistical computing [Internet]. Vienna, Austria; 2014. 2017.
38. Aye IL, Singh AT, Keelan JA. Transport of lipids by ABC proteins: interactions and implications for cellular toxicity, viability and function. Chemico-Biol Interactions. 2009;180:327–39. https://doi.org/10.1016/j.cbi.2009.04.012.
39. Davis W Jr, Boyd JT, Ile KE, Tew KD. Human ATP-binding cassette transporter-2 (ABCA2) positively regulates low-density lipoprotein receptor expression and negatively regulates cholesterol esterification in Chinese hamster ovary cells. Biochim Biophys Acta. 1683;2004:89–100. https://doi.org/10.1016/j.bbalip.2004.04.009.
40. Davis W Jr. The ATP-binding cassette transporter-2 (ABCA2) regulates cholesterol homeostasis and low-density lipoprotein receptor metabolism in N2a neuroblastoma cells. Biochim Biophys Acta. 1811;2011:1152–64. https://doi.org/10.1016/j.bbalip.2011.07.010.
41. Gu HM, Wang FQ, Zhang DW. Caveolin-1 interacts with ATP binding cassette transporter G1 (ABCG1) and regulates ABCG1-mediated cholesterol efflux. Biochim Biophys Acta. 1841;2014:847–58. https://doi.org/10.1016/j.bbalip.2014.02.002.
42. Phillips MC. Molecular mechanisms of cellular cholesterol efflux. J Biol Chem. 2014;289:24020–9. https://doi.org/10.1074/jbc.R114.583658.
43. Adorni MP, Zimetti F, Billheimer JT, Wang N, Rader DJ, Phillips MC, et al. The roles of different pathways in the release of cholesterol from macrophages. J Lipid Res. 2007;48:2453–62. https://doi.org/10.1194/jlr.M700274-JLR200.
44. Brown MS, Goldstein JL. The SREBP pathway: regulation of cholesterol metabolism by proteolysis of a membrane-bound transcription factor. Cell. 1997;89:331–40.
45. Horton JD, Shah NA, Warrington JA, Anderson NN, Park SW, Brown MS, et al. Combined analysis of oligonucleotide microarray data from transgenic and knockout mice identifies direct SREBP target genes. Proceed Nat Acad Sci USA. 2003;100:12027–32. https://doi.org/10.1073/pnas.1534923100.
46. Ye J, DeBose-Boyd RA. Regulation of cholesterol and fatty acid synthesis. Cold Spring Harbor Perspectives Biol. 2011;3 https://doi.org/10.1101/cshperspect.a004754.
47. Huber MD, Vesely PW, Datta K, Gerace L. Erlins restrict SREBP activation in the ER and regulate cellular cholesterol homeostasis. J Cell Biol. 2013;203: 427–36. https://doi.org/10.1083/jcb.201305076.
48. Goldstein JL, Brown MS. A century of cholesterol and coronaries: from plaques to genes to statins. Cell 2015;161:161–72. doi: https://doi.org/10.1016/j.cell.2015.01.036.
49. Raatz SK, Bibus D, Thomas W, Kris-Etherton P. Total fat intake modifies plasma fatty acid composition in humans. J Nutr. 2001;131:231–4.
50. Horton JD, Bashmakov Y, Shimomura I, Shimano H. Regulation of sterol regulatory element binding proteins in livers of fasted and refed mice. Proceed Nat Acad Sci USA. 1998;95:5987–92.

Permissions

All chapters in this book were first published in G&N, by BioMed Central; hereby published with permission under the Creative Commons Attribution License or equivalent. Every chapter published in this book has been scrutinized by our experts. Their significance has been extensively debated. The topics covered herein carry significant findings which will fuel the growth of the discipline. They may even be implemented as practical applications or may be referred to as a beginning point for another development.

The contributors of this book come from diverse backgrounds, making this book a truly international effort. This book will bring forth new frontiers with its revolutionizing research information and detailed analysis of the nascent developments around the world.

We would like to thank all the contributing authors for lending their expertise to make the book truly unique. They have played a crucial role in the development of this book. Without their invaluable contributions this book wouldn't have been possible. They have made vital efforts to compile up to date information on the varied aspects of this subject to make this book a valuable addition to the collection of many professionals and students.

This book was conceptualized with the vision of imparting up-to-date information and advanced data in this field. To ensure the same, a matchless editorial board was set up. Every individual on the board went through rigorous rounds of assessment to prove their worth. After which they invested a large part of their time researching and compiling the most relevant data for our readers.

The editorial board has been involved in producing this book since its inception. They have spent rigorous hours researching and exploring the diverse topics which have resulted in the successful publishing of this book. They have passed on their knowledge of decades through this book. To expedite this challenging task, the publisher supported the team at every step. A small team of assistant editors was also appointed to further simplify the editing procedure and attain best results for the readers.

Apart from the editorial board, the designing team has also invested a significant amount of their time in understanding the subject and creating the most relevant covers. They scrutinized every image to scout for the most suitable representation of the subject and create an appropriate cover for the book.

The publishing team has been an ardent support to the editorial, designing and production team. Their endless efforts to recruit the best for this project, has resulted in the accomplishment of this book. They are a veteran in the field of academics and their pool of knowledge is as vast as their experience in printing. Their expertise and guidance has proved useful at every step. Their uncompromising quality standards have made this book an exceptional effort. Their encouragement from time to time has been an inspiration for everyone.

The publisher and the editorial board hope that this book will prove to be a valuable piece of knowledge for researchers, students, practitioners and scholars across the globe.

List of Contributors

Shamjeet Singh
Department of Pre-Clinical Sciences, Faculty of Medical Sciences, The University of the West Indies, St. Augustine Campus, St. Augustine, Trinidad and Tobago, West Indies

D. Dan Ramdath
Department of Pre-Clinical Sciences, Faculty of Medical Sciences, The University of the West Indies, St. Augustine Campus, St. Augustine, Trinidad and Tobago, West Indies
Guelph Food Research Centre, Agriculture and Agri-Food Canada, 93 Stone Road West, Guelph, ON N1G 5C9, Canada

Thomas Netticadan
Canadian Centre for Agri-Food Research in Health and Medicine, 351 Taché Avenue, Winnipeg, Manitoba, Canada

Małgorzata Knapik-Czajka and Anna Gawędzka
Department of Analytical Biochemistry, Faculty of Pharmacy, Jagiellonian University Medical College, Krakow, Poland

Jagoda Drąg
Department of Analytical Biochemistry, Faculty of Pharmacy, Jagiellonian University Medical College, Krakow, Poland
Andrzej Frycz Modrzewski Krakow University, 1 G. Herlinga-Grudzińskiego St., 30-705 Krakow, Poland

Anna Goździalska and Jerzy Jaśkiewicz
Faculty of Health and Medical Sciences, Andrzej Frycz Modrzewski Krakow University, Krakow, Poland

Katarzyna Gawlik
Department of Diagnostics, Chair of Clinical Biochemistry, Jagiellonian University Medical College, Krakow, Poland

K. A. Szcześniak, A. Ciecierska, P. Ostaszewski and T. Sadkowski
Department of Physiological Sciences, Faculty of Veterinary Medicine, Warsaw University of Life Sciences-SGGW, Nowoursynowska 159, 02-776 Warsaw, Poland

Tiande Zou, Bing Yu, Jie Yu, Xiangbing Mao, Ping Zheng, Jun He, Zhiqing Huang, Yue Liu and Daiwen Chen
Key Laboratory for Animal Disease-Resistant Nutrition of the Ministry of Education of China, Animal Nutrition Institute, Sichuan Agricultural University, Cheng du, China

Raffaella Comitato, Barbara Guantario, Maria Beatrice Ronci, Raffaella Canali and Fabio Virgili
Council for Agricultural Research and Economics - Food and Nutrition Research Centre (C.R.E.A.-AN), via Ardeatina 546, 00178 Rome, Italy

Guido Leoni
Department of Physics, Sapienza University of Rome, Piazzale Aldo Moro 5, 00185 Rome, Italy

Kalanithi Nesaretnam
Malaysian Palm Oil Board, 6 Persiaran Institusi, Bandar Baru Bangi, 4300 Selangor, Malaysia

Abhijit Ghadge, Abhay Harsulkar and Aniket Kuvalekar
Nutrigenomics and Functional Foods Laboratory, Interactive Research School for Health Affairs (IRSHA), Bharati Vidyapeeth Deemed University, Pune-Satara Road, Pune, Maharashtra 411043, India

Manjiri Karandikar
Department of Pathology, Bharati Vidyapeeth Medical College, Bharati Vidyapeeth Deemed University, Pune-Satara Road, Pune, Maharashtra 411043, India

Vijaya Pandit
Department of Pharmacology, Bharati Vidyapeeth Medical College, Bharati Vidyapeeth Deemed University, Pune-Satara Road, Pune, Maharashtra 411043, India

Magdalena Ogłuszka, Agnieszka Szostak, Ewa Poławska, Paweł Urbański, Tadeusz Blicharski, Edyta Juszczuk-Kubiak, Jarosław O. Horbańczuk and Mariusz Pierzchała
Institute of Genetics and Animal Breeding of the Polish Academy of Sciences, Postępu 36A, 05-552 Jastrzębiec, Poland

Marinus F. W. te Pas
Breeding and Genomic Centre, Wageningen UR Livestock Research, 6700 AH Wageningen, The Netherlands

Chandra S. Pareek
Division of Functional Genomics in Biological and Biomedical Research, Centre for Modern Interdisciplinary Technologies, Nicolaus Copernicus University, 87-100 Torun, Poland

Jenelle R. Dunkelberger
Department of Animal Science, Iowa State University, 2255 Kildee Hall, Ames, IA 50011, USA

Stella Aslibekyan, Howard W. Wiener and Bertha A. Hidalgo
Department of Epidemiology, University of Alabama at Birmingham, Birmingham, AL, USA

Hemant K. Tiwari
Department of Biostatistics, University of Alabama at Birmingham, Birmingham, AL, USA

Laura K. Vaughan
Department of Biostatistics, University of Alabama at Birmingham, Birmingham, AL, USA
Department of Biology, King University, Bristol, TN, USA

Dominick J. Lemas
Department of Health Outcomes and Policy, College of Medicine, University of Florida, Gainesville, FL, USA

Diane M. O'Brien, Scarlett E. Hopkins and Bert B. Boyer
Center for Alaska Native Health Research, Institute of Arctic Biology, University of Alaska Fairbanks, Fairbanks, AK, USA

Kimber L. Stanhope and Peter J. Havel
Departments of Molecular Biosciences and Nutrition, University of California at Davis, Davis, CA, USA

Kenneth E. Thummel
Department of Pharmaceutics, University of Washington, Seattle, WA, USA

Majdi Nagara and Sahar Elouej
Laboratory of Biomedical Genomics and Oncogenetics, Institut Pasteur de Tunis, BP 74, 13 Place Pasteur, 1002 Tunis, Tunisia

Yosra Ben Halima, Rym Kefi and Chokri Nouali
Laboratory of Biomedical Genomics and Oncogenetics, Institut Pasteur de Tunis, BP 74, 13 Place Pasteur, 1002 Tunis, Tunisia
Université de Tunis El Manar, 2092 El Manar I, Tunis, Tunisia

Marco Sazzini, Cristina Giuliani, Sara De Fanti, Giacomo Mengozzi and Donata Luiselli
Laboratory of Molecular Anthropology and Centre for Genome Biology, Department of Biological, Geological and Environmental Sciences (BiGeA), University of Bologna, 40126 Bologna, Italy

Abdelmajid Abid, Henda Jamoussi and Sonia Abdelhak
Laboratory of Biomedical Genomics and Oncogenetics, Institut Pasteur de Tunis, BP 74, 13 Place Pasteur, 1002 Tunis, Tunisia
Department of external consultation, National Institute of Nutrition and Food Technology, Tunis, Tunisia

Lotfi Chouchane
Laboratory of Genetic Medicine and Immunology, Weill Cornell Medical College in Qatar, Qatar Foundation, Doha, Qatar

Giovanni Romeo
Medical Genetics Unit, Department of Medical and Surgical Sciences, Polyclinic S. Orsola-Malpighi, University of Bologna, Bologna, Italy

George Hindy, Inês G. Mollet, Gull Rukh, Ulrika Ericson and Marju Orho-Melander
Department of Clinical Sciences in Malmö, Lund University, Skåne University Hospital, Jan Waldenströms gata 35, SE-205 02 Malmö, Sweden

Agnieszka Szostak, Magdalena Ogłuszka, Ewa Poławska, Paweł Urbański, Edyta Juszczuk-Kubiak, Tadeusz Blicharski, Jarosław O. Horbańczuk and Mariusz Pierzchała
Institute of Genetics and Animal Breeding, Polish Academy of Science, Jastrzębiec, Poland

Marinus F. W. te Pas
Animal Breeding and Genetics Centre, Wageningen UR Livestock Research, Lelystad, The Netherlands

Chandra Shekhar Pareek
Functional Genomics Laboratory, Faculty of Biology and Environment Protection, Nicolaus Copernicus University, Toruń, Poland

Jenelle R. Dunkelberger
Department of Animal Science, Iowa State University, Ames, IA, USA

Seong-Yeop Jeong
Department of R&D, Microbial Institute for Fermentation Industry, Sunchang, South Korea

Suna Kang, Cao Shi Hua, Zhang Ting and Sunmin Park
Department of Food & Nutrition, Obesity/Diabetes Center, Hoseo University, 165 Sechul-Ri, BaeBang-Yup, Asan-Si, ChungNam-Do 336-795, South Korea

Giuseppe Iacomino, Paola Russo, Ilaria Stillitano, Fabio Lauria, Pasquale Marena and Alfonso Siani
Institute of Food Sciences, CNR, Via Roma, 64, 83100 Avellino, Italy

Wolfgang Ahrens
Leibniz Institute for Prevention Research and Epidemiology - BIPS, Bremen, Germany

Institute of Statistics, Faculty of Mathematics and Computer Science, University Bremen, Bremen, Germany

Pasquale De Luca
BioGeM, Ariano Irpino, Italy

Juliana Frossard Ribeiro Mendes and Sandra Fernandes Arruda
Postgraduate Program in Human Nutrition, Faculty of Health Sciences, University of Brasília, Campus Universitário Darcy Ribeiro, Brasília, DF, Brazil
Instituto de Ciências Biológicas, Departamento de Biologia Celular, Laboratório de Bioquímica da Nutrição, Universidade de Brasília, Campus Universitário Darcy Ribeiro, Bloco J, 1 Andar. Asa Norte, Brasília, Distrito Federal CEP: 70910-900, Brasil

Egle Machado de Almeida Siqueira
Cell Biology Department of Biological Sciences Institute, University of Brasília, Campus Universitário Darcy Ribeiro, Brasília, DF, Brazil

João Gabriel Marques de Brito e Silva
3Nutrition Department of Health Sciences Faculty, University of Brasília, Campus Universitário Darcy Ribeiro, Brasília, DF, Brazil

Tamio Furuse, Ikuko Yamada, Tomoko Kushida, Misho Kashimura, Kimio Kobayashi, Hideki Kaneda and Shigeharu Wakana
Japan mouse clinic, RIKEN BRC, 3-1-1 Koyadai, Tsukuba, Ibaraki 305-0074, Japan

Kunio Miyake, Takae Hirasawa and Takeo Kubota
Department of Epigenetic Medicine, University of Yamanashi, 1110 Shimokato, Chuo, Yamanashi 409-3898, Japan

Takashi Kohda and Fumitoshi Ishino
Department of Epigenetics, Medical Research Institute, Tokyo Medical and Dental University, 1-5-45 Yushima, Bunkyoku, Tokyo 113-8510, Japan

Maja Klapper and Frank Döring
Institute of Human Nutrition and Food Science, Molecular Prevention, Christian-Albrechts University of Kiel, Heinrich-Hecht-Platz 10, 24118 Kiel, Germany

Daniel Findeis
Institute of Genetics, TU Braunschweig, 38106 Braunschweig, Germany

Harald Koefeler
ZMF—Center for Medical Research, University of Graz, Core Facility for Mass Spectrometry, Lipidomics and Metabolomics, A-8010 Graz, Austria
Omics Center Graz, A-8010 Graz, Austria

David C. Merritt, Joseph Jamnik and Ahmed El-Sohemy
Department of Nutritional Sciences, University of Toronto, 150 College Street, Room 350, Toronto, Ontario M5S 3E2, Canada

Franco Miglietta
Institute of Biometeorology (IBIMET), National Research Council (CNR), Via Giovanni Caproni, 8, 50145 Florence, FI, Italy

Francesco Vitali and Duccio Cavalieri
Institute of Biometeorology (IBIMET), National Research Council (CNR), Via Giovanni Caproni, 8, 50145 Florence, FI, Italy
Department of Biology, University of Florence, Via Madonna del Piano, 6, 50019 Sesto F, FI, Italy

Rosario Lombardo
The Microsoft Research - University of Trento Centre for Computational and Systems Biology (COSBI), Piazza Manifattura, 1, I-38068 Rovereto, TN, Italy

Nathalie De Cock and Carl Lachat
Department of Food Technology, Safety and Health, Ghent University, Coupure links 653, 9000 Ghent, Belgium

Damariz Rivero
Department of Biology, University of Florence, Via Madonna del Piano, 6, 50019 Sesto F, FI, Italy

Pietro Franceschi
Food Quality and Nutrition Department, Research and Innovation Centre, Edmund Mach Foundation, Via Edmund Mach, 1, 38010 San Michele all'Adige, TN, Italy

Fulvio Mattivi
Food Quality and Nutrition Department, Research and Innovation Centre, Edmund Mach Foundation, Via Edmund Mach, 1, 38010 San Michele all'Adige, TN, Italy
Center Agriculture Food Environment, University of Trento, San Michele all'Adige, Italy.

Alessandra Bordoni, Alessia Trimigno and Francesco Capozzi
Department of Agri-Food Sciences and Technologies, University of Bologna, Piazza Goidanich 60, Cesena, FC, Italy

Giovanni Felici and Francesco Taglino
Institute for Systems Analysis and Computer Science (IASI), National Research Council (CNR), Via dei Taurini, 19, 00185 Rome, RM, Italy

Bernard De Baets
KERMIT, Department of Data Analysis and Mathematical Modelling, Ghent University, Coupure links 653, 9000 Ghent, Belgium

Guy De Tré
Department of Telecommunications and Information Processing, Ghent University, Coupure links 653, 9000 Ghent, Belgium

Mariona Pinart, Katharina Nimptsch and Tobias Pischon
Molecular Epidemiology Research Group, Max Delbrück Center for Molecular Medicine, Berlin, Germany

Jildau Bouwman
Microbiology and Systems Biology, TNO, Utrechtseweg 48, 3704HE Zeist, The Netherlands

Xiyuan Zhang
Pediatric Oncology Branch (POB), National Cancer Institute (NCI), National Institute of Health (NIH), Bethesda, MD 20892, USA

Guanying Bianca Xu
Department of Food Science and Human Nutrition, University of Illinois Urbana-Champaign, 461 Bevier Hall, MC-182, 905 South Goodwin Avenue, Urbana, IL 61801, USA

Yuan-Xiang Pan
Department of Food Science and Human Nutrition, University of Illinois Urbana-Champaign, 461 Bevier Hall, MC-182, 905 South Goodwin Avenue, Urbana, IL 61801, USA
Division of Nutritional Sciences (DNS), University of Illinois Urbana-Champaign, 461 Bevier Hall, MC-182, 905 South Goodwin Avenue, Urbana, IL 61801, USA
Illinois Informatics Institute, University of Illinois at Urbana-Champaign, 461 Bevier Hall, MC-182, 905 South Goodwin Avenue, Urbana, IL 61801, USA

Dan Zhou
Hongqiao International Institute of Medicine, Shanghai Tongren Hospital/Faculty of Public Health, Shanghai Jiao Tong University School of Medicine, Shanghai 200025, China

Sunniva V. Larsen, Inger Ottestad and Stine M. Ulven
Department of Nutrition, Institute for Basic Medical Sciences, University of Oslo, Blindern, 0317 Oslo, Norway

Kirsten B. Holven
Department of Nutrition, Institute for Basic Medical Sciences, University of Oslo, Blindern, 0317 Oslo, Norway
Norwegian National Advisory Unit on Familial Hypercholesterolemia, Department of Endocrinology, Morbid Obesity and Preventive Medicine, Oslo University Hospital, Nydalen, 0424 Oslo, Norway

Kine N. Dagsland and Mari C. W. Myhrstad
Department of Health, Nutrition and Management, Faculty of Health Sciences, Oslo and Akershus University College of Applied Sciences, St. Olavs plass, 0130 Oslo, Norway

Index

www.ingramcontent.com/pod-product-compliance
Lightning Source LLC
LaVergne TN
LVHW060557210926
848485LV00005B/1330
* 9 7 8 1 6 3 2 4 1 8 9 1 3 *